Sellar and Parasellar Tumors

Diagnosis, Treatments, and Outcomes

Thieme

Sellar and Parasellar Tumors

Diagnosis, Treatments, and Outcomes

Edward R. Laws Jr., MD, FACS
Professor of Neurosurgery
Harvard Medical School
Director
Pituitary–Neuroendocrine Program
Department of Neurosurgery
Brigham and Women's Hospital
Boston, Massachusetts

Jason P. Sheehan, MD, PhD, FACS
Alumni Professor
Department of Neurological Surgery
University of Virginia
Charlottesville, Virginia

Thieme
New York · Stuttgart

Thieme Medical Publishers, Inc.
333 Seventh Ave.
New York, NY 10001

Executive Editor: Kay Conerly
Managing Editor: Lauren Henry
Editorial Assistant: Yasmine Kasi
Editorial Director, Clinical Reference: Michael Wachinger
Production Editor: Kenneth L. Chumbley
International Production Director: Andreas Schabert
Vice President, International Marketing and Sales: Cornelia Schulze
Vice President, Finance and Accounts: Sarah Vanderbilt
President: Brian D. Scanlan
Compositor: Kenneth L. Chumbley, Publisher
Printer: Leo Paper Group

Library of Congress Cataloging-in-Publication Data
Sellar and parasellar tumors / [edited by] Edward R. Laws Jr., Jason Sheehan.
p. ; cm.
Includes bibliographical references.
ISBN 978-1-60406-421-6 (hardback)
1. Sella turcica—Tumors. 2. Pituitary gland—Tumors. 3. Skull base—Tumors. I. Laws, Edward R. II. Sheehan, Jason P.
[DNLM: 1. Adenoma—surgery. 2. Pituitary Neoplasms—surgery. 3. Neurosurgical Procedures—methods. 4. Pituitary Neoplasms—pathology. 5. Sella Turcica—pathology. 6. Sella Turcica—surgery. WK 585]
RC280S45 2011
616.99'447—dc23 2011018947

Printed in China

5 4 3 2 1

ISBN 978-1-60406-421-6

Contents

Foreword vii

Preface ix

Contributors xi

1 Introduction and Historical Perspective 1
Edward R. Laws Jr. and Zachary N. Litvack

2 Anatomy of the Sellar and Parasellar Region 8
Albert L. Rhoton Jr.

3 Radiologic Evaluation and Diagnosis for Pathology in the Sellar and Parasellar Region 50
Prashant Raghavan and Max Wintermark

4 Medical Evaluation and Management 61
Mary Lee Vance

5 Ophthalmologic Evaluation and Management 65
Steven A. Newman

6 Surgical Treatment of Pituitary Adenomas 124
Soriya Motivala, Yakov Gologorsky, Joshua Bederson, and Kalmon D. Post

7 Surgical Treatment of Meningiomas 135
Ossama Al-Mefty and Ian F. Dunn

8 Surgical Treatment of Craniopharyngiomas 145
R. Michael Scott and Edward R. Smith

9 Surgical Treatment of Chordomas and Chondrosarcomas 155
Devyani Lal, Nancy J. Fischbein, and Griffith R. Harsh IV

10 Surgical Treatment of Rathke Cleft Cysts 170
Erin N. Kiehna, Spencer C. Payne, and John A. Jane Jr.

11 Transsphenoidal Approaches to the Sellar and Parasellar Area 177
Daniel M. Prevedello

12 Transcranial Approaches to the Sellar and Parasellar Area 187
Bradley N. Bohnstedt, Todd Eads, R. Shane Tubbs, and Aaron A. Cohen-Gadol

13 Radiation Therapy 199
Itai Pashtan, Kevin S. Oh, and Jay S. Loeffler

14 Stereotactic Radiosurgery 216
Ricky Medel, Brian Williams, and Jason P. Sheehan

15 Intracavitary Radiation for Cystic Craniopharyngiomas 229
L. Dade Lunsford, Ajay Niranjan, Hideyuki Kano, Peter Kang, and Douglas Kondziolka

16 Chemotherapy Options for Sellar and Parasellar Tumors 236
Arnaldo Neves Da Silva and David Schiff

Index 247

Foreword

The unique association of vascular, neural, and endocrine anatomy within the central skull base that comprises the sellar and parasellar region and the varieties of pathologies that arise in this part of the skull base provide considerable challenges to the neurosurgeon. Management of lesions in this region continues to generate considerable controversy, as there is often a fine balance between treatment-outcome related to the pathology and the morbidity produced by the management.

With this book, Edward Laws Jr. and Jason Sheehan have edited the first comprehensive guide to the management of the large varieties of pathologies that arise in the sellar and parasellar area. Over the past two decades, changes in management practices have been underpinned by a better understanding of the nature of the pathology, improved imaging, and a refinement of both surgical and radiation therapy techniques. The location of the sellar and parasellar region has challenged neurosurgeons (and radiotherapists) to develop innovative, refined approaches to the region, often using the best of skull base, endoscopic, and microsurgical techniques. These have been utilized within the context of an improved understanding of the pathology, with the imperative that the treatment (or therapy) must optimize control of the pathology, while minimizing morbidity.

This book collects the leaders in the various facets of the management options that have evolved over the past two decades. It covers the broad topics involved with evaluation of the pathology and the variety of treatment options. It is highly recommended to all neurosurgeons and radiotherapists involved in the management of patients with sellar and parasellar pathology.

Andrew H. Kaye, MB BS, MD, FRACS
James Stewart Professor of Surgery
Head, Department of Surgery
The University of Melbourne
Director, Department of Neurosurgery
The Royal Melbourne Hospital
Melbourne, Australia

Preface

Since 1912, when Harvey Cushing published his seminal work *The Pituitary Body and Its Disorders*, physicians have had a high degree of interest in the management of sellar and parasellar tumors. Certainly, the histopathology of tumors in this area is broader than that of pituitary adenomas alone. A variety of other tumors may arise from this area of the skull base. This compact intracranial space contains critical vascular, neuronal, and endocrine structures. Thus, when a pathologic entity affects the sellar and parasellar region, pronounced clinical problems can arise. The critical structures and their function similarly make the diagnosis and treatment of such patients extremely challenging.

Diagnosis and management of the sellar and parasellar tumors require a thorough knowledge of the anatomy, approaches, and therapeutic options available. In contemporary practice, patients with a sellar or parasellar tumor frequently receive care from a variety of specialists, including neurological surgeons, otolaryngologists, endocrinologists, radiologists, ophthalmologists, endocrine surgeons, radiation oncologists, and medical oncologists.

The diagnostic and therapeutic algorithm for patients with sellar and parasellar tumors is complex and intricate. For some patients, single modality treatment may be sufficient. For others, however, multimodality treatment will be required to achieve long-term control of the tumor, while at the same time hopefully achieving neurological and hormonal preservation or improvement.

This book focuses on the diagnosis and management of tumors in the sellar and parasellar regions of the skull base. We wish to thank the authors of the chapters for contributing to this work. In addition, we appreciate the support and assistance of Thieme Medical Publishers, with particular gratitude to Kay Conerly and Lauren Henry.

Our sincerest appreciation must be given to our wives, Peggy and Diane, along with our families for support and patience throughout this academic endeavor.

Contributors

Ossama Al-Mefty, MD, FACS
Instructor in Neurosurgery
Harvard Medical School
Department of Neurosurgery
Brigham and Women's Hospital
Boston, Massachusetts

Joshua Bederson, MD
Professor and Chairman
Department of Neurosurgery
Mount Sinai Medical Center
New York, New York

Bradley N. Bohnstedt, MD
Resident
Goodman Campbell Brain and Spine
Indiana University
Department of Neurological Surgery
Indianapolis, Indiana

Aaron A. Cohen-Gadol, MD, MSc
Neurosurgeon
Goodman Campbell Brain and Spine
Assistant Professor
Indiana University
Department of Neurological Surgery
Indianapolis, Indiana

Arnaldo Neves Da Silva, MD
Senior Resident
Department of Neurology
University of Chicago
Chicago, Illinois

Ian F. Dunn, MD
Instructor in Neurosurgery
Harvard Medical School
Department of Neurosurgery
Brigham and Women's Hospital
Boston, Massachusetts

Todd Eads, MD
Resident
Goodman Campbell Brain and Spine
Indiana University
Department of Neurological Surgery
Indianapolis, Indiana

Nancy J. Fischbein, MD
Associate Professor of Radiology and (by courtesy) Otolaryngology–Head and Neck Surgery, Neurology, and Neurosurgery
Department of Radiology
Stanford University Medical Center
Stanford, California

Yakov Gologorsky, MD
Senior Resident
Department of Neurosurgery
Mount Sinai Hospital
New York, New York

Griffith R. Harsh IV, MD
Professor and Vice-Chair
Department of Neurosurgery
Stanford University
Palo Alto, California

John A. Jane Jr., MD
Associate Professor of Neurosurgery and Pediatrics
Department of Neurosurgery
University of Virginia Health System
Charlottesville, Virginia

Peter Kang, BA
Medical Student
School of Medicine
University of Pittsburgh
Pittsburgh, Pennsylvania

Hideyuki Kano, MD, PhD
Research Assistant Professor
Department of Neurological Surgery
University of Pittsburgh
Pittsburgh, Pennsylvania

Erin N. Kiehna, MD
Chief Resident
Department of Neurosurgery
University of Virginia
Charlottesville, Virginia

Douglas Kondziolka, MD, MSc, FRCSC, FACS
Peter J. Jannetta Professor and Vice-Chairman of Neurological Surgery
Professor of Radiation Oncology
Director, Center for Brain Function and Behavior
Co-Director, Center for Image-Guided Neurosurgery
University of Pittsburgh
Pittsburgh, Pennsylvania

Devyani Lal, MD
Assistant Professor
Department of Otolaryngology
Mayo Clinic
Phoenix, Arizona

Edward R. Laws Jr., MD, FACS
Professor of Neurosurgery
Harvard Medical School
Director
Pituitary–Neuroendocrine Program
Department of Neurosurgery
Brigham and Women's Hospital
Boston, Massachusetts

Zachary N. Litvack, MD, MCR
Assistant Professor
Department of Neurosurgery
George Washington University Medical Center
Washington, DC

Jay S. Loeffler, MD, FACR, FASTRO
Chief
Department of Radiation Oncology
Massachusetts General Hospital
Herman and Joan Suit Professor
Harvard Medical School
Boston, Massachusetts

L. Dade Lunsford, MD, FACS
Lars Leksell Professor of Neurological Surgery
Distinguished Professor of Neurological Surgery
The University of Pittsburgh
Director
Center for Image Guided Neurosurgery
Director
Neurosurgery Residency Program
Chair
Technolology and Innovative Practice Committee
Pittsburgh, Pennsylvania

Ricky Medel, MD
Resident
Department Neurosurgery
University of Virginia Health System
Charlottesville, Virginia

Soriya Motivala, MD
Resident
Department of Neurosurgery
Mount Sinai School of Medicine
New York, New York

Ajay Niranjan, MD, MBA
Associate Professor of Neurological Surgery
Director of Radiosurgery Research
Director of Brain Mapping Center
University of Pittsburgh
Pittsburgh, Pennsylvania

Steven A. Newman, MD
Professor of Ophthalmology
University of Virginia Health System
Charlottesville, Virginia

Kevin S. Oh, MD
Assistant Professor of Radiation Oncology
Massachusetts General Hospital
Harvard Medical School
Boston, Massachusetts

Itai Pashtan, MD
Resident
Harvard Radiation Oncology Program
Boston, Massachusetts

Spencer C. Payne, MD
Assistant Professor
Department of Otolaryngology–Head and Neck Surgery
University of Virginia Health System
Charlottesville, Virginia

Kalmon D. Post, MD
Chairman Emeritus
Leonard I. Malis, MD/Corinne and Joseph Graber Professor
Department of Neurosurgery
Professor
Department of Medicine
Mount Sinai School of Medicine
New York, New York

Daniel M. Prevedello, MD
Assistant Professor
Department of Neurological Surgery
Director
Minimally Invasive Cranial Surgery Program
The Ohio State University
Columbus, Ohio

Prashant Raghavan, MD
Assistant Professor of Radiology
Division of Neuroradiology
University of Virginia Health System
Charlottesville, Virginia

Albert L. Rhoton Jr., MD
R. D. Keene Family Professor and Chairman Emeritus
Department of Neurosurgery
University of Florida College of Medicine
Gainesville, Florida

David Schiff, MD
Harrison Distinguished Professor
Neuro-Oncology Center
Departments of Neurology, Neurological Surgery, and Medicine
University of Virginia
Charlottesville, Virginia

R. Michael Scott, MD
Neurosurgeon-in-Chief
Department of Neurosurgery
The Children's Hospital
Professor of Surgery
Harvard Medical School
Boston, Massachusetts

Jason P. Sheehan, MD, PhD, FACS
Alumni Professor
Department of Neurological Surgery
University of Virginia
Charlottesville, Virginia

Edward R. Smith, MD
Director
Cerebrovascular Surgery
Department of Neurosurgery
The Children's Hospital
Associate Professor
Harvard Medical School
Boston, Massachusetts

R. Shane Tubbs, MS, PA-C, PhD
Director of Research
Pediatric Neurosurgery
Children's Hospital
Birmingham, Alabama

Mary Lee Vance, MD
Professor of Medicine and Neurosurgery
University of Virginia School of Medicine
Charlottesville, Virginia

Brian Williams, MD
Resident
Department of Neurosurgery
University of Virginia Health System
Charlottesville, Virginia

Max Wintermark, MD, MAS
Associate Professor of Radiology, Neurology, Neurosurgery, and Biomedical Engineering
Chief
Division of Neuroradiology
University of Virginia Health System
Charlottesville, Virginia

1 Introduction and Historical Perspective

Edward R. Laws Jr. and Zachary N. Litvack

"As is true of all difficult operative procedures, the performance becomes progressively simplified by the combined suggestion and experience of many."
Harvey Cushing, 1912[1]

Ever since Pierre Marie recognized acromegaly as a pituitary-related syndrome in 1886, intense vigor has characterized the search for knowledge related to the anatomy, physiology, and pathology of the pituitary gland.[2] Interdisciplinary research and collaboration have allowed a dramatic transformation in the management of pathology of the sellar and parasellar region. Over the past century, collaborative efforts have resulted in medical and surgical advances that allow us to preserve normal function, restore vision, and restore to health a group of patients who were once uniformly condemned to disability and death.

◆ Early Approaches to the Sellar and Parasellar Region

Initial attempts at the surgical management of pituitary lesions were made primarily in patients with large lesions who presented either with the characteristic visual loss associated with compression of the optic chiasm or with symptoms and stigmata of acromegaly. The first published cases of treatment with craniotomy by Sir Victor Horsley and others were not uniformly encouraging.[3] Because surgeons were unaware of the intricacies of the hypothalamic-pituitary axis and unable to properly visualize the sella, early procedures were blunt and largely blind attempts to perform what would "generously" be called hypophysectomy. Horsley's early attempts at subfrontal approaches were plagued by complications secondary to the extent of cerebral retraction necessary to visualize the sella. In 1893, under the encouragement of Horsley, Caton and Paul in Liverpool used a subtemporal approach in a patient with acromegaly[4] (**Fig. 1.1**). It would be another 15 years before Schloffer attempted to use a more direct transnasal transsphenoidal route to the sella, which resulted in the patient's death due to cerebrospinal fluid leak and meningitis.[5] Not discouraged by this early result, surgeons developed a variety of more successful transsphenoidal approaches nearly simultaneously in the early 1900s. Kanavel and Kocher introduced the sublabial approach, which Cushing popularized while he was at Johns Hopkins[6–8] (**Fig. 1.2**). Oskar Hirsch, then in Vienna, developed a transnasal transseptal approach, which became the basis for every subsequent endonasal operation for pituitary lesions.[6]

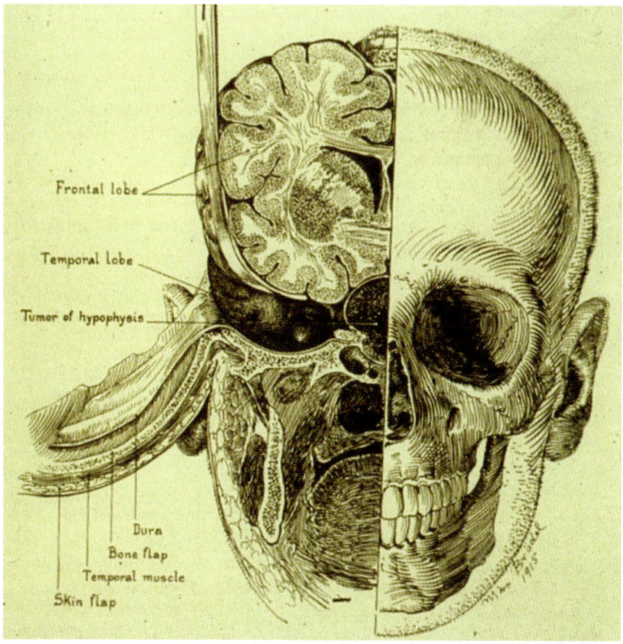

Fig. 1.1 Example of the subtemporal approach originally reported by Caton and Paul, and later refined by Walter Dandy. (Illustration by Max Brödel, 1915. From the personal collection of Dr. Edward R. Laws Jr.)

In 1927, near the end of his tenure at the Peter Bent Brigham Hospital in Boston, Cushing abandoned the transsphenoidal approach for craniotomy for most of these lesions (**Fig. 1.3**). In 1933, Hirsch relocated to Boston, continuing to use the transnasal transsphenoidal approach long after much of the growing neurosurgical community had followed Cushing's lead.[9] Hirsch recognized the limitations of both transsphenoidal and transcranial operations in completely resecting pituitary tumors. With great prescience, in 1910 Hirsch used local irradiation with an endonasal radium bomb under roentgenographic guidance as adjuvant therapy, thus beginning both image guidance and radiosurgery for sellar lesions[10] (**Fig. 1.4**).

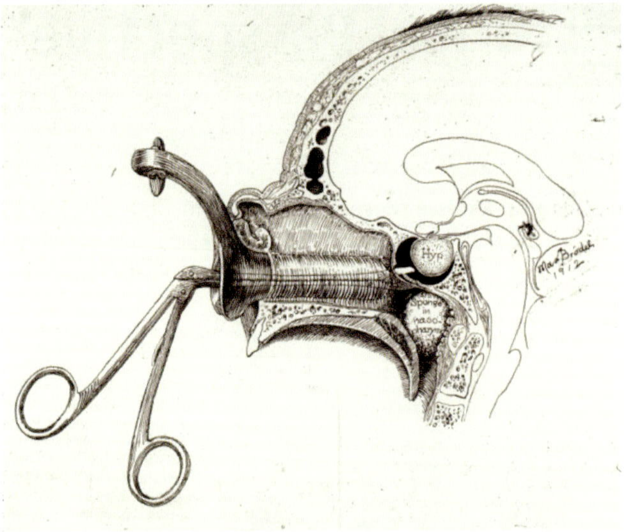

Fig. 1.2 Example of the sublabial transsphenoidal approach popularized by Harvey Cushing. (Illustration by Max Brödel, 1912. From the personal collection of Dr. Edward R. Laws Jr.)

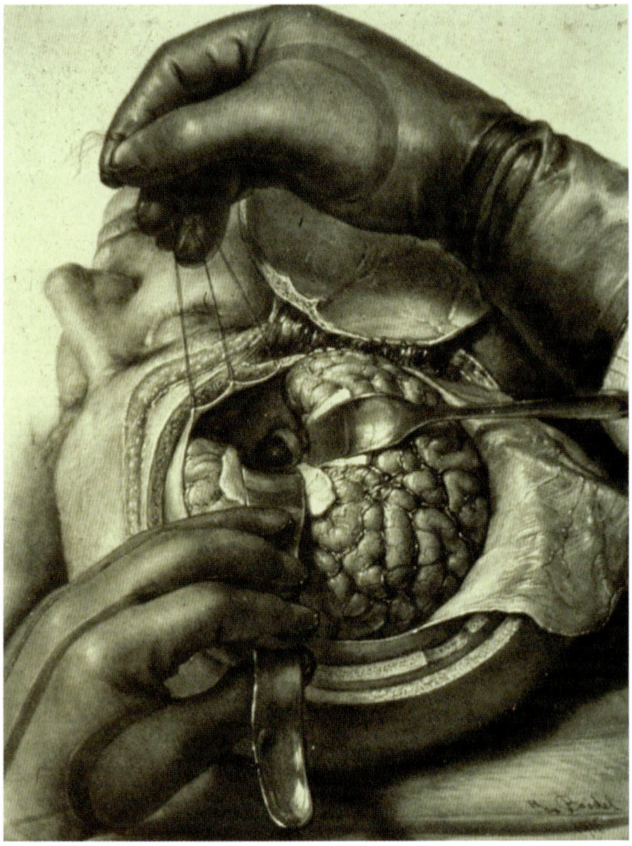

Fig. 1.3 Example of the frontotemporal approach popularized by Harvey Cushing. (Illustration by Max Brödel, 1915. From the personal collection of Dr. Edward R. Laws Jr.)

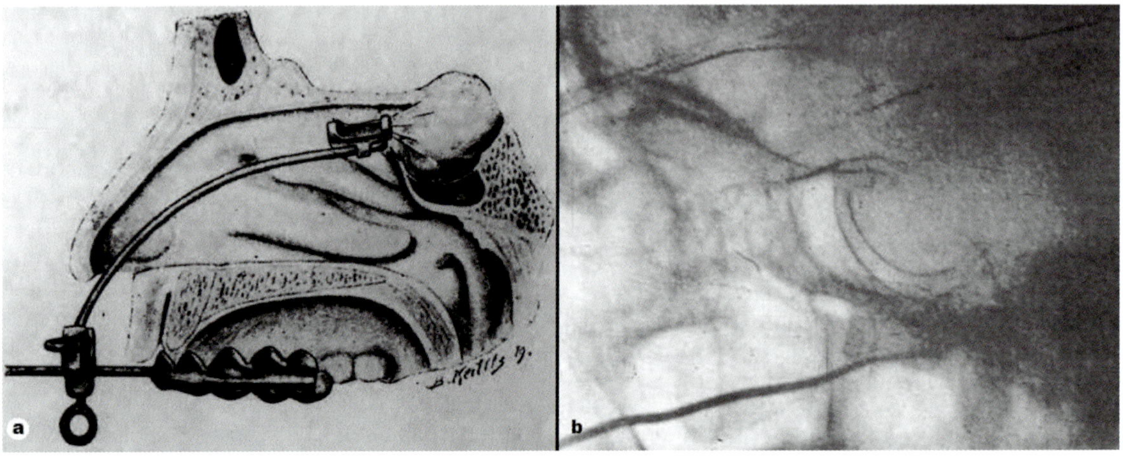

Fig. 1.4 **(A)** Hirsch's original schema for transnasal delivery of radium therapy to the sella. **(B)** Lateral skull X-ray as used by Oskar Hirsch for image-guided delivery of a radium bomb to the sella. (From Hirsch O. Symptoms and treatment of pituitary tumors. AMA Arch Otolaryngol 1952;55(3):268–306. Roentgenogram from the personal collection of Dr. Edward R. Laws Jr. Reprinted with permission.)

◆ The Birth of Microneurosurgery

As surgeons across the globe struggled to visualize the pituitary from both the transsphenoidal and transcranial routes, a quiet revolution was beginning in Stockholm. In 1921, Carl Nylén, an otolaryngologist at the University Clinic in Stockholm, performed the first microsurgery with a monocular dissecting microscope[11] (**Fig. 1.5**). A year later, Gunnar Holmgren, Nylén's chief, attached a light source to a binocular microscope. This allowed three-dimensional depth perception, and the external light source made it possible to work at even higher magnification than ambient light would.[12] In 1938, two otolaryngologists, Tullio and Calicetti, working in Parma, Italy, overcame two more limitations; they mounted the microscope on a counterweighted base to minimize vibrations and mounted a prism beam splitter in the optical pathway, which allowed two surgeons to work with the same field of view. These and other refinements were ultimately incorporated in the first generation of operative microscopes in the early 1950s, when commercial production for use in otolaryngology and ophthalmology began.[12]

Microneurosurgery as we know it was born on August 1, 1957, when Theodore Kurze at the University of Southern California, encouraged by William House's feats of microscopic middle ear surgery, brought a microscope into the operating room to assist with resection of a facial nerve schwannoma.[13] One year later, the first interdisciplinary microsurgical laboratory was established by R. M. P. Donaghy in Burlington, VT.[14] Over the next decade, collaboration between neurosurgeons and vascular surgeons, building on the early experience of ophthalmologists and otologists, resulted in new instrumentation and techniques. These were taught to M. Gazi Yaşargil, who returned to Zurich in 1967 after a year in Donaghy's laboratory to perform the first cerebrovascular bypass.[15]

With the newly found ability to illuminate and visualize deep structures, neurosurgeons and otolaryngologists began to approach the sellar and parasellar region with bravado. In the 1950s and 1960s, Smith and Ketcham's reports of combined transfacial and transcranial approaches to the paranasal sinuses re-ignited interest in radical resection of tumors in this region.[16] Parkinson reported one of the first successful microsurgical approaches to the cavernous carotid.[17] Over the next 20 years, the field of microscopic neurosurgery of the skull base underwent a period of exponential growth and popularity. Aided by the anterior and middle fossa approaches described by innovators such as Dolenc, Sekhar, and Al-Mefty, and the transfacial approaches described by Smith, Ketcham, VanBuren, and others, surgeons were no longer impotent in addressing complex lesions of the sellar and parasellar regions via transcranial and transfacial approaches.[18,19]

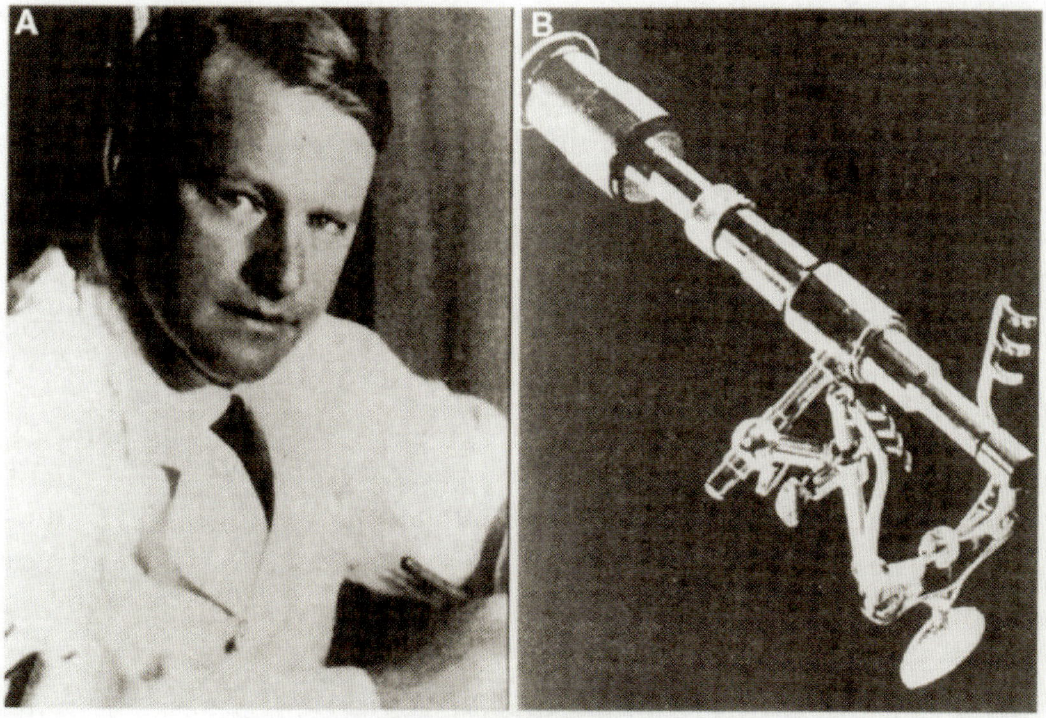

Fig. 1.5 **(A)** Carl Nylén and **(B)** his original operative monocular microscope. (From Kriss TC, Kriss VM. History of the operating microscope: from magnifying glass to microneurosurgery. Neurosurgery 1998;42(4):899–907. Reprinted with permission.)

◆ The Resurgence of Transsphenoidal Surgery

Norman Dott returned to Edinburgh after spending 1923–1924 in Cushing's clinic and surgical theater at the Brigham. In contrast to most surgeons, who followed Cushing's lead in abandoning the transsphenoidal approach, Dott continued to practice and refine it over the next 30 years[20] and demonstrated its virtues in the mid 1950s to his pupil, Gerard Guiot of France. Guiot was an extraordinary innovator, and he designed new instrumentation, including an endoscope, to facilitate the operation. However, he abandoned the endoscope because of its poor illumination and visualization compared with the operative microscope. Guiot adapted intraoperative fluoroscopy, using air and contrast to localize instruments in the sagittal plane and visualize the extent of tumor resection[21] (**Fig. 1.6**). This allowed him and his brilliant pupil, Jules Hardy of Montreal, to safely and accurately work above the sella under indirect visualization. This marked the beginning of real-time image guidance in pituitary surgery, which continues to evolve today.

While working with Guiot, Hardy began to use the operating microscope and microtechnique in pituitary surgery. In another example of simultaneous advancement, Hardy reported the use of the operating microscope for selective hypophysectomy in 1965—the same year Leonard Malis, at Mount Sinai Hospital in New York, used the operating microscope to completely resect a craniopharyngioma in a patient with a prefixed chiasm.[22,23] The advancements in microsurgery introduced by Yasargil and Malis—namely, bipolar electrocautery for hemostasis and microsurgical techniques—were adapted by Hardy for pituitary surgery. Hardy's demonstration in the late 1960s that one could do selective operations to remove pituitary microadenomas, while preserving the normal pituitary gland, was a revolutionary concept and led to renewed interest in transsphenoidal microsurgery for the treatment of pituitary tumors.[24,25]

◆ Radiosurgery of the Pituitary and Surrounding Areas

The development of roentgenography in 1896 and its ability to visualize the bony structures in the region of the sella became not only a key factor in the anatomic diagnosis of pituitary disease but also the basis for the radiosurgical treatment of many pituitary disorders. In 1901, Oppenheim reported the first use of roentgenography to diagnose a pituitary tumor. By 1907, the same year that Schloeffer attempted the first transsphenoidal pituitary operation, physicians were beginning to use X-ray therapy to treat acromegaly. In 1909, Gramegna, in Venice, reported his 2-year experience treating a patient with acromegaly by directing X-rays transorally to the sella.[26] That same year, Béclère reported a case in which the enlarged sella of a 16-year-old giant was irradiated with X-rays, and after the patient's vision improved and headaches abated with irradiation alone, Béclère abandoned his plans for craniotomy.[27] External beam radiation therapy was demonstrated to be a viable alternative to surgery when he reported the patient's 5-year symptom-free follow-up in 1913.

With the Curies' discovery of polonium and radium as sources of ionizing radiation, surgeons began to experiment with crude forms of brachytherapy. In 1912, Hirsch reported his use as early as 1910 of a radium "bomb" placed transnasally, with image guidance, to treat a pituitary tumor.[6,10] Cushing's case logs for the decade from 1914 through 1923 reveal several cases in which he used brachytherapy, although he was not enthusiastic about the results.[28]

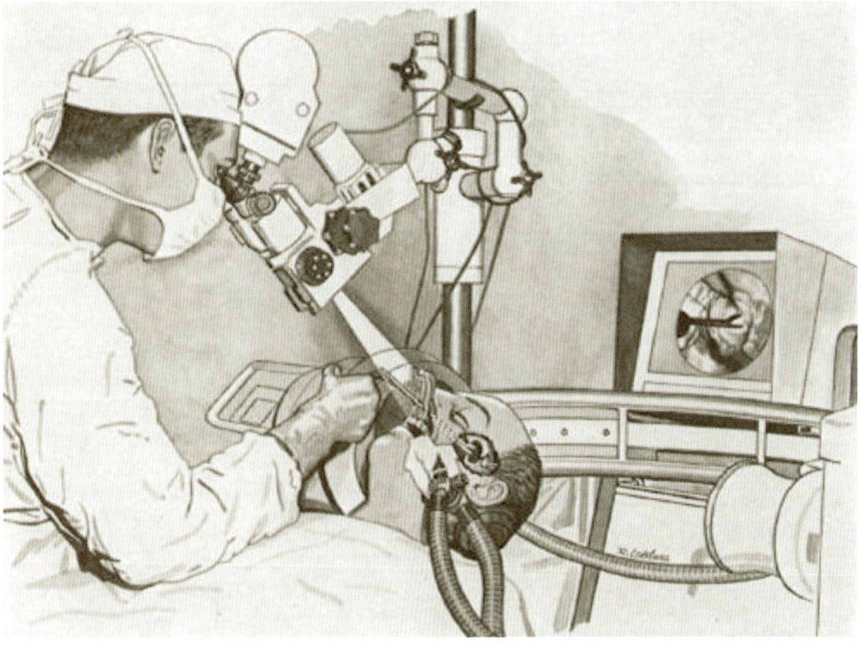

Fig. 1.6 Operative setup as originally reported by Gerard Guiot and later refined by Jules Hardy. (From Hardy J. Transsphenoidal hypophysectomy. J Neurosurg 1971;34:582–594. Reprinted with permission.)

The end of World War II also brought several scientific and technologic advances to medicine. The cyclotron, developed by Ernest Lawrence at Berkley National Laboratory, provided not only a sustainable source of fissile material for military purposes but also a new source of high-energy protons and helium ions for use in external beam radiotherapy. Lawrence's brother John began experimental treatments with the synchrocyclotron in patients in the early 1950s.[29] These treatments of neurosurgical disease were expanded upon in the early 1960s by Kjellberg at Massachusetts General in Boston, who treated patients in the Harvard cyclotron.[30] (**Fig. 1.7**).

The end of the war also brought a new exchange of ideas, such as the fateful discussion in 1947 between Sir Hugh Cairns and Lars Leksell at the first meeting of the Scandinavian Neurosurgical Society in Oslo. Encouraged by Cairns, Leksell proceeded to develop a polar-coordinate stereotactic frame for arc-based neurosurgery.[31] After early experiments, Leksell was dissatisfied with the collateral damage and imprecise therapy delivered by coupling his frame with existing X-ray and proton sources.

The delivery of the first production gamma knife in 1968 to the Karolinska Institute in Stockholm ushered in the era of "radiosurgery," a term coined by Leksell to suggest the idea of an operation in which the surgeon used a single dose of radiation as precisely as a knife to "excise" (or in this case inactivate) a lesion.[31 (p 4)] Over the years, stereotactic radiosurgery (gamma knife in the late 1960s, LINAC [linear accelerator] in the early 1980s, CyberKnife in the 1990s) has become an indispensable tool in both the primary and the adjuvant therapy of sellar and parasellar lesions.

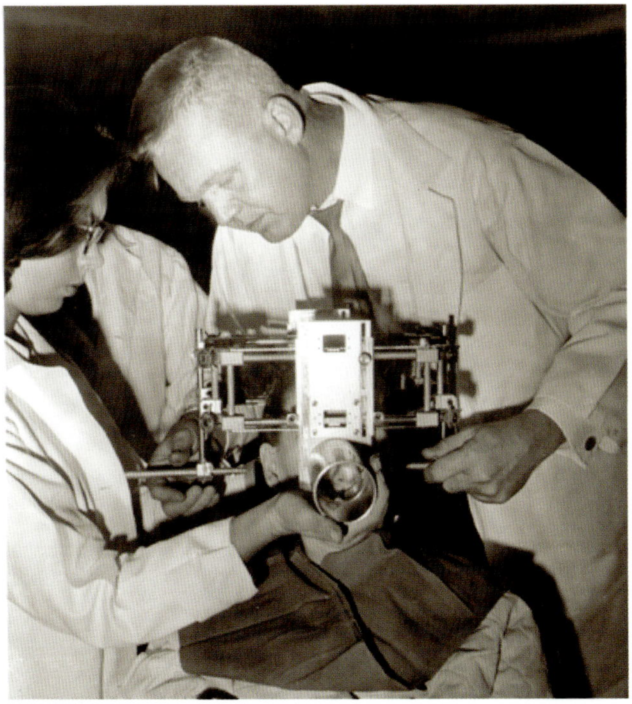

Fig. 1.7 Raymond Kjellberg fitting a patient with a stereotactic frame for proton beam therapy at the Harvard Cyclotron ca. 1960. (From Wilson R. A Brief History of the Harvard University Cyclotrons. Harvard University Press; 2004:104–105. Reprinted with permission.)

◆ The Rise of Endoscopic Skull Base Surgery

Although the endoscope was used with varying success as early as 1910 for intraventricular surgery, its resolution (and therefore utility) was limited in both cranial and endonasal surgery until the mid 20th century.[32] Two dramatic design advances in the 1950s—the Hopkins rod-lens and Storz "cold" illumination—suddenly allowed surgeons to see with the same clarity as did an operative microscope.[33] As the resolution and illumination of endoscopes improved, they were rapidly adopted by rhinologists for use in sinus surgery. A whole armamentarium of instruments and techniques was developed and refined by otorhinolaryngologists working in relative isolation from neurosurgeons until the mid 1990s, when, as with microsurgery in the 1950s, collaboration between the two disciplines launched a new era in surgical technique.

In the late 1970s, the first reports of endoscopically assisted transsphenoidal surgery emerged.[34,35] Over the ensuing years, improvements in lighting and digital cameras allowed the development of endoscopes with visualization besting that of a galilean instrument. Angled lenses allowed surgeons to look off axis, and combined with angled sinus instrumentation, they allowed surgeons to work in areas previously unreachable from an endonasal approach. These technologic advances made possible additional work on the suprasellar portion of tumors, as noted by Apuzzo et al in the late 1970s and by Fries and Perneczky in the late 1980s.[35,36] However, most neurosurgeons continued to consider the endoscope a replacement for angled mirrors and relegated its use to augmenting the operating microscope.

By the early 1990s, collaboration between neurosurgeons and otorhinolaryngologists resulted in the first reports of purely endoscopic approaches to the sella. Jho and Carrau in Pittsburgh are credited with demonstrating the safety and efficacy of a purely endoscopic approach for pituitary adenoma[37,38] (**Fig. 1.8**). In a recapitulation of the evolution of microsurgery, they described initial attempts as single-nostril single-surgeon approaches. Nearly simultaneously, Cappabianca, de Divittis, and colleagues in Naples, Italy, reported their initial experiences with the Jho-Carrau technique, taking a rigorously scientific approach to designing improved instrumentation and addressing the limitations of the techniques.[39,40] Soon thereafter, reports from Kassam, Snyderman, and Carrau also described a binasal three- to four-hand technique that restored the neurosurgeon's ability to perform bimanual microneurosurgery.[41] In the early 2000s, the combined experience of many surgeons allowed exponential improvement in the purely endoscopic technique over a relatively short time. Today, surgeons are able to attack disease from the olfactory bulb rostrally to the odontoid process caudally and as far laterally as the foramen ovale from a purely endonasal endoscopic approach.

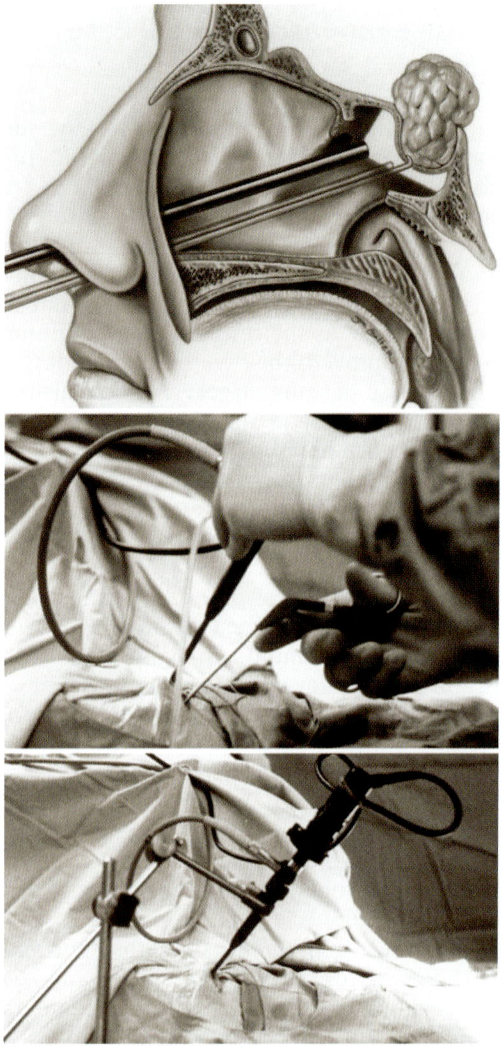

Fig. 1.8 (A–C) Schematic and example of operative setup for a purely endoscopic single-nostril endonasal approach to the sella as originally reported by Jho and Carrau. (From Jho H, Carrau RL. Endoscopic endonasal transsphenoidal surgery: experience with 50 patients. J Neurosurg 1997;87(1):44–51.)

◆ Conclusion

The surgeon who treats these disorders now can choose an optimal approach tailored to the patient and the disease. It may be traditional transsphenoidal microsurgery, precise craniotomy based on skull base concepts, minimally invasive eyebrow exposure, or any of the straightforward or extended endoscopic anterior skull base techniques.

Although radiation therapy is much less often used as adjunctive treatment for pituitary tumors, many tumors, particularly those that are invasive of surrounding structures or recurrent, will eventually require this modality of treatment. The major advance has been the development of stereotactic radiosurgery and its application to suitable pituitary and parasellar tumors as both primary and adjuvant therapy.

Further advances in all these treatment modalities will continue. Within our lifetime, the surgical treatment of pituitary lesions will become as foreign to us as our current techniques would have been to the forefathers of pituitary surgery. Versatility is one of the most important factors in the successful surgical management of sellar and parasellar pathology. A disease-oriented approach by a multispecialty team is the key to optimal management for patients with these difficult and challenging disorders.

Suggested Readings

History of Transsphenoidal Surgery

Gandhi CD, Christiano LD, Eloy JA, Prestigiacomo CJ, Post KD. The historical evolution of transsphenoidal surgery: facilitation by technological advances. Neurosurg Focus 2009;27(3):E8

Liu JK, Cohen-Gadol AA, Laws ER, et al. Harvey Cushing and Oskar Hirsch: early forefathers of modern transsphenoidal surgery. J Neurosurg 2005;103(6):1096–1104

Liu JK, Das K, Weiss MH, Laws ER, Couldwell WT. The history and evolution of transsphenoidal surgery. J Neurosurg 2001;95(6):1083–1096

History of Microneurosurgery

Kriss TC, Kriss VM. History of the operating microscope: from magnifying glass to microneurosurgery. Neurosurgery 1998;42(4):899–907, discussion 907–908

History of Radiosurgery

Laws ER, Vance ML. Radiosurgery for pituitary tumors and craniopharyngiomas. Neurosurg Clin N Am 1999;10(2):327–336

Lederman M. The early history of radiotherapy: 1895-1939. Int J Radiat Oncol Biol Phys 1981;7(5):639–648

History of Endoscopic Pituitary Surgery

Pettorini BL, Tamburrini G. Two hundred years of endoscopic surgery: from Philipp Bozzini's cystoscope to paediatric endoscopic neurosurgery. Childs Nerv Syst 2007;23(7):723–724

Prevedello DM, Doglietto F, Jane JA, et al. History of endoscopic skull base surgery: its evolution and current reality. J Neurosurg 2007;107(1):206–213

References

1. Cushing H. The Pituitary Body and Its Disorders: Clinical States Produced by Disorders of the Hypophysis Cerebri. J. B. Lippincott Company; 1912
2. Marie P. Sur deux cas d'acromégalie. Rev Med (Paris) 1886;6: 297–333

3. Pollock JR, Akinwunmi J, Scaravilli F, Powell MP. Transcranial surgery for pituitary tumors performed by Sir Victor Horsley. Neurosurgery 2003;52(4):914–925, discussion 925–926
4. Caton R, Paul F. Subtemporal decompression in an acromegalic. BMJ 1893;2:1421–1423
5. Lindholm J. A century of pituitary surgery. Neurosurgery 2007;61(4):865–868
6. Liu JK, Cohen-Gadol AA, Laws ER, et al. Harvey Cushing and Oskar Hirsch: early forefathers of modern transsphenoidal surgery. J Neurosurg 2005;103(6):1096–1104
7. Kanavel A. The removal of tumors of the pituitary body by an infranasal route. A proposed operation and description of the technique. JAMA 1909;53:1704–1707
8. Cushing H. The Wier Mitchell lecture: surgical experiences with pituitary disorders. JAMA 1914;63:1515–1525
9. Couldwell WT. Transsphenoidal and transcranial surgery for pituitary adenomas. J Neurooncol 2004;69(1–3):237–256
10. Lederman M. The early history of radiotherapy: 1895–1939. Int J Radiat Oncol Biol Phys 1981;7(5):639–648
11. Nylen CO. The microscope in aural surgery, its first use and later development. Acta Otolaryngol Suppl 1954;116:226–240
12. Uluç K, Kujoth GC, Başkaya MK. Operating microscopes: past, present, and future. Neurosurg Focus 2009;27(3):E4
13. Kriss TC, Kriss VM. History of the operating microscope: from magnifying glass to microneurosurgery. Neurosurgery 1998; 42(4):899–907, discussion 907–908
14. Donaghy RM. The history of microsurgery in neurosurgery. Clin Neurosurg 1979;26:619–625
15. Yasargil M. Microsurgery: Applied to Neurosurgery. Thieme; 2006
16. Donald PJ. History of skull base surgery. Skull Base Surg 1991; 1(1):1–3
17. Parkinson D. Transcavernous repair of carotid cavernous fistula. Case report. J Neurosurg 1967;26(4):420–424
18. Shah JP. Skull base surgery: the first 50 years. Eur Arch Otorhinolaryngol 2007;264(7):711–712
19. Maroon JC. Skull base surgery: past, present, and future trends. Neurosurg Focus 2005;19(1):E1
20. Liu JK, Das K, Weiss MH, Laws ER, Couldwell WT. The history and evolution of transsphenoidal surgery. J Neurosurg 2001;95(6):1083–1096
21. Gandhi CD, Christiano LD, Eloy JA, Prestigiacomo CJ, Post KD. The historical evolution of transsphenoidal surgery: facilitation by technological advances. Neurosurg Focus 2009;27(3):E8
22. Hardy J, Wigser SM. Trans-sphenoidal surgery of pituitary fossa tumors with televised radiofluoroscopic control. J Neurosurg 1965;23(6):612–619
23. Malis LI. Base of skull: history and philosophy. Skull Base Surg 1992;2(2):69–75
24. Hardy J. Transsphenoidal microsurgery of the normal and pathological pituitary. Clin Neurosurg 1969;16:185–217
25. Hardy J. Transsphenoidal hypophysectomy. J Neurosurg 1971; 34(4):582–594
26. Gramegna A. Un cas d'acromégalie traité par la radiothérapie. Rev Neurol 1909;xvii:15–17
27. Béclère A. The radio-therapeutic treatment of tumours of the hypophysis, gigantism, and acromegaly. Arch Roentgen Ray 1909;14:142–150
28. Schulder M, Loeffler JS, Howes AE, Alexander E, Black PM. Historical vignette: The radium bomb: Harvey Cushing and the interstitial irradiation of gliomas. J Neurosurg 1996;84(3): 530–532
29. Lawrence JH, Tobias CA, Born JL. Acromegaly. Trans Am Clin Climatol Assoc 1962;73:176–185
30. Wilson R. A Brief History of the Harvard University Cyclotrons. Harvard University Press; 2004:104–105
31. Germano IM. Linac and Gamma Knife Radiosurgery. Thieme; 2000:4
32. Pettorini BL, Tamburrini G. Two hundred years of endoscopic surgery: from Philipp Bozzini's cystoscope to paediatric endoscopic neurosurgery. Childs Nerv Syst 2007;23(7):723–724
33. Prevedello DM, Doglietto F, Jane JA, et al. History of endoscopic skull base surgery: its evolution and current reality. J Neurosurg 2007;107(1):206–213
34. Bushe KA, Halves E. [Modified technique in transsphenoidal operations of pituitary adenomas. Technical note (author's translation).] Acta Neurochir (Wien) 1978;41(1–3):163–175
35. Apuzzo ML, Heifetz MD, Weiss MH, Kurze T. Neurosurgical endoscopy using the side-viewing telescope. J Neurosurg 1977;46(3):398–400
36. Fries G, Perneczky A. Endoscope-assisted brain surgery: part 2–analysis of 380 procedures. Neurosurgery 1998;42(2):226–231, discussion 231–232
37. Jho H, Carrau RL. Endoscopic endonasal transsphenoidal surgery: experience with 50 patients. J Neurosurg 1997;87(1):44–51
38. Carrau RL, Jho HD, Ko Y. Transnasal-transsphenoidal endoscopic surgery of the pituitary gland. Laryngoscope 1996;106(7): 914–918
39. Cappabianca P, Alfieri A, Thermes S, Buonamassa S, de Divitiis E. Instruments for endoscopic endonasal transsphenoidal surgery. Neurosurgery 1999;45(2):392–395, discussion 395–396
40. Cappabianca P, Alfieri A, de Divitiis E. Endoscopic endonasal transsphenoidal approach to the sella: towards functional endoscopic pituitary surgery (FEPS). Minim Invasive Neurosurg 1998;41(2):66–73
41. Carrau RL, Kassam AB, Snyderman CH. Pituitary surgery. Otolaryngol Clin North Am 2001;34(6):1143–1155, ix

2 Anatomy of the Sellar and Parasellar Region

Albert L. Rhoton Jr.

This chapter focuses on the anatomic basis of the microsurgical and endoscopic approaches to the sellar and parasellar regions.

◆ Subcranial Relationships

The pituitary gland and sella are located in the cranial base below the center of the brain (**Fig. 2.1**). Access to the sella is limited from above by the optic nerves and chiasm and the circle of Willis, from the sides by the cavernous sinuses and internal carotid arteries, and from behind by the brainstem and basilar artery. Because of the vital structures blocking superior, lateral, and posterior access to the sella, the preferred surgical route to most sellar tumors is from below, through the nasal cavity and sphenoid sinus. These subcranial approaches are being expanded with the aid of the endoscope to include other areas bordering the sella, including the cavernous sinus, Meckel's cave, and the adjacent parts of the anterior, middle, and posterior cranial fossae. This section focuses on the sella and sphenoid sinus and their subcranial relationships.

Nasal Cavity

The sella can be reached by several routes through the nasal cavity.[1,2] The nasal cavity, wider below than above, is bounded above by the anterior cranial fossa, laterally by the ethmoid and maxillary sinuses and orbits, and below by the hard palate (**Figs. 2.2** and **2.3**). This cavity is divided sagittally by the nasal septum, which is formed anteriorly and superiorly by the perpendicular plate of the ethmoid and inferiorly and posteriorly by the vomer; an anterior bony deficiency is occupied by septal cartilage. The nasal cavity opens anteriorly onto the face through the anterior nasal aperture and posteriorly into the nasopharynx by way of the posterior nasal apertures. Each posterior nasal aperture, measuring ~25 mm vertically and 13 mm transversely, is bordered above by the anterior aspect of the sphenoid body, below by the posterior margin of the hard palate formed by the horizontal plate of the palatine bones, medially by the part of the nasal septum formed by the vomer, and laterally by the medial pterygoid plate and perpendicular plate of the palatine bone.

Fig. 2.1 The pituitary gland and its relationships. **(A)** Anterior view of pituitary gland. The gland is located below the optic nerves and chiasm and between the cavernous segments of the internal carotid arteries. The right optic nerve has been elevated to expose the pituitary stalk. The superior hypophyseal arteries arise from the medial side of the supraclinoid portion of the internal carotid arteries and pass medially to the pituitary stalk and optic chiasm. **(B)** Superior view of pituitary gland. In this case, the diaphragm was largely absent, so that the subarachnoid space extended across and was separated from the top of the anterior lobe only by arachnoid membrane. The right half of the dorsum sellae has been removed to expose the posterior lobe, which was hidden under the dorsum. The inferior hypophyseal artery travels medially from the intracavernous carotid to the posterior lobe. **(C,D)** Superior and inferior surfaces of a gland in which the anterior and posterior lobes form a relatively ovoid structure. The pars tuberalis wraps partially around the stalk. **(E)** The anterior and posterior lobes have been separated. The stalk joins the anterosuperior surface of the posterior lobe and is partially surrounded by the pars tuberalis. **(F)** Midsagittal section of the sella extending through the anterior and posterior lobes and sphenoid sinus. The intracavernous carotid produces prominences in the lateral wall of the sphenoid sinus below and anterior to the gland. The sella extends forward to the anterior edge of the intracavernous carotid only if greatly expanded by tumor. The intercavernous sinuses course along the anterior and posterior margins of the diaphragm. The basilar sinus, located on the back of the dorsum, is the largest connection across the midline between the posterior edge of the paired cavernous sinuses. The inferior hypophyseal artery arises from the posterior bend of the intracavernous carotid and is directed medially toward the posterior lobe. **(G)** Anterior view of another gland. The optic nerves and chiasm have been elevated to expose the pituitary stalk and the superior hypophyseal and ophthalmic arteries. The superior hypophyseal arteries arise from the medial side of the supraclinoid carotid and pass to the chiasm and stalk. **(H)** Another gland and sella viewed superiorly. The diaphragm partially covers the upper surface of the gland, but the opening in the diaphragm is larger than the pituitary stalk. The posterior lobe (not shown) was entirely hidden below the dorsum sellae. An intercavernous sinus passes across the upper anterior surface of the gland. **(I)** Superior view of another gland exposed below a large natural opening in the diaphragm.

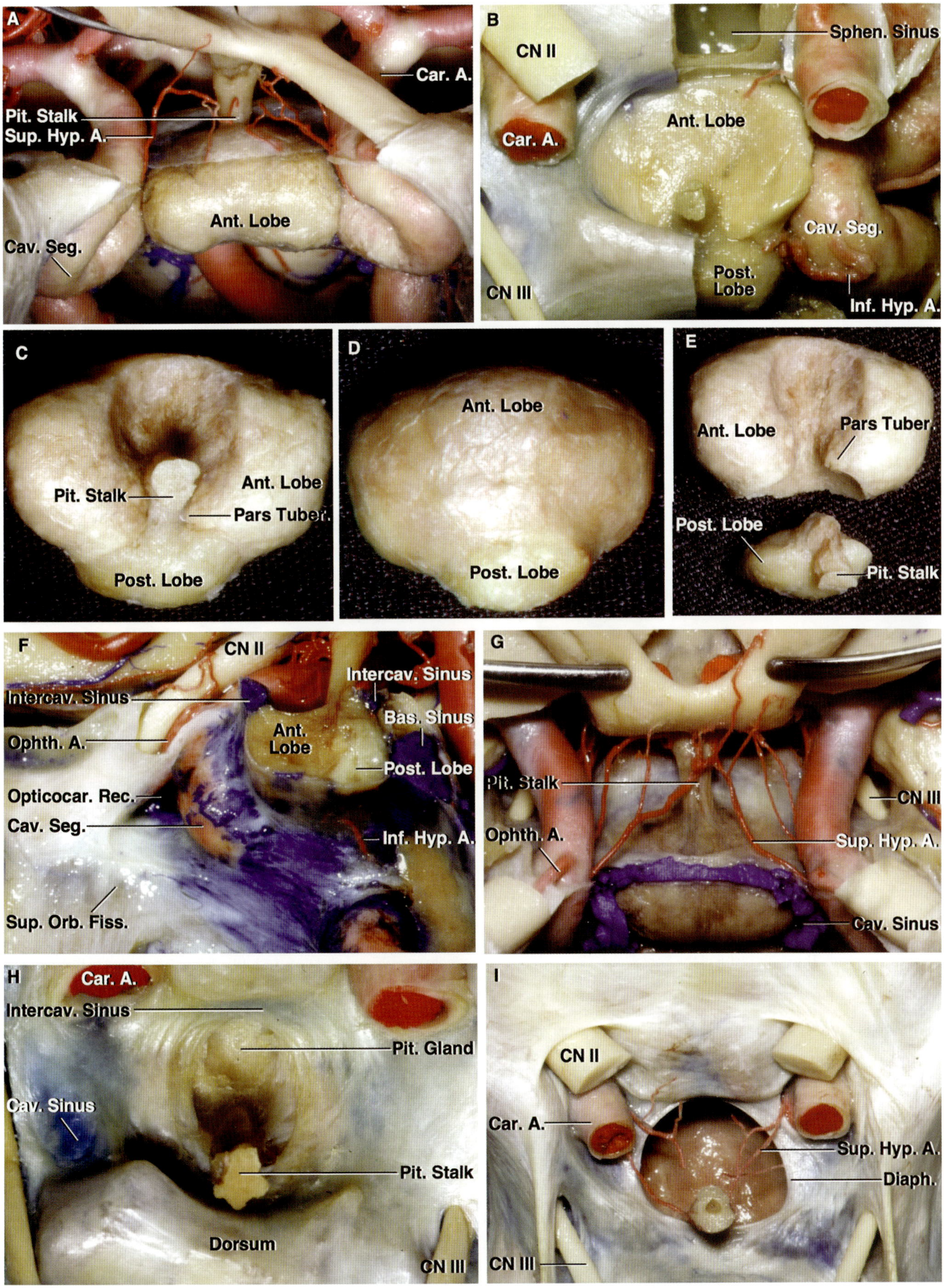
A
Car. A.
Pit. Stalk
Sup. Hyp. A.
Ant. Lobe
Cav. Seg.
B
CN II
Sphen. Sinus
Car. A.
Ant. Lobe
Cav. Seg.
Post. Lobe
CN III
Inf. Hyp. A.
C
Pit. Stalk
Ant. Lobe
Pars Tuber.
Post. Lobe
D
Ant. Lobe
Post. Lobe
E
Ant. Lobe
Pars Tuber.
Post. Lobe
Pit. Stalk
F
CN II
Intercav. Sinus
Intercav. Sinus
Bas. Sinus
Ophth. A.
Ant. Lobe
Post. Lobe
Opticocar. Rec.
Cav. Seg.
Inf. Hyp. A.
Sup. Orb. Fiss.
G
Pit. Stalk
CN III
Ophth. A.
Sup. Hyp. A.
Cav. Sinus
H
Car. A.
Intercav. Sinus
Pit. Gland
Cav. Sinus
Pit. Stalk
Dorsum
CN III
I
CN II
Car. A.
Sup. Hyp. A.
Diaph.
CN III

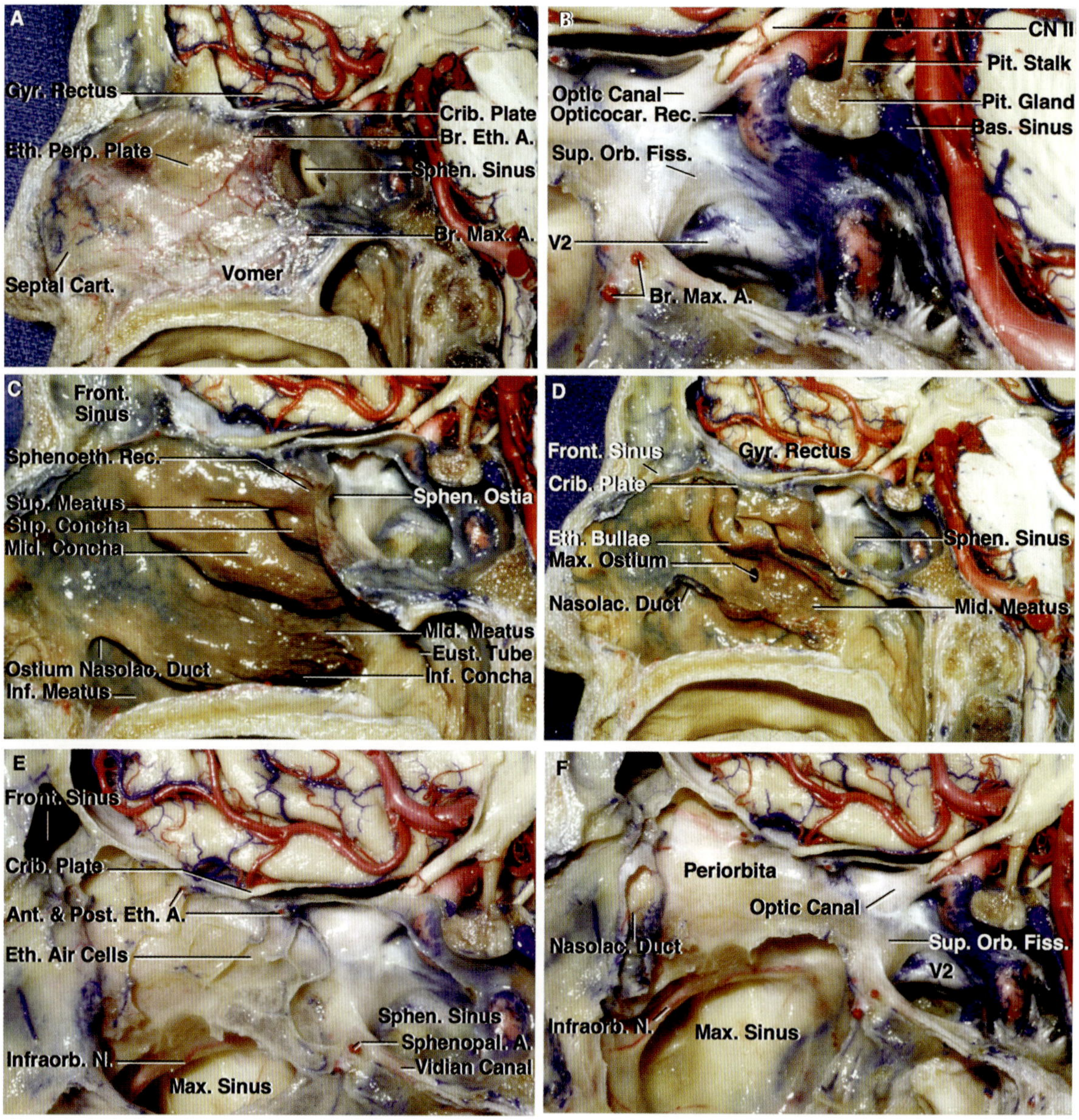

Fig. 2.2 Stepwise dissection of the nasal pathway along which the transsphenoidal surgery is directed. **(A)** Sagittal section to the left of the midline and nasal septum. The nasal septum is formed anteriorly by the septal cartilage, above by the perpendicular plate of the ethmoid, and below and posteriorly by the vomer. The posterior inferior part of the septum is supplied by the branches of the sphenopalatine artery, a terminal branch of the maxillary artery. The upper part of the septum, below the cribriform plate, is supplied by the branches of the ethmoidal arteries, which arise from the ophthalmic artery. A septum divides the sphenoid sinus near the midline. The optic chiasm, optic and oculomotor nerves, third ventricle, and pituitary stalk are located above the pituitary gland. The gyrus rectus of the frontal lobe is located above the cribriform plate and olfactory tract. **(B)** Midsagittal section of the sphenoid sinus and pituitary gland. Prominences overlie the optic canal, internal carotid artery, superior orbital fissure, and maxillary nerve in the wall of the sphenoid sinus. The opticocarotid recess extends laterally between the optic nerve, internal carotid artery, and the prominence medial to the superior orbital fissure, and it extends into the optic strut, which separates the optic canal from the superior orbital fissure. The serpiginous prominence overlying the internal carotid artery is located anterior to and below the pituitary gland. **(C)** The lateral wall of the nasal cavity is constituted below by the nasal surface of the maxilla and above by the nasal surface of the ethmoid sinuses. The inferior concha (turbinate) is an independent bone that articulates with the nasal surface of the maxilla and perpendicular plate of the palatine bone. The middle and superior conchae are appendages of the ethmoid bone. The lacrimal duct opens below the anterior part of the inferior concha. The inferior, middle, and superior nasal meati are located below their respective conchae. The superior meatus is located between the middle and superior conchae. The sphenoethmoidal recess, a narrow cleft located above the superior concha, separates the superior concha from the anterior surface of the sphenoid sinus and is the site of the ostium communicating the sphenoid sinus and nasal cavity. The eustachian tube opens into the nasopharynx behind the medial pterygoid plate and below the sphenoid sinus. **(D)** The concha has been removed. The maxillary and frontal sinuses drain into the middle meatus. The lacrimal duct opens below the inferior turbinate into the inferior meatus. The ethmoid bullae are rounded prominences overlying the ethmoidal air cells. The anterior ethmoidal air cells drain into the superior meatus. The posterior ethmoidal air cells and the sphenoid sinus drain into the sphenoethmoidal recess. **(E)** The medial wall of the maxillary sinus has been removed to expose the sinus roof, which forms the orbital floor. The infraorbital sulcus and canal, which transmit the infraorbital nerve, are situated in the floor of the orbit, forming a prominence in the roof of the maxillary sinus. The anterior and posterior ethmoidal arteries arise from the ophthalmic artery and pass through the anterior and posterior ethmoidal canals to reach the floor of the anterior fossa beside the cribriform plate, where they again penetrate the bone to reach the walls of the nasal cavity. The vidian canal is the site of passage of the vidian nerve to the pterygopalatine ganglion. The vidian nerve is formed by parasympathetic fibers from the greater petrosal nerve and sympathetic fibers from the deep petrosal branch of the carotid plexus. The frontal sinus is situated at the upper anterior part of the medial wall. **(F)** Removing the lateral wall of the ethmoid air cells, which forms the medial wall of the orbit, exposes the periorbita. The medial wall of the nasolacrimal duct has been removed to expose the interior of the duct.

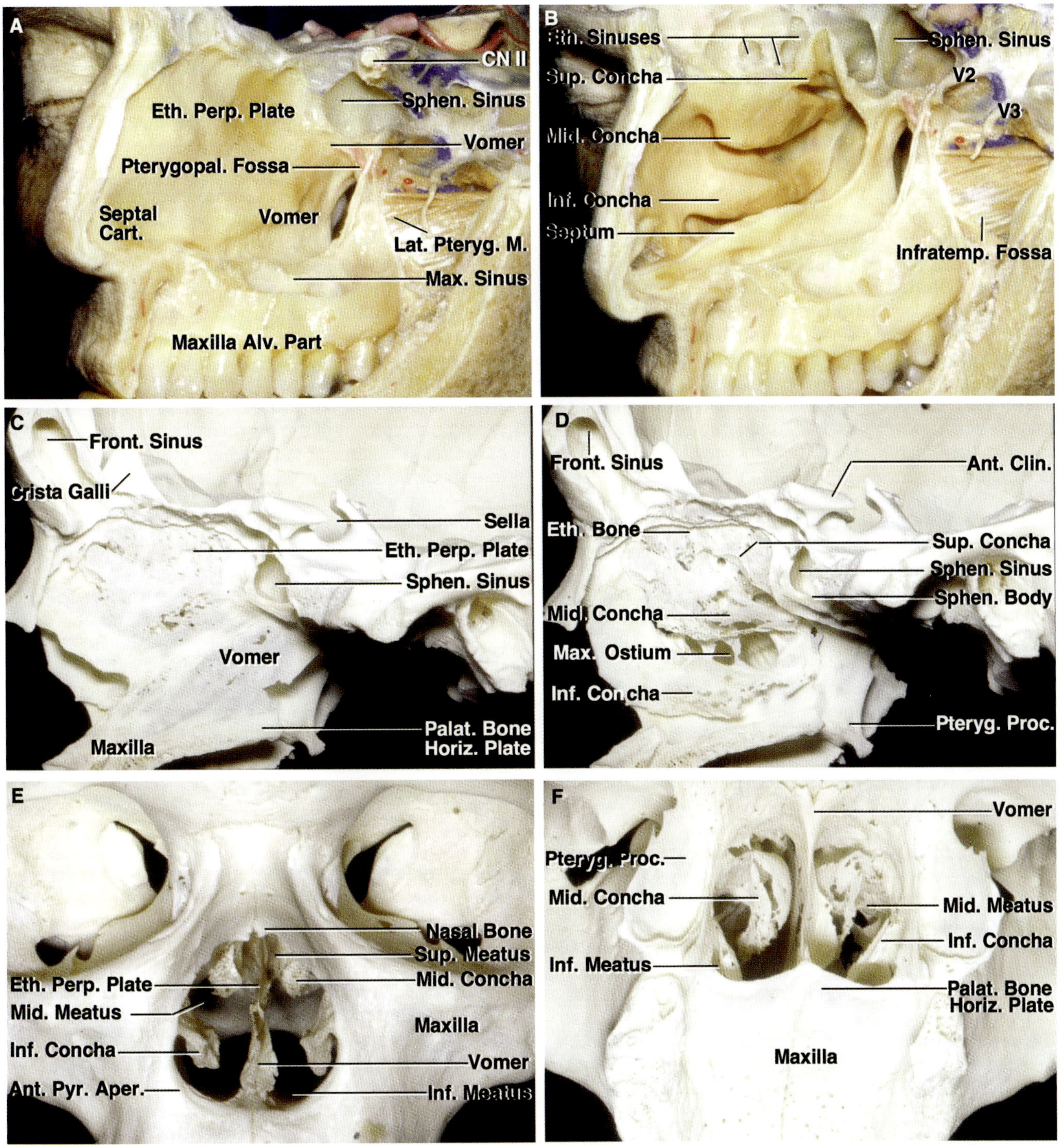

Fig. 2.3 (A–D) Comparison of osseous and mucosal structures in the nasal septum and conchae. (E–F) Osseous relationships along the transsphenoidal and endonasal approaches to the sella. (A) The structures anterior to the left orbital apex and the portion of the maxilla above the alveolar process have been removed to expose the nasal septum, which is formed posteriorly by the vomer, above by the perpendicular plate of the ethmoid, and anteriorly by the septal cartilage. (B) The nasal septum and anterior wall of the sphenoid sinus have been removed. This exposes the superior, middle, and inferior conchae and a midline septum within the sphenoid sinus. The ethmoid air cells are exposed in the medial wall of the right orbit. The part of the sphenoid sinus medial to and below the orbital apex has been opened. (C) The left half of facial skeleton, including the left half of the maxilla and orbit, has been removed to expose the left side of the nasal septum, which is formed above by the perpendicular plate of the ethmoid bone and below by the vomer. The palate is formed anteriorly by the maxilla and posteriorly by the horizontal plate of the palatine bone. (D) The nasal septum has been removed. The inferior concha is a separate bone, which protrudes into the nasal cavity from the maxilla. The middle and superior conchae are appendages of the ethmoid bone. The maxillary ostium is located between the perpendicular plate of the palatine bone behind, the ethmoid superiorly, and the medial maxillary wall below. The maxillary and frontal sinuses and the anterior ethmoid air cells drain into the middle meatus and the posterior ethmoid air cells drain into the superior meatus. (E) The anterior nasal aperture is formed above by the nasal bones, and laterally and below by the maxilla. The anterior part of the osseous nasal septum is formed above by the perpendicular ethmoid plate and below by the vomer. The inferior concha, a separate bone, and the middle concha, an appendage of the ethmoid bone, are visible through the aperture. (F) Posterior view of the posterior nasal aperture. The floor of the posterior aperture is formed by the horizontal plate of the palatine bone. The lateral margin is formed by the medial plate of the pterygoid process and is joined anteriorly by the perpendicular plate of the palatine bone, which forms the part of the lateral nasal wall between the maxilla and the medial pterygoid plate. Posteriorly, the middle concha is much more prominent than the inferior concha and often must be displaced laterally in the transsphenoidal approach to the sphenoid sinus and sella. The vomer extends from the upper surface of the hard palate to the body of the sphenoid bone and separates the paired nasal cavities at the posterior aperture.

The lateral nasal wall has three medially directed projections—the superior, middle, and inferior nasal conchae—below which are the corresponding superior, middle, and inferior nasal meati (**Figs. 2.2** and **2.3**). The paired sphenoethmoidal recesses, located above and behind the superior nasal conchae, are the site of the paired sphenoid ostia, which communicate between the nasal cavity and the sphenoid sinus. The upper half of the lateral nasal wall, composed anteriorly to posteriorly of the frontal process of the maxilla, lacrimal bone, and ethmoid bone with its air cells, separate the nasal cavity from the orbit. The nasolacrimal groove and canal, the site of the lacrimal sac and nasolacrimal duct, respectively, pass downward in front of the anterior end of the middle nasal concha and open into the inferior nasal meatus. The frontoethmoidal suture, located at the junction of the roof and medial orbital wall, is situated at the level of the roof of the nasal cavity and the cribriform plate. The anterior and posterior ethmoidal foramina, through which the anterior and posterior ethmoidal arteries and nerves enter the ethmoidal canals, are located on the medial orbital wall at or just above the frontoethmoidal suture. These arteries and nerves exit the orbit by passing through the ethmoidal canals to enter the anterior cranial fossa at the lateral edge of the cribriform plate. The anterior ethmoidal artery, a terminal branch of the ophthalmic artery, supplies the mucosa of the anterior and middle ethmoid sinuses, the dura covering the cribriform plate and planum sphenoidale, and the upper part of the nasal spectrum. It gives rise to the anterior falcine artery intracranially. The posterior ethmoidal artery, usually smaller than the anterior ethmoidal artery and absent in up to 30% of orbits, feeds the mucosa of the posterior ethmoid sinus, adjacent part of the nasal spectrum, and dura of the planum sphenoidale. The average distance between the anterior lacrimal crest of the frontal process of the maxilla and the anterior ethmoidal foramen is 22 to 24 mm; between the anterior and posterior ethmoidal foramina, 12 to 15 mm; and between the posterior ethmoidal foramen and the optic canal, 3 to 7 mm.[2] In transfacial procedures, these arteries may be divided between the periorbita and the medial orbital wall. Care should be taken to prevent damaging the optic nerve, which is sometimes located immediately behind the posterior ethmoidal foramen.

The lower part of the lateral nasal wall is formed anteriorly to posteriorly by the maxilla, the perpendicular plate of the palatine bone, and the medial pterygoid plate. The eustachian tube opens into the nasopharynx along the posterior edge of the medial pterygoid plate. The middle nasal concha, an appendage of the ethmoid bone, attaches to the lateral nasal wall at the level of the orbit floor and roof of the maxillary sinus. Thus, the medial wall of the maxillary sinus is bounded medially by the middle and inferior nasal meati and the inferior nasal concha (**Figs. 2.2** and **2.3**). The maxillary sinus communicates with the middle nasal meatus through an opening located in the medial sinus wall just below the sinus roof.

The pterygopalatine fossa, situated just outside the lateral wall of the nasal cavity, is positioned between the posterior wall of the maxillary sinus anteriorly, the pterygoid process posteriorly, and the perpendicular plate of the palatine bone medially (**Figs. 2.2, 2.3,** and **2.4**). The pterygopalatine fossa contains the pterygopalatine ganglion, which receives the vidian nerve (nerve of the pterygoid canal), the segment of the maxillary nerve and its branches located just anterior to the foramen rotundum, and the internal maxillary artery and its terminal branches. This fossa communicates laterally with the infratemporal fossa through the pterygomaxillary fissure and medially with the nasal cavity via the sphenopalatine foramen, through which pass the corresponding nerve and vessels, which provide the predominant supply to the turbinates and nasal septum. The maxillary artery exits the infratemporal fossa to enter the pterygopalatine fossa by passing through the pterygomaxillary fissure. The greater and lesser palatine arteries and nerves arise from the maxillary artery and nerve and descend in the greater and lesser palatine canals, which are separated medially from the nasal cavity by the perpendicular plate of the palatine bone.

Sphenoid Bone

The sphenoid bone is located in the center of the cranial base[3–5] (**Figs. 2.3** and **2.5**). Because of the intimate contact of the body of the sphenoid bone with the nasal cavity below and the pituitary gland above, the transsphenoidal route is the operative approach of choice for most pituitary tumors. The neural relationships of the sphenoid bone are among the most complex of any bone: the olfactory tracts, gyrus rectus, and posterior part of the frontal lobe rest against the smooth upper surface of the lesser wing; the temporal lobe rests against the inner surface of the greater wing; the pons and mesencephalon lie posterior to the clival portion; and the optic chiasm lies posterior to the chiasmatic sulcus. Additionally, the second through sixth cranial nerves are intimately related to the sphenoid bone, and all exit the skull through the optic canal, superior orbital fissure, or foramen rotundum or ovale, all of which are located in the sphenoid bone (**Fig. 2.6**).

Fig. 2.4 Transnasal route to the sphenoid sinus and sella. **(A)** The cross-section extends across the nasal cavity, the superior and middle turbinates, the maxillary sinuses, the orbits near the apex, and the ethmoid sinuses in front of the sphenoid sinus. The zygomatic and infraorbital nerves arise from the maxillary nerve in the pterygopalatine fossa, which is located behind the posterior maxillary wall. The nasal septum is formed above by the perpendicular ethmoid plate, below by the vomer, and anteriorly by the cartilaginous septum. **(B)** The concha and posterior ethmoid air cells have been removed to expose the vomer and the anterior wall of the sphenoid sinus and the sphenoid ostia. The nasolacrimal duct descends along the lateral wall of the nasal cavity. **(C)** Enlarged view. The perpendicular ethmoid plate joins the anterior sphenoid face, and the vomer extends upward to join the inferior sphenoid wall, both in the midline. The posterior ethmoid air cells are located anterior to the lateral part of the sphenoid face and overlap the superolateral margins of the sphenoid ostia. **(D)** The anterior face of the sphenoid has been removed to expose the multiseptate sphenoid sinus and the anterior wall of the sella. The bony prominences over the optic canals are situated in the superolateral margins of the sinus. **(E)** The anterior wall of the sella and the lateral wall of the sphenoid sinus have been removed

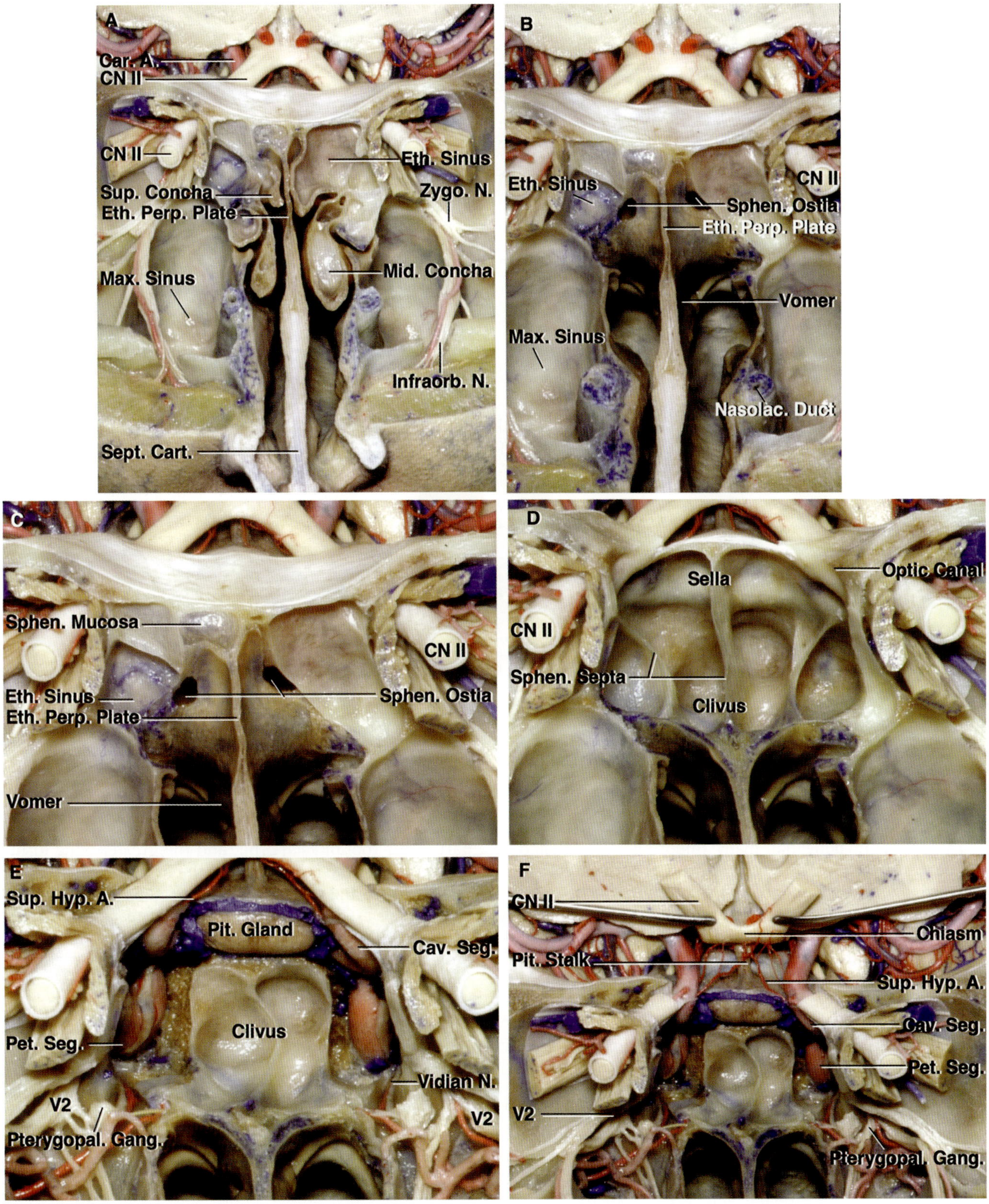

Fig. 2.4 *(Continued)* to expose the petrous and cavernous segments of the carotid artery and the pituitary gland. The posterior wall of the maxillary sinus has been removed to expose the maxillary nerve and artery and the pterygopalatine ganglion in the pterygopalatine fossa. The branches of the maxillary artery penetrate the lateral wall of the nasal cavity to course along the sphenoid face. The maxillary nerve sends communicating rami to the sphenopalatine ganglion. The vidian nerve enters the posterior aspect of the sphenopalatine ganglion. The pituitary gland is surrounded by the cavernous sinuses laterally and an anterior intercavernous sinus above. **(F)** The optic nerves have been elevated to show the suprasellar area and the relationships between the orbital apex, optic canals, nasal cavity, pterygopalatine fossa, and the petrous and intracavernous segments of the internal carotid artery. The superior hypophyseal arteries pass to the lower margin of the optic chiasm and the pituitary stalk.

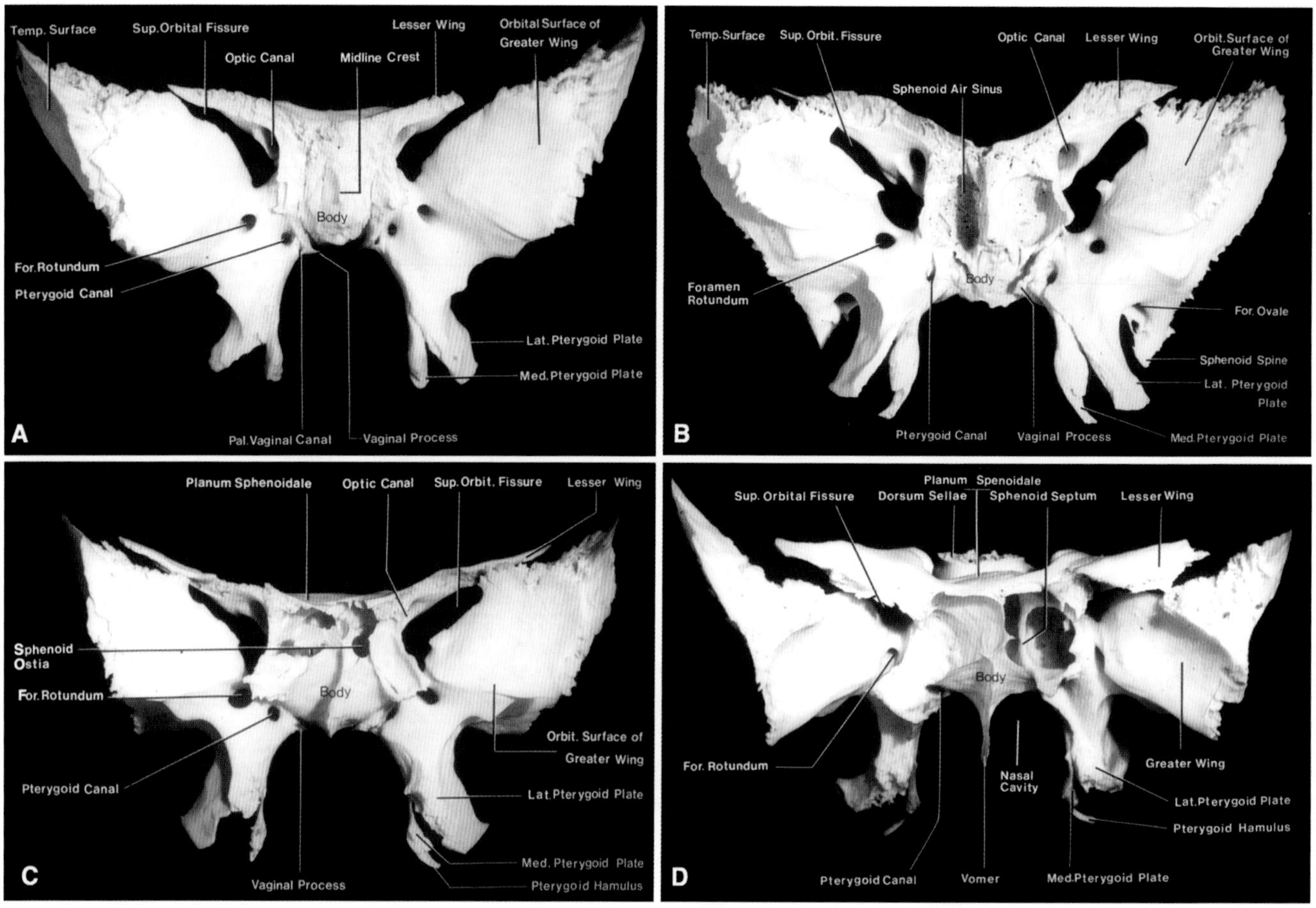

Fig. 2.5 Types of sphenoid bone. Anterior views. **(A)** Conchal type of sphenoid bone. **(B)** Bone with presellar type of sphenoid sinus. **(C)** Bone with sellar type of sphenoid sinus and well-defined sphenoid ostia. **(D)** Bone with sellar type of sphenoid sinus with poorly defined sphenoid ostia and obliquely oriented sphenoidal septa.

The sphenoid bone has many important arterial and venous relationships: the carotid arteries form a groove on each side of the sphenoid bone and often form a serpiginous prominence in the lateral wall of the sphenoid sinus; the basilar artery rests against its posterior surface; the circle of Willis is located above its central portion; and the middle cerebral artery courses parallel to the sphenoid ridge of the lesser wing. The cavernous sinuses rest against the sphenoid bone, and intercavernous venous connections line the walls of the pituitary fossa and dorsum sellae.

In the anterior view, the sphenoid bone resembles a bat with wings outstretched (**Fig. 2.5**). It has a central portion called the body; two lesser wings, which spread outward from the superolateral part of the body; two greater wings, which spread upward from the lower part of the body; and two pterygoid processes, whose medial and lateral pterygoid plates are directed downward from the body. The body of the sphenoid bone is more or less cubical and contains the sphenoid sinus. The superior orbital fissure, through which the oculomotor, trochlear, abducens, and ophthalmic nerves pass, is formed on its inferior and lateral margins by the greater wing and on its superior margin by the lesser wing. The lesser wing forms the posterior part of the roof of each orbit, and the greater wing forms a large part of the lateral wall of the orbit, the floor of the middle fossa, and the roof of the infratemporal fossa. The optic canals are situated above and are separated from the superomedial margin of the superior orbital fissure by the optic strut, a bridge of bone that extends from the lower margin of the base of the anterior clinoid process to the body of the sphenoid. The narrowest part of the optic canal is closer to the orbital than to the intracranial end. The optic canals average 5 mm in length and are of a conical configuration, tapering to a narrow waist near the orbit end. The sphenoid ostia communicate the nasal cavity with the sinus. The infratemporal crest on the inferior surface of the greater wing is positioned above the junction of the temporal and infratemporal fossae. The lateral pterygoid muscles arise from the lower surface of the greater wing between the infratemporal crest and the lateral pterygoid plate. The area lateral to the infratemporal crest gives origin to the temporalis muscle. The pterygoid (vidian) canal courses posteriorly to anteriorly through the junction of the pterygoid process and the sphenoid body and may be exposed under the mucosa lining the sinus floor by a bony dehiscence.

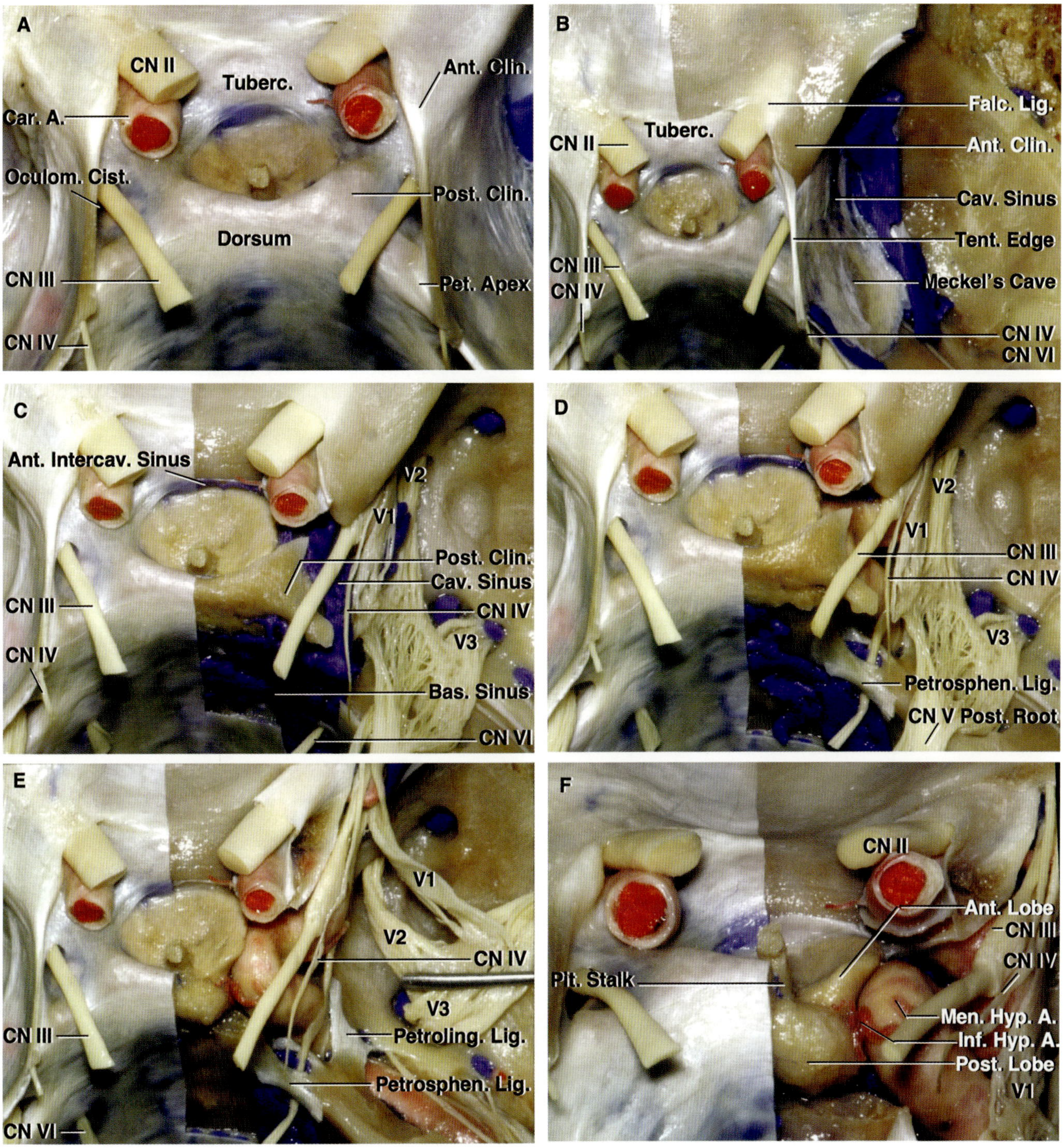

Fig. 2.6 Superior view of sellar region. **(A)** The sella is located between the cavernous sinuses. The diaphragm, which usually separates the sella from the suprasellar cisterns, is absent in this case. The oculomotor nerves enter the roof of the cavernous sinus, where there is a narrow cistern around the nerve. The oculomotor triangle, the triangular patch of dura through which the oculomotor nerve enters the dura in the cavernous sinus roof, is positioned between the anterior and posterior clinoid processes and the petrous apex. The roof of the cavernous sinus extends forward under the anterior clinoid process. **(B)** The dura covering the anterior clinoid process and optic canal has been removed. The outer layer of dura in the lateral wall of the cavernous sinus has been removed to expose the thin inner layer of the lateral sinus wall and the lateral surface of Meckel's cave. The falciform ligament, the dural fold extending above the optic nerve proximal to the entrance of the nerve into the optic canal, extends from the anterior clinoid to the tuberculum. **(C)** The inner layer of the lateral wall of the cavernous sinus has been removed to expose the nerves coursing in the wall of the cavernous sinus and middle fossa. The dura covering the dorsum sellae, basilar sinus, and posterior clinoid process has been removed. The oculomotor nerve passes forward lateral to the posterior clinoid and below the anterior clinoid. An abnormal bony projection extends laterally from the right posterior clinoid below the oculomotor nerve toward the petrous apex. The basilar sinus crosses the back of the dorsum and upper clivus and communicates widely with the posterior edge of the paired cavernous sinuses. The abducens nerve passes through the lower margin of the basilar sinus. An anterior intercavernous sinus passes along the anterior margin of the sella. **(D)** The anterior clinoid process has been removed to expose the clinoid segment of the internal carotid artery, defined by the upper and lower dural rings. The upper ring is formed by the dura extending medially from the upper surface of the anterior clinoid. The lower dural ring is formed by the dura, which extends medially from the lower margin of the anterior clinoid and separates the lower clinoid margin from the oculomotor nerve. **(E)** Posterosuperior view of the sella. The dorsum and posterior clinoid have been removed to expose the posterior lobe of the pituitary, which was hidden below the dorsum. The abducens nerve passes through Dorello's canal, which is roofed by the petrosphenoid ligament. The trigeminal nerve has been reflected forward to expose the petrolingual ligament, which extends above the internal carotid artery just proximal to the entry of the artery into the cavernous sinus. **(F)** Enlarged view. The carotid artery protrudes medially to deform the lateral surface of the anterior lobe of the pituitary gland. A tongue of anterior lobe extends laterally above the intercavernous carotid. The inferior hypophyseal branch of the meningohypophyseal artery passes medially to reach the posterior lobe.

In the superior view, the pituitary fossa occupies the central part of the body and is bounded anteriorly by the tuberculum sellae and posteriorly by the dorsum sellae (**Figs. 2.1** and **2.6**). The chiasmatic groove (sulcus), a shallow depression between the paired optic foramina, is bounded posteriorly by the tuberculum sellae and anteriorly by the planum sphenoidale. The frontal lobes and the olfactory tracts rest against the smooth upper surface of the lesser wings and the planum sphenoidale. The posterior margin of the lesser wing forms a free edge, the sphenoid ridge, which projects into the sylvian fissure to separate the frontal and temporal lobes. The anterior clinoid processes are located at the medial end of the lesser wings, the middle clinoid processes are lateral to the tuberculum sellae, and the posterior clinoid processes are situated at the superolateral margin of the dorsum sellae. The dorsum sellae is continuous below with the clivus. The upper part of the clivus is formed by the sphenoid bone and the lower part by the occipital bone.

The depth of the sella turcica is the greatest distance between the floor and a perpendicular line connecting the tuberculum and dorsum. Sellar length is defined as the greatest anteroposterior diameter of the pituitary fossa, which may occur at the level of the tuberculum sellae or below. Sellar width is defined as the width of the horizontal plateau of the sellar floor between the carotid sulci. The volume is calculated by applying the simplified mathematical formula for the volume of an ellipsoid: volume (mm^3) = 0.5 (length × width × depth [mm])/1000. The upper limit of normal depth is 13 mm; length, 17 mm; width, 15 mm; and volume, 1100 mm^3.[6]

The superior surface of each greater wing is concave upward and filled by the pole of each temporal lobe. The foramen rotundum, foramen ovale, and foramen spinosum, anteriorly to posteriorly, are located near the junction of the body and greater wing. When viewed from the inferior aspect, the vomer, a separate bone forming the lower part of the osseous nasal septum, frequently remains attached to the lower surface of the anterior half of the body of the sphenoid.

The pterion and the "keyhole" are two important anatomic landmarks in the region of the greater wing in the lateral view. The pterion is located over the upper part of the greater wing and approximates the site of the lateral end of the sphenoid ridge. The "keyhole" is located behind the junction of the temporal line and the zygomatic process of the frontal bone several centimeters anterior to the pterion. A burr hole placed over the pterion will be located near the lateral end of the sphenoid ridge. A burr hole placed at the keyhole will expose the periorbita in its lower part, the frontal dura in its upper part, and the orbital roof in its midportion. The placement of the keyhole burr hole is reviewed elsewhere.[7]

Sphenoid Sinus

The sphenoid sinus is positioned in the sphenoid body between the paired cavernous sinuses, internal carotid arteries, and optic, extraocular, and trigeminal nerves. In addition, the sinus sits between the pituitary gland and the nasal cavity. The sphenoid sinus varies considerably in size and shape and in the degree of pneumatization[8,9] (**Figs. 2.5, 2.7,** and **2.8**). It is present as minute cavities at birth, but its main development takes place after puberty. In early life, it extends backward into the presellar area and subsequently expands into the area below and behind the sella turcica, reaching full size during adolescence. As the sinus enlarges, it may partially encircle the optic and vidian canals and extend into the roots of the pterygoid processes, greater wings of the sphenoid bone, anterior clinoid processes, and clival part of the occipital bone. With advancing age, the sinus frequently undergoes further enlargement associated with absorption of its bony walls. Occasionally, there are gaps in its bone, with the mucous membrane lying directly against the dura mater.

There are three types of sphenoid sinus in adults: conchal, presellar, and sellar, based on the extent of sinus pneumatized (**Fig. 2.5**). In the conchal type, the sphenoid body below the sella is a solid block of bone without an air cavity. In the presellar type of sinus, the air cavity does not penetrate beyond a vertical plane parallel to the anterior sellar wall. In the sellar type of sphenoid sinus, the most common type, the air cavity extends into the sphenoid body below the sella and as far posteriorly as the clivus. In our previous study in adult cadavers, this sinus was of the presellar type in 24% and of the sellar type in 76%.[6] The conchal type is most common in children before the age of 12 years, at which time pneumatization begins within the sphenoid sinus. In the conchal type, which is infrequent in adults, the thickness of bone separating the sella from the sphenoid sinus is at least 10 mm.

The depth of the sphenoid sinus is defined as the distance from the ostium of the sphenoid sinus to the closest part of the sella (**Fig. 2.8**). In the adult, the average depth is 17 mm (range, 12–23 mm).[8] This measurement defines the length of the path within the sinus through which instruments must be passed to reach the sellar wall and is important when instruments are selected for transsphenoidal surgery. The speculum most commonly used for transsphenoidal surgery is 9 cm in length, and its tip should be placed anterior to the sphenoid sinus. In reaching the floor of the sella turcica, the depth of the sphenoid sinus (≥ 2 cm) is added to the 9-cm length of the speculum. Thus, after traversing a distance of 11 to 12 cm, the dissecting instruments must enter the sella turcica and be able to reach above the sella if a suprasellar tumor is present. The distance may be greater in the presence of acromegaly; therefore, it is important that transsphenoidal instruments have shafts at least 12 cm in length. The fact that important neural and vascular structures are exposed either in the lateral sinus wall, directly lateral to the sella, or above the diaphragma sellae, especially if the latter is defective, has led this writer to prefer blunt rather than sharp ring curettes for dissection and tumor removal. Another measurement important in transsphenoidal surgery is the thickness of the anterior sellar wall and sellar floor. In the sellar type of sinus, the thickness of the anterior sellar wall ranged from 0.1 to 0.7 mm (mean, 0.4 mm), compared with 0.3 to 1.5 mm (mean, 0.7 mm) for the presellar type. The thickness of bone covering the sinus was defined at the planum sphenoidale, tuberculum sellae, anterior

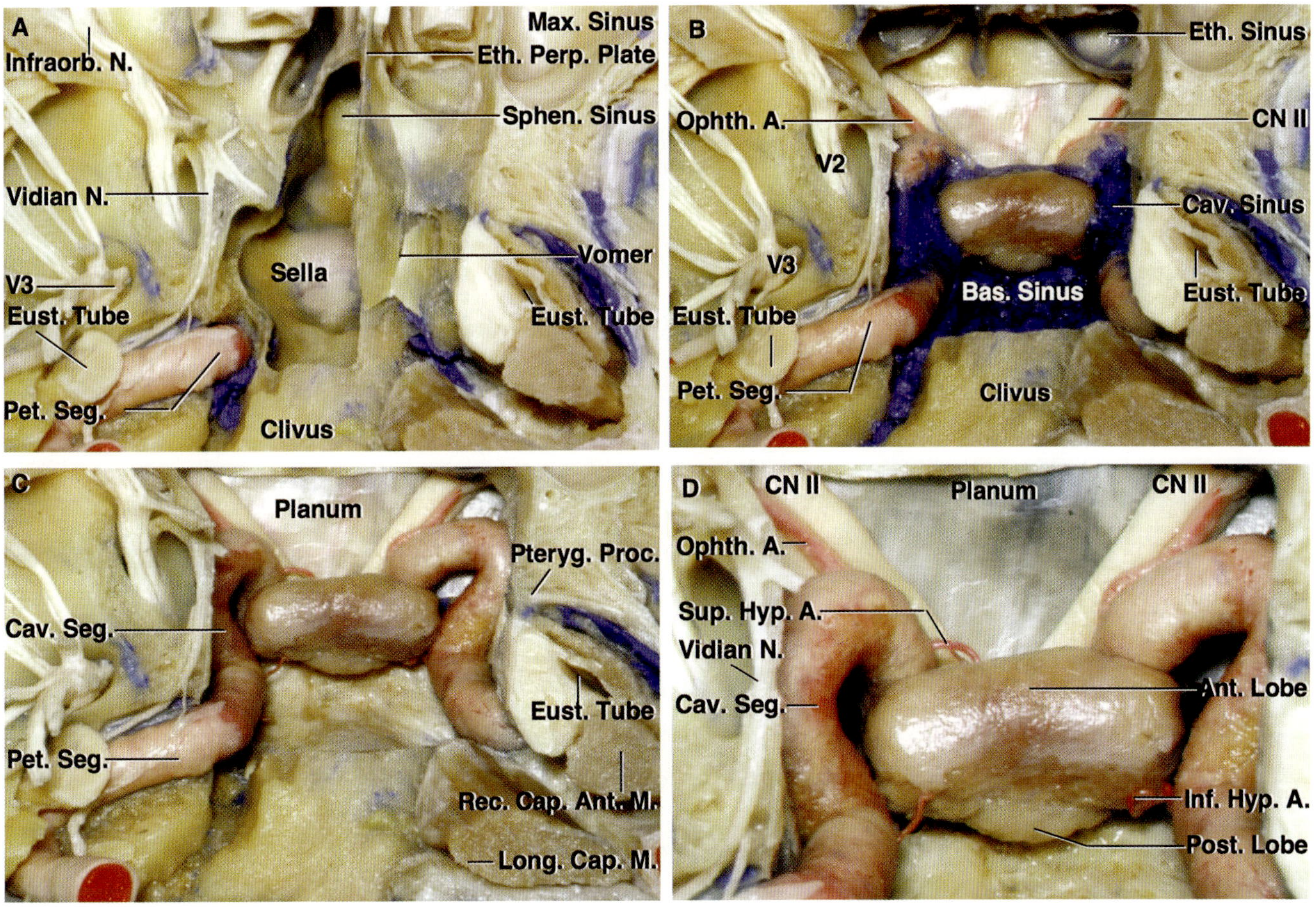

Fig. 2.7 (A–D) Inferior view of the sellar region and surrounding skull base. (A) The right half of the floor of the sphenoid sinus has been removed to expose the sellar floor and the part of the sphenoid sinus below the planum and tuberculum. On the left side of the specimen, the eustachian tube, pterygoid process, and posterior part of the maxillary sinus have been preserved. On the right side, the medial portion of the eustachian tube and the pterygoid process have been removed. This exposes the right mandibular nerve exiting the foramen ovale and the maxillary nerve exiting the foramen rotundum and passing forward as the infraorbital nerve. The pterygopalatine ganglion is located in the pterygopalatine fossa behind the maxillary sinus in the lateral wall of the nasal cavity. The right pterygoid process has been removed to expose the vidian canal, in which the vidian nerve travels to reach the pterygopalatine ganglion. The bone below the petrous carotid has been removed up to the point where the artery turns upward to enter the posterior part of the cavernous sinus. (B) Part of the vomer, perpendicular ethmoid plate, and floor of the sphenoid sinus have been removed to expose the cavernous sinus, intracavernous carotid, and pituitary gland. The floors of the optic canals have been removed to expose the ophthalmic arteries coursing below the optic nerves. The cavernous sinus surrounds the intracavernous carotid. An anterior intercavernous sinus crosses the anterior margin of the gland. Some of the upper clivus has been removed to expose the basilar sinus, which sits on the back of the dorsum and is the largest connection between the cavernous sinuses. (C) The venous spaces around the pituitary gland have been cleared to expose the petrous and intracavernous carotid segments. (D) Enlarged view of the pituitary gland, intracavernous carotid, and optic nerves and ophthalmic arteries. The inferior hypophyseal arteries pass to the posterior lobe. The superior hypophyseal arteries arise in the chiasmatic cistern and pass medially to reach the stalk and chiasm.

sellar wall, sellar floor, and clivus. The thickest bone was found at the clivus and tuberculum sellae and the thinnest along the anterior sellar wall.[4,6]

The septa within the sphenoid sinus vary greatly in size, shape, thickness, location, completeness, and relation to the sellar floor (**Fig. 2.9**). The cavities within the sinus are seldom symmetric from side to side and are often subdivided by irregular minor septa. The septa are often located off the midline as they cross the floor of the sella. In our previous study, a single major septum separated the sinus into two large cavities in only 68% of specimens, and even in these cases the septa were often located off the midline or deflected to one side.[6] The most common type of sphenoid sinus has multiple small cavities in the large paired sinuses. The smaller cavities may be separated by septa oriented in all directions. Computed tomography (CT) or magnetic resonance imaging (MRI) of the sella provides the definition of the relationship of the septa to the floor of the sella needed for transsphenoidal surgery. Major septa may be found as far as 8 mm off the midline.[6] The septa are not to be used as a guide to the midline but may be used as landmarks based on where preoperative CT and MRI show them to be located in relation to the sella and the tumor.

The internal carotid artery rests directly against the lateral surface of the body of the sphenoid bone, and its course is marked by a groove in the bone, the carotid sulcus, which defines the course of the intracavernous portion of the carotid artery. As the sinus expands and its walls are resorbed, the carotid sulcus produces a prominence within the sinus wall below the floor and along the

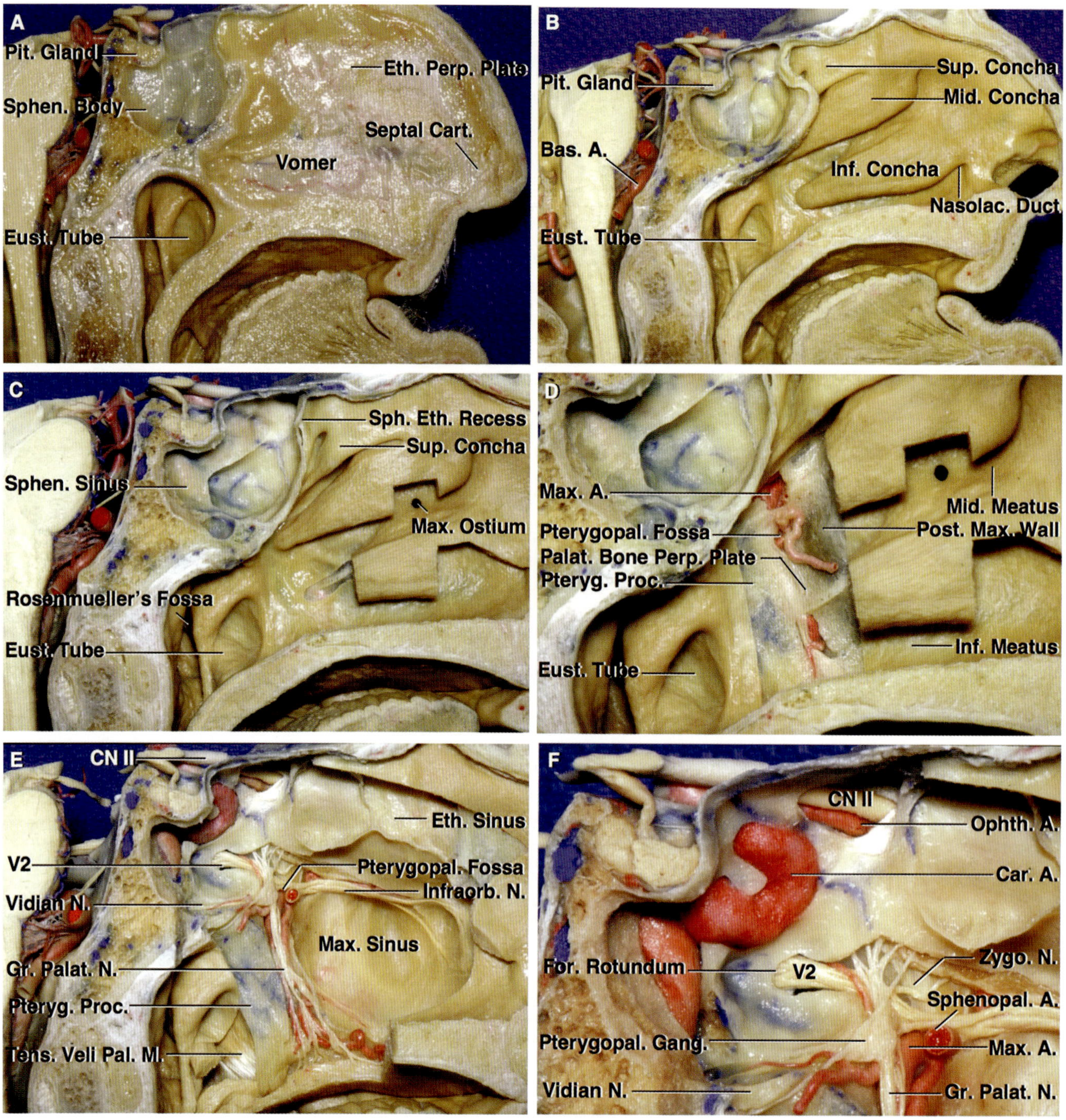

Fig. 2.8 Nasal pathway to the sphenoid sinus. Stepwise dissections showing the structures that form the lateral limit of the transnasal route to the sphenoid sinus and sella. **(A)** Sagittal section to the right of midline. The nasal septum, along which the transsphenoidal approach is directed, is formed above by the perpendicular plate of the ethmoid, anteriorly by the nasal septal cartilage, and below by the vomer. The vomer articulates with the anterior-inferior part of the sphenoid body, and the perpendicular plate articulates with the anterior face. The sphenoid sinus is located in the body of the sphenoid bone. **(B)** The sagittal section has been extended to the right of midline. The nasal conchae and meati and the eustachian tubes are in the lateral margin of the exposure. **(C)** A portion of the middle and inferior turbinates has been removed. The ostia of the maxillary and frontal sinuses open into the middle meatus, located below the middle turbinate. The nasolacrimal duct opens below the lower turbinate into the inferior meatus. Rosenmuller's fossa is located behind the eustachian tube. **(D)** The mucosa in the lateral margin of the nasal cavity and the posterior part of the inferior and middle turbinates have been removed to expose the pterygoid process and posterior maxillary wall, which form the posterior and anterior boundaries of the pterygopalatine fossa, respectively. The eustachian tube opens into the nasopharynx at the posterior edge of the pterygoid process. The terminal branches of the maxillary artery pass through the pterygopalatine fossa, located between the posterior maxillary wall and the pterygoid process, and give rise to the sphenopalatine artery, which enters the posterior superior part of the nasal cavity by passing through the sphenopalatine foramen. The medial wall of the pterygopalatine fossa is formed by the perpendicular plate of the palatine bone. **(E)** The medial wall of the maxillary sinus has been opened to expose the infraorbital nerve, which arises in the pterygopalatine fossa and passes forward in the sinus roof. The maxillary nerve passes through the foramen rotundum to enter the pterygopalatine fossa, where it gives rise to the infraorbital, zygomatic, and greater palatine nerves, plus communicating rami to the pterygopalatine ganglion. **(F)** Enlarged view. The bone and dura covering the optic canal in the superolateral part of the sphenoid sinus have been opened to expose the optic nerve and ophthalmic artery in the optic canal. The junction of the petrous and cavernous carotid limits the exposure below the level of the sella. Terminal branches of the maxillary artery intermingle with the neural structures in the pterygopalatine fossa and exit the fossa to supply structures within and bordering the nasal cavity.

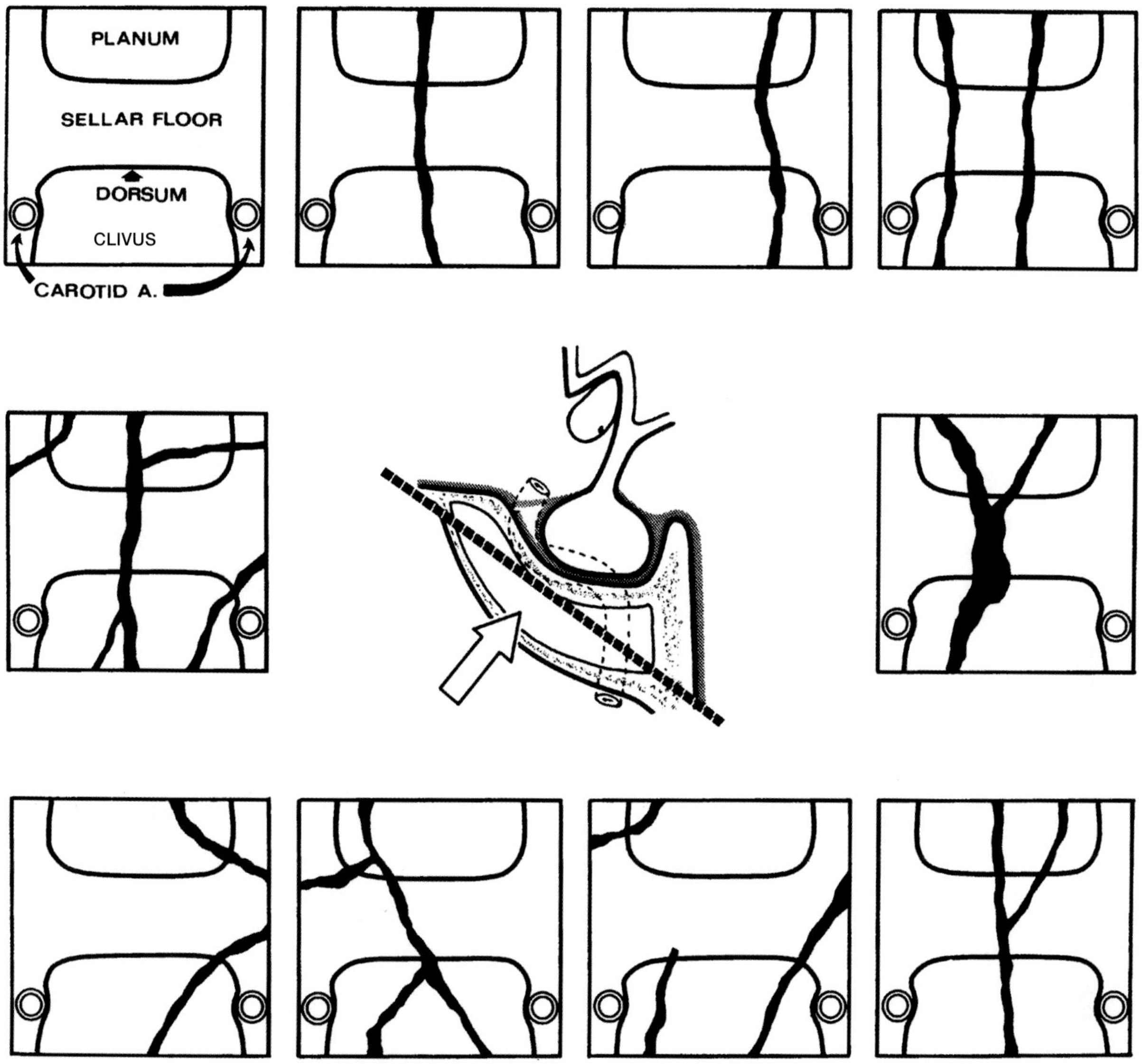

Fig. 2.9 Septa in the sphenoid sinus. The *heavy broken line* on the central diagram shows the plane of the section of each specimen from which the drawings were taken, and the *large arrow* shows the direction of view. The planum is above, the dorsum and clivus are below, and the sella is in an intermediate position on each diagram. The *heavy dark lines* on the drawings show the location of the septa in the sphenoid sinus. A wide variety of septa separate the sinus into cavities that vary in size and shape and are seldom symmetric from side to side.

anterior margin of the sella[6,8] (**Figs. 2.6, 2.8,** and **2.10**). This prominence is most pronounced with maximal pneumatization of the sphenoid and varies from a small focal bulge to a serpiginous elevation marking the full course of the carotid artery along the lateral sinus wall. The intrasinus carotid prominence can be divided into three parts: the retrosellar, infrasellar, and presellar segments. The first part, the retrosellar segment, is located in the posterolateral part of the sinus. This segment of the prominence is present only in well-pneumatized sellar-type sinuses in which the air cavity extends laterally in the area below the dorsum. The second part, the infrasellar segment, is located below the sellar floor. The third part, the presellar segment, is located anterolateral to the anterior sellar wall. Of the 50 specimens we examined, 98% had presellar, 80% had infrasellar, and 78% had retrosellar prominences.[1,6] Any part of the prominence may be present and the others absent. If all three parts are present and connected, they form a serpiginous bulge marking the full course of the carotid artery along the lateral wall of the sinus. In the normal sinus, the presellar part courses anterolateral to the anterior sellar wall. The anterior sellar wall bulges forward of the carotid prominence only when the sella is greatly expanded by tumor.

Only the presellar part of the carotid prominence is present in a presellar type of sphenoid sinus, and it is this part that is also most frequently present in the sellar type of sinus. The corresponding arterial segments are slightly longer than the segments of the prominence because of tortuosity of the artery. This tortuosity, although present, is limited by the dural walls of the cavernous sinus, particularly if the artery is encircled by a ring of bone formed by the union of the anterior and middle clinoid processes. Serial coronal scans through the cavernous sinus show that the artery does not always nestle into the bony carotid sulcus on the intracranial surface of the sphenoid

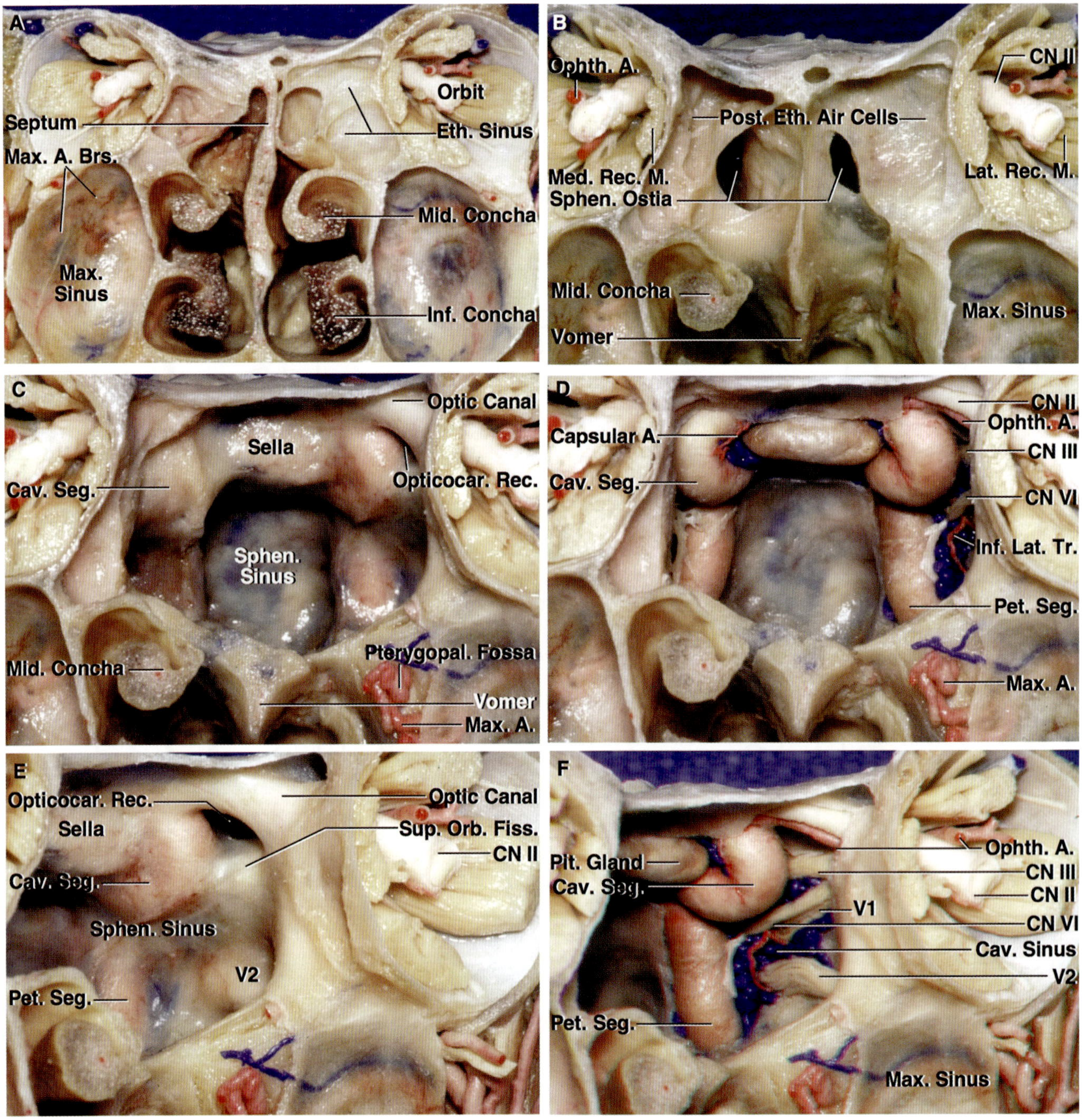

Fig. 2.10 Anterior view of a coronal section in front of the sphenoid sinus, through the nasal cavity, orbits, and ethmoid and maxillary sinuses. **(A)** The upper part of the nasal cavity is separated from the orbits by the ethmoid sinuses. The lower part of the nasal cavity is bounded laterally by the maxillary sinuses. The middle concha projects medially from the lateral nasal wall at the junction of the maxillary and ethmoid sinuses. The posterior ethmoid air cells are located in front of the lateral part of the face of the sphenoid sinus. **(B)** The middle and inferior nasal conchae on the left side and the nasal septum and the posterior ethmoid sinuses on both sides have been removed to exposed the posterior nasopharyngeal wall, the anterior aspect of the sphenoid body, and the sphenoid ostia. The posterior ethmoid air cells overlap the lateral margin of the sphenoid ostia. **(C)** The anterior wall of the sphenoid sinus has been opened, and the sphenoid septum has been removed to expose the anterior sellar wall in the midline and the prominences over the optic canals and carotid arteries in the lateral walls of this well-pneumatized sphenoid sinus. The medial part of the posterior wall of the left maxillary sinus has been removed to expose branches of the maxillary artery in the pterygopalatine fossa. The opticocarotid recesses extend laterally between the prominences over the carotid arteries and optic nerves. **(D)** The pituitary gland, intracavernous carotids, optic nerves, ophthalmic arteries, and cavernous sinuses have been exposed by removing the bone of the sinus wall. The inferolateral trunk passes above and lateral to the abducens nerve. The shortest distance between the paired carotid arteries is usually located just below the tuberculum sellae. A capsular artery arises from the intracavernous carotid and passes upward and medially. **(E)** Oblique view. The bony prominences overlying the optic canal, superior orbital fissure, intracavernous carotid artery, and maxillary nerve are exposed in the lateral wall of the sphenoid sinus. The bony depression between the carotid prominence and the optic canal, the opticocarotid recess, extends into the medial end of the optic strut. The broad, round prominence below the opticocarotid recess is produced by the structures passing through the superior orbital fissure. **(F)** Oblique view. The pituitary gland, intracavernous carotid artery, ophthalmic artery, and optic, ophthalmic, maxillary, oculomotor, and abducens nerves have been exposed. The abducens nerve courses medial to the ophthalmic nerve.

bone, but is separated from it by an extension of the cavernous sinus.

The bone separating the artery and the sphenoid sinus is thinner over the anterior than over the posterior parts of the carotid prominence and is thinnest over the part of the artery just below the tuberculum sellae. A layer of bone less than 0.5 mm thick separates the artery and sinus in nearly 90% of sinuses, and areas of absence of bone between the artery and the sinus are present in nearly 10%.[8] Only the dura covering the intracranial surface of the sphenoid bone and the sinus mucosa separate the air cavity and carotid arteries if there is a dehiscence of bone along the carotid prominences.

The proximity of the carotid prominences to the midline is important in pituitary surgery. The transverse separation between the carotid prominences of each side was measured at the level of the tuberculum sellae, anterior sellar wall, sellar floor, dorsum sellae, and clivus. The shortest distance between the prominences was located just below the tuberculum in 72%, at the level of the sellar floor in 20%, and adjacent the clivus in 8% of our specimens[8] (**Figs. 2.4, 2.7,** and **2.10**).

The optic canals protrude into the superolateral portion of the sinus, and there are areas where no bone separates the optic sheath and sinus mucosa (**Figs. 2.2, 2.4, 2.8, 2.10,** and **2.11**). The superior orbital fissure produces a smooth, wide prominence in the midlateral sinus wall below the optic canal, and the maxillary nerve underlies a prominence in the inferolateral part. A bone thickness of 0.5 mm or less separates 80% of optic nerves from the sinus. Care must be taken to avoid damage to the nerves in the transsphenoidal approach if a dehiscence of the bone covering exposes them in the sinus.[10,11]

A pneumatized diverticulum of the sinus, the opticocarotid recess, often extends laterally into the optic strut between the prominences along the optic canal, carotid artery, and superior orbital fissure (**Figs. 2.2, 2.10,** and **2.11**). This pneumatization may extend through the optic strut into the anterior clinoid process, thus creating a channel through which cerebrospinal fluid (CSF) can leak into the sinus after an anterior clinoidectomy, with resulting CSF rhinorrhea.

There is frequently a prominence in the lateral sinus wall overlying the maxillary branch of the trigeminal nerve just proximal to the extracranial end of the foramen rotundum, especially if the sinus is well pneumatized. There also may be areas where no bone separates the nerve from the sinus mucosa, and the presence of a bone thickness of less than 0.5 mm separating the nerve from the sinus is common. The length of maxillary division bulging into the sinus ranges from 7.0 to 15.0 mm (mean, 10.9 mm).[8] The sphenoid sinus may also extend laterally below the maxillary nerve into the medial part of the greater sphenoid wing and partially surround the foramen ovale. The prominences overlying the optic canal, superior orbital fissure, and maxillary nerve located in the lateral part of the presellar portion of the sphenoid sinus are not normally visible with the operating microscope; however, they are easily identified with the use of straight and angled endoscopes.

Removing the mucosa and bone from the lateral wall of the sinus exposes the dura mater covering the medial surface of the cavernous sinus and optic canals (**Figs. 2.10** and **2.11**). Opening this dura may expose the carotid artery and the nerves passing through the optic canal, superior orbital fissure, cavernous sinus, and foramen rotundum. The abducens nerve is located between the lateral side of the carotid artery and the medial side of the first trigeminal division. The second and third trigeminal divisions are seen in the lower margin of the opening through the lateral wall of sphenoid sinus. In half of the cases, the optic and trigeminal nerves and the carotid arteries have areas where bone 0.5 mm or less in thickness separates them from the mucosa of the sphenoid sinus, and in a few cases the bone separating these structures from the sinus is absent[6,12] (**Figs. 2.2, 2.8,** and **2.10**). The absence of such bony protection within the walls of the sinus may explain some of the cases of cranial nerve deficits and carotid artery injury after transsphenoidal operations.[10] Placing the speculum in the sinus, as has been advocated, also increases the risk for damaging other structures in the wall of the sinus, including the maxillary nerves and the nerves passing through the superior orbital fissure.[13] Vigorous curettage of the walls of the sphenoid sinus can also cause damage to the nerves passing through the optic canal, superior orbital fissure, and foramen rotundum and to the carotid arteries.[8]

The carotid arteries always project anterior to the plane of the anterior sellar wall unless the sella has been greatly expanded anteriorly by tumor. The bone overlying the carotid arteries at the lateral edges of the anterior sellar wall is often thinner than the bone anterior to the pituitary gland. The bulge of the sellar floor is usually identifiable, unless the sinus is of a presellar or conchal type, in which case the sellar bulge may not be apparent. However, the floor of the sella turcica should be directly ahead of the long axis of the transsphenoidal exposure if the blades of the speculum have been positioned correctly, with the vertical crest on the face of the sphenoid positioned between the tips of the speculum blades (**Fig. 2.12**). The prominences overlying the carotid arteries are frequently exposed at the lateral edge of the anterior sellar wall and are not to be confused with the prominence overlying a tumor (**Figs. 2.2, 2.8,** and **2.10**).

Excessive spreading of the bivalve speculum has been reported to cause a fracture of the medial orbital wall with visual loss.[14] The distance between the optic nerves at the coronal plane through the anterior wall of the sphenoid sinus averages 2.93 cm (range, 2.71–3.09 cm).[15] This distance, measured 5 and 10 mm behind the anterior sinus wall and inside the sinus, decreases to an average of 2.62 cm (range, 2.47–2.71 cm) and 1.58 cm (range, 1.39–1.74 cm), respectively. Care should be taken in opening the speculum at the anterior wall of the sphenoid sinus beyond 2.5 cm. This distance between the optic nerves may narrow to less than 1.5 cm if the speculum is advanced 10 mm into the sinus. It is important to remember that the blades of the speculum are pushing several millimeters of soft and osseous tissue from the turbinates and nasal wall laterally ahead of the tips of the blades. The transsphenoidal speculum usually encounters the firm resistance of the middle turbinates and the lateral nasal wall as it is opened, so that the extent of opening the blades is limited. Displacement of the speculum contralaterally by the middle turbinate places the tip of the blades near the contralateral optic nerve and may be associated with optic nerve injury with lesser de-

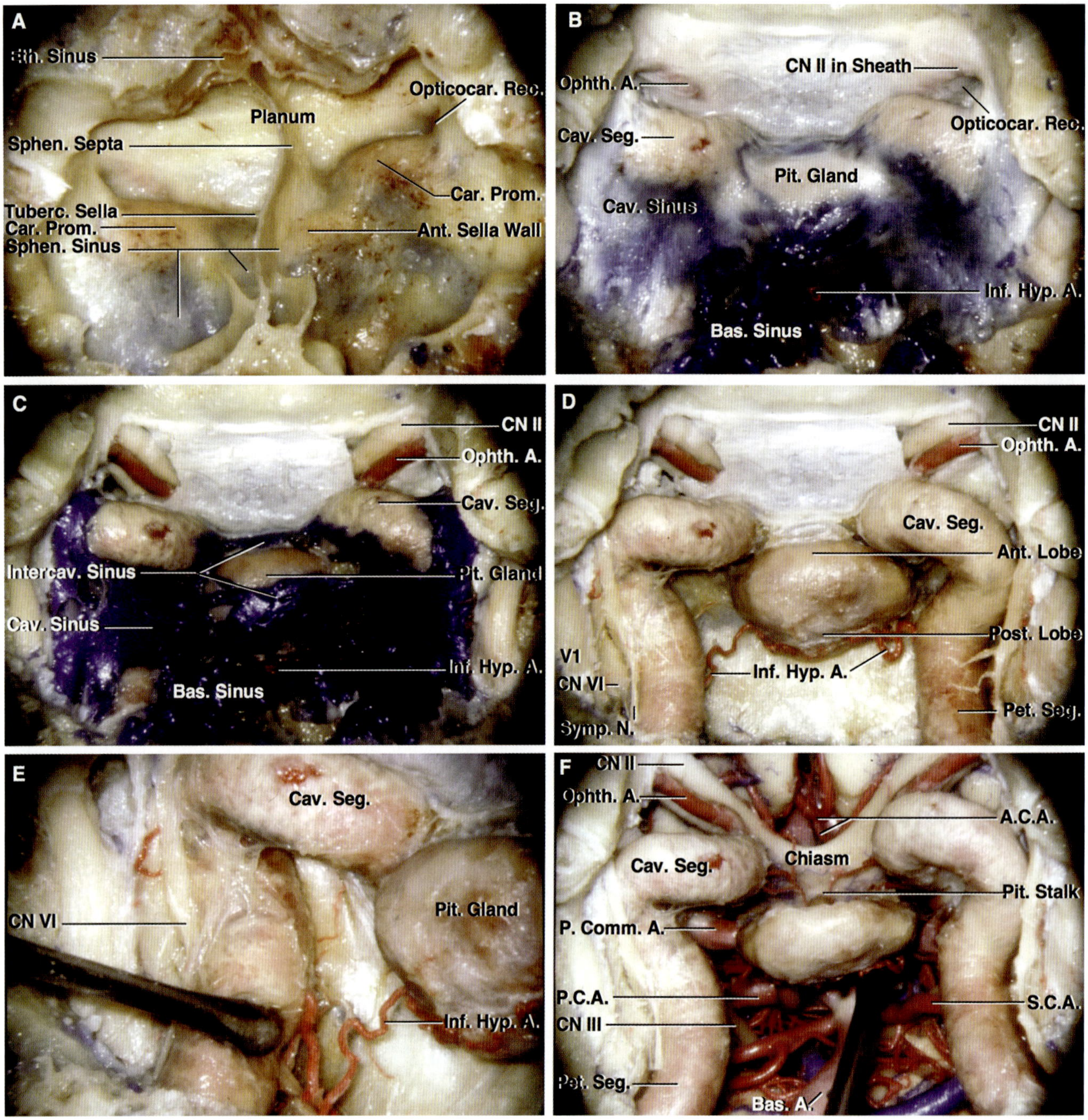

Fig. 2.11 Stepwise dissection examining the relationship of the sphenoid sinus to the pituitary fossa, cavernous sinus, and sellar region. **(A)** Anterior view into a sphenoid sinus with the mucosa removed to show the relationships of the structures that can be exposed by the transsphenoidal approach. The structures in the exposure include the major sphenoidal septum, anterior sellar wall, and prominences over the carotid arteries and optic canals. The tuberculum sellae and planum sphenoidale are located above the anterior sellar wall. The opticocarotid recess extends laterally between the carotid artery and optic canal. **(B)** The bone in the walls of the sphenoid sinus has been removed while the dura is preserved. The optic nerves, intracavernous carotids, and pituitary gland are seen through the dura. The anterior bend of the intracavernous carotid bulges forward inside the dura immediately below the optic canals. The basilar sinus, which forms the largest connection between the paired cavernous sinuses, is situated behind the clivus and dorsum sellae. The inferior hypophyseal artery passes to the capsule of the posterior lobe. The optic nerve and ophthalmic artery can be seen through the optic sheath. **(C)** The dura forming the medial and lower walls of the cavernous sinuses has been removed. Intercavernous sinuses connect the paired cavernous sinuses across the midline. The dura in the floor of the optic canals has been opened to expose the ophthalmic arteries and optic nerves. The basilar sinus sits on the dorsum sellae and clivus and interconnects the posterior end of the paired cavernous sinuses. **(D)** The venous space has been cleared to expose the intracavernous carotid and the anterior and posterior pituitary lobes. The inferior hypophyseal arteries arise from the meningohypophyseal branch of the intracavernous carotid and pass to the capsule of the posterior lobe. Sympathetic nerves ascend on the carotid arteries. The abducens nerve passes through the cavernous sinus on the lateral side of the internal carotid artery and medial to the ophthalmic nerve. **(E)** Oblique view of the intracavernous carotid showing the inferior hypophyseal artery passing to the capsule of the posterior lobe. **(F)** The dura has been removed to expose the intradural structures. The anterior cerebral arteries are situated above and the pituitary gland is situated below the optic chiasm. The basilar apex is located behind the gland. The oculomotor nerve passes forward between the posterior cerebral and superior cerebellar arteries.

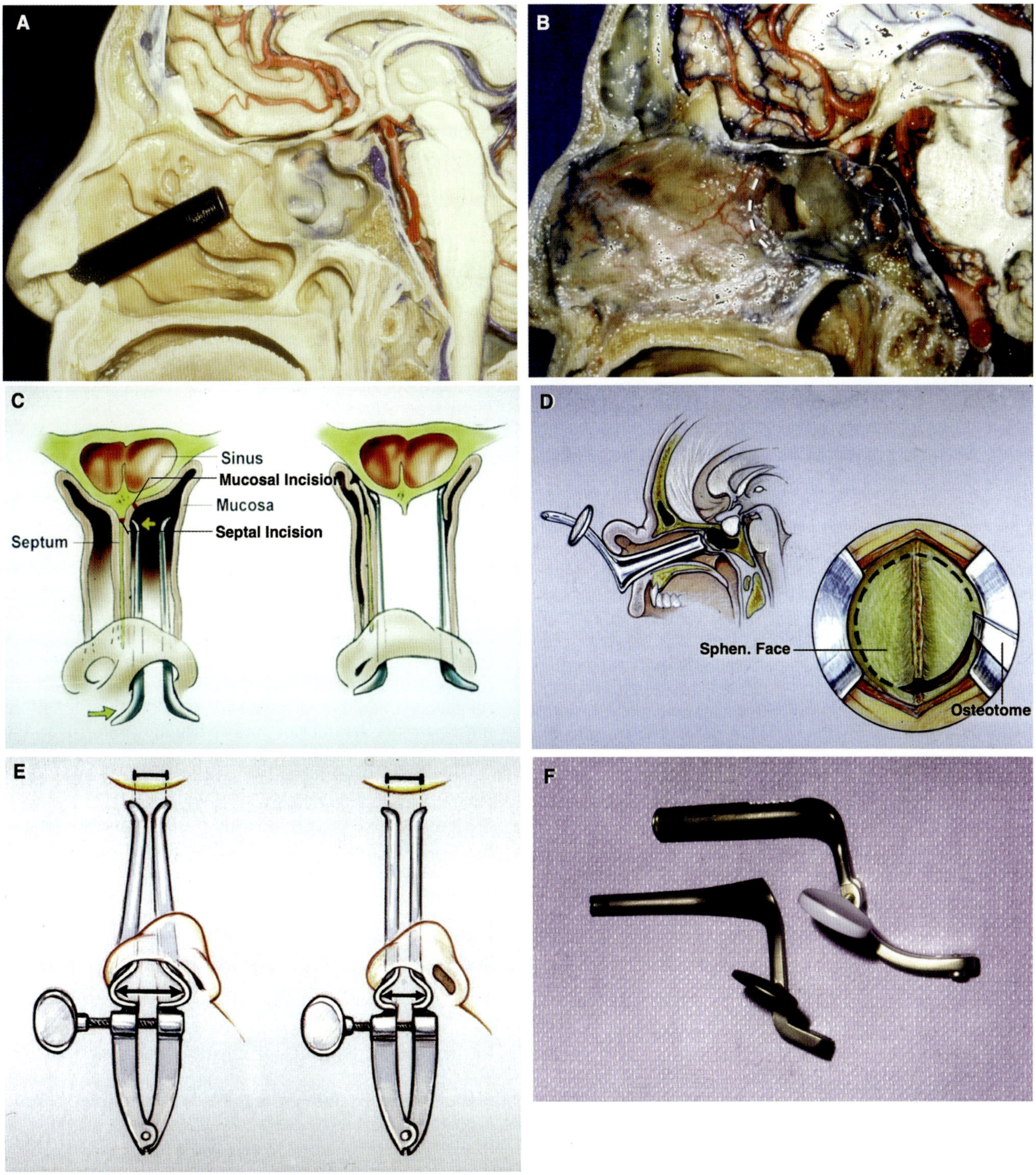

Fig. 2.12 Endonasal approaches to the sphenoid sinus. **(A)** The Rhoton endonasal transsphenoidal speculum has been inserted along the route of the endonasal transsphenoidal approach directed through one nostril, between the conchae laterally and the nasal septum medially. **(B)** The *broken line* shows the area where the posterior septum is separated from the face of the sphenoid sinus. **(C)** Superior view of the nasal cavity (left side). The speculum is advanced in one nostril between the septum and turbinates to the sphenoid face. The mucosa is opened on the sphenoid face to the left of the septum (*arrow*), and the mucosa is elevated and the posterior septum separated from the face of the sphenoid (*red arrow,* right side). The speculum blades have been advanced submucosally along the face of the sphenoid sinus. The speculum is positioned so that the crest on the face of the sphenoid is in the midline between the tips of the blades of the speculum. **(D)** Upper left, lateral view of the endonasal exposure of the sphenoid sinus. Lower right, a small osteotome is used to open the face of the sphenoid. No bone is removed from the septum, and the bone taken from the face of the sphenoid is preserved to serve as a stent for closing the anterior sellar wall. **(E)** Variations of transsphenoidal specula. The speculum on the left has blades that are tapered so that the opening at the nostril is greater than the exposure obtained at the sphenoid face. The Rhoton speculum on the right was designed for endonasal transsphenoidal surgery. It has parallel blades that open so that the exposure at the sphenoid face is slightly greater than the opening of the speculum at the anterior nasal aperture. **(F)** The upper right shows the thicker, wider blades on the traditional transsphenoidal speculum. The lower left shows the Rhoton modified endonasal speculum with smaller, thinner blades that open like the parallel blades shown in **(E)**.

grees of speculum opening. This natural resistance, which tends to limit speculum opening, may be absent in some cases of reduced bone strength due to extensive erosion of bone by tumor, reoperation after extensive bone removal, and softening of osteoporotic bone associated with Cushing disease and long-standing steroid use. In these cases, the speculum should be opened gently.

Several routes through the nasal cavity have been used to reach the sphenoid sinus (**Fig. 2.12**). The sublabial approach is directed under the lip and submucosally along the nasal septum to the sphenoid sinus. The transseptal approach avoids the oral cavity because it is directed through a small incision along one side of the columella and submucosally along the septum. The direct endonasal approach, used in recent years by the author, is directed through one nostril, between the conchae laterally and the nasal septum medially, and does not require an incision in the nose before the anterior face of the sphenoid is reached and opened[16] (**Fig. 2.12**). No incision is needed in the anterior part of the nasal cavity, and nasal packing is uncommonly needed at the end of the procedure. In the direct endonasal approach, a handheld nasal speculum inserted into one nostril between the conchae and nasal septum is opened to compress the conchae and septum sufficiently that the endonasal transsphenoidal speculum can be advanced through one nostril to the sphenoid face. Removal of the conchae is not required. The junction of the crest in the sphenoid face at the attachment of the septum is the most reliable anatomic landmark for maintaining the exposure in the midline. The sphenoid ostia are situated on each side of the perpendicular ethmoid plate, which forms the upper part of the nasal septum and marks the upper limit of the sinus opening for most pituitary tumors.

The sinus mucosa should be preserved if possible because the ciliary action of the normal mucosa aids in clearing secretions from the sinus. A sinus devoid of mucosa lacks normal drainage, becomes easily infected, and may be the source of a patient experiencing a foul odor following surgery.

Diaphragma Sellae

The diaphragma sellae forms the roof of the sella turcica (**Fig. 2.1**). It covers the pituitary gland, except for a small central opening in its center, which transmits the pituitary stalk. The diaphragma is more rectangular than circular, tends to be convex or concave rather than flat, and is thinner around the infundibulum and somewhat thicker at the periphery. It frequently is a thin, tenuous structure that would not be an adequate barrier for protecting the suprasellar structures during a transsphenoidal operation. In a prior anatomic study, Renn and Rhoton[17] found that the diaphragma was at least as thick as one layer of dura in 38% of cases, and in these cases it furnishes an adequate barrier during transsphenoidal hypophysectomy. In the remaining 62%, the diaphragma was extremely thin over some portion of the pituitary gland. It was concave when viewed from above in 54% of the specimens, convex in 4%, and flat in 42%. Even when flat, it lies below the plane of the upper surface of the anterior clinoid process, so that a medially projecting supradiaphragmatic lesion, such as an aneurysm, may appear on neuroradiologic studies to be located below the anterior clinoid and within the cavernous sinus when it is above the diaphragm in the subarachnoid space.

The opening in the center of the diaphragm is large compared with the size of the pituitary stalk. The diaphragmatic opening was 5 mm or greater in 56% of our cases, and in these, it would not have formed a barrier during transsphenoidal pituitary surgery. The opening was round in 54% of the cases and elliptic, with the short diameter of the ellipse oriented in an anteroposterior direction, in 46%. A deficiency of the diaphragma sellae is assumed to be a precondition to the formation of an empty sella. An outpouching of the arachnoid protruded through the central opening in the diaphragma in about half of the sellae. This outpouching, if opened, represents a potential source of postoperative CSF leakage.[10]

Pituitary Gland

When exposed from above by opening the diaphragma, the superior surface of the posterior lobe of the pituitary gland is lighter in color than the anterior lobe (**Figs. 2.1** and **2.6**). The anterior lobe wraps around the lower part of the pituitary stalk to form the pars tuberalis.[4,17] The posterior lobe is softer, almost gelatinous, and more densely adherent to the posterior sellar wall. The anterior lobe is firmer and more easily separated from the sellar walls. The width of the gland is equal to or greater than its depth or length in most patients. Its inferior surface usually conforms to the shape of the sellar floor, but its lateral and superior margins vary in shape because these walls are composed of soft tissue rather than bone. If there is a large opening in the diaphragma, the gland tends to be concave superiorly in the area around the stalk. The superior surface may become triangular as a result of being compressed laterally and posteriorly by the carotid arteries. As the anterior lobe is separated from the posterior lobe, there is a tendency for the pars tuberalis to be retained with the posterior lobe. Small intermediate lobe cysts may be encountered during separation of the anterior and posterior lobes.

Pituitary Gland and Carotid Artery

The distance separating the medial margin of the carotid artery and the lateral surface of the pituitary gland is an important consideration in transsphenoidal surgery (**Figs. 2.6, 2.7,** and **2.10**). There is often a separation between the lateral surface of the gland and the carotid artery. In the cases in which the artery did not indent the gland, the distance between the gland and artery varied from 1 to 7 mm (average, 2.3 mm); however, in about one in four cases, the artery will indent the medial wall of the cavernous sinus and the gland[6,18] (**Fig. 2.6F**). In these cases, the gland loses its spherical shape and conforms to the wall of the artery, often developing protrusions above or below the artery that may be confused with extensions of tumor. Intrasellar tumors are subjected to the same forces, which prevent them from being spherical, and the increased pressure within a tumor increases the degree to which the tumor insinuates into surrounding crevices and tissue planes. Separation of these extensions from the main mass of a tumor during surgery may explain cases in which the tumor and elevated pituitary hormone levels persist or recur after adenoma removal.

The proximity of the carotid arteries to the midline is extremely important in pituitary surgery. In a previous study, the shortest distance between the two carotid arteries was found in the supraclinoid area in 82% of the cases, in the cavernous sinus along the lateral sellar margin in 14%, and in the sphenoid sinus in 4%.[6] Arterial bleeding during transsphenoidal surgery has been reported as due to carotid artery injury, but it may also have arisen from a tear in an arterial branch of the carotid, such as the inferior hypophyseal artery, or by avulsion of a small capsular artery from the carotid artery.[10] It is best to avoid using a pointed knife blade to open the dura in the corners of the sellar opening because of the proximity of the carotid arteries to these corners. It is best to begin the dural opening with a short vertical midline incision in the dura, after which a small, blunt, right-angled ring curette is inserted through the small vertical dural opening and the dura is separated from the anterior surface of the gland or tumor. After the dura has been freed, a 45-degree-angle alligator scissor, rather than a knife, is selected to open the dura in an x-shaped cut from corner to corner because a pointed knife may damage the carotid arteries in the far lateral corners of the exposure.

Intercavernous Venous Connections

Venous sinuses that interconnect the paired cavernous sinuses may be found in the margins of the diaphragma and around the gland[6] (**Figs. 2.1, 2.6, 2.11,** and **2.13**). The intercavernous connections within the sella are named on the basis of their relationship to the pituitary gland; the anterior intercavernous sinuses pass anterior to the hypophysis, and the posterior intercavernous sinuses pass behind the gland. Actually, these intercavernous connections can occur at any site along the anterior, inferior, or posterior surface of the gland, or all connections between the two sides may be absent. The anterior intercavernous sinus may cover the whole anterior wall of the sella. The

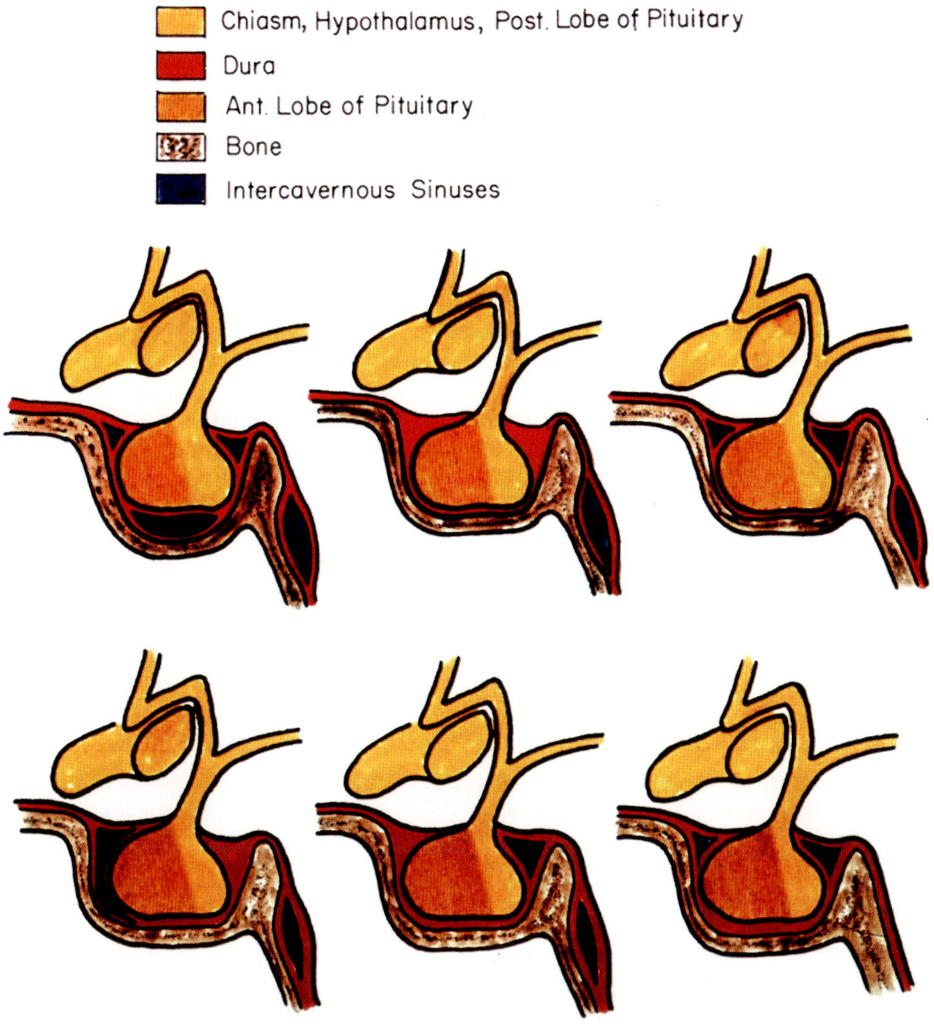

Fig. 2.13 Six sagittal sections of the sellar region showing variations in the intercavernous venous connections within the dura. The variations shown include combinations of anterior, posterior, and inferior intercavernous connections and the frequent presence of a basilar sinus posterior to the dorsum. Either the anterior (lower center) or posterior (lower left) intercavernous connections or both (top center) may be absent. The anterior intercavernous sinus may extend along the whole anterior margin of the gland (lower left). The basilar sinus may be absent (lower right).

anterior sinus is usually larger than the posterior sinus, but either or both may be absent. If the anterior and posterior connections coexist, the whole structure constitutes the "circular sinus." Entering an anterior intercavernous connection that extends downward in front of the gland during transsphenoidal operation may produce brisk bleeding. However, this usually stops with temporary compression of the channel with hemostatic foam or with light bipolar coagulation, which serves to glue the walls of the channel together.

A large intercavernous venous connection called the basilar sinus passes posterior to the dorsum sellae and upper clivus, connecting the posterior aspect of both cavernous sinuses (**Figs. 2.6, 2.7,** and **2.11**). The basilar sinus is the largest and most constant intercavernous connection across the midline. The superior and inferior petrosal sinuses join the basilar sinus. The abducens nerve often enters the posterior part of the cavernous sinus by passing through the basilar sinus or the junction of the inferior petrosal and basilar sinus.

Extensions of the Sellar Type of Sphenoid Sinus

There are several variations in the extensions of pneumatization of the sellar type of sphenoid sinus that may facilitate entry into areas bordering the sphenoid sinus[19,20] (**Figs. 2.14** and **2.15**). These extensions or recesses act as "windows" opening from the sinus in different areas of the skull base that may facilitate minimally invasive access to lesions involving the cavernous sinus, Meckel's cave, middle cranial fossa, planum sphenoidale, suprasellar region, and clivus. These variations in the sellar type of sinus have been classified into six basic types. (1) Sphenoid body type: the pneumatization does not progress beyond the body of sphenoid bone. (2) Lateral type: the sinus extends lateral to a line connecting the medial edge of the anterior opening of vidian canal and the extracranial end of the foramen rotundum (VR line). (3) Clival type: the posterior wall of the sphenoid sinus extends beyond the vertical coronal plane of the posterior wall of pituitary fossa. (4) Lesser wing type: the pneumatization extends into the lesser sphenoid wing and possibly into the anterior clinoid process. (5) Anterior type: the anterior wall of the sinus extends anterolaterally beyond the vertical coronal plane of the sinus side of the sphenoid crest. (6) Combined type: more than one type of extension appears in the same sinus. Among the sellar type of sinuses, the combined type was the most common (59.2%), and the lesser wing type was the least common.

The lateral type, present in 46% of lateral sinus walls, extends into either the greater wing or pterygoid process, or both. It is referred to as a greater wing type if it extends only into the greater wing, as a pterygoid type if it extends into only the pterygoid process, and a full lateral type if it extends into both the greater wing and pterygoid process. In the endoscopic view from inside the sphenoid sinus, the lateral recess is a quadrangular area bordered by four prominences in the sinus wall: the maxillary nerve superiorly, the vidian nerve inferiorly, the petrous segment of the carotid artery posteriorly, and the part of the sinus wall between the foramen rotundum and vidian canal anteriorly. A prominence in the lateral sinus wall overlying cranial nerve V_3 can be seen when the lateral recess extends to the foramen ovale.

A clival type of sinus was identified when it had a clival recess in which the posterior wall of the sphenoid sinus extended posteriorly beyond the vertical coronal plane of the posterior wall of the pituitary fossa. A clival recess, present in 68% of the sinuses, may extend superiorly into the dorsum sellae and/or inferiorly to the basilar part of the occipital bone. Three types of clival recesses were found: dorsum type, which extends above the horizontal plane of the floor of the pituitary and into the dorsum sellae; subdorsum type, which lies between the horizontal plane of the floor of pituitary fossa and the horizontal plane passing through the anterior opening of vidian canals; and occipital type, which extends inferiorly below the horizontal plane crossing the anterior opening of the paired vidian canals. Of the clival-type sinuses, 24% were of the dorsum type, 63% subdorsum type, 2% occipital type, and 9% combined dorsum-occipital type. The subdorsum type is seen directly ahead as the sinus is entered, whereas the dorsum type may be partially hidden behind the pituitary fossa and the clival type may be partially hidden below the floor of the sphenoid sinus. Approximately, 10% of the sellar-type sinuses had pneumatization of the anterior clinoid process, referred to as lesser wing type. Every specimen with pneumatization of the anterior clinoid process also had optic strut aeration, but optic strut aeration did not always extend into the anterior clinoid process.

An anterior recess originating from the lateral portion of anterior wall of the sphenoid sinus was identified when the recess extended anteriorly beyond a line directed from side to side along the sinus side of the sphenoid crest on the axial CT. An anterior recess, found in anterior-type sinuses, present either unilaterally or bilaterally in 25% of sinuses, extends in an inferolateral direction and is separated from the maxillary sinus by a thin bony plate.

Fig. 2.14 Lateral extensions of the sphenoid sinuses. Anterior view of the sphenoid sinus illustrating the pneumatized extensions of the sphenoid sinus. Structures surrounding the sinus, such as the sella, carotid artery, and the optic, vidian, and the trigeminal divisions, may underlie prominences and recesses inside the sinus. The lateral extensions of the sinus extend beyond the VR line directed along the medial edge of the anterior end of the vidian canal and the extracranial end of the foramen rotundum. **(A)** Body type of sphenoid sinus. The pneumatization is confined to the body of the sphenoid bone and does not extend beyond the VR line. **(B)** Lesser wing type. The sinus pneumatizes through the optic strut (*arrow*) and into the anterior clinoid process. **(C–E)** Lateral type. The lateral wall of the sinus extends laterally beyond the VR line, which crosses the medial edge of the foramen rotundum and vidian canal. Three lateral subtypes were found: greater wing, pterygoid, and full lateral types. **(C)** Greater wing type. The pneumatization extends laterally between the foramen rotundum and vidian canal into the greater wing. **(D)** Pterygoid type. The pneumatization extends laterally between the foramen rotundum and vidian canal and inferiorly into the pterygoid process. **(E)** Full lateral type. The sinus extends laterally into both the greater wing and the pterygoid process.

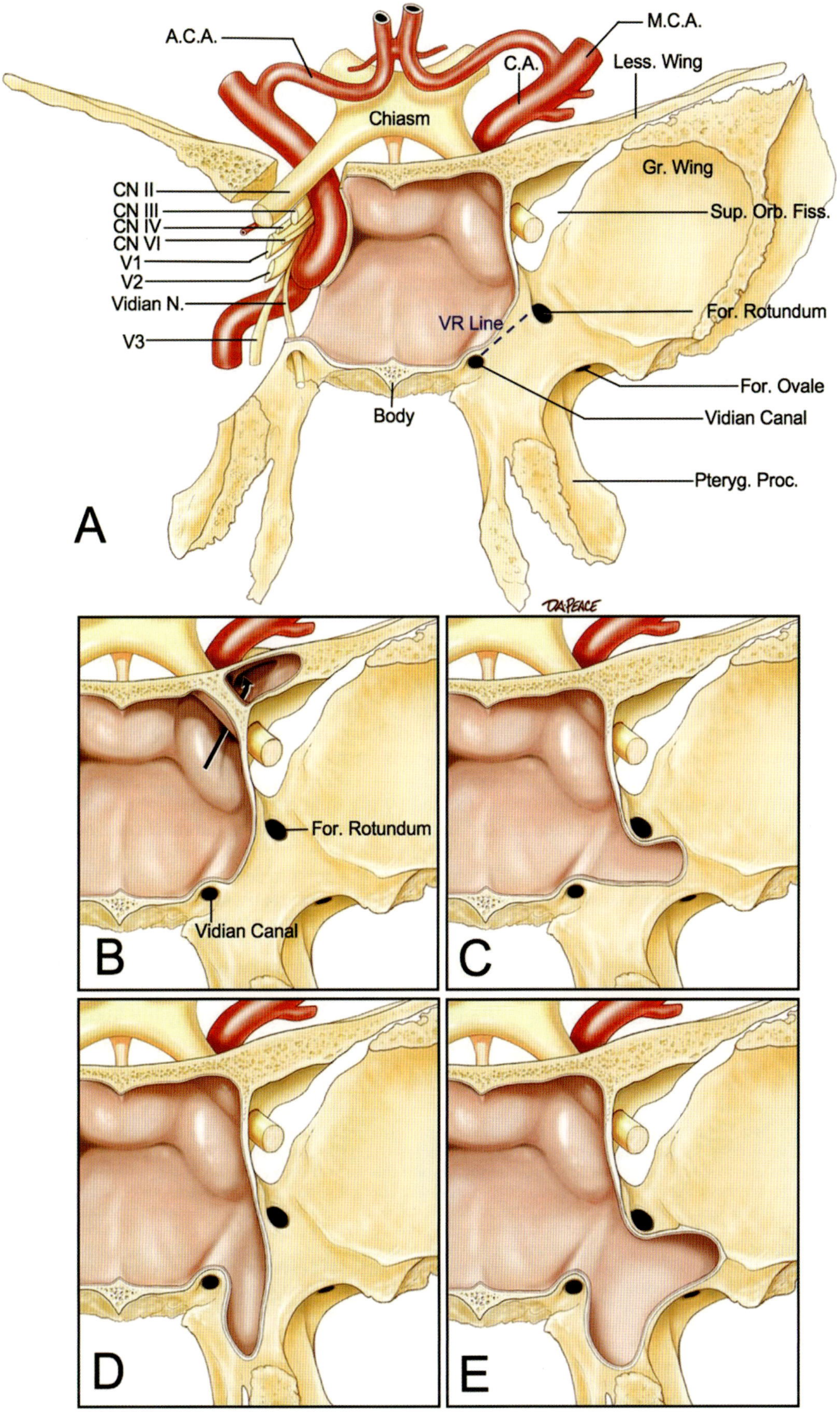
A.C.A.
M.C.A.
C.A.
Less. Wing
Chiasm
Gr. Wing
CN II
CN III
CN IV
CN VI
V1
V2
Vidian N.
V3
Sup. Orb. Fiss.
For. Rotundum
VR Line
For. Ovale
Vidian Canal
Body
Pteryg. Proc.
A
B
For. Rotundum
Vidian Canal
C
D
E

Fig. 2.14

The lateral type of sphenoid sinus, divided into greater wing, pterygoid process, and full lateral types, facilitates approaches to the cavernous sinus, middle cranial fossa, and petrous apex. The clival type of sinus, divided into dorsum, subdorsum, occipital, and dorsum-occipital types, depending on the direction of pneumatization, may facilitate access to the dorsum, posterior clinoids, petrous apex, the entire clivus down to the anterior lip of the foramen magnum and odontoid process, and the anterior brainstem and adjacent cisterns. The lesser wing type provides an easier surgical corridor to the lateral suprasellar area than do the other types. The recesses that guide the approach to the various surrounding areas are not as distinct if the sphenoid sinus is not well pneumatized, and removing the bone in poorly pneumatized areas carries an elevated risk for injury to the adjacent neurovascular structures even though intraoperative navigation may be used to confirm the surgical targets.

◆ The Parasellar Region

The parasellar region includes the cavernous sinuses and adjacent part of the middle cranial fossae.[21,22] The paired cavernous sinuses have dural walls that surround a venous space through which a segment of the internal carotid artery courses. Each sinus extends from the superior orbital fissure in front to the area lateral to the dorsum sellae behind (**Figs. 2.16** and **2.17**). Its anterior edge is attached to the margins of the superior orbital fissure, and its posterior wall is located between the dorsum sellae medially and the ostium of Meckel's cave laterally. The oculomotor, trochlear, and ophthalmic nerves course in the lateral wall. The abducens nerve courses on the medial side of the ophthalmic nerve between it and the internal carotid artery. The lateral wall faces the temporal lobe, the roof faces the basal cisterns, the medial wall faces the sella, pituitary gland, and body of the sphenoid bone, and the lower edge is located below the horizontal portion of the intracavernous segment of the internal carotid artery.

The sinus is the site of a venous confluence that receives the terminal end of multiple veins draining the orbit, sylvian fissure, and middle and anterior fossae, and it has free communication with the basilar, superior and inferior petrosal, and intercavernous sinuses. Over all, it is shaped like a boat, with its narrow keel located at the superior orbital fissure and its broader bow (posterior wall) located lateral to the dorsum sellae above the petrous apex. It has four walls: a roof and lateral, medial, and posterior walls. The deck or roof of the sinus, which is narrow anteriorly and wide posteriorly, faces upward. The lower edge, formed at the junction of the medial and lateral walls below the intracavernous segment of the internal carotid artery, gives the sinus a triangular shape in cross-section (**Fig. 2.17**). The roof is formed by the dura lining the lower margin of the anterior clinoid process anteriorly and the patch of dura, called the oculomotor triangle, between the anterior and posterior clinoid processes and the petrous apex through which the oculomotor nerve penetrates the sinus roof. The medial edge of the oculomotor triangle is formed by the interclinoid dural fold, which extends from the anterior to the posterior clinoid process; the lateral margin by the anterior petroclinoid fold, which extends from the anterior clinoid process to the petrous apex; and the posterior margin by the posterior petroclinoid fold, which extends from the posterior clinoid process to the petrous apex.

The lateral wall extends from the medial edge of Meckel's cave posteriorly to the lateral margin of the nerves passing through the superior orbital fissure anteriorly, and from the anterior petroclinoid dural fold above to the lower margin of the carotid sulcus below. The carotid sulcus is the groove on the lateral aspect of the body of the sphenoid along which the internal carotid artery courses (**Fig. 2.18**). The sheet of dura forming the posterior part of the lateral wall of the sinus also forms the upper third of the medial wall of Meckel's cave, which is located lateral to and is separated from the posterior part of the cavernous sinus by their shared dural wall. The medial wall is formed by the dura that constitutes the lateral wall of the sella turcica and covers the lateral surface of the body of the sphenoid bone. The medial wall extends from the lateral edge of the dorsum sellae posteriorly to the medial edge of the superior orbital fissure anteriorly, and from the interclinoid dural fold above to the lower margin of the carotid sulcus below. Anteriorly, the lower edge of the sinus, where the medial and lateral walls meet, is located just below where the ophthalmic nerve courses in the lateral sinus wall, and proceeding posteriorly it is located medial to the junction of the upper and middle thirds of the gas-

Fig. 2.15 Clival extensions of the sphenoid sinus. Sagittal section. **(A)** Body type of sinus without a clival extension. In the body type of sinus, the posterior wall of the sphenoid sinus does not extend beyond a vertical line directed along the posterior wall of the pituitary fossa (line 1). **(B–E)** Clival type of sinuses. The posterior wall of the sphenoid sinus extends beyond the vertical coronal plane of the posterior wall of the pituitary fossa (line 1). There are four types of clival extensions: subdorsum, dorsum, occipital, and combined dorsum-occipital types. **(B)** Subdorsum type. The sinus extends posterior to a line directed along the posterior wall of the sella but not into the dorsum sellae or into the clivus below the level of the vidian canal. **(C)** Occipital type. The expansion of the sinus behind the posterior wall of the sella (line 1) extends inferiorly below the level of the horizontal plane directed along the upper edge of the paired vidian canals (line 3). **(D)** Dorsum type. The sinus extends above the line directed along the floor of the sella (line 2) and into the dorsum sellae. **(E)** Combined dorsum-occipital type. The sinus extends superiorly into the dorsum and downward below the horizontal plane directed along the upper edge of the vidian canals. **(F)** Superior view of a cross-section extending through an anterior type of sphenoid sinus. The sinus has an anterolateral protrusion that extends anterior to a transverse line crossing the sphenoid sinus side of the sphenoid crest to form an anterior recess facing the maxillary sinus. The sphenomaxillary plate separates the sphenoid and maxillary sinuses in this anterior type of recess. This type of sinus extends anteriorly above the sphenopalatine artery and foramen. **(G)** Superior view of an oblique axial section showing the angle between the midline plane at the anterior nasal spine and the most lateral point of the sphenoid sinus, which averaged 16.7 degrees (range, 10.1–32.1 degrees). The angle from the midline plane to the sphenopalatine foramen averaged 12.2 degrees (range, 7.0–18.6 degrees). The sphenopalatine artery passes through the sphenopalatine foramen to enter the lateral wall of the nasal cavity.

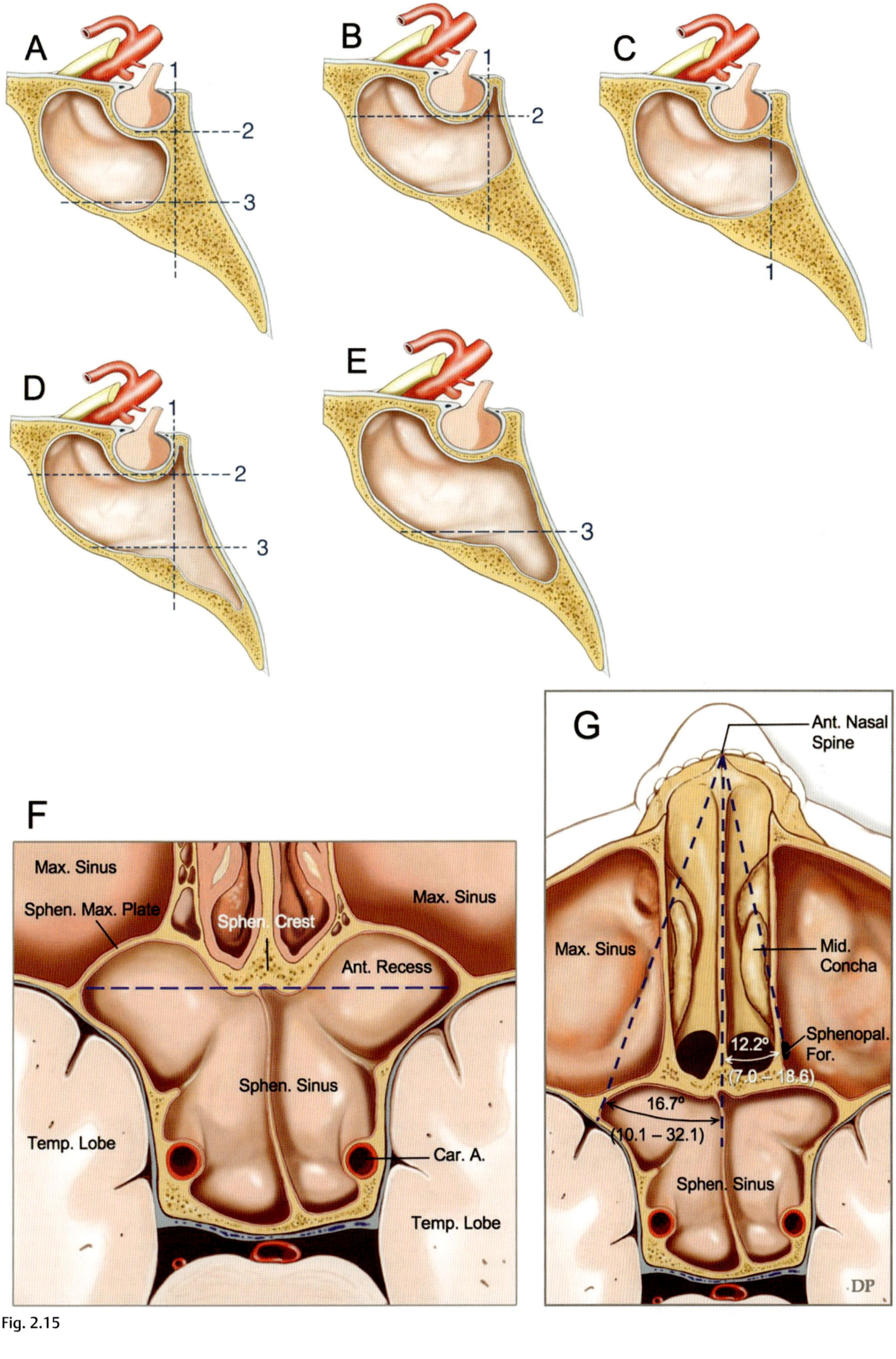

A
1
2
3
B
1
2
C
1
D
1
2
3
E
3
F
Max. Sinus
Sphen. Max. Plate
Max. Sinus
Sphen. Crest
Ant. Recess
Sphen. Sinus
Temp. Lobe
Car. A.
Temp. Lobe
G
Ant. Nasal Spine
Max. Sinus
Mid. Concha
12.2°
Sphenopal. For.
(7.0 – 18.6)
16.7°
(10.1 – 32.1)
Sphen. Sinus
DP

Fig. 2.15

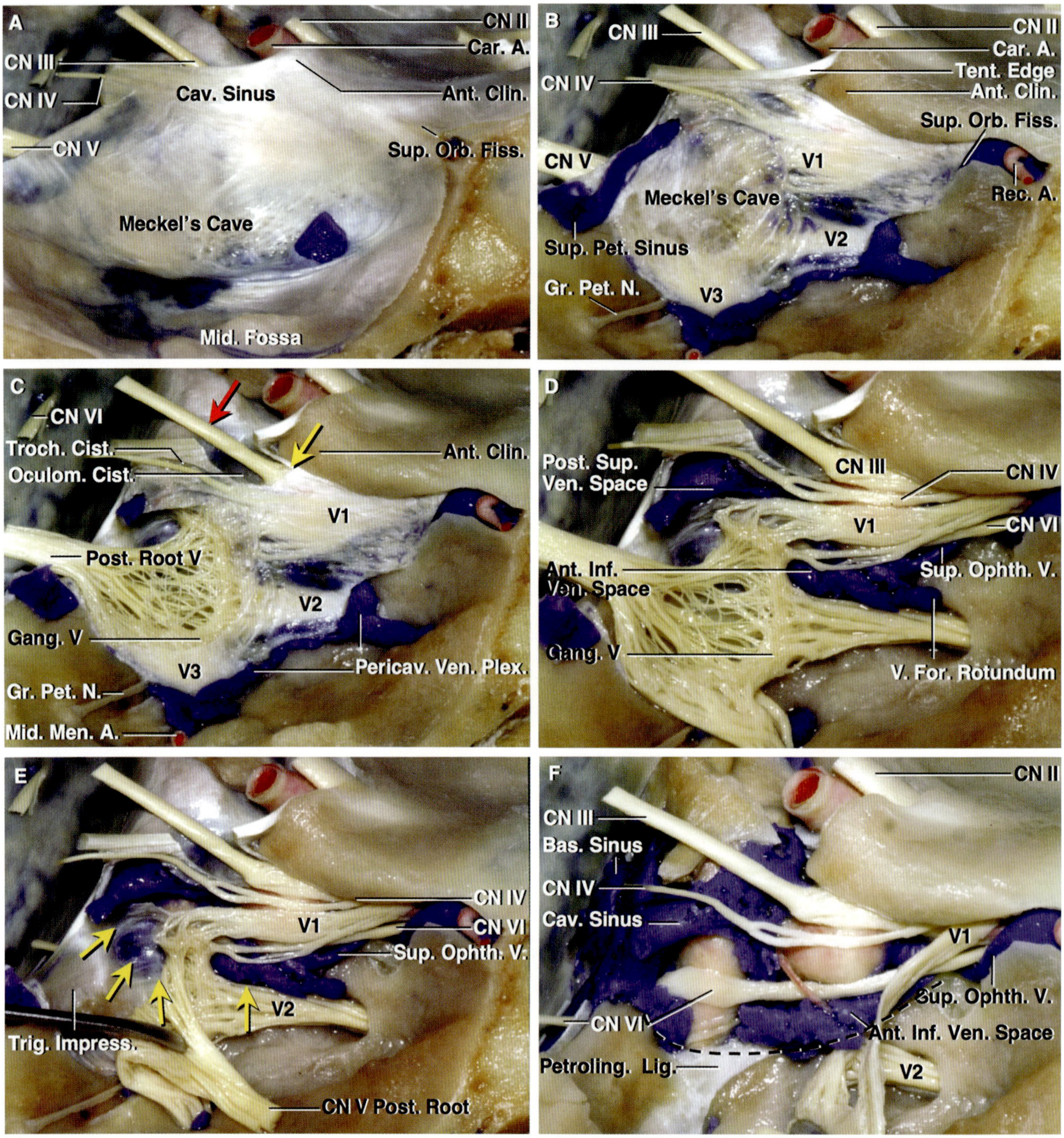

Fig. 2.16 Stepwise dissection of the right cavernous sinus. **(A)** The lateral wall of the cavernous sinus extends downward from the tentorial edge and blends into the dura covering Meckel's cave and the middle fossa. The oculomotor and trochlear nerves enter the roof of the cavernous sinus. The carotid artery exits the cavernous sinus on the medial side of the anterior clinoid process. **(B)** The outer layer of dura has been peeled away from the lateral wall of the cavernous sinus and Meckel's cave. This exposes the oculomotor and trochlear nerves entering the roof of the cavernous sinus and passing forward through the superior orbital fissure. The thin layer covering Meckel's cave consists in part of the arachnoid membrane extending forward from the posterior fossa and surrounding trigeminal nerve to the level of the trigeminal ganglion. The superior petrosal sinus passes above the ostium of Meckel's cave and joins the posterior part of the cavernous sinus. **(C)** The oculomotor nerve enters a short cistern in the sinus roof (*red arrow*) and does not become incorporated into the lateral wall until it reaches the lower margin of the anterior clinoid process (*yellow arrow*). The arachnoid covering of Meckel's cave, which extends forward around the posterior trigeminal root to the level of the midportion of the ganglion, has been removed. The cavernous sinus extends from the superior orbital fissure to the petrous apex. It is located medial to the upper third of the gasserian ganglion. The pericavernous venous plexus surrounds the maxillary and mandibular nerves in the region of the foramen rotundum and foramen ovale. **(D)** The remaining dura covering the lateral wall has been removed. The oculomotor, trochlear, and ophthalmic nerves pass forward to converge on the superior orbital fissure. The segment of the superior petrosal sinus above the posterior trigeminal root has been removed. **(E)** The posterior trigeminal root has been reflected forward to expose the posterior part of the lower margin of the cavernous sinus (*yellow arrow*) in the area medial to the trigeminal impression on the petrous apex, in which Meckel's cave sits. The superior ophthalmic vein exits the orbit through the superior orbital fissure and passes posteriorly below the ophthalmic nerve to enter the cavernous sinus. **(F)** The trigeminal nerve and its three divisions have been reflected forward to expose the venous spaces of the cavernous sinus. The lower margin of the cavernous sinus (*broken line*) is located at the site where the internal carotid artery exits the carotid canal by passing below the petrolingual ligament. The venous spaces in the cavernous sinus communicate posteriorly with the inferior and superior petrosal and basilar sinuses. In addition, the cavernous sinus communicates with the superior ophthalmic veins and the venous plexus around the maxillary and mandibular nerves and the pituitary gland.

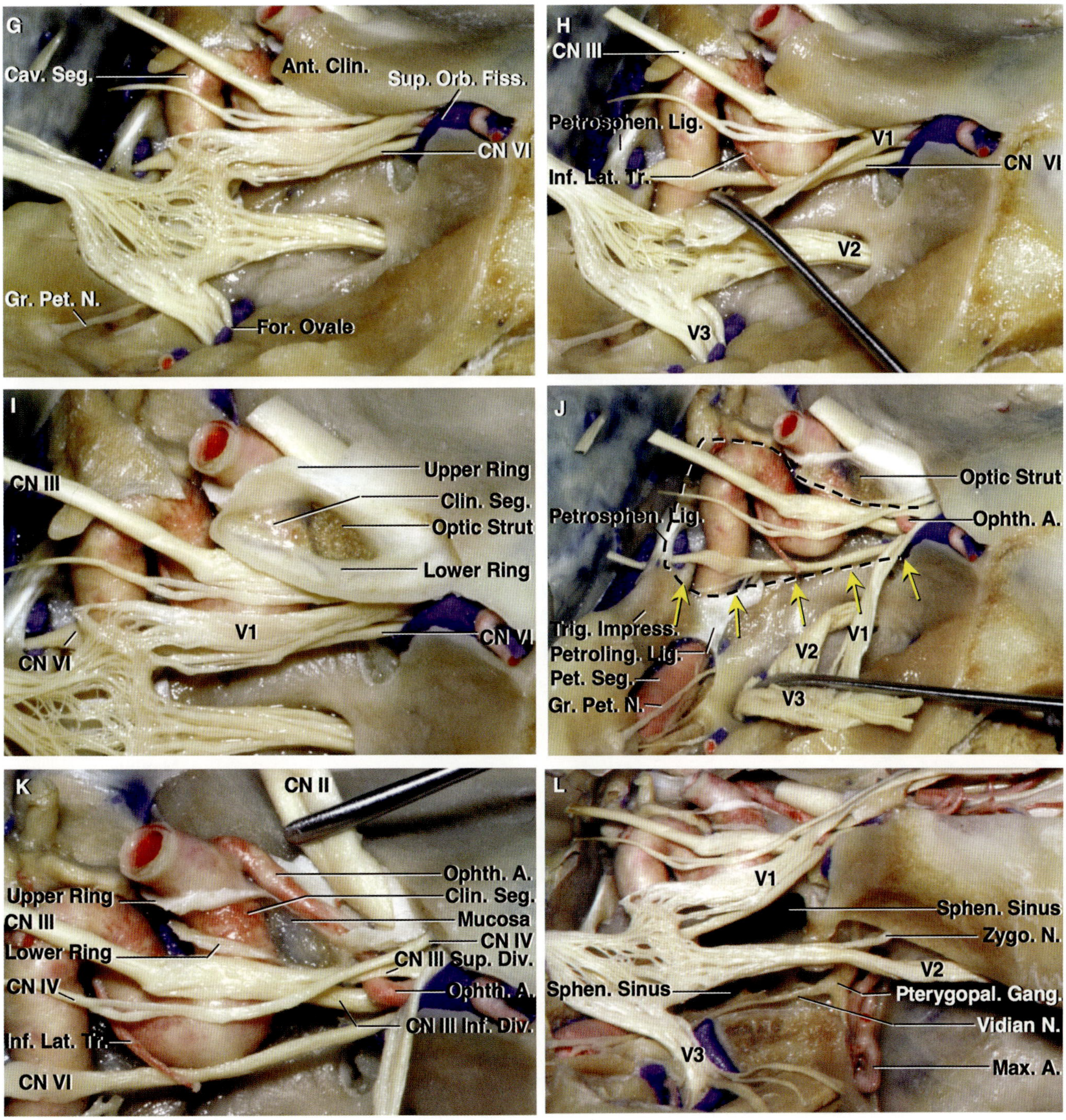

Fig. 2.16 *(Continued)* Stepwise dissection of the right cavernous sinus. **(G)** The venous plexus surrounding the nerves has been removed to expose the trigeminal divisions and the nerves coursing in the wall of the cavernous sinus. **(H)** The ophthalmic nerve has been depressed to expose the abducens nerve, which passes under the petrosphenoid ligament roofing Dorello's canal and courses medial to the ophthalmic nerve. The abducens nerve crosses laterally below the ophthalmic nerve as it passes through the superior orbital fissure. **(I)** The anterior clinoid process has been removed. The optic strut separates the optic canal and superior orbital fissure. The dura extending medially off the upper surface of the anterior clinoid forms the upper dural ring around the internal carotid artery, and the dura lining the lower margin of the clinoid extends medially to form the lower dural ring. The clinoid segment of the carotid artery, located between the upper and lower rings, is enclosed in the dura sheath, referred to as the carotid collar. **(J)** The trigeminal nerve has been folded downward to expose the petrolingual ligament, which extends above the internal carotid artery, just proximal to where the artery enters the cavernous sinus. The abducens nerve passes around the internal carotid artery and courses medial to the ophthalmic nerve in the lower part of the cavernous sinus. The margins of the cavernous sinus are shown with a *broken line*. The cavernous sinus does not extend laterally into the area of the trigeminal impression where Meckel's cave sits. **(K)** Enlarged view. The optic nerve has been elevated to expose the ophthalmic artery coursing within the optic sheath. At the orbital apex, the artery penetrates the optic sheath and enters the orbital apex on the lateral side of the optic nerve. Removal of additional optic strut exposes the mucosa lining the sphenoid sinus on the medial side of the optic strut. **(L)** The bone between the first and second and the second and third trigeminal divisions has been drilled to expose the lateral wing of the sphenoid sinus. The vidian nerve, which passes forward to enter the sphenopalatine ganglion in the pterygopalatine fossa, is exposed between the second and third trigeminal divisions. *(Continued on page 32)*

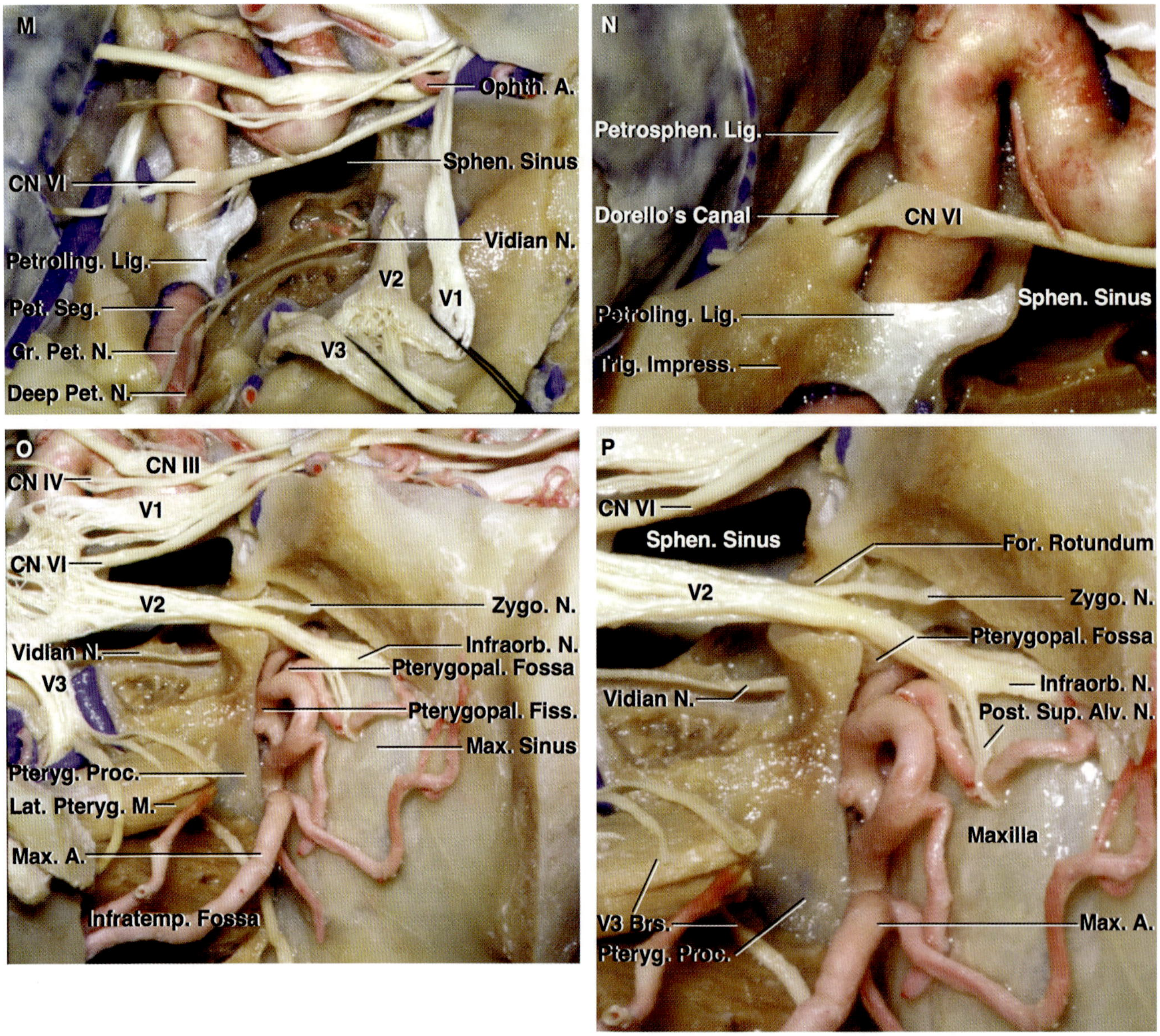

Fig. 2.16 *(Continued)* Stepwise dissection of the right cavernous sinus. **(M)** The trigeminal nerve has been reflected forward to expose the opening into the lateral wing of the sphenoid sinus. The vidian nerve, formed by the union of the greater and deep petrosal nerves, courses forward in the vidian canal to reach the pterygopalatine fossa. **(N)** Enlarged view of the petrolingual and petrosphenoid ligaments. The petrosphenoid ligament extends from the lower part of the lateral margin of the dorsum sellae above the abducens nerve to the petrous apex. The lower margin of the posterior wall of the cavernous sinus is located at the lower margin of Dorello's canal. Anteriorly, the lower margin of the cavernous sinus is located at the level at which the internal carotid artery exits the area below the petrolingual ligament and enters the posterior part of the cavernous sinus. **(O)** The exposure has been extended down to the infratemporal and pterygopalatine fossae. The infratemporal fossa contains branches of the mandibular nerve and maxillary artery, the pterygoid muscles, and the pterygoid venous plexus. The maxillary nerve passes through the foramen rotundum to enter the pterygopalatine fossa. **(P)** Enlarged view. The pterygopalatine fossa is located between the posterior maxillary wall and the pterygoid process. The vidian nerve penetrates the upper part of the pterygoid process and the area below the foramen rotundum to enter pterygopalatine fossa. The maxillary nerve gives rise to the zygomatic, infraorbital, and posterosuperior alveolar nerves, and branches and rami to the pterygopalatine ganglion.

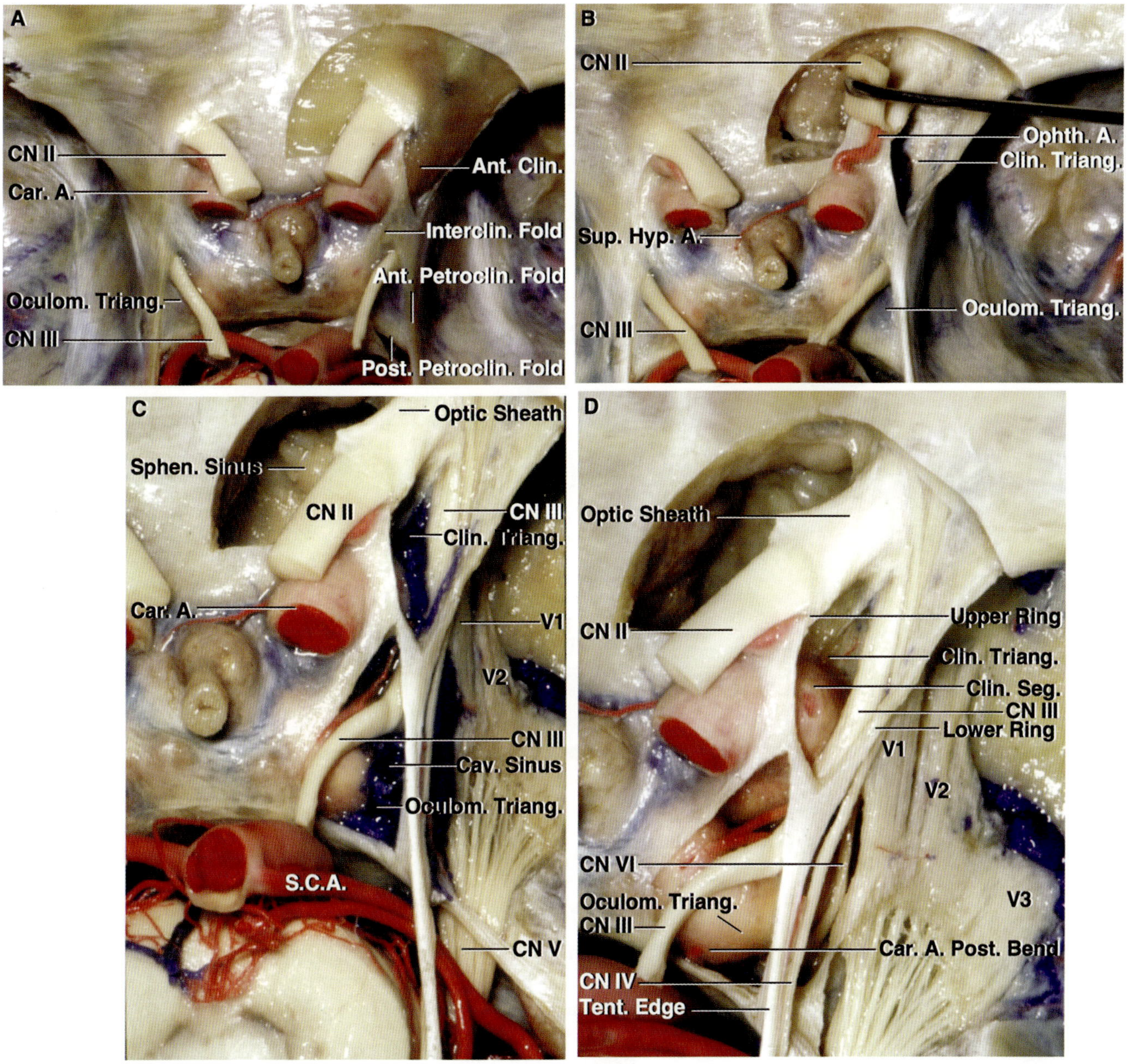

Fig. 2.17 Stepwise dissection of the roof of the cavernous sinus. **(A)** Superior view. The dura covering the upper surface of the right anterior clinoid process, optic canal, and adjacent part of the planum has been removed. The roof of the cavernous sinus is formed anteriorly by the dura lining the lower margin of the anterior clinoid and posteriorly by the dura covering the oculomotor triangle, located between the anterior and posterior petroclinoidal and intraclinoidal dural folds. The oculomotor nerve enters the roof of the cavernous sinus through the oculomotor triangle. **(B)** The anterior clinoid and roof of the optic canal have been removed. The optic nerve has been elevated to expose the ophthalmic artery entering the optic foramen. Removing the anterior clinoid exposes the floor of the clinoidal triangle located between the optic and oculomotor nerves. The dura separating the lower surface of the clinoid from the oculomotor nerve and extending medially around the carotid artery, referred to as the carotid-oculomotor membrane, forms the floor of the clinoidal triangle and the anterior part of the roof of the cavernous sinus. The dura extending medially off the upper surface of the clinoid forms the upper dural ring, and the carotid-oculomotor membrane extending medially from the lower surface of the clinoid forms the lower dural ring. **(C)** The dura in the floor of the clinoidal triangle and roof of the oculomotor triangle, which together form the roof of the cavernous sinus, have been removed to expose the upper part of the cavernous sinus. The dura has been elevated from the lateral wall of the cavernous sinus and middle fossa floor to expose the nerves coursing in the lateral wall of the cavernous sinus. **(D)** The sinus has been cleared to expose the clinoid segment of the internal carotid artery in the clinoidal triangle and the posterior bend of the intercavernous carotid below the oculomotor triangle. The anterior part of the roof is formed by the dura that separates the anterior clinoid and oculomotor nerve and that extends medially to form the lower dural ring. The posterior part of the roof consists of the dura forming the oculomotor triangle.

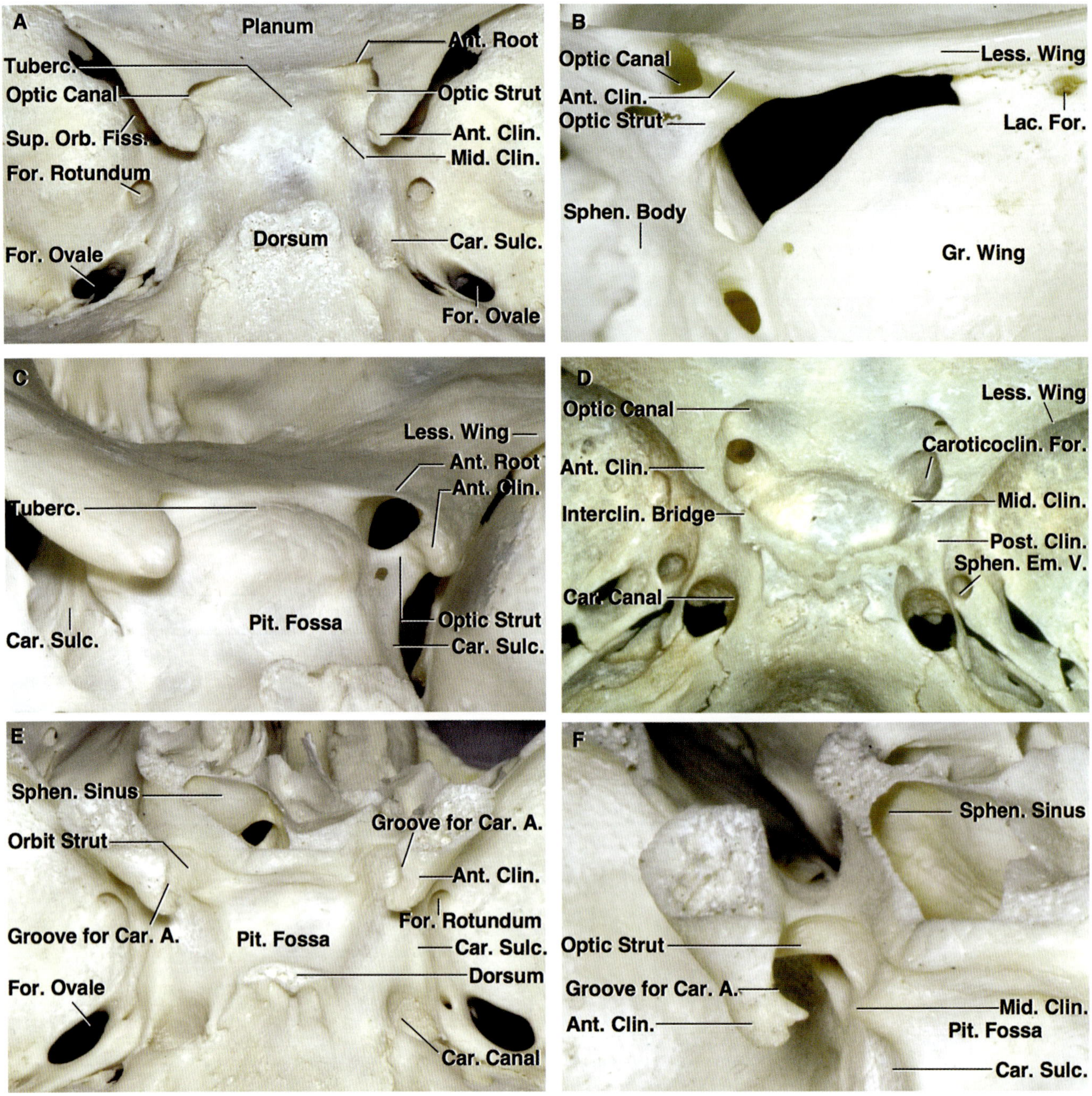

Fig. 2.18 Osseous relationships of the cavernous sinus and carotid collar. **(A)** Superior view. The osseous structures, which nearly encircle the clinoid segment of the internal carotid artery, include the anterior clinoid laterally, the optic strut anteriorly, and the carotid sulcus medially. The carotid sulcus begins lateral to the dorsum sellae at the intracranial end of the carotid canal, extends forward just below the sellar floor, and turns upward along the posterior surface of the optic strut. The anterior clinoid process projects backward from the lesser wing of the sphenoid bone, often overlapping the lateral edge of the carotid sulcus. The anterior root of the lesser sphenoid wing extends medially to form the roof of the optic canal. The posterior root of the lesser wing, referred to as the optic strut, extends from the inferomedial aspect of the anterior clinoid to the sphenoid body. The bony collar around the carotid artery, formed by the anterior clinoid, optic strut, and carotid sulcus, is inclined downward as it slopes medially from the upper surface of the anterior clinoid to the carotid sulcus. Another small prominence, the middle clinoid process, situated on the medial side of the carotid sulcus at the level of the tip of the anterior clinoid process, projects upward and laterally. In some cases, there is an osseous bridge extending from the tip of the middle clinoid to the tip of the anterior clinoid. In well-pneumatized sphenoid bones, the carotid sulcus is seen as a prominence in the lateral wall of the sphenoid sinus just below the floor of the sella. **(B)** Posterior view of the optic strut, optic canal, and superior orbital fissure. The optic strut separates the optic canal and superior orbital fissure and forms the floor of the optic canal and the superomedial part of the roof of the superior orbital fissure. The posterior surface of the strut is shaped to accommodate the anterior wall of the clinoid segment. The artery courses along and may form a groove in the medial half of the lower aspect of the anterior clinoid before turning upward along the medial edge of the clinoid. The air cells in the sphenoid sinus may extend into the optic strut and anterior clinoid. In this case, the sphenoid sinus has pneumatized to a degree that bone is absent over the anterior part of the carotid sulcus, just medial to where the optic strut attaches to the body of the sphenoid bone. The maxillary strut is the bridge of bone separating the

serian ganglion; finally, at the posterior part it slopes upward medial to the upper part of Meckel's cave (**Fig. 2.16**). Behind the site where the ophthalmic nerve arises from the trigeminal ganglion, the lower edge of the medial and lateral walls of the sinus come together at the lateral edge of the carotid sulcus on the medial side of the upper part of Meckel's cave. Only the upper part of the medial wall of Meckel's cave and the upper part of the gasserian ganglion are located directly lateral to the cavernous sinus; thus, the lower two-thirds of Meckel's cave is located below and lateral to the posterior part of the cavernous sinus in the medial part of the middle fossa (**Fig. 2.16**). Meckel's cave extends forward from the posterior fossa, where its ostium is located between the medial part of the petrous ridge below, the superior petrosal sinus above, and the lateral edge of the cavernous sinus medially. The subarachnoid space extends forward within Meckel's cave to approximately the level of the midportion of the gasserian ganglion. The terminal part of the petrous carotid exits the carotid canal and passes below the trigeminal nerve and the petrolingual ligament, where it turns upward to enter the posterior part of the cavernous sinus. It is only after the artery exits the region of the foramen lacerum and turns upward after traveling below the petrolingual ligament to reach the carotid sulcus on the lateral surface of the sphenoid body that it becomes enclosed in the dural envelope of the cavernous sinus (**Fig. 2.16**).

The maxillary nerve does not course in the lateral wall of the dural envelope of the sinuses, as does the ophthalmic nerve. It courses beneath the dura of the middle fossa below the level where the medial and lateral walls of the cavernous sinus join at the lower edge of the ophthalmic nerve. As the dura is elevated from the floor of the middle fossa, it can be stripped upward off of the lateral aspect of both of the maxillary and ophthalmic nerves, but only the ophthalmic nerve has the venous space of the cavernous sinus on its medial side. The medial side of the maxillary nerve sits against the bone and is located below the lower edge of the anterior part of the sinus.

The carotid sulcus is the shallow groove on the lateral aspect of the body of the sphenoid bone along which the internal carotid courses in the cavernous sinus. The intracavernous carotid sits against and is separated from the carotid sulcus by the dura of the medial sinus wall (**Fig. 2.18**). The carotid sulcus begins below and lateral to the dorsum sellae at the intracranial end of the carotid canal, turns forward to form a groove in the body of the sphenoid immediately below the lateral edge of the floor of the sella, and turns upward to end medial to the anterior clinoid process. The segment of the internal carotid artery that courses along the medial side of the clinoid is referred to as the clinoid segment. The carotid sulcus, in well-pneumatized sphenoid bones, forms a serpiginous prominence that can be seen in the lateral wall of the sphenoid sinus below and anterior to the pituitary fossa. The bone in the lateral wall of the sphenoid sinus may be thin or even absent in some areas, allowing the artery to be observed through the sinus wall.

Anterior and Middle Clinoid Processes

The anterior clinoid process projects posteriorly from the lesser wing of the sphenoid bone above the anterior part of the roof of the sinus (**Fig. 2.18**). The base of the clinoid has three sites of continuity with the adjacent part of the sphenoid bone. The base is attached anteriorly at the medial edge of the sphenoid ridge, formed by the lesser sphenoid wing, and medially to the anterior and posterior roots of the lesser wing. The anterior root of the lesser wing extends medially from the base of the anterior clinoid to the body of the sphenoid bone and forms the roof of the optic canal. The posterior root of the lesser wing, called the optic strut, extends medially below the optic nerve to the sphenoid body and forms the floor of the optic canal. The base of the anterior clinoid forms the lateral margin of the optic canal. The segment of the internal carotid artery that courses along the medial aspect of, and is exposed by removal of the anterior clinoid, is referred to as the clinoid segment. The clinoid segment courses below the medial half of the lower margin of the clinoid, where it forms a grooves in the bone before coursing upward along the medial edge of the clinoid (**Fig. 2.18F**). The medial edge of the clinoid, just behind the base, is frequently the site of a shallow, rounded indention that accommodates the lateral surface of the clinoid segment. The posterior tip of the clinoid often projects posteriorly lateral to the lateral part of the clinoid segment. The anterior clinoid is the site of attachment of the anteromedial part of the tentorium and the anterior petroclinoid and interclinoid dural folds. Another dural fold, the falciform ligament, extends from the base of the clinoid across

Fig. 2.18 *(Continued)* superior orbital fissure from the foramen rotundum. **(C)** Oblique posterior view of the right optic strut. The lateral part of the bony collar around the clinoid segment is formed by the anterior clinoid, and the anterior part is formed by the posterior surface of the optic strut and the part of the carotid sulcus located medial to the anterior clinoid process. The posterior surface of the optic strut is wider medially adjacent to the carotid sulcus than it is laterally at the site of attachment to the anterior clinoid process. The optic strut slopes downward from its lateral end so that the medial part of the bony collar is located below the level of the part of the collar joining the anterior clinoid. The inferomedial aspect of the right anterior clinoid has a groove formed by the artery. **(D)** Superior view of a specimen with bilateral caroticoclinoidal foramina and interclinoidal osseous bridges. An osseous bridge connects the tips of the anterior and middle clinoid processes bilaterally, thus creating a bony ring around the artery, called a caroticoclinoidal foramen, on each side. There is also an interclinoidal osseous bridge connecting the anterior and posterior clinoid processes on both sides. **(E)** Superior view of another specimen, in which the lesser sphenoid wings and the base of the anterior clinoids and roof of the optic canals have been removed. The remaining part of the anterior clinoid is held in place by its attachment to the optic strut. The medial side of the anterior clinoid is grooved to accommodate the clinoid segment. **(F)** Enlarged view of the left half of **(E)**. The posterior face of the optic strut is shaped to accommodate the anterior surface, and the medial aspect of the anterior clinoid is grooved to accommodate the lateral surface of the clinoid segment. The tip of the anterior clinoid process is the site of a small bony projection directed toward the middle clinoid process, with the anterior and middle clinoids nearly completing a ring around the clinoid segment at the level of the cavernous sinus roof. The sphenoid sinus may pneumatize through the optic strut into the anterior clinoid.

the roof of the optic canal to the planum sphenoidale. The chiasmatic sulcus is a shallow trough on the upper surface of the sphenoid bone between the intracranial end of the optic canals. The tuberculum sellae is located in the midline along the ridge forming the posterior margin of the chiasmatic sulcus. The anterior clinoid has a dense surface of cortical bone and a weak diploe of cancellous bone that is sometimes crossed by small venous channels that communicate with the cavernous sinus and the diploic veins of the orbital roof. The air cells in the sphenoid sinus may also extend through the optic strut into the anterior clinoid.

There is another small prominence, the middle clinoid process, that projects upward on the medial side of the terminal part of the carotid sulcus and medial to the tip of the anterior clinoid process (**Fig. 2.18**). An osseous bridge may extend from the tip of the middle clinoid to the tip of the anterior clinoid, thus converting the roof of the anterior part of the cavernous sinus into a bony ring or foramen, referred to as a caroticoclinoidal foramen, through which the internal carotid artery passes (**Fig. 2.18D**). This type of variant may infrequently occur bilaterally.[23] There may also be interclinoidal osseous bridges that extend from the anterior to the posterior clinoid unilaterally or bilaterally (**Fig. 2.18D**). Such bridges make it difficult to remove the anterior clinoid process.

Optic Strut

The optic strut (posterior root of the lesser wing) is a small bridge of bone that extends from the inferomedial aspect of the base of the anterior clinoid process to the body of the sphenoid just in front of the carotid sulcus[24] (**Figs. 2.16** and **2.18**). The strut, from its junction with the clinoid, slopes gently downward as it approaches the body of the sphenoid. The strut separates the optic canal and superior orbital fissure. The superior surface of the strut, which slopes downward and forward from its intracranial edge, forms the floor of the optic canal. The inferior surface of the optic strut forms the medial part of the roof of the superior orbital fissure and the anterior part of the roof of the cavernous sinus. The strut sits at the junction of the orbital apex anteriorly with the superior orbital fissure and optic canal posteriorly. The anterior edge of the strut is a narrow ridge located at the junction of its superior and inferior surfaces. The posterior face of the optic strut, which faces slightly downward, is shaped to accommodate the anterior surface of the anterior bend of the intracavernous carotid, which rests against the posterior surface of the optic strut as it ascends on the medial side of the anterior clinoid process. The site at which the strut blends into the sphenoid body is marked in the sphenoid sinus by a recess, the opticocarotid recess, that extends laterally from the superolateral part of the sphenoid sinus between the prominences in the sinus wall overlying the carotid sulcus and optic canal. This recess may extend deeply into the strut, so that the strut is partially or completely aerated by a lateral extension of the sphenoid sinus. The aeration may extend through the strut into the anterior clinoid process. Venous channels connecting the cavernous sinus with diploic veins of the orbital roof and anterior clinoid process may extend into or through the optic strut.

Dural Relationships

The dural relationships of the anterior clinoidal process are especially important in planning surgical approaches to the area (**Figs. 2.16, 2.17, 2.18,** and **2.19**). The dura extends medially from the upper surface of the anterior clinoid to surround the carotid artery and form a dural ring, referred to as the upper or distal ring, at the upper margin of the clinoid segment of the carotid.[25] The dura forming the lateral part of the upper ring extends forward and medially below the optic nerve to line the upper surface of the optic strut and posteriorly at the level of the upper part of the carotid sulcus to form the medial part of the upper ring. Further medially, the dura forming the upper ring blends into the diaphragma sellae. The dura extending medially above the optic nerve from the clinoid process to line the anterior root of the lesser wing and attaching to the posterior edge of the planum sphenoidale is located at the horizontal level of the upper surface of

Fig. 2.19 Triangles in the region of the cavernous sinus and middle fossa formed by the convergence and divergence of the cranial nerves. **(A,B)** Lateral aspect of brainstem and posterior fossa showing the brainstem origin of the cranial nerves, which form the margins of the cavernous sinus and middle fossa triangles. The tentorial edge was preserved in **(A)** and removed in **(B)**. There are four cavernous sinus triangles, four middle fossa triangles, and two paraclival triangles. The cavernous sinus triangles are the clinoidal, oculomotor, supratrochlear, and infratrochlear triangles. The clinoidal triangle, exposed by removing the anterior clinoid process, is situated in the interval between the optic and oculomotor nerves. The optic strut is in the anterior part, the clinoid segment is in the midportion, and the thin roof of the cavernous sinus is in the posterior part of this triangle. The oculomotor triangle is the triangular patch of dura through which the oculomotor nerve enters the roof of the cavernous sinus. The posterior margin of this triangle is formed by the posterior petroclinoid dural fold, which extends from the petrous apex to the posterior clinoid process. The lateral margin is formed by the anterior petroclinoid dural fold, which extends from the petrous apex to the anterior clinoid process. The medial margin is formed by the intraclinoid dural fold, which extends from the anterior to the posterior clinoid. The supratrochlear triangle is situated between the lower surface of the oculomotor nerve and the upper surface of the trochlear nerve, and a line joining the points of entrance of these nerves into the dura is its third margin. This triangle is very narrow. The infratrochlear triangle (Parkinson's triangle) is located between the lower margin of the trochlear nerve and the upper margin of the ophthalmic nerve, and a third margin is formed by a line connecting the point of entry of the trochlear nerve into the dura to the site where the trigeminal nerve enters Meckel's cave. The posterior bend of the carotid artery and the origin of the meningohypophyseal trunk are located in this triangle. The middle fossa triangles are the anteromedial, anterolateral, posterolateral, and posteromedial triangles. The anteromedial triangle is situated between the lower margin of the ophthalmic and the upper margin of the maxillary nerves, and a third edge is formed by a line connecting the point where the ophthalmic nerve passes through the superior orbital fissure and the maxillary nerve passes through the foramen rotundum. Removing bone in the medial wall of this triangle will create an opening into the sphenoid sinus. The anterolateral triangle is located between the lower surface of the maxillary nerve, the upper surface of the mandibular nerve, and a line connecting the foramen ovale and rotundum. Opening the bone in the medial wall of this triangle exposes the sphenoid sinus. The posterolateral triangle (Glasscock's triangle) is formed on the anterolateral side by the lateral surface of the mandibular nerve distal to the point at which the greater petrosal nerve crosses below the lateral surface of the

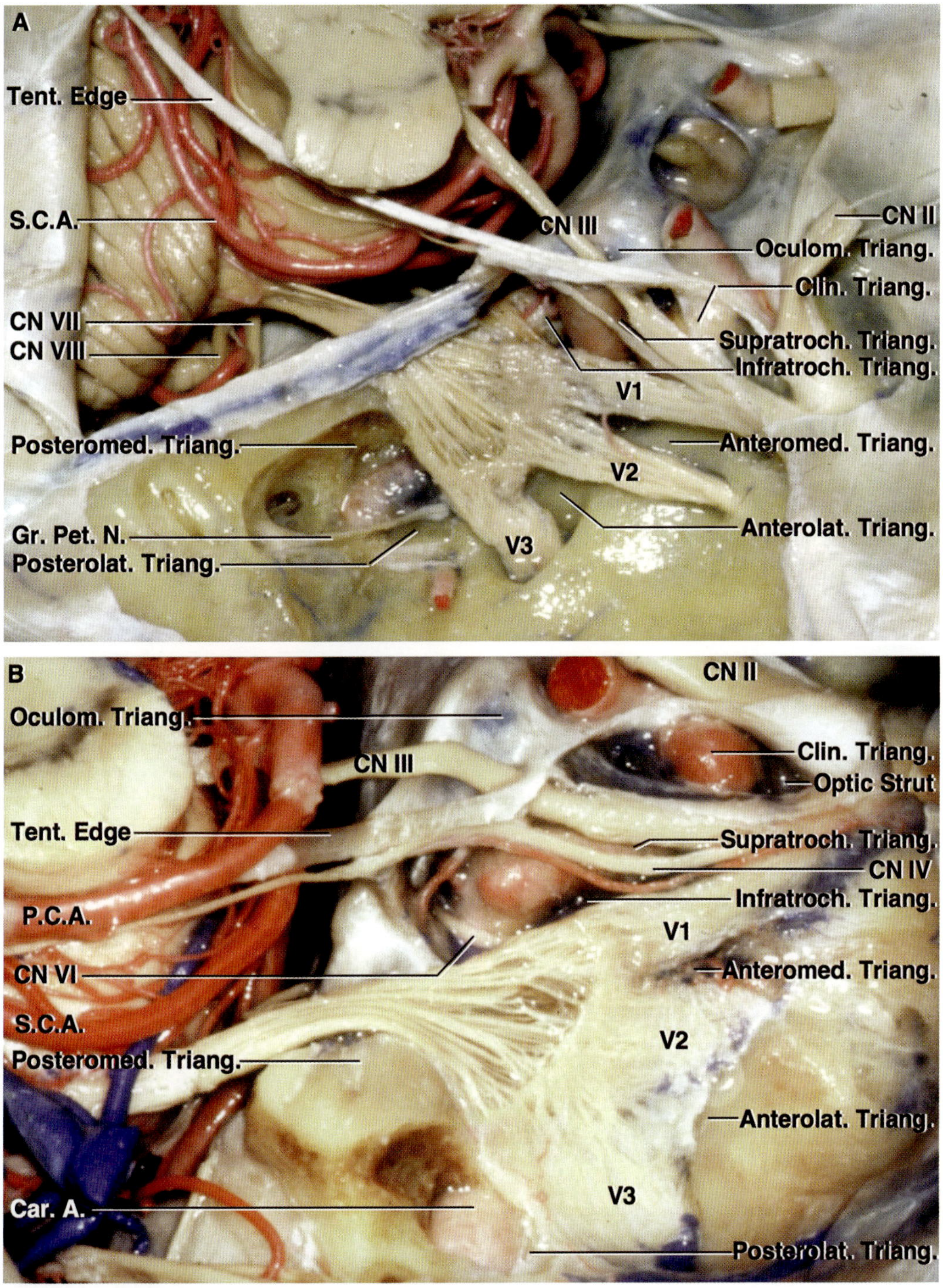

Fig. 2.19 *(Continued)* trigeminal nerve; on the posterolateral side it is formed by the anterior margin of the greater petrosal nerve. This triangle encompasses the floor of the middle cranial fossa between these two structures. The middle meningeal artery passes through the foramen spinosum in this triangle. Opening the floor of the middle fossa in this triangle exposes the infratemporal fossa. The posteromedial triangle (Kawase's triangle) is located between the greater petrosal nerve and the lateral edge of the trigeminal nerve behind the point where the greater petrosal nerve passes below the lateral edge of the trigeminal nerve, and a line along the connecting hiatus fallopii to the dural ostium of Meckel's cave. The petrous carotid crosses the anterior margin of this triangle. The cochlea is located below the floor of the middle fossa in the lateral apex of the triangle. Drilling the bony floor of the triangle in the area behind the internal carotid artery and medial to the cochlea exposes the lateral edge of the clivus. The paraclival triangles are the inferomedial and inferolateral triangles. The inferolateral paraclival triangle is located on the posterior surface of the clivus and temporal bone. The medial margin is formed by a line connecting the dural entry sites of the trochlear and abducens nerves; the upper margin extends from the dural entrance of the trochlear nerve to the point at which the first petrosal vein lateral to Meckel's cave joins the superior petrosal sinus (removed), and the lower margin is formed by a line connecting the point at which the abducens nerve enters the dura to the site at which the first petrosal vein, lateral to the trigeminal nerve, joins the superior petrosal sinus. The porus, through which the posterior trigeminal root enters Meckel's cave, is situated in the center of the inferolateral paraclival triangle. The inferomedial paraclival triangle is formed above by a line extending from the posterior clinoid process to the dural entrance of the trochlear nerve, laterally by a line connecting the dural entrances of the trochlear and abducens nerves, and medially by a line extending from the dural entrance of the abducens nerve to the posterior clinoid process. The dura in this triangle forms the posterior wall of the cavernous sinus. *(Continued on page 38)*

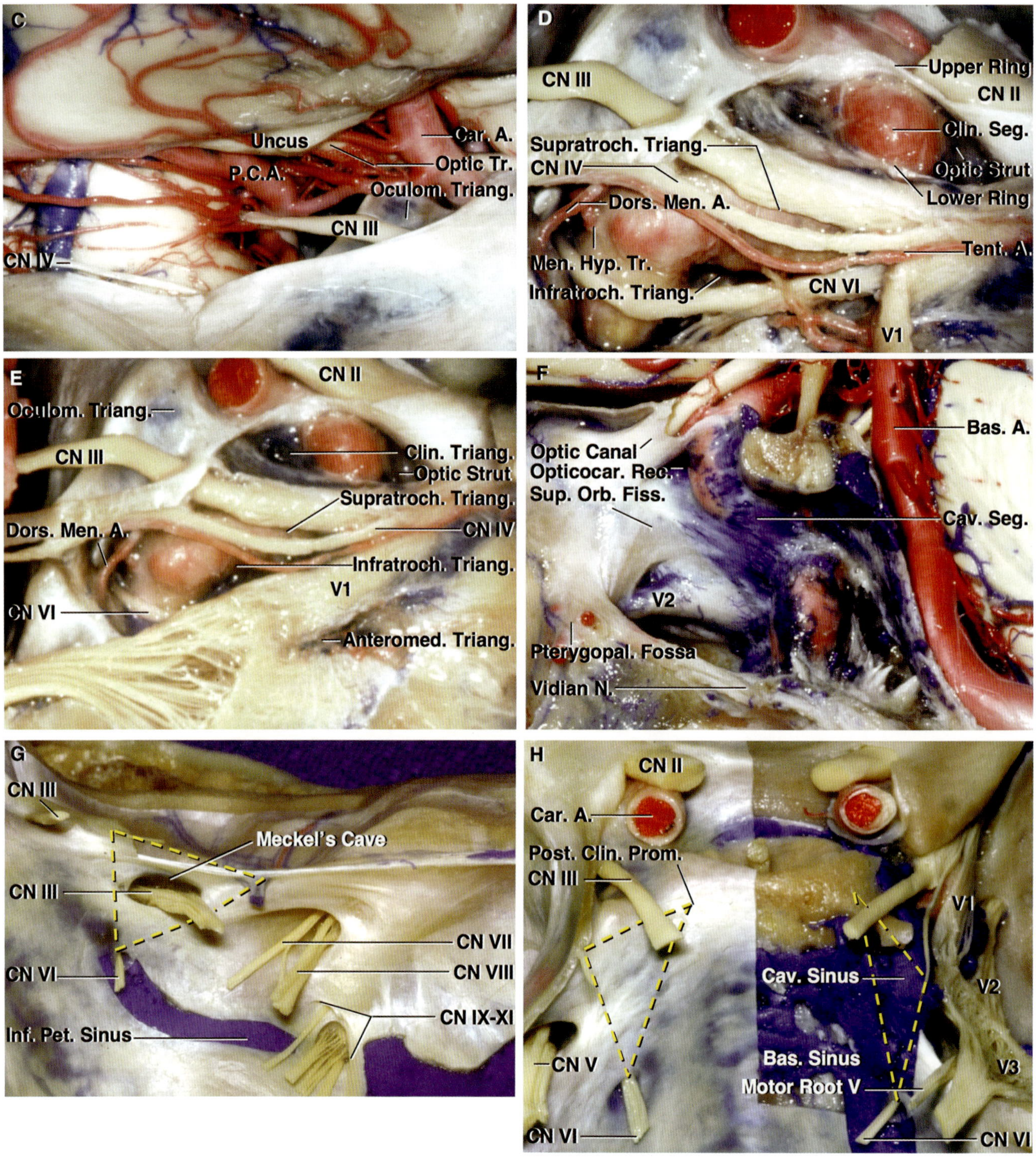

Fig. 2.19 *(Continued)* Triangles in the region of the cavernous sinus and middle fossa formed by the convergence and divergence of the cranial nerves. **(C)** Lateral view of the parasellar area and the oculomotor triangle. The temporal lobe has been elevated to expose the oculomotor and trochlear nerves as they enter the roof of the cavernous sinus. The oculomotor triangle is the triangular patch of dura through which the oculomotor nerve enters the roof of the cavernous sinus. The optic tract passes backward on the medial side of the uncus. **(D)** Enlarged view of the clinoidal, oculomotor, supratrochlear, and infratrochlear cavernous sinus triangles. The optic strut is exposed in the anterior part of the clinoidal triangle, the clinoid segment is exposed in the midportion, and the roof of the cavernous sinus is exposed in the posterior part. The upper margin of the clinoid segment is surrounded by the upper dural ring, which is formed by the dura extending medially from the upper surface of the anterior clinoid. The lower margin of the clinoid segment is defined by the lower dural ring, which is formed by the dura extending medially from the lower margin of the anterior clinoid. The dura on the lower margin of the anterior clinoid, referred to as the carotid-oculomotor membrane, separates the lower surface of the anterior clinoid from the upper surface of the oculomotor nerve and extends medially to form the lower dural ring. The posterior bend of the internal carotid artery and the origin of the meningohypophyseal trunk, which gives rise to the tentorial and dorsal meningeal arteries, are exposed in the infratrochlear triangle. The abducens nerve passes through Dorello's canal and between the lateral surface of the intracavernous carotid and the medial side of the ophthalmic nerve. The inferolateral trunk arises from the horizontal segment of the intracavernous carotid and passes above the abducens nerve. **(E,F)** Side-by-side comparison of

the clinoid. However, the dura that extends medially off the upper surface of the clinoid to line the upper surface of the optic strut and form the upper dural ring slopes downward as it proceeds medially, so that the medial part of the upper dural ring actually lies at the level of the lower rather than the upper surface of the anterior clinoid and optic canal.

The layer of dura that lines the lower margin of the anterior clinoid and extends medially to form the lower or proximal dural ring is called the carotid-oculomotor membrane because it separates the lower margin of the clinoid from the oculomotor nerve and extends medially around the carotid artery (**Figs. 2.16** and **2.19**). This membrane extends medially and forward to line the lower surface of the optic strut. The segment of the internal carotid artery located between the upper and lower dural rings, which is exposed by removing the anterior clinoid process, is referred to as the clinoid segment. It may be necessary to divide the dural rings to mobilize the carotid artery in the management of tumors and aneurysms arising at the level of the roof of the cavernous sinus.

Neural Relationships

The location of the nerves in the sinus wall or sinus, superiorly to inferiorly, are the third nerve followed by the trochlear, ophthalmic, and abducens nerves[18,26,27] (**Figs. 2.16, 2.17,** and **2.19**). The oculomotor, trochlear, and ophthalmic nerves course in the inner part of the lateral sinus wall. The abducens courses medial to the ophthalmic nerve and is adherent to the lateral surface of the intracavernous carotid medially, but it also is adherent laterally to the medial surface of the ophthalmic nerve and the inner part of the lateral sinus wall.

The oculomotor nerve pierces the roof of the cavernous sinus near the center of the oculomotor triangle, and the fourth nerve enters the dura at the posterolateral edge of the triangle. A short length of both the trochlear and oculomotor nerves is surrounded by a dural and arachnoid cuff, to create the oculomotor and trochlear cisterns, as they pass through the roof of the cavernous sinus and below the anterior clinoid process. Both nerves are situated medial to, and slightly beneath, the level of the free edge of the tentorium at their point of entry.

The oculomotor nerve enters the cavernous sinus slightly lateral and anterior to the dorsum sellae, almost directly above the origin of the meningohypophyseal trunk from the intracavernous carotid, and courses along the lower margin of the anterior clinoid and the carotid-oculomotor membrane. The oculomotor nerve pierces the sinus roof between 2 and 7 mm posterior to the initial supraclinoid segment of the carotid artery; the average separation is 5 mm.[18]

The trochlear nerve enters the roof of the sinus posterolateral to the third nerve and courses below the oculomotor nerve in the posterior part of the lateral wall. Anteriorly, below the base of the anterior clinoid process, it passes upward along the lateral surface of the oculomotor nerve. From there, the trochlear nerve passes medially between the oculomotor nerve and dura lining the lower margin of the anterior clinoid and optic strut to reach the medial part of the orbit and the superior oblique muscle.

The ophthalmic nerve is the smallest of the three trigeminal divisions. It is inclined upward as it passes forward near the medial surface of the dura forming the lower part of the lateral wall of the cavernous sinus to reach the superior orbital fissure. It is flattened in the wall of the cavernous sinus, but at the superior orbital fissure it takes on an oval configuration. The ophthalmic nerve splits into the lacrimal, frontal, and nasociliary nerves as it approaches the superior orbital fissure.

The superior petrosal sinus passes above the posterior root of the trigeminal root to form the upper margin of the ostium of Meckel's cave, the dural and subarachnoid cavern that communicates with the subarachnoid space in the posterior fossa (**Fig. 2.16**). The cave extends forward around the posterior trigeminal root to the midportion of the ganglion. The motor root of the trigeminal nerve courses on the medial side of the sensory fibers at the level of Meckel's cave.

The abducens nerve pierces the dura forming the lower part of the posterior wall of the sinus at the upper border of the petrous apex and enters a dural cave, referred to as Dorello's canal; here it passes below the petrosphenoid ligament (Gruber's ligament), which extends from the lower part of the lateral edge of the dorsum sellae to the petrous apex, to enter the cavernous sinus (**Figs. 2.6** and **2.16**). The nerve bends laterally around the proximal portion of the intercavernous carotid and gently ascends as it passes forward inside the cavernous sinus medial to the ophthalmic nerve and on the lateral side of the internal carotid artery and below and medial to the nasociliary nerve. It has the most medial site of entry of the nerves coursing in the si-

Fig. 2.19 *(Continued)* the medial and lateral aspects of the cavernous sinus. **(E)** Lateral view of cavernous sinus. **(F)** View, through the sphenoid sinus, of the medial side of the cavernous sinus. The optic nerve is exposed at the upper margin of the clinoidal triangle and above the optic strut. On the sphenoid sinus side of the specimen, the optic canal is seen above the opticocarotid recess, which leads into the optic strut. The clinoid segment rests against the posterior aspect of the optic strut in both views. In the lateral view, the superior orbital fissure, through which the ophthalmic, trochlear, and abducens nerves pass, is seen below the optic strut. In the view through the sphenoid sinus, the medial edge of the superior orbital fissure produces a wide, rounded prominence below the optic strut, and the maxillary nerve produces a prominence in the lower part of the sphenoid sinus just distal to the foramen rotundum. The lateral wing of the sphenoid sinus extends laterally under the maxillary nerve into the medial part of the floor of the middle fossa. Opening the middle fossa floor in the anteromedial and anterolateral triangles exposes the sphenoid sinus. **(G)** Posterior view of the inferolateral triangle. The medial edge of the inferolateral triangle extends between the dural entrances of cranial nerves IV and V. The inferior limb extends from cranial nerve VI to where the first vein lateral to Meckel's cave joins the superior petrosal sinus and the superior limb extends from that vein to the dural entrance of cranial nerve IV. The ostium of Meckel's cave is located within the inferolateral triangle. **(H)** Posterior view of the inferomedial triangles. The medial limb of the inferomedial triangle extends from the posterior clinoid to the dural entrance to the abducens nerve. The lateral limb extends between the dural entrances of nerves IV and VI, and the superior limb extends from nerve IV to the posterior clinoid. On the right side, there is an abnormal projection of the posterior clinoid process that extends below the oculomotor nerve toward the petrous apex.

nus wall and maintains that position in its course through the sinus. The nerve usually enters the sinus as a single bundle but may persist as two bundles in the subarachnoid space. After entering the sinus, it may split into as many as five rootlets as it courses between the internal carotid artery and ophthalmic nerve. In a study of 50 sinuses, the intracavernous segment of the nerve consisted of a single rootlet in 34 specimens, two in 13, three in two, and five in one.[18]

Sympathetic fiber bundles large enough to be recognized without a surgical microscope travel on the surface of the carotid as it emerges from the foramen lacerum. Some of the bundles join the sixth nerve within the sinus before ultimately being distributed to the first trigeminal division, which sends sympathetic fibers that reach the pupillodilator through the long ciliary nerves and pass through the ciliary ganglion.[28,29] Some sympathetic fibers pass directly from the carotid plexus to the ciliary ganglion, and others may travel along the ophthalmic artery to the globe.[30]

Parasellar Triangles

The parasellar region is the site of several significant triangular relationships formed by the convergence and divergence of the cranial nerves in the region of the cavernous sinus and middle fossa. The four triangles in the cavernous sinus, four in the middle fossa lateral to the cavernous sinus, and two in the paraclival area are helpful in understanding and planning approaches to the cavernous sinus (**Fig. 2.19**). The cavernous sinus triangles are formed by the optic, oculomotor, trochlear, and ophthalmic nerves converging on the optic canal and superior orbital fissure. The middle fossa triangles are formed by the trigeminal divisions diverging as they pass from the gasserian ganglion to reach their foramina.[27]

Cavernous Sinus Triangles

1. Clinoidal triangle. This triangle is situated in the interval between the optic and oculomotor nerves. It is exposed by removing the anterior clinoid process. The optic strut is in the anterior part, the clinoid segment of the internal carotid artery is in the midportion, and the thin roof of the cavernous sinus is in the posterior part of this triangle (**Fig. 2.19**).
2. Oculomotor triangle. This triangle is formed by the triangular patch of dura through which the oculomotor nerve enters the roof of the cavernous sinus. Two margins of the triangle are formed by the anterior and posterior petroclinoidal dural folds, which extend, respectively, from the anterior and posterior clinoid processes to the petrous apex; the third side is formed by the interclinoidal dural fold, which extends from the anterior to the posterior clinoid process.
3. Supratrochlear triangle. This triangle is situated between the lower surface of the oculomotor nerve and the upper surface of the trochlear nerve; a line joining the points of entrance of these nerves into the dura is its third margin. This triangle is very narrow.
4. Infratrochlear triangle (Parkinson's triangle). This triangle is located between the lower margin of the trochlear nerve and the upper margin of the ophthalmic nerve, and a third margin is formed by a line connecting the point of entry of the trochlear nerve into the dura to the site where the trigeminal nerve enters Meckel's cave. The posterior bend of the internal carotid artery and the origin of the meningohypophyseal trunk from the posterior bend are located in this triangle, except when the carotid artery is elongated and tortuous, in which case the origin may be pushed upward into the oculomotor triangle. Parkinson first described the surgical exposure of the intercavernous portion of the carotid artery through this triangle for the treatment of carotid cavernous fistulas.[29,31,32] In a prior study, we found that the superior margin of the triangle formed by the lower margin of the fourth cranial nerve averaged 13 mm (range, 8–20 mm); the inferior margin formed by the upper margin of the fifth cranial nerve averaged 14 mm (range, 5–24 mm); the posterior margin represented by the slope of the dorsum and clivus averaged 6 mm (range, 3–14 mm). The average triangle measured 13 × 14 × 6 mm; however, it can be very small, measuring only 8 × 5 × 3 mm, and may not be large enough to provide a good surgical exposure of all of the arterial branches within the sinus.[18] Parkinson, through an incision starting 4 mm beneath the dural entrance of the third nerve and extending anteriorly ~2 cm parallel to the slope of the third and fourth nerves, exposed the meningohypophyseal trunk and the artery of the inferior cavernous sinus.[29] The sixth nerve at the bottom edge of the exposure was seen upon retraction of the superior aspect of the trigeminal nerve.

Middle Fossa Triangles

1. Anteromedial middle fossa triangle. This triangle is situated between the lower margin of the ophthalmic nerve and the upper margin of the maxillary nerve, and a third edge is formed by a line connecting the point where the ophthalmic nerve passes through the superior orbital fissure and the maxillary nerve passes through the foramen rotundum (**Fig. 2.19**). Removing bone in the triangular space between the ophthalmic and maxillary nerves creates an opening into the sphenoid sinus.
2. Anterolateral middle fossa triangle. This triangle is located between the lower surface of the maxillary nerve, the upper surface of the mandibular nerve, and a line connecting the foramen ovale and foramen rotundum. Opening the bone in the medial wall of this triangle exposes the lateral wing of the sphenoid sinus.
3. Posterolateral middle fossa triangle (Glasscock's triangle). This triangle is formed on the antero-

medial side by the lateral surface of the mandibular nerve distal to the point at which the greater petrosal nerve crosses below the lateral surface of the trigeminal nerve, and on the posterolateral side by the anterior margin of the greater petrosal nerve. This triangle opens laterally to encompass the midportion of the floor of the middle cranial fossa. The middle meningeal artery passes through the foramen spinosum in this triangle. Opening the floor of the middle fossa in this triangle exposes the infratemporal fossa, which is the site of the pterygoid muscles and venous plexus, branches of the mandibular nerve, and a segment of the maxillary artery.

4. Posteromedial middle fossa triangle (Kawase's triangle). This triangle is located between the greater petrosal nerve, the lateral edge of the trigeminal nerve behind the point where the greater petrosal nerve passes below its lateral surface, and a line along the connecting hiatus fallopii to the dural ostium of Meckel's cave. The petrous segment of the internal carotid artery crosses the anterior margin of this triangle. Removing the bone in the lateral part of the posteromedial triangle exposes the cochlea and anterior wall of the internal auditory canal, and in the medial part of the posteromedial triangle exposes the side of the clivus and the inferior petrosal sinus.

Paraclival Triangles

1. Inferolateral paraclival triangle. This triangle is located on the posterior surface of the clivus and temporal bone between the lines connecting the dural entry sites of the trochlear and abducens nerves and the point at which the abducens nerve enters the dura to the site where the first petrosal vein, lateral to the trigeminal nerve, joins the superior petrosal sinus. The porus through which the posterior trigeminal root enters Meckel's cave is situated in the center of the inferolateral paraclival triangle.
2. Inferomedial paraclival triangle. This triangle is located between the lines connecting the posterior clinoid process and the dural entrance of the trochlear nerve. The abducens nerve enters the cavernous sinus at the lower edge of this triangle. This triangle extends along the posterior sinus wall. Opening the dura in the medial part of the inferomedial triangle exposes the lateral edge of the dorsum sellae, the upper end of the petroclival suture, and the sixth nerve passing below Gruber's ligament.

Arterial Relationships

The internal carotid artery exits the foramen lacerum lateral to the posterior clinoid process, where it passes under the petrolingual ligament and turns abruptly forward to course along the carotid sulcus and lateral part of the body of the sphenoid (**Figs. 2.16, 2.17, 2.18,** and **2.19**). It passes forward in a horizontal direction for ~2 cm and terminates by passing upward along the medial side to the anterior clinoid process and the posterior surface of the optic strut, where it penetrates the roof of the cavernous sinus. The clinoid segment of the carotid artery is tightly surrounded by the anterior clinoid process laterally, the optic strut anteriorly, and the carotid sulcus medially, with only a narrow space left between the bone and the artery. The dura lining the surface of these osseous structures facing the clinoid segment forms the carotid collar around the clinoid segment. The intracavernous carotid is relatively fixed by the bony ring, but despite this, large extensions of pituitary tumor may produce lateral displacement of the artery.

Just proximal to the cavernous sinus in the foramen lacerum, the artery lies beneath the trigeminal nerve.[18] In surgical approaches to the trigeminal nerve directed through the middle cranial fossa, there is a tendency to assume that the carotid artery is distant from the trigeminal nerve. However, nearly 85% of carotid arteries are exposed under some portion of Meckel's cave and the trigeminal nerve, with only dura, and no bone, separating the nerve from the artery[18] (**Figs. 2.16** and **2.19**). In the remainder, the bone separating the nerve and artery is often paper-thin. The region without bone over the carotid often extends to the lateral edge of the trigeminal nerve, and in more than one-third, the bone covering the carotid is defective lateral to the edge of the third division. The maximum length of artery exposed lateral to the nerve was 7 mm in our study.

The branches of the intracavernous carotid are the meningohypophyseal trunk, the largest branch, present in 100% of our specimens; the artery of the inferior cavernous sinus, present in 84%; and McConnell's capsular arteries, present in 28%[21,33] (**Figs. 2.1, 2.11,** and **2.19**). Less frequent branches of the intracavernous carotid were the ophthalmic artery (8%) and the dorsal meningeal artery (6%).[18] The meningohypophyseal trunk, the most proximal intracavernous branch, arises at or just before the apex of the first curve of the intracavernous carotid, where it turns forward after leaving the foramen lacerum (**Fig. 2.19**). The meningohypophyseal trunk typically gives rise to three branches: (1) the tentorial artery, also called the artery of Bernasconi-Cassinari,[34] which courses lateral to the tentorium; (2) the inferior hypophyseal artery, which travels medially to supply the posterior pituitary capsule; and (3) the dorsal meningeal artery, which enters the dura of the posterior sinus wall and supplies the clival dura and cranial nerve VI. The artery of the inferior cavernous sinus, also called the inferolateral trunk, may infrequently arise from the meningohypophyseal trunk.[18] The tentorial artery, the most constant branch of the meningohypophyseal trunk, present in 100% of instances, passes forward to the roof of the cavernous sinus and then posterolaterally along the free edge of the tentorium. The dorsal meningeal artery arises from the meningohypophyseal trunk in 90% of cavernous sinuses. It passes posteriorly through the cavernous sinus with the abducens nerve to reach the dura over the dorsum and clivus. The inferior hypophyseal artery, the least frequent of the three common branches of the meningohypophyseal trunk, arises from the meningohypophyseal trunk in 80% of cavernous sinuses.[18,26] It passes medial to the posterior pituitary capsule and lobe and anastomoses with its mate of the opposite side after supplying the dura of the sellar floor. The dorsal meningeal and inferior hypophyseal arteries that do not arise from the meningohypophyseal artery usually arise directly from the intracavernous carotid.

The inferolateral trunk (artery of the inferior cavernous sinus) arises from the lateral side of the midportion of the horizontal segment of the intracavernous carotid ~5 to 8 mm distal to the origin of the meningohypophyseal trunk. It arises directly from the carotid artery in 84% of cavernous sinuses and from the meningohypophyseal artery in another 6%.[18,26] It passes above or below the sixth nerve and downward medial to the first trigeminal division to supply the dura of the inferior lateral wall of the cavernous sinus and the area of the foramen rotundum and foramen ovale.

McConnell's capsular arteries arise from the medial side of the carotid artery and pass to the capsule of the gland or the dura lining the anterior wall and floor of the sella. They are frequently absent, found in approximately a quarter of cavernous sinuses.[18]

The ophthalmic artery commonly arises just above the upper ring from the medial half of the anterior wall of the internal carotid artery, but it may also arise in the cavernous sinus, in which case it usually passes through the superior orbital fissure. It may rarely arise from the middle meningeal artery.[35]

◆ Suprasellar and Third Ventricular Region

This section deals with neural, arterial, and venous relationships in the suprasellar and third ventricular regions that are important in the management of tumors that extend upward from the sella into these areas.

Ventricular and Cisternal Relationships

Tumors arising in the sella often extend upward into the suprasellar cisterns to compress the optic nerves and chiasm and floor of the third ventricle, and to involve the circle of Willis[36] (**Fig. 2.20**). The area involved by those tumors arising in the sella corresponds to the anterior incisural space located between the free edges of the tentorium and the front of the midbrain. The anterior incisural space corresponds roughly to the suprasellar area. From the front of the midbrain, it extends obliquely forward and upward around the optic chiasm to the subcallosal area. It opens laterally into the sylvian fissure and posteriorly between the uncus and the brainstem.

The part of the anterior incisural space located below the optic chiasm has posterior and posterolateral walls.[37,38] The posterior wall is formed by the cerebral peduncles and walls of the interpeduncular cistern. The posterolateral wall is formed by the anterior one-third of the uncus, which extends medially above the free edge of the tentorium and oculomotor nerve. The infundibulum of the pituitary gland crosses the anterior incisural space to reach the opening in the diaphragma sellae. The part of the anterior incisural space situated above the optic chiasm is limited superiorly by the rostrum of the corpus callosum, posteriorly by the lamina terminalis, and laterally by the part of the medial surfaces of the frontal lobes located below the frontal horns.

The anterior incisural space opens laterally into the part of the sylvian fissure situated below the anterior perforated substance. The anterior limb of the internal capsule, the head of the caudate nucleus, and the anterior part of the lentiform nucleus are located above the anterior perforated substance. The interpeduncular cistern, which sits in the posterior part of the anterior incisural space between the cerebral peduncles and the dorsum sellae, communicates anteriorly with the chiasmatic cistern, which is located below the optic chiasm. The interpeduncular and chiasmatic cisterns are separated by Liliequist's membrane, an arachnoidal sheet extending from the dorsum sellae to the mamillary bodies. The chiasmatic cistern communicates around the optic chiasm with the cisterna laminae terminalis, which lies anterior to the lamina terminalis.

Cranial Nerves

The optic and oculomotor nerves and the posterior part of the olfactory tracts pass through the suprasellar region and anterior incisural space (**Figs. 2.16, 2.17, 2.19,** and **2.20**). Each olfactory tract runs posteriorly and splits just above the anterior clinoid process to form the medial and lateral olfactory striae, which course along the anterior margin of the anterior perforated substance.

The optic nerves and chiasm and the anterior part of the optic tracts cross the anterior incisural space. The optic nerves emerge from the optic canals medial to the anterior clinoid processes and are directed posteriorly, superiorly, and medially toward the optic chiasm. From the chiasm, the optic tracts continue in a posterolateral direction around the cerebral peduncles toward the lateral geniculate bodies. The optic nerve proximal to its entrance into the optic canal is covered by a reflected leaf of dura mater, the falciform process, which extends medially from the anterior clinoid process across the top of the optic nerve. The length of nerve covered only by the dura of the falciform process at the intracranial end of the optic canal may vary from less than 1 mm to as much as 1 cm.[6] Coagulation of the dura above the optic nerve just proximal to the optic canal on the assumption that bone separates the dura mater from the nerve can lead to nerve injury. Compression of the optic nerve against the sharp edge of the falciform process may result in a visual field deficit even if the compressing lesion does not damage the nerve enough to cause visual loss.[6,8]

The optic chiasm is situated at the junction of the anterior wall and floor of the third ventricle (**Figs. 2.20** and **2.21**). The anterior cerebral and anterior communicating arteries, the lamina terminalis, and the third ventricle are located above the chiasm. The tuber cinereum and the infundibulum are posterior to, the internal carotid arteries are lateral to, and the diaphragma sellae and pituitary gland are below the optic chiasm. The suprachiasmatic recess of the third ventricle is located between the chiasm and lamina terminalis. The infundibular recess extends into the base of the pituitary stalk behind the optic chiasm. The relationship of the chiasm to the sella is an important determinant of the ease with which the pituitary fossa can be exposed

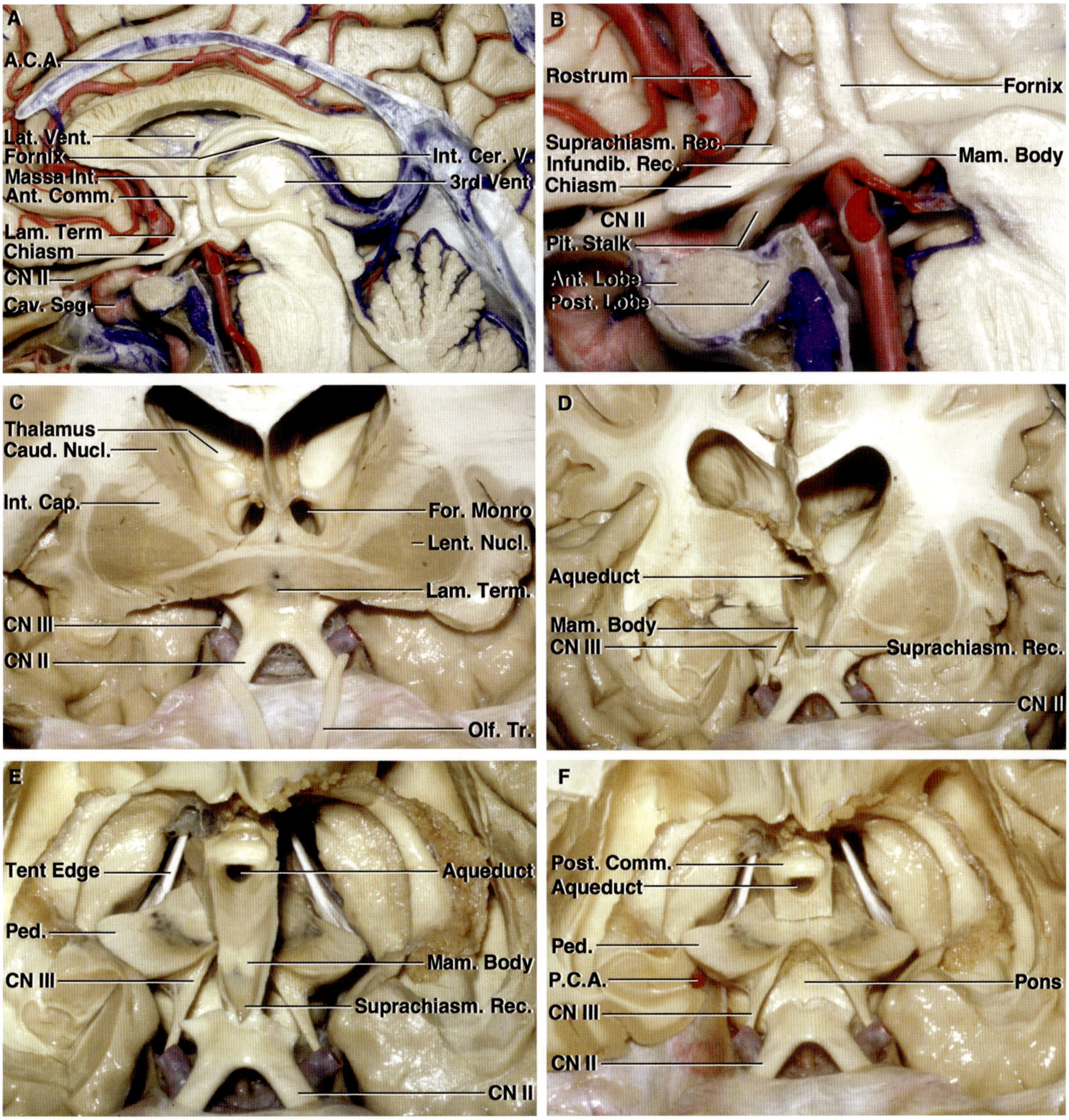

Fig. 2.20 Neural relationships in the suprasellar area. **(A)** Midsagittal section of the sella, pituitary gland, sphenoid sinus, and third ventricle. The anterior part of the third ventricle is located above the sella. The columns of the fornix descend along the superior and anterior margins of the foramen of Monro to reach the mamillary bodies. The optic chiasm and stalk are located above the sella. The internal cerebral veins course in the roof of the third ventricle. **(B)** Enlarged view. The suprachiasmatic recess of the third ventricle is located between the lamina terminalis and the chiasm. The infundibular recess extends into the stalk in the area behind the chiasm. The lamina terminalis extends upward and is continuous with the rostrum of the corpus callosum. The thin part of the third ventricular floor between the chiasm and the mamillary bodies is suitable for a third ventriculostomy. The anterior commissure crosses the wall of the third ventricle in front of the columns of the fornix. The massa intermedia crosses the midportion of the third ventricle. **(C)** The anterior part of the hemisphere has been removed to expose the lateral ventricles and suprasellar area. The optic nerve and chiasm are located above the sella. The chiasm cistern is located below the optic chiasm and opens upward between the optic nerves to the area in front of the lamina terminalis. The anterior commissure crosses the anterior wall of the third ventricle above the lamina terminalis. The anterior part of the third ventricle is located above the sella. The body of the lateral ventricle is situated above the third ventricle. The columns of the fornix form the superior and anterior margins of the foramen of Monro. The olfactory tracts pass above the optic nerves, and the optic tracts pass above the oculomotor nerves. **(D)** The cross-section on the right hemisphere has been extended backward to the midportion of the temporal horn and thalamus. This exposes the oculomotor nerve arising on the medial surface of the cerebral peduncle and passing below the floor of the third ventricle and lateral to the sella. The crural cistern is located between the uncus and the cerebral peduncle. The mamillary bodies are positioned in the floor of the third ventricle. The posterior commissure sits above the aqueduct. **(E)** The full length of the floor of the third ventricle has been exposed by removing the thalami bilaterally. The mamillary bodies are located at the junction of the anterior and middle thirds of the floor. The floor behind the mamillary bodies is formed by the upper midbrain. The floor in front of the mamillary bodies is very thin and serves as a suitable site for third ventriculostomy. **(F)** Anterior-superior view. The upper part of the left thalamus has been removed to expose the optic tract, which extends backward above the oculomotor nerve in the lateral part of the suprasellar area to reach the lateral geniculate body. The chiasm and posterior part of the optic nerves are located directly above the sella. The anterior cerebral arteries pass above the chiasm. The left anterior cerebral artery is hypoplastic.

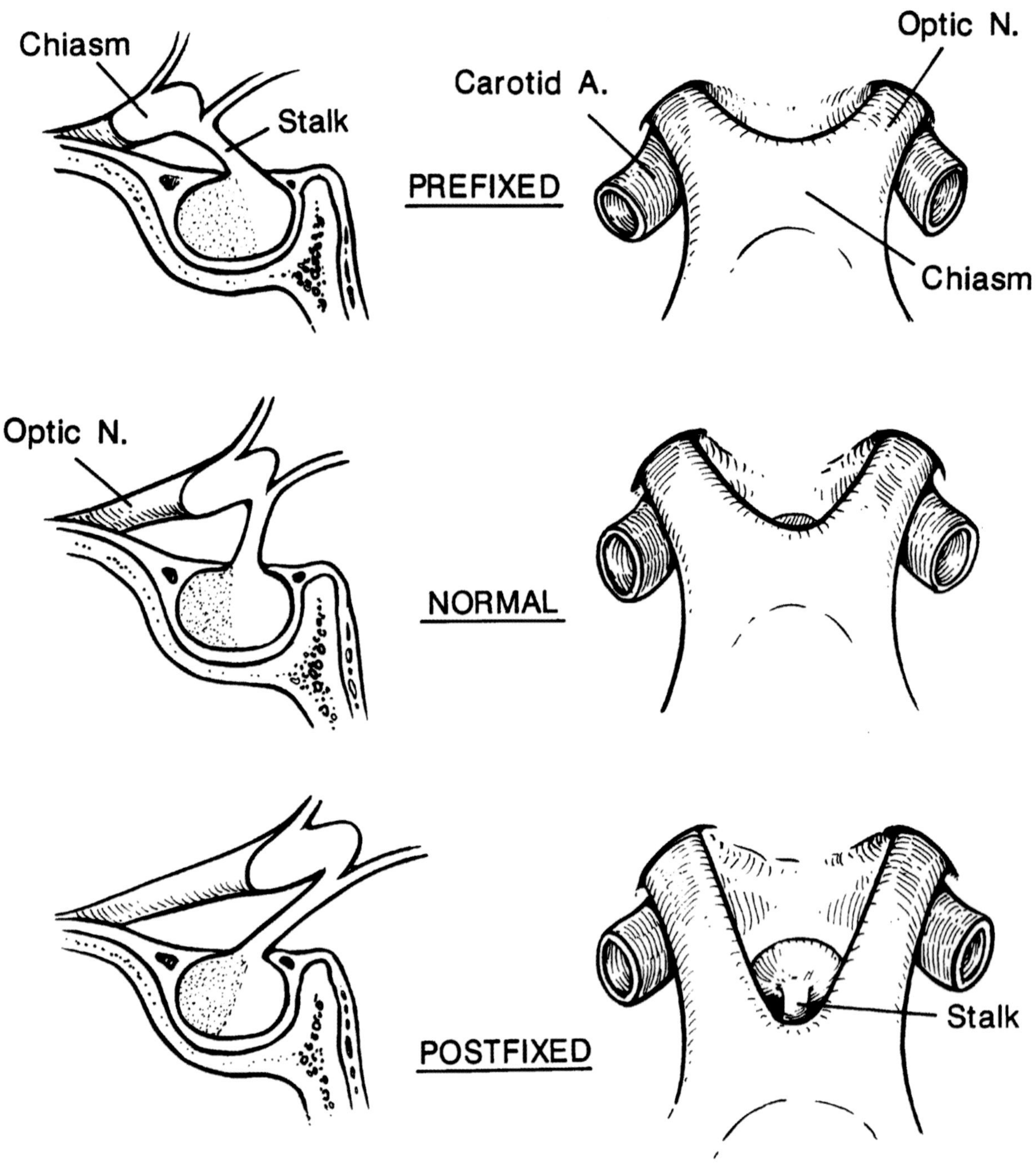

Fig. 2.21 Sagittal sections and superior views of the sellar region showing the optic nerve and chiasm and the carotid artery. The prefixed chiasm is located above the tuberculum. The normal chiasm is located above the diaphragma. The postfixed chiasm is situated above the dorsum.

by the transfrontal surgical route (**Fig. 2.21**). The normal chiasm overlies the diaphragma sellae and the pituitary gland, the prefixed chiasm overlies the tuberculum, and the postfixed chiasm overlies the dorsum. In ~70% of cases, the chiasm is in the normal position. Of the remaining 30%, about half are "prefixed" and half "postfixed."[6]

A prominent tuberculum sellae may restrict access to the sella even in the presence of a normal chiasm. The tuberculum may vary from almost flat to protruding upward as much as 3 mm, and it may project posteriorly to the margin of a normal chiasm[6] (**Fig. 2.18**). A prefixed chiasm, a normal chiasm with a small area between the tuberculum and the chiasm, and a superior protruding tuberculum sellae do not limit exposure by the transsphenoidal approach, but they do limit the access to the suprasellar area provided by the transcranial approach. There are several methods of gaining access to the suprasellar area when these variants are present. One is to expose the sphenoid sinus from above by opening through the tuberculum and planum sphenoidale, thus converting the approach to a transfrontal-transsphenoidal exposure. If the chiasm is prefixed and the tumor is seen through a thin, stretched anterior wall of the third ventricle, the lamina terminalis may be opened to expose the tumor, but this exposure is infrequently used for pituitary adenomas and more commonly for craniopharyngiomas and gliomas involving the third ventricle. If the space between the carotid artery and the optic nerve has been enlarged by a lateral or parasellar extension of tumor, the tumor may be removed through this space.[17]

An understanding of the relationships of the carotid artery, optic nerve, and anterior clinoid process is fundamental to all surgical approaches to the sellar and parasellar areas (**Figs. 2.6, 2.16,** and **2.17**). The carotid artery and the optic nerve are medial to the anterior clinoid process. The artery exits the cavernous sinus beneath and slightly lateral to the optic nerve. The optic nerve pursues a posteromedial course toward the chiasm, and the carotid artery pursues a posterolateral course toward its bifurcation below the anterior perforated substance.

The oculomotor nerve arises in the interpeduncular cistern from the midbrain on the medial side of the cerebral peduncle and courses between the posterior cerebral and superior cerebellar arteries (**Fig. 2.19**). The oculomotor nerve courses in the lateral wall of the interpeduncular cistern and forms the pillars to which the lateral edge of Liliequist's membrane attaches. Liliequist's membrane extends upward from the arachnoid membrane covering the dorsum sellae and separates the chiasmatic and interpeduncular cisterns. The uncus of the temporal lobe is situated lateral to the oculomotor nerve. The oculomotor nerve pierces the roof of the cavernous sinus and slopes downward in the superolateral corner of the cavernous sinus.

The trochlear nerve is the longest and thinnest cranial nerve (**Figs. 2.6, 2.16,** and **2.19**). The trochlear nerve arises from the midbrain below the inferior colliculus and passes around the brainstem near the junction of the midbrain and pons to reach the lower margin of the tentorial edge. The trochlear nerve pierces the medial edge of the tentorium and enters the roof of the cavernous sinus just behind the anterior tentorial attachment.

The abducens nerve arises at the lower margin of the pons and passes above or below or is split into two bundles by the anterior inferior cerebellar artery (**Figs. 2.16** and **2.19**). It passes upward in the prepontine cistern, then turns forward at the upper border of the petrous apex, where it pierces the dura and passes below the petrosphenoid (Gruber's) ligament to enter the posterior part of the cavernous sinus.

The trigeminal nerve arises in the posterior fossa from the midpons. The posterior root passes above the petrous apex to enter Meckel's cave, a cavern in the subarachnoid space located lateral to the cavernous sinus. Meckel's cave extends forward to the level of the trigeminal ganglion.

Arterial Relationships

The arterial relationships in the suprasellar area are among the most complex in the head because this area contains all the components of the circle of Willis (**Figs. 2.22** and **2.23**). Numerous arteries, including the internal carotid and basilar arteries and the circle of Willis and its branches, may be stretched around tumors in this area. The posterior part of the circle of Willis and the apex of the basilar artery are located in the anterior incisural space below the floor of the third ventricle; the anterior part of the circle of Willis and the anterior cerebral and anterior communicating arteries are intimately related to the anterior wall of the third ventricle; both the anterior and posterior cerebral arteries send branches into the roof of the third ventricle; the internal carotid, anterior choroidal, anterior and posterior cerebral, and anterior and posterior communicating arteries give rise to perforating branches that reach the walls of the third ventricle and anterior incisural space; and all the arterial components of the circle of Willis and the adjacent segments of the carotid and basilar arteries and their perforating branches may be stretched around suprasellar extensions of pituitary tumors.[1]

The internal carotid artery exits the cavernous sinus along the medial surface of the anterior clinoid process to reach the anterior incisural space (**Figs. 2.16, 2.17,** and **2.19**). After entering this space it courses posteriorly, superiorly, and laterally to reach the site of its bifurcation below the anterior perforated substance. It is first below and then lateral to the optic nerve and chiasm. It sends perforating branches to the optic nerve, chiasm, and tract and to the floor of the third ventricle. These branches pass across the interval between the internal carotid artery and the optic nerve and may be an obstacle to the operative approaches directed through the triangular space between the internal carotid artery, the optic nerve, and the anterior cerebral artery. The internal carotid artery also gives off the superior hypophyseal artery, which runs medially below the floor of the third ventricle to reach the tuber cinereum and joins its mate of the opposite side to form a ring around the infundibulum.

The ophthalmic artery, the first branch of the internal carotid artery above the cavernous sinus, usually arises and enters the optic canal below the optic nerve (**Figs. 2.16, 2.17,** and **2.23**). Its origin and proximal segment may be visible below the optic nerve without retraction of the nerve, although elevation of the optic nerve away from the carotid artery is usually required to see the segment proximal to the optic foramen. The artery arises from the supraclinoid segment of the carotid artery in most cases, but in some cases, it arises within the cavernous sinus or rarely as a branch of the middle meningeal artery.[6,18,26,39]

The posterior communicating artery arises from the posterior wall of the internal carotid artery and courses posteromedially below the optic tracts and the floor of the third ventricle to join the posterior cerebral artery (**Figs. 2.22** and **2.23**). Its branches penetrate the floor of the third ventricle between the optic chiasm and the cerebral peduncle and reach the thalamus, hypothalamus, subthalamus, and internal capsule. Its posterior course varies depending on whether the artery provides the major supply to the distal posterior cerebral artery. If it is normal, with the posterior cerebral artery arising predominantly from the basilar artery, it is directed posteromedially above the oculomotor nerve toward the interpeduncular fossa. If the posterior cerebral artery has a fetal type of configuration, in which it

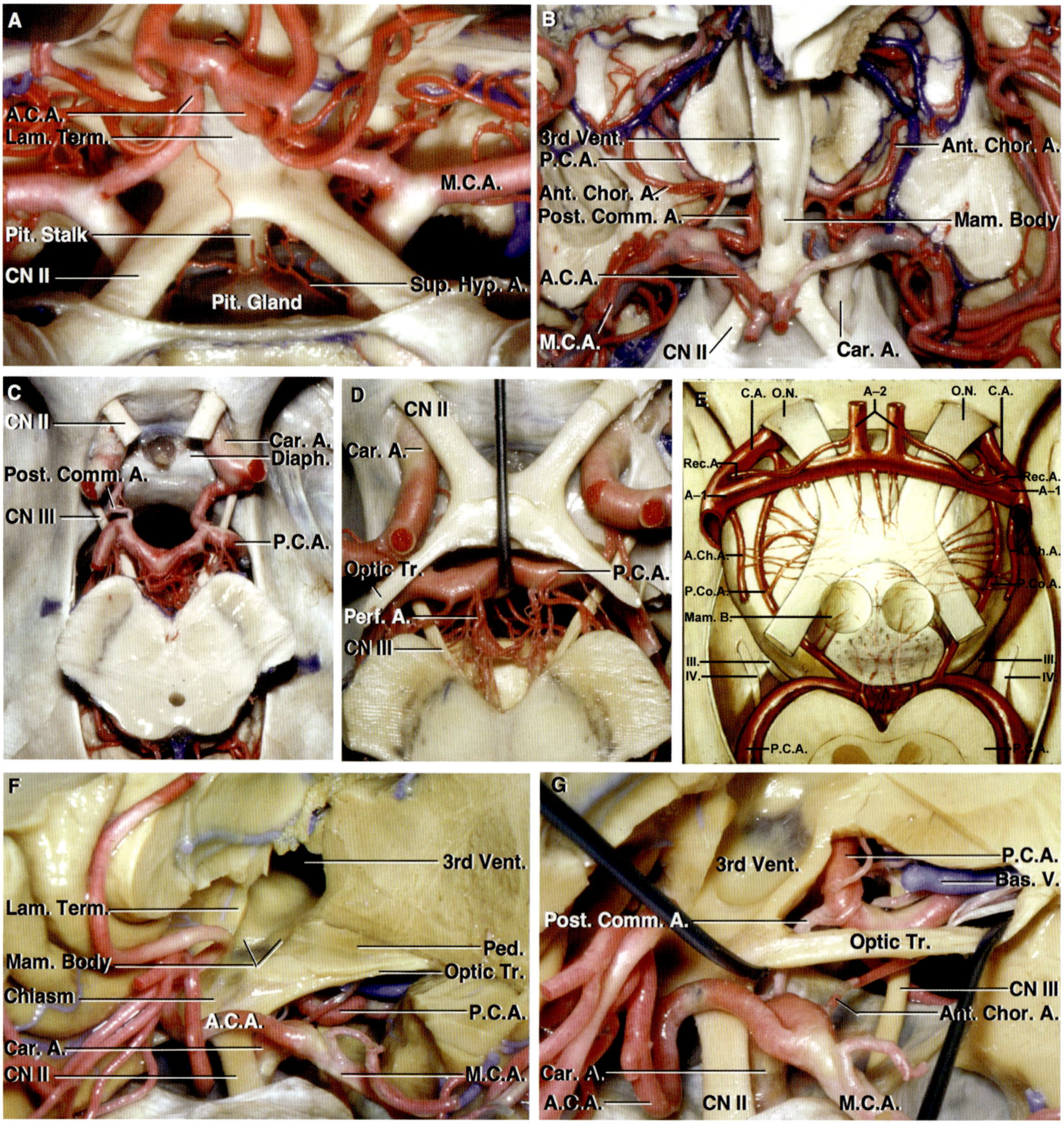

Fig. 2.22 Vascular relationships in the suprasellar area. **(A)** The anterior cerebral arteries course above the optic chiasm and in front of the lamina terminalis. The carotid arteries exit the cavernous sinus and pass upward in the lateral margins of the suprasellar area. The superior hypophyseal arteries cross the chiasmatic cistern to reach the lower margin of the chiasm and pituitary stalk. **(B)** Superior view of the suprasellar region. The floor of the third ventricle has been exposed from the suprachiasmatic recess anteriorly to the level of the aqueduct posteriorly. The anterior cerebral arteries pass above the chiasm. The posterior communicating arteries pass backward below the floor of the third ventricle. The basilar artery bifurcates into the posterior cerebral arteries below the floor of the third ventricle. **(C)** Superior view of the suprasellar region. The carotid arteries course along the lateral margin of the chiasmatic cistern. The basilar bifurcation is located above and behind the sella. The posterior communicating arteries travel backward across the dorsum to join the posterior cerebral arteries. The posterior communicating arteries usually course above and medial to the oculomotor nerves. **(D)** The optic chiasm is positioned above the diaphragm and sella. The optic tracts extend backward and laterally above the posterior cerebral arteries and oculomotor nerves toward the lateral geniculate bodies. The basilar bifurcation has been retracted forward to show the perforating arteries entering the midbrain, which can be damaged in the transsphenoidal approach if the posterior wall of the capsule of a pituitary adenoma is opened. **(E)** Diagrammatic view of the arteries in the suprasellar area, which can be stretched over the margin of a large tumor with suprasellar extension. All the components of the circle of Willis and their perforating branches can be stretched over the dome of these tumors. **(F)** Superolateral view of the left optic nerve, optic chiasm, and left optic tract and the floor of the third ventricle. The optic tract extends backward from the optic chiasm, around the upper edge of the cerebral peduncle, and above the posterior cerebral artery. The anterior cerebral arteries pass in front of the lamina terminalis and around the corpus callosum. **(G)** Some of the anterior part of the left cerebral peduncle has been removed while the optic tract is preserved. The posterior cerebral artery and terminal part of the posterior communicating artery can be seen through the interval between the floor of the third ventricle and the optic tract.

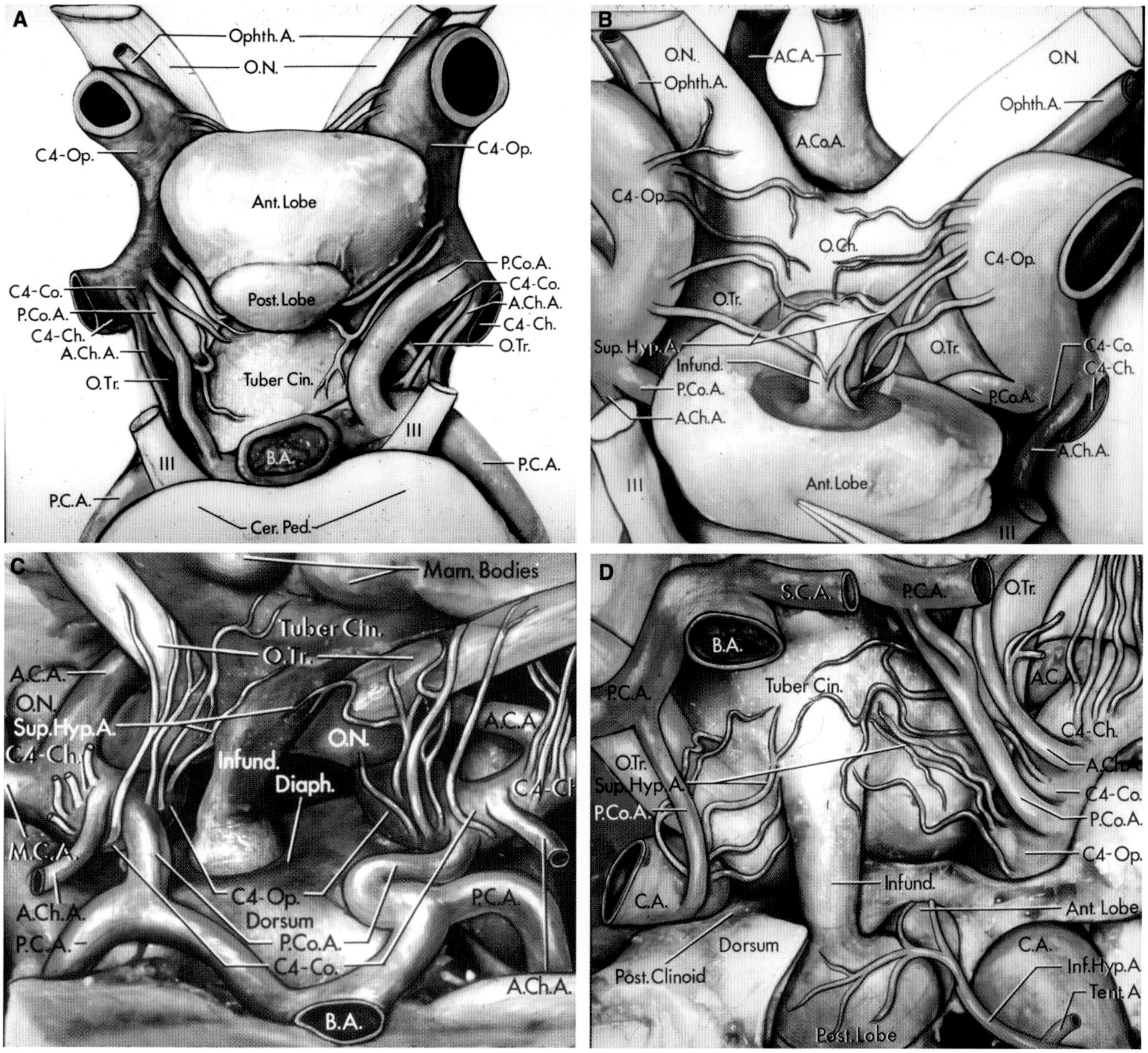

Fig. 2.23 Relationships in the sellar and suprasellar areas. **(A)** Inferior view. The supraclinoid portion of the carotid artery is divided into three segments based on the site of origin of its major branches; the ophthalmic segment extends from the origin of the ophthalmic artery to the origin of the posterior communicating artery, the communicating segment extends from the origin of the posterior communicating artery to the origin of the anterior choroidal artery, and the choroidal segment extends from the origin of the anterior choroidal artery to the bifurcation of the carotid artery. The optic nerves are above the ophthalmic arteries. The optic chiasm and optic tracts are above the anterior and posterior lobes of the pituitary gland. The tuber cinereum is anterior to the apex of the basilar artery. The posterior cerebral arteries pass around the cerebral peduncles above the oculomotor nerves. The perforating branches arising from the ophthalmic segment pass to the anterior lobe, optic nerve and chiasm, and the anterior part of the tuber cinereum. A single perforating branch arises from the communicating segment on each side and passes upward to the optic tract and floor of the third ventricle. **(B)** The pituitary gland has been reflected backward to show the superior hypophyseal arteries passing from the ophthalmic segments to the infundibulum. The anterior cerebral and anterior communicating arteries pass above the optic chiasm. **(C)** Posterior view. The basilar artery and brainstem have been divided and the floor of the third ventricle elevated to provide this posterior view of the arteries in the suprasellar area. The tuber cinereum and mamillary bodies are exposed between the optic tracts. **(D)** The right half of the dorsum and the right posterior clinoid process have been removed to expose the anterior and posterior lobes of the pituitary gland. The basilar, posterior cerebral, and superior cerebellar arteries have been elevated to expose the pituitary stalk and floor of the third ventricle. The inferior hypophyseal and tentorial arteries arise from the carotid artery.

arises predominantly from the carotid artery, the posterior communicating artery is directed posterolaterally above or lateral to the oculomotor nerve.

The anterior choroidal artery arises from the posterior surface of the internal carotid artery above the origin of the posterior communicating artery (**Figs. 2.22** and **2.23**). It is directed posterolaterally below the optic tract between the uncus and cerebral peduncle. It passes through the choroidal fissure behind the uncus to supply the choroid plexus in the temporal horn, sending branches into the optic tract and posterior part of the third ventricular floor that reach the optic radiations, globus pallidus, internal capsule, midbrain, and thalamus.

The anterior cerebral artery arises from the internal carotid artery below the anterior perforated substance and courses anteromedially above the optic nerve and chiasm to reach the interhemispheric fissure, where it is joined to the opposite anterior cerebral artery by the anterior communicating artery (**Figs. 2.22** and **2.23**). The junction of the anterior communicating artery with the right and left A1 segments is usually above the chiasm rather than above the optic nerves. The shorter A1 segments are stretched tightly over the chiasm, and the larger ones pass anteriorly over the nerves. Visual loss caused by elevation of the chiasm against these arteries may occur before visual loss caused by direct compression of the tumor on the visual pathways. The arteries with a more forward course are often tortuous and elongated, and some may course forward and rest on the tuberculum sellae or planum sphenoidale. The anterior cerebral and anterior communicating arteries give rise to perforating branches that terminate in the whole anterior wall of the third ventricle and reach the adjacent parts of the hypothalamus, fornix, septum pellucidum, and striatum. The recurrent branch of the anterior cerebral artery, frequently encountered in the area, arises from the anterior cerebral artery in the region of the anterior communicating artery, courses laterally above the bifurcation of the internal carotid artery, and enters the anterior perforated substance.

The bifurcation of the basilar artery into the posterior cerebral arteries is located in the posterior part of the suprasellar area below the posterior half of the floor of the third ventricle (**Figs. 2.11, 2.22,** and **2.23**). A high basilar bifurcation may indent the ventricular floor. The posterior cerebral artery courses laterally around the cerebral peduncle and above the oculomotor nerve, and then passes between the uncus and the cerebral peduncle to reach the ambient and quadrigeminal cisterns. Its branches reach the floor, roof, and posterior and lateral walls of the third ventricle. The thalamoperforating arteries are a pair of larger perforating branches that arise from the proximal part of the posterior cerebral artery in the suprasellar region and enter the brain through the posterior part of the floor and lateral walls of the third ventricle. The author is aware of several cases in which damage to the thalamoperforating branches occurred during transsphenoidal surgery after the posterosuperior part of the tumor capsule was opened, with resulting coma and death.

Venous Relationships

Veins do not pose a formidable obstacle to operative approaches to the suprasellar area and lower part of the third ventricle, as they do in the region of the roof and posterior third ventricle, because the veins in the suprasellar region are small. The suprasellar area is drained, almost totally, by tributaries of the basal vein. The basal veins are formed by the union of veins draining the suprasellar area and proceed posteriorly between the midbrain and the temporal lobes to empty into the internal cerebral or great vein. The internal cerebral veins course in the roof of the third ventricle and are only infrequently involved in sellar tumors. They originate just behind the foramen of Monro and course posteriorly within the velum interpositum. They join above or posterior to the pineal body to form the great vein.

◆ Conclusion

The treatment of pathologic entities in the parasellar and sellar regions requires exquisite knowledge of neuroanatomy. The anatomy of the normal state is complex. Variations in anatomy related to pathologic conditions make this region even more challenging.

References

1. Barrow DL, Tindall GT. Loss of vision after transsphenoidal surgery. Neurosurgery 1990;27(1):60–68
2. Bernasconi V, Cassinari V. Caratteristische Angiografiche dei Meningiomi del Tentorio. Radiol Med (Torino) 1957;43:1015–1026
3. Fujii K, Chambers SM, Rhoton AL Jr. Neurovascular relationships of the sphenoid sinus. A microsurgical study. J Neurosurg 1979;50(1):31–39
4. Fujii K, Lenkey C, Rhoton AL Jr. Microsurgical anatomy of the choroidal arteries: lateral and third ventricles. J Neurosurg 1980;52(2):165–188
5. Garcia AS, Rhoton AL Jr. Speculum opening in transsphenoidal surgery. Neurosurgery 2006; 59(1, Suppl 1):ONS35–ONS40
6. Gibo H, Lenkey C, Rhoton AL Jr. Microsurgical anatomy of the supraclinoid portion of the internal carotid artery. J Neurosurg 1981;55(4):560–574
7. Hardy J. Transsphenoidal hypophysectomy. J Neurosurg 1971; 34(4):582–594
8. Harris FS, Rhoton AL Jr. Anatomy of the cavernous sinus. A microsurgical study. J Neurosurg 1976;45(2):169–180
9. Hitotsumatsu T, Matsushima T, Rhoton AL Jr. Surgical anatomy of the midface and the midline skull base. In: Spetzler RF. Operative Techniques in Neurosurgery. WB Saunders; 1999:160–180
10. Inoue T, Rhoton AL Jr, Theele D, Barry ME. Surgical approaches to the cavernous sinus: a microsurgical study. Neurosurgery 1990;26(6):903–932
11. Johnston JA, Parkinson D. Intracranial sympathetic pathways associated with the sixth cranial nerve. J Neurosurg 1974;40(2):236–243
12. Laws ER Jr, Kern EB. Complications of trans-sphenoidal surgery. Clin Neurosurg 1976;23:401–416
13. Liu Q, Rhoton AL Jr. Middle meningeal origin of the ophthalmic artery. Neurosurgery 2001;49(2):401–406, discussion 406–407
14. McConnell EM. The arterial blood supply of the human hypophysis cerebri. Anat Rec 1953;115(2):175–203

15. Ono M, Rhoton AL Jr, Barry M. Microsurgical anatomy of the region of the tentorial incisura. J Neurosurg 1984;60(2):365–399
16. Osawa S, Rhoton AL Jr, Seker A, Shimizu S, Fujii K, Kassam AB. Microsurgical and endoscopic anatomy of the vidian canal. Neurosurgery 2009;64(5, Suppl 2):385–411, discussion 411–412
17. Renn WH, Rhoton AL Jr. Microsurgical anatomy of the sellar region. J Neurosurg 1975;43(3):288–298
18. Parkinson D. A surgical approach to the cavernous portion of the carotid artery. Anatomical studies and case report. J Neurosurg 1965;23(5):474–483
19. Parkinson D. Carotid cavernous fistula: direct repair with preservation of the carotid artery. Technical note. J Neurosurg 1973; 38(1):99–106
20. Parkinson D. Surgical anatomy of the lateral sellar compartment (cavernous sinus). Clin Neurosurg 1990;36:219–239
21. Parkinson D. Transcavernous repair of carotid cavernous fistula. Case report. J Neurosurg 1967;26(4):420–424
22. Rhoton AL Jr, Hardy DG, Chambers SM. Microsurgical anatomy and dissection of the sphenoid bone, cavernous sinus and sellar region. Surg Neurol 1979;12(1):63–104
23. Rhoton AL Jr, Harris FS, Renn WH. Microsurgical anatomy of the sellar region and cavernous sinus. Clin Neurosurg 1977;24:54–85
24. Rhoton AL Jr, Maniscalco JE. Microsurgery of the sellar region. In: Glaser JS, ed. Neuro-Ophthalmology. CV Mosby; 1977:106–127
25. Rhoton AL Jr, Natori Y. Neural structures. In: Rhoton AL Jr, Natori Y. The Orbit and Sellar Region: Microsurgical Anatomy and Operative Approaches. Thieme; 1996:28–77, 70–77
26. Rhoton AL Jr, Natori Y. The skull. In: Rhoton AL Jr, Natori Y. The Orbit and Sellar Region: Microsurgical Anatomy and Operative Approaches. Thieme; 1996:4–25
27. Rhoton AL Jr, Yamamoto I, Peace DA. Microsurgery of the third ventricle: Part 2. Operative approaches. Neurosurgery 1981; 8(3):357–373
28. Rhoton AL Jr. The sellar region. Neurosurgery 2002;51:335–374
29. Rhoton AL Jr. Anatomy of the pituitary gland and sellar region. In: Thapar K, Kovacs K, Scheithauer BW, Lloyd RV, eds. Diagnosis and Management of Pituitary Tumors. Humana Press; 2000:13–40
30. Rhoton AL Jr. Microsurgical anatomy of the region of the third ventricle. In: Apuzzo ML, ed. Surgery of the Third Ventricle. Williams & Wilkins; 1987:92–166
31. Rhoton AL Jr. Tentorial incisura. Neurosurgery 2000;47(3, Suppl):S131–S153
32. Rhoton AL Jr. The cavernous sinus, the cavernous venous plexus, and the carotid collar. Neurosurgery 2002;51(4, Suppl):S375–S410
33. Rhoton AL Jr. The anterior and middle cranial base. Neurosurgery 2002;51(4, Suppl):S273–S302
34. Seoane ER, Rhoton AL Jr, de Oliveira E. Microsurgical anatomy of the dural collar (carotid collar) and rings around the clinoid segment of the internal carotid artery. Neurosurgery 1998;42(4):869–884, discussion 884–886
35. Shimizu S, Tanriover N, Rhoton AL Jr, Yoshioka N, Fujii K. MacCarty keyhole and inferior orbital fissure in orbitozygomatic craniotomy. Neurosurgery 2005;57(1, Suppl):152–159
36. Sunderland S, Hughes ESR. The pupillo-constrictor pathway and the nerves to the ocular muscles in man. Brain 1946;69(4): 301–309
37. Tindall GT, Barrow DL. Pituitary surgery. In: Tindall GT, Barrow DL, eds. Disorders of the Pituitary. CV Mosby; 1986:349–400
38. Wang J, Bidari S, Inoue K, Yang H, Rhoton AL Jr. Extensions of the sphenoid sinus: a new classification. Neurosurgery 2010; 66(4):797–816
39. Yamamoto I, Rhoton AL Jr, Peace DA. Microsurgery of the third ventricle: Part I. Microsurgical anatomy. Neurosurgery 1981; 8(3):334–356

3 Radiologic Evaluation and Diagnosis for Pathology in the Sellar and Parasellar Region

Prashant Raghavan and Max Wintermark

The complex anatomy of the sella turcica and parasellar skull base lends itself to the occurrence of a diverse array of pathologic processes. Imaging plays a key role in the diagnosis and mapping of the anatomic extent of these lesions. This chapter focuses primarily on the imaging of pituitary glandular neoplasms and nonvascular parasellar processes that are amenable to surgical or radiation treatment

◆ Imaging Strategies

Modern imaging of central skull base pathology is almost entirely performed with magnetic resonance imaging (MRI). Computed tomography (CT) may be useful in conjunction with MRI when evaluation of the osseous anatomy is of importance. CT is performed at our institution only when a contraindication to MRI exists. When information about the integrity of the sellar floor or the presence of intralesional calcification is desired, CT offers excellent visualization of such detail.[1]

CT images acquired at a thickness of 0.625 mm after the administration of intravenous (i.v.) contrast enable the depiction of most macroadenomas; however, MR remains superior to CT in characterizing lesional morphology and establishing its extent.[2]

All MR examinations of the skull base at our institution are performed after the administration of i.v. contrast unless there are contraindications to the use of gadolinium-based agents, such as significant renal impairment or pregnancy.[3] It is possible, however, to detect microadenomas on unenhanced images, especially when narrow window settings are used (**Fig. 3.1**). Such a strategy may be useful in those situations in which contrast cannot be administered. Most microadenomas are best revealed on postcontrast images when thin (3-mm) coronal and sagittal T1-weighted sections are employed. The addition of fat saturation pulses and use of a volumetric spoiled gradient (SPGR) acquisition may also be beneficial.[4] We have found the latter sequence to be especially useful in a setting of Cushing disease. When conventional contrast-enhanced MRI fails to depict a microadenoma and clinical suspicion is strong, a dynamic study with rapid acquisition of a set of coronal T1-weighted images (T1WIs) after administration of a bolus of contrast may be helpful. Typical scanning times for a set of such images through the sella on most modern scanners are on the order of 10 to 12 seconds. On such sequences, the gland is seen to exhibit a characteristic pattern of centrifugal enhancement, with the stalk and the site of its insertion enhancing first. Kucharczyk et al,[5] using a dynamic keyhole MR technique, reported an increased sensitivity for adenoma detection compared with conventional MRI. Tabarin et al,[6] however, warn of the false-positive interpretations that may occur with this technique if the pattern of glandular enhancement is not well understood.

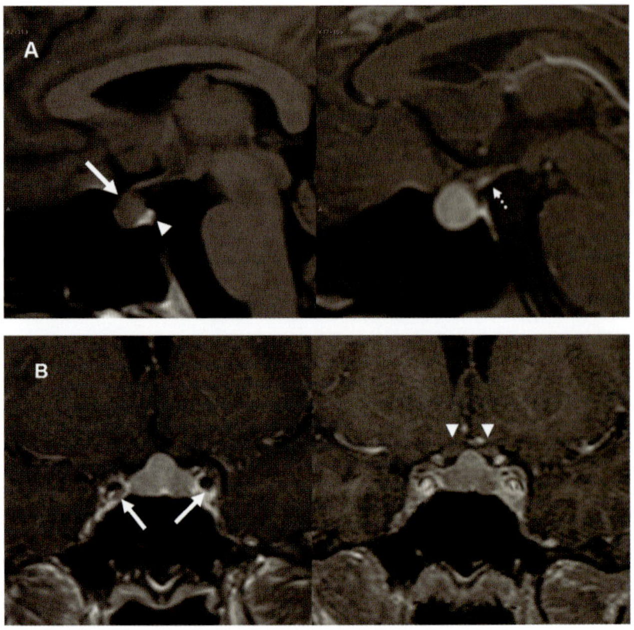

Fig. 3.1 Normal MRI anatomy. **(A)** The isointense adenohypophysis and the hyperintense neurohypophysis (*long arrow* and *arrowhead*, respectively) are clearly identified on the sagittal unenhanced T1-weighted image. The uniform enhancement and the smoothly tapered appearance of the stalk are also evident. **(B)** Postcontrast coronal T1WI SPGR image. Note the more heterogeneous enhancement pattern in the latter. The convex superior contour of the gland is normal in this 22-year-old female patient. The cavernous internal carotid arteries (*solid arrows*) and the optic chiasm (*arrowheads*) are seen.

Other novel MR techniques that may be used to study the pituitary gland include diffusion-weighted imaging (DWI) and MR spectroscopy. Pierallini et al[7] suggested that adenomas may be classified into soft and hard groups based on their apparent diffusion coefficient values obtained by DWI. This information may be of surgical importance and help determine if suction or fragmentation and curettage are required for an adenoma to be removed. Stadlbauer et al[8] in a study of 37 patients with pituitary adenomas concluded that MR spectroscopy may provide insights that can help predict proliferative potential and detect the presence of intratumoral hemorrhage. These techniques, however, are difficult to implement in routine practice and may be limited by artifacts that arise from the osseous skull base and air in the sinus cavities.

Heavily T2-weighted volumetric sequences are often used in skull base imaging and provide exquisite depiction of cranial nerve anatomy. When radiosurgery is considered, MR scans at our institution are performed with a contrast-enhanced volumetric T1-weighted sequence to enable accurate registration. The addition of fat saturation, we have observed, greatly increases target conspicuity. A typical MRI protocol for the sella/skull base at our institution is presented in **Table 3.1**.

Inferior petrosal sinus sampling (IPSS) is performed when noninvasive studies fail to depict an adenoma whose presence is strongly suspected clinically. Complication rates are less than 1% with this procedure. It is a sensitive and specific test for accurately diagnosing Cushing disease and differentiating it from ectopic ACTH (adrenocorticotropic hormone) syndrome.[9]

Table 3.1 Sella Protocol for 3.0-Tesla Magnetic Resonance Imaging

Precontrast
Sagittal TSE T1: 2 mm, 10% gap, 220 FOV. Minimum of 19 slices to ensure adequate brainstem coverage.
Axial TSE T2: Whole-brain coverage, 5 mm thick, 30–40% gap. R→L phase direction.
Coronal TSE T1: 2 mm, 10% gap, 160 FOV, perpendicular to floor of sella, making adjustments as needed for a particularly large lesion.
Postcontrast
Coronal TSE T1 dynamic: 350 TR, 7 slices, 2 mm, 210 FOV. Slices should be centered just over the sella. Scan is 6 measurements, 21 seconds each.
Coronal T1 SPGR postcontrast: Match precontrast coronal T1 coverage: 1.2 mm, 0 gap, 160 FOV.
Coronal TSE T1 postcontrast: Match precontrast coronal T1 coverage: 2 mm, 160 FOV, making adjustments as needed for a particularly large lesion.
Sagittal TSE T1 fat-saturated: Match coverage of precontrast sagittal T1: 3 mm, 10% gap, 220 FOV. Note that a coronal saturation pulse should be placed posteriorly over the sagittal sinus. This will prevent pulsatile flow artifact from obscuring visualization of the sella postcontrast.
Axial 3D FLASH T1: 1.2–1.4 mm thick (for stereotactic radiosurgery planning): Cover entire brain, extending slices above vertex into air. Include ears, nose, and chin within FOV. Coronal reconstructions of the whole brain (thickness of 5 mm at distance of 6.5 mm) are obtained from these images.

Abbreviations: 3D, three-dimensional; FLASH, fast low-angle shot; FOV, field of view; SPGR, spoiled gradient; TR, repetition time; TSE, turbo spin echo.

◆ Imaging Anatomy

It is important to be aware of the age-dependent variability in the contour and size of the pituitary gland when MR examinations are interpreted. Elster's rule that the pituitary gland measures 6 mm in height in infants and children, 8 mm in men and postmenopausal women, 10 mm in women of childbearing age, and 12 mm in pregnant and postpartum women is useful to keep in mind.[10] The adenohypophysis is isointense to brain parenchyma on all sequences, whereas the neurohypophysis demonstrates a characteristic hyperintensity on T1-weighted imaging (**Fig. 3.1**). The neonatal adenohypophysis, possibly because of lactotrope hyperplasia, can be hyperintense on T1WI. The precise reason for the neurohypophyseal hyperintensity is unknown, but it is possibly due to the presence of neurophysin, a vasopressin-associated carrier protein. Absence of this bright spot may be seen with central diabetes insipidus but is a normal finding in a small percentage of the population. Any cause of stalk interruption may result in the bright spot occupying an "ectopic" position proximally in the stalk or in the hypothalamus.[11] The normal pituitary stalk does not exceed 4 mm in thickness and demonstrates a smoothly tapered insertion into the gland. It enhances fairly homogeneously.

The optic chiasm, which is isointense to white matter on all sequences, is best evaluated on the coronal images. The cavernous sinuses are visualized as paired parasellar structures that enhance heterogeneously. Their lateral, thicker dural walls are consistently seen, whereas depiction of the more gracile medial wall is more problematic. The cavernous internal carotid arteries are more easily visible as paired flow voids on spin-echo images and demonstrate flow-related enhancement on SPGR images. The cranial nerves in the lateral walls of the cavernous sinuses are inconstantly seen. The demonstration of the cisternal segments of these nerves is easily achieved by using volumetric, heavily T2-weighted sequences. The skull base foramina in the middle cranial fossa are best seen on thin-section CT, ideally when bone reconstruction algorithms are used.

◆ Tumors

Pituitary Neoplasms

Adenomas

Close scrutiny of unenhanced coronal images may reveal the presence of an adenoma, especially if narrow window settings are used. The majority of microadenomas are isointense to hypointense with respect to the remainder of the gland on T1WI. The presence of T1 hyperintensity may indicate hemorrhage. The signal intensity on T2WI is more variable. No definite characteristics exist that enable one to differentiate between the different types of adenoma. It has been suggested that adenomas producing ACTH, thyroid-stimulating hormone (TSH), or follicle-stimulating hormone/luteinizing hormone (FSH/LH) have a tendency to occur in the central gland, whereas prolactinomas and gonadotropic hormone (GH)–producing adenomas prefer the glandular periphery.

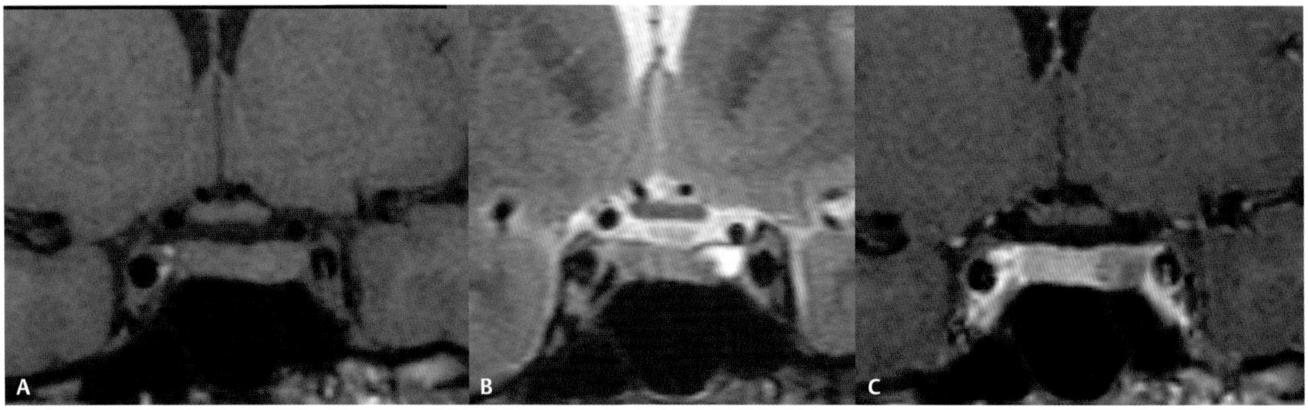

Fig. 3.2 Typical microadenoma. The coronal unenhanced T1WI to the left reveals a subtle contour abnormality in the left half of the gland. On the coronal T2WI in the middle, the adenoma is hyperintense. On the postcontrast coronal spin-echo T1WI, the adenoma enhances to a lesser degree than the remainder of the gland.

It has also been proposed that densely granulated GH adenomas have a propensity for infrasellar extension, possibly owing to a tendency to thicken the diaphragma and cause osteopenia of the sellar floor, and perhaps owing to a sella-enlarging effect of growth hormone itself.[12]

The presence of a microadenoma may be inferred on the basis of a glandular contour deformity, focal remodeling of the sellar floor, or stalk deviation. The latter is an overrated sign and may be encountered in the normal population. The stalk may even be deviated toward an adenoma.[13] It must also be remembered that a convex superior glandular contour may be normal in women of reproductive age and in the peripartum period.

Most microadenomas enhance to a lesser degree than normal gland (**Fig. 3.2**). They are best identified on coronal postcontrast T1WIs and SPGR images. The latter are often useful in detecting small ACTH-producing adenomas[4] (**Fig. 3.3**), but one must be aware of the slightly higher false-positive rate with this sequence because the gland tends to enhance more inhomogeneously than with conventional T1WI. Small foci of normal glandular inhomogeneity may be misinterpreted as microadenomas. A dynamic technique as described above may be employed as a problem-solving technique, but its routine use is unnecessary (**Fig. 3.4**). The overall sensitivity for MRI in the detection of adenomas is in excess of 90%. False-positive results may arise from artifacts (**Fig. 3.10B**), volume averaging with prominent clinoid processes, or mistaking cysts for adenomas. The site of insertion of the sphenoid sinus septum in the sellar floor may produce a small susceptibility artifact that can mimic a microadenoma.

The diagnosis of pituitary microadenomas is reliant on two important findings—a determination that the lesion in question arises from the gland and, when present, a smooth expansion of the sella. Sellar expansion enables differentiation from other aggressive processes—such as infection, inflammation, and malignancy—that either do not expand the sella or, when they do, are associated with bone destruction. Macroadenomas demonstrate a wide range of signal intensities on MRI. A high T2 signal may indicate liquefactive change. T1 hyperintensity may indicate the presence of hemorrhage. Apoplectic adenomas may contain blood-fluid levels. Gradient-echo sequences are highly sensitive to intratumoral hemorrhage. Blood products of any age appear profoundly hypointense on such sequences.[14]

Perhaps the most important task of the radiologist evaluating macroadenomas is to determine the presence of

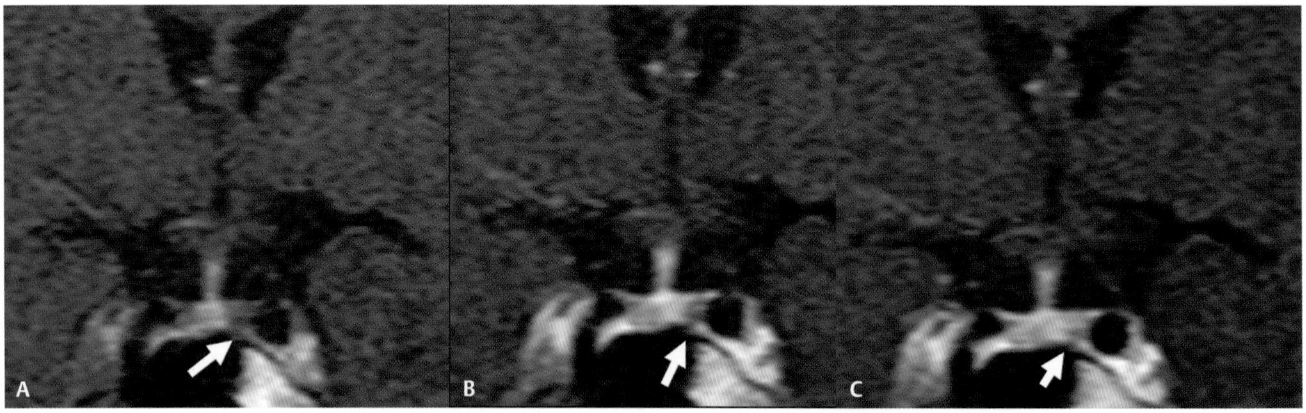

Fig. 3.3 Dynamic MRI. Three images from a dynamic MR set obtained at the level of the infundibulum.The subtle focus of decreased enhancement in the extreme periphery of the gland corresponded to a tiny microadenoma found at surgery. Note the centrifugal pattern of glandular enhancement.

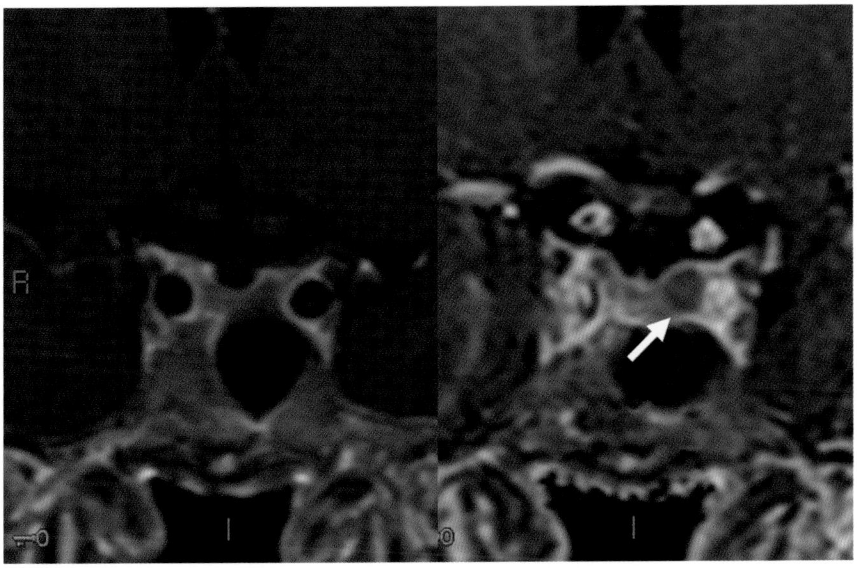

Fig. 3.4 Value of SPGR imaging. This ACTH-producing microadenoma is nearly imperceptible on the postcontrast spin-echo T1WI (left). It is readily evident on the postcontrast SPGR image on the right (*white arrow*).

cavernous sinus invasion (**Fig. 3.5**). The only reliable sign of cavernous sinus invasion on MRI is the presence of tumor on both sides of the cavernous and internal carotid artery.[15] The medial wall of the cavernous sinus is not well seen on MRI. This wall may be displaced, or the tumor may lie embedded within it or may have invaded through it. None of these are confidently predicted with MRI except when, as mentioned above, tumor is evident encasing the internal carotid artery, a finding that is 100% specific for invasion. Several authors have proposed numerous criteria for cavernous sinus invasion, with varying degrees of specificity and sensitivity. Of these, perhaps the most helpful are the presence of tumor beyond a line drawn tangential to the lateral walls of the supraclinoid and cavernous internal carotid arteries and the presence of tumor in the medial compartment of the cavernous sinus inferomedial to the internal carotid artery, which have reported positive predictive values of 95% and 85%, respectively. If the degree of circumferential encasement of the internal carotid artery was greater than 67%, invasion was found to be certain, whereas if it was less than 25%, the negative predictive value was 100%. It must, however, be noted that constriction of the internal carotid artery is uncommon, even with large macroadenomas, and is more likely to be a feature of meningiomas in the cavernous sinus, although exceptions to this certainly exist. The optic chiasm and its relationship to the tumor are best seen on coronal images. The presence of abnormal optic nerve T2 signal intensity due to tumor compression has been shown to correlate with the degree of visual acuity impairment.[16] A case of optic tract hemorrhage following pituitary apoplexy has also been reported.[17]

Other Pituitary Tumors

Uncommon neoplasms of the pituitary gland include pituicytomas and granular cell tumors. These are usually indistinguishable from macroadenomas, but a tendency to affect the posterior gland and stalk (as a consequence of which the bright spot may be ectopic) and intense enhancement may provide clues to the diagnosis. True astrocytomas may rarely arise from the pituitary gland.[18,19] Metastatic deposits may occasionally be seen in the gland, usually from breast and lung primaries. About 1 to 5% of patients with these cancers harbor pituitary metastatic

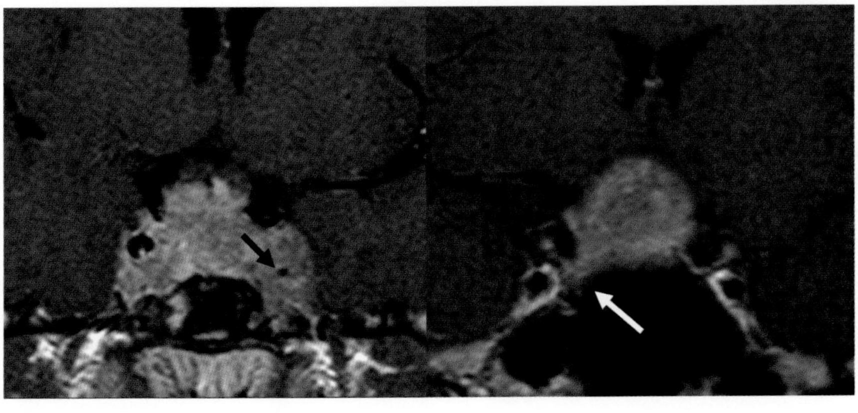

Fig. 3.5 Patterns of cavernous sinus invasion. In the image to the left, the macroadenoma encases the cavernous ICAs circumferentially, a finding that unequivocally indicates cavernous sinus invasion. The constriction of the lumen of the left ICA (*black arrow*) is a highly unusual finding and more often seen with meningiomas. In the image to the left, a tongue of tumor (*white arrow*) protrudes into the medial venous compartment. Cavernous sinus invasion was present at surgery.

deposits. Symptomatic metastatic disease usually presents with diabetes insipidus due to stalk involvement. Imaging, however, cannot distinguish between metastases and adenomas reliably.[20] Primary lymphoma of the pituitary gland is exceedingly rare, and lymphoma is more likely to be seen as a secondary phenomenon. The presence of low T2 signal intensity due to the dense cellularity of lymphoma may indicate the diagnosis.[21] About 1.4% of patients with systemic leukemia have pituitary involvement. Langerhans cell histiocytosis involves the infundibulum in ~50% of cases. The stalk thickening and enhancement seen in histiocytosis are not specific for this entity. Similar findings may be seen with sarcoidosis and tuberculosis (**Fig. 3.9A**). The diagnosis can, however, be made if lytic bone lesions and pineal, white matter, choroid plexus, or dentate nucleus involvement are simultaneously seen.[11]

Cystic Sellar/Suprasellar Lesions

Craniopharyngiomas

Craniopharyngiomas present on imaging as complex suprasellar/sellar solid-cystic masses. The two histologic subtypes—the papillary and adamantinomatous varieties—may sometimes be distinguished on imaging. The adamantinomatous subtype seen in children and younger adults usually manifests as a mixed solid-cystic or mainly cystic lobulated suprasellar/intrasellar tumor with large, nonenhancing, T1-hyperintense cysts (**Fig. 3.6**). The papillary variety is more likely to present in older individuals as a solid enhancing tumor, although a mixed solid-cystic pattern with T1-hypointense cysts may be seen.[22] The dense calcific component of these lesions is better defined on CT scans. However, the true extent of these lesions, the nature of the cystic contents, the presence of vascular encasement, and the status of the optic apparatus are all better demonstrated on MRI.

Rathke Cleft, Arachnoid, and Pars Intermedia Cysts

Rathke cleft cysts present as sellar/suprasellar discrete nonenhancing lesions on MRI. The signal intensities of the contents of these cysts are largely a function of protein concentration. Cysts with watery content are T1-hypointense and T2-hyperintense on MRI. The T1 signal intensity increases as protein concentration increases, whereas T2 signal intensity usually decreases. The presence of a mural nodule representing inspissated desquamated de-

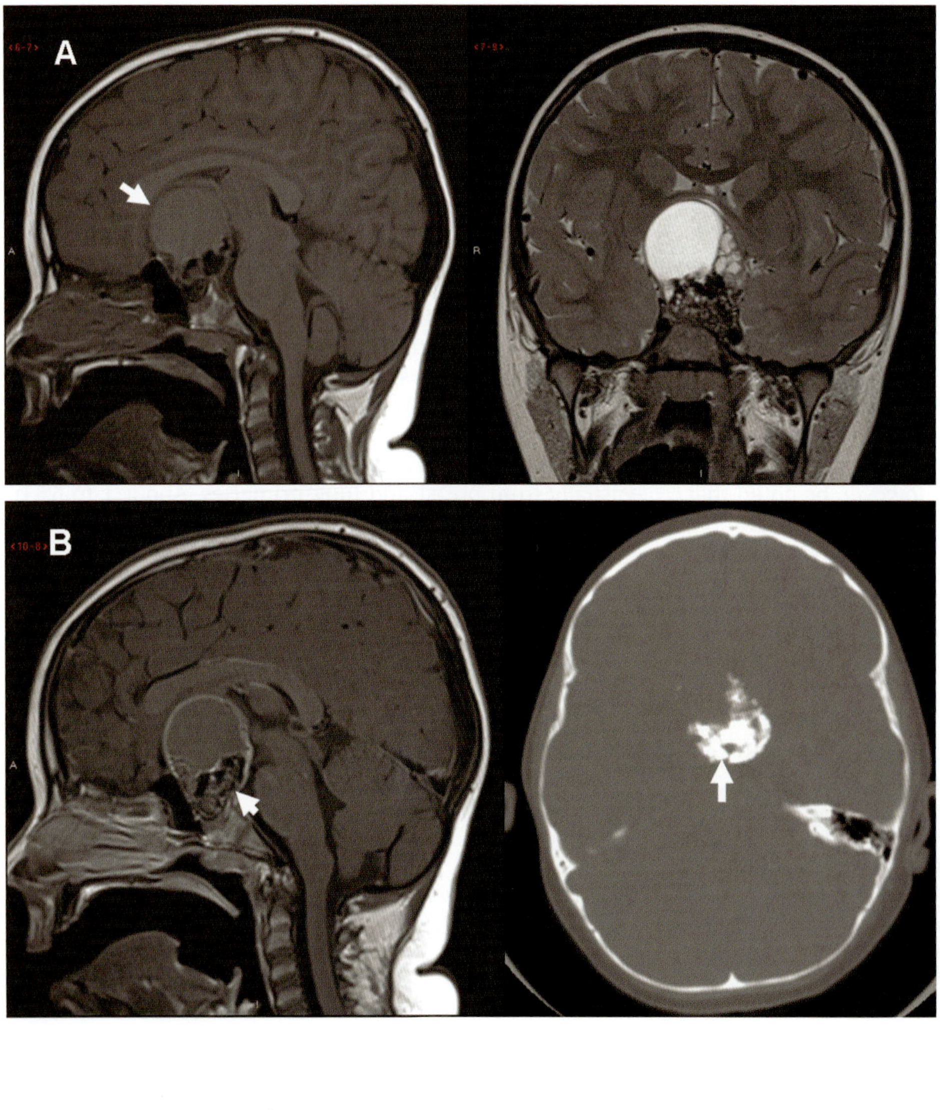

Fig. 3.6 Typical adamantinomatous craniopharyngioma. **(A)** A mixed solid cystic lesion containing T1 hyperintense fluid is seen on the sagittal unenhanced T1WI (*arrow*). On the coronal T2WI to the left, the cystic component is hyperintense. The hypointense foci inferior to the cyst is dense calcification. **(B)** The cystic component enhances peripherally. The dense calcification is confirmed on the CT image to the left (*arrows*).

bris has been described as highly specific for these cysts[23] (**Fig. 3.7A**). Rathke cleft cysts may coexist with adenomas. Pars intermedia cysts are located between the adenohypophysis and neurohypophysis and are often incidental findings. They usually demonstrate T1 hypointensity and T2 hyperintensity on MRI and do not enhance. Arachnoid cysts of the suprasellar cistern arise from incomplete perforation of the membrane of Liliequist. Unless hemorrhage has occurred, they demonstrate signal intensity identical to that of cerebrospinal fluid (CSF) on all imaging sequences.

Epidermoid and Dermoid Cysts

These developmental lesions may occur in the suprasellar cistern or parasellar region and can be recognized based on their characteristic MR signal intensities. Epidermoid tumors are hyperintense on T2-weighted and FLAIR (fluid-attenuated inversion recovery) images and demonstrate characteristic hyperintensity on DWI. This latter finding enables distinction from an arachnoid cyst (**Fig. 3.7B**). Dermoid cysts, owing to their fat content, are hyperintense on T1WI and occur usually in the suprasellar cistern. Fat-

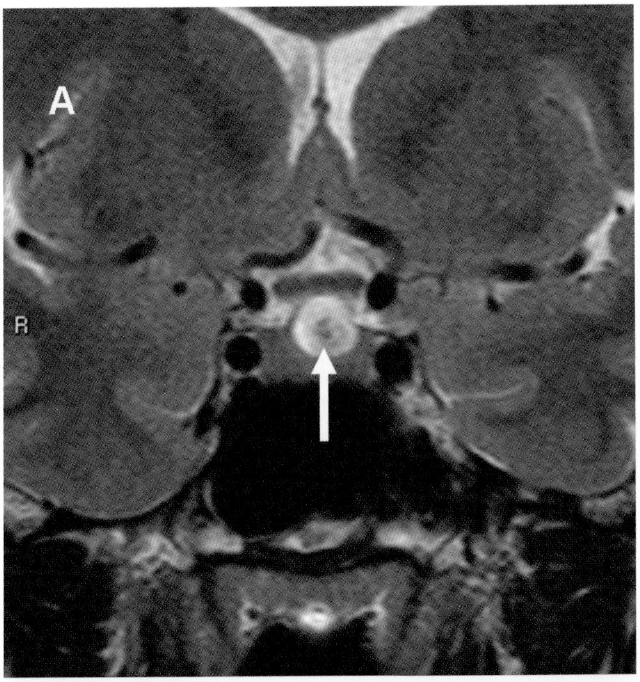

Fig. 3.7 Cystic lesions. (A) Rathke cleft cyst. The discrete margins and the intracystic nodule (*arrow*) are features typical of this entity. (B) Sellar-suprasellar epidermoid demonstrating characteristic lack of enhancement on the sagittal T1WI to the left and typical hyperintensity on the DWI to the right.

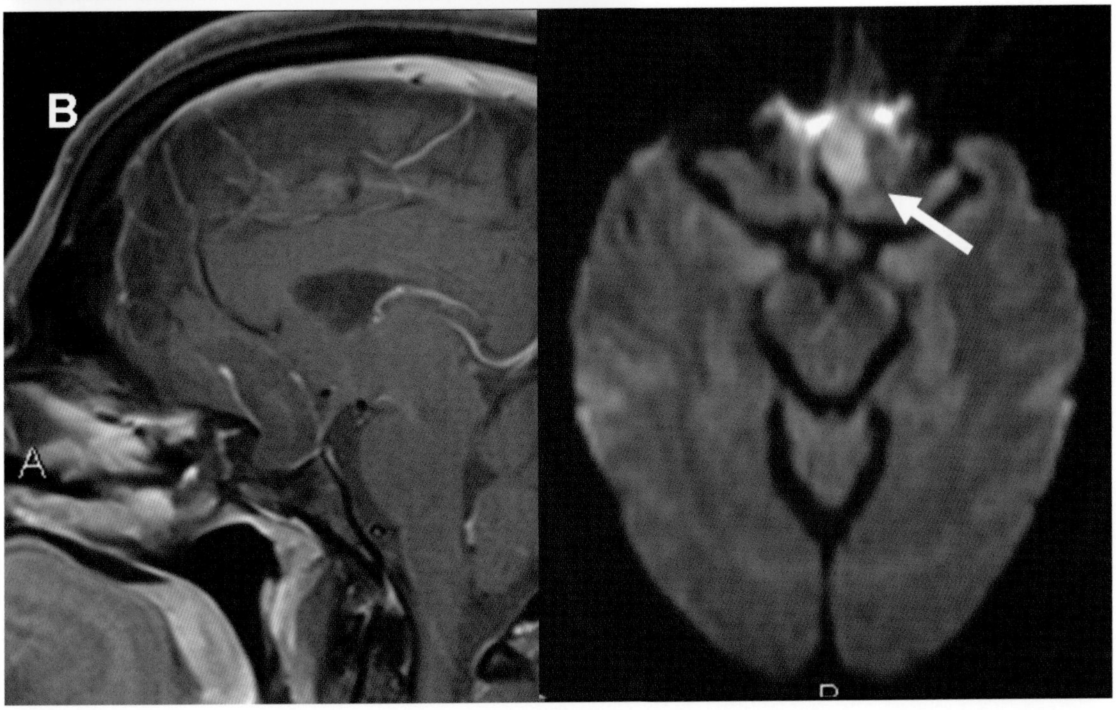

suppressed sequence, by eliminating this hyperintense signal, may be of value in the diagnosis. Rupture of a dermoid cyst can result in chemical meningitis, best seen on unenhanced MRI as foci of high T1 signal intensity, representing fat droplets in the subarachnoid spaces.[24]

Meningiomas and Schwannomas

Approximately 10% of intracranial meningiomas occur in the parasellar region. They arise from the dura overlying the planum sphenoidale, diaphragma sellae, lesser and greater sphenoid wings, cavernous sinus, and optic nerve sheaths. They may extend into the sella and displace or engulf the pituitary gland. They are best recognized on contrast-enhanced MRI as intensely enhancing extra-axial masses with a broad dural attachment, a dural tail, and a cleft of CSF separating them from adjacent brain parenchyma (**Fig. 3.8A**). Densely calcified meningiomas are markedly hypointense on T2WI and may not enhance substantially. When a significant intrasellar component is present, differentiation from an adenoma can be made by the frequent absence of sellar expansion in the former. When meningiomas involve the cavernous sinus and encircle the cavernous internal carotid artery, they tend to constrict it, as opposed to macroadenomas, in which constriction is not usually a feature. Meningiomas confined to the cavernous sinus may mimic schwannomas, most often of the trigeminal nerve. Schwannomas usually enhance uniformly with gadolinium but can demonstrate foci of cystic change or hemorrhage. They often demonstrate a tubular shape, conforming to the nerve of origin (**Fig. 3.8B**).[11,25] Occasionally, perineural tumor spread from oropharyngeal or sinonasal cancers may result in enhancing masses in the cavernous sinus that mimic meningiomas or schwannomas.

Germ Cell Tumors

Approximately 20% of intracranial germ cell tumors occur in the suprasellar cistern. They may arise as primary tumors in these regions or may arise from leptomeningeal metastatic dissemination from a pineal primary. A midline enhancing solid suprasellar lesion in a young person, especially with a coexistent pineal lesion, is almost certainly a germinoma (**Fig. 3.9B**). One must also be wary of the so-called occult neurohypophyseal germinoma, a germ cell tumor in a young patient with diabetes insipidus that may be inapparent on initial imaging. A follow-up MRI may reveal its presence and is therefore warranted.[26]

Chordomas and Chondrosarcomas

These tumors arise from the clivus and petrous temporal bones and may present as parasellar masses or secondarily invade the sella. Chondrosarcomas have a tendency to be centered at the petroclival fissure. CT is useful in demonstrating the arcs and whorls of calcification that are typical of chondroid tumors. On MRI, they are significantly hyperintense on T2WI and tend to enhance variably. Chordomas are more midline in location. The bone destruction and tumoral calcifications of chordomas are best seen on CT. On MRI, heterogeneous signal intensity due to the presence of hemorrhage, calcification, and proteinaceous material is visible.[27] On T2WI, these, like chondrosarcomas, are hyperintense. Distinguishing between these may be difficult, but a more lateral location favors a chondrosarcoma (**Fig. 3.8C,D**).

◆ Infectious/Inflammatory Disorders of the Pituitary Gland

Infection of the pituitary gland is a rare phenomenon. Bacterial pituitary abscess due to Gram-positive cocci may be caused by hematogenous seeding, extension from sphenoid sinusitis, cavernous sinus thrombophlebitis, or meningitis. Prior transsphenoidal surgery, an underlying pituitary lesion, and an immunosuppressed state are known preexisting factors. The presence of a ring-enhancing lesion in a setting of meningitis and sphenoid sinusitis, especially when gas is present, must point to the diagnosis.[28]

Lymphocytic adenohypophysitis (LAH), with or without infundibular involvement (**Fig. 3.9C**), and lymphocytic infundibuloneurohypophysitis (LIN) are autoimmune diseases with distinct clinical presentations. LAH is seen most often in the postpartum state and presents with pituitary insufficiency, whereas LIN presents as diabetes insipidus. LAH manifests on MRI as diffuse enlargement and enhancement of the gland with or without stalk thickening and enhancement. The latter, when present, enables distinction from an adenoma. Also, the sella in LAH is of normal size. Local meningeal enhancement and extension into the cavernous sinus have been reported. LIN presents as thickening and enhancement of the stalk and loss of the normal posterior pituitary bright spot, findings that are entirely nonspecific.[29]

◆ Miscellaneous Disorders of the Pituitary Gland

Intracranial Hypotension

A prominent pituitary gland with a convex superior surface has been described as an imaging finding in the syndrome of intracranial hypotension. This is known to occur owing to venous hyperemia in an attempt to maintain intracranial volume in compliance with the Monro-Kellie hypothesis. This finding is often mistaken for an adenoma or hyperplasia. The coexistence of tonsillar descent, an effaced suprasellar cistern, and smooth dural enhancement over the cerebral convexities with or without subdural effusions should point to the correct diagnosis[30] (**Fig. 3.10A**).

Pituitary Apoplexy

Pituitary apoplexy may occur spontaneously or less commonly be associated with precipitating factors such as bromocriptine therapy, recent surgery, pregnancy, gamma knife radiation, or coagulopathy. On histopathology, hem-

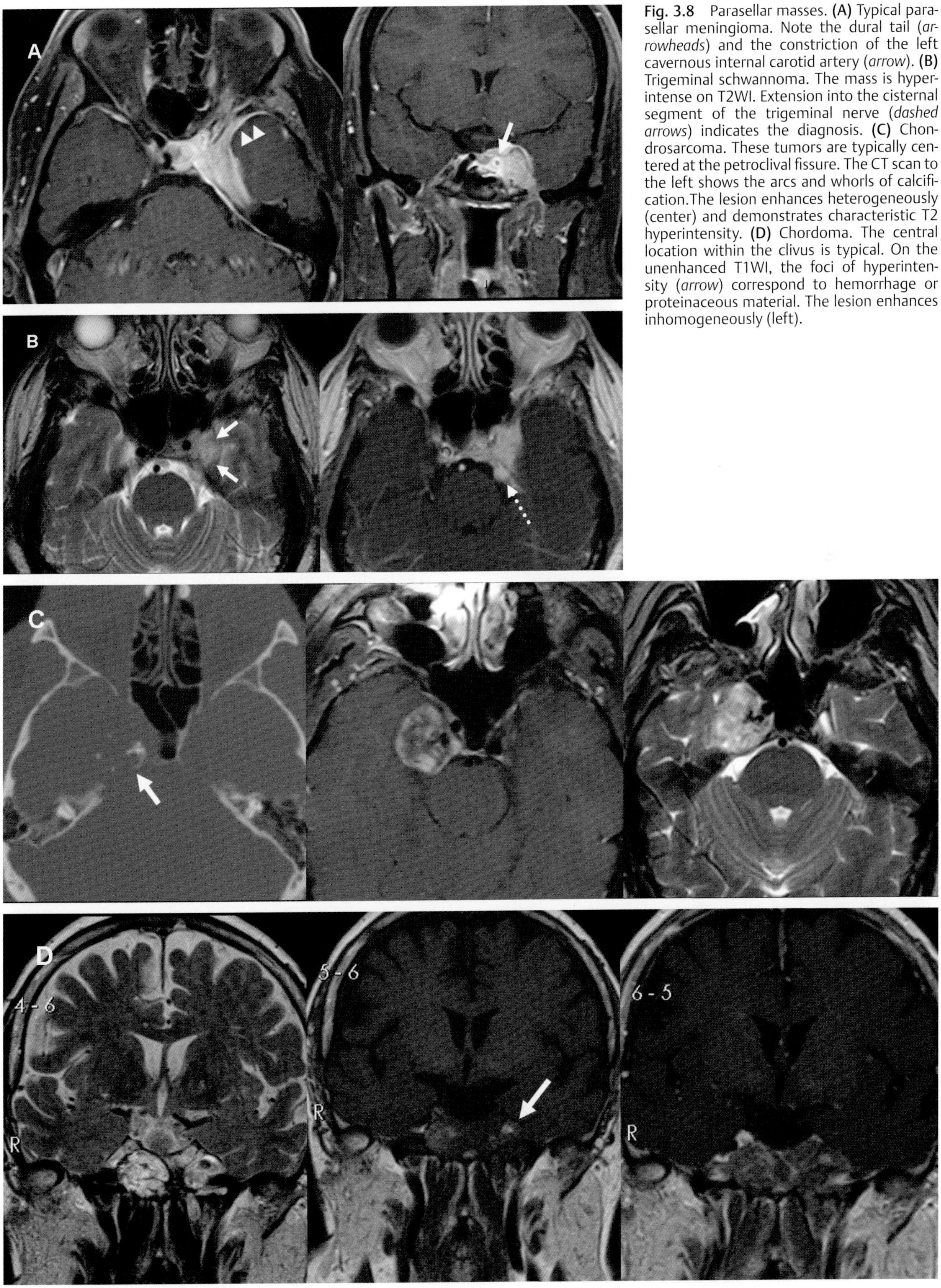

Fig. 3.8 Parasellar masses. **(A)** Typical parasellar meningioma. Note the dural tail (*arrowheads*) and the constriction of the left cavernous internal carotid artery (*arrow*). **(B)** Trigeminal schwannoma. The mass is hyperintense on T2WI. Extension into the cisternal segment of the trigeminal nerve (*dashed arrows*) indicates the diagnosis. **(C)** Chondrosarcoma. These tumors are typically centered at the petroclival fissure. The CT scan to the left shows the arcs and whorls of calcification.The lesion enhances heterogeneously (center) and demonstrates characteristic T2 hyperintensity. **(D)** Chordoma. The central location within the clivus is typical. On the unenhanced T1WI, the foci of hyperintensity (*arrow*) correspond to hemorrhage or proteinaceous material. The lesion enhances inhomogeneously (left).

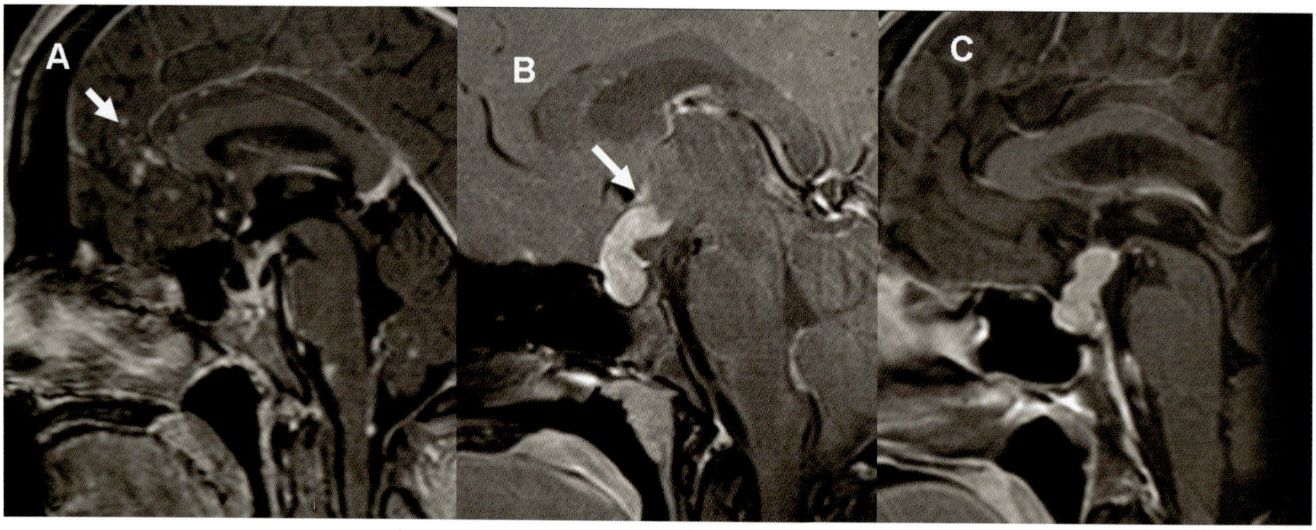

Fig. 3.9 Pituitary stalk lesions. (A) Neurosarcoid. Note the thickening and enhancement of the stalk and hypothalamus. Nodular and linear leptomeningeal enhancement (*arrow*) is evident. (B) Germ cell tumor. The gland and stalk demonstrate diffuse thickening and enhancement. The lack of sellar expansion argues against a macroadenoma. The enhancement of the hypothalamus and in the supraoptic recess are worrisome for an aggressive process (*arrow*). (C) Lymphocytic adenohypophysitis with stalk involvement. Again, note the lack of sellar expansion.

orrhage or hemorrhagic infarction is observed. The signal intensity of an apoplectic adenoma depends on the degree and duration of the hemorrhage. Adenomas that have undergone infarction demonstrate only a thin rim of peripheral enhancement. An acutely infarcted adenoma may appear hyperintense on DWI.. Predominantly hemorrhagic adenomas demonstrate complex signal intensities. T1 hyperintensity due to the presence of methemoglobin and, less commonly, a hematocrit effect with blood-fluid levels may be seen (**Fig. 3.11**). As mentioned earlier, gradient-echo imaging may be able to demonstrate subtle foci of hemorrhage as areas of profound hypointensity.[31,32] A profoundly gradient- and T2-hypointense gland may also be seen with hemochromatosis.

The "Empty" Sella

An "empty" sella is usually the consequence of a developmental defect in the diaphragma sellae that has resulted in the herniation of arachnoid and CSF into the sella. It may be encountered incidentally but may also be a consequence of chronically raised intracranial pressure, as in pseudotumor cerebri. The presence of flat optic discs and distended optic nerve sheaths in conjunction with an empty sella enables a diagnosis of pseudotumor cerebri to be made in the appropriate clinical setting. In this setting, it has been observed to reverse with treatment.[33] An intrasellar arachnoid cyst can mimic an empty sella but is more likely to deform the pituitary stalk.

The Post-treatment Sella

The interpretation of CT or MR studies of the post-treatment sella is often a challenging process. A postoperative sella may contain any combination of residual/recurrent tumor, fat packing, fluid, hemorrhage, Gelfoam, and native gland. Fat packing, which tends to involute with time, is easily recognizable as foci of T1 hyperintensity that disappear on fat-suppressed imaging. Gelfoam is more variable in appearance but most often contains a T1- and T2-hy-

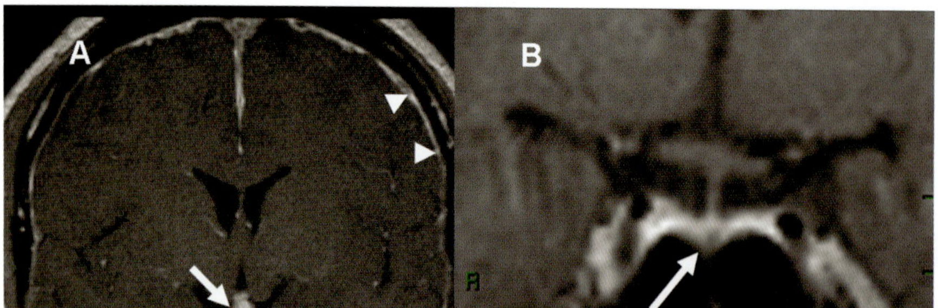

Fig. 3.10 False-positive diagnoses of pituitary disease. (A) The enlarged appearance of the pituitary gland is secondary to intracranial hypotension. The smooth enhancement of the convexity dura (*arrowheads*) clinches the diagnosis. (B) The small focus of glandular hypoenhancement represents a susceptibility artifact at the sphenoid septum insertion and must not be mistaken for a microadenoma.

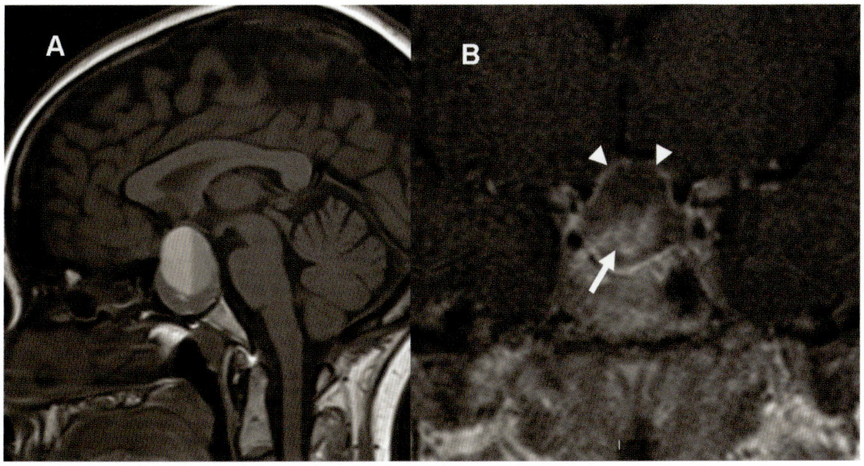

Fig. 3.11 Apoplectic adenomas. **(A)** Hemorrhagic pituitary macroadenoma. Note the blood-fluid level. **(B)** Predominantly infarcted adenoma. Note the faint peripheral enhancement (*arrowheads*). A few small areas of hemorrhage are also present (*arrow*).

pointense core. Methylmethacrylate can also be used to pack the sella and is dark on all sequences. Following the stalk to its insertion enables identification of the native gland (**Fig. 3.12**). Residual/recurrent tumor and granulation tissue may be indistinguishable. The only true sign of tumor is its growth as observed on serial scans.[11] MRI is also useful to monitor complications arising from stereotactic radiosurgery to the sella and parasellar regions, such as temporal lobe necrosis and optic neuropathy.

◆ Conclusion

Modern sellar imaging is highly reliant on MRI. CT has a useful supplementary role. A vast number of disease processes involve the sellar and parasellar region. Knowledge of key imaging findings analyzed in conjunction with the underlying clinical picture enables a specific diagnosis in most cases.

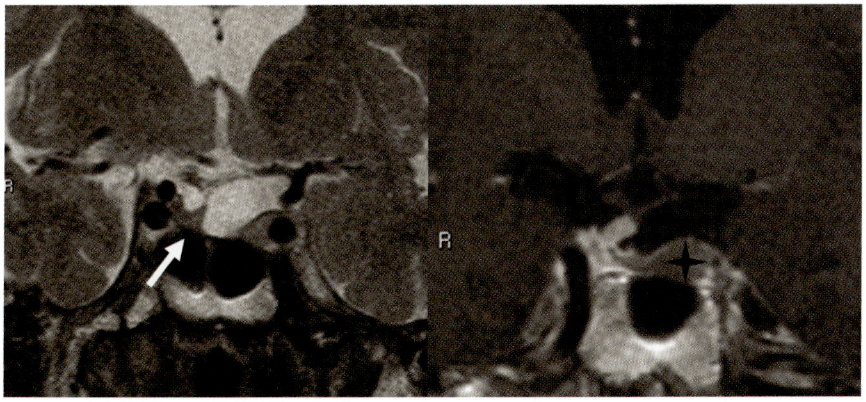

Fig. 3.12 Postoperative sella. Coronal T2WI (left) demonstrates two foci of soft tissue on either side of the midline. The stalk inserts into the homogeneously enhancing focus (*arrow*) on the right, which represents residual native pituitary gland. The relatively hypoenhancing soft tissue on the right (*star*) is residual tumor. The signal intensities of the sellar contents after surgery may be confusing. Often, the only reliable means of identifying tumor is to demonstrate serial growth on follow-up MR studies.

References

1. Webb SM, Ruscalleda J, Schwarzstein D, et al. Computerized tomography versus magnetic resonance imaging: a comparative study in hypothalamic-pituitary and parasellar pathology. Clin Endocrinol (Oxf) 1992;36(5):459–465
2. Davis PC, Hoffman JC Jr, Spencer T, Tindall GT, Braun IF. MR imaging of pituitary adenoma: CT, clinical, and surgical correlation. AJR Am J Roentgenol 1987;148(4):797–802
3. Sadowski EA, Bennett LK, Chan MR, et al. Nephrogenic systemic fibrosis: risk factors and incidence estimation. Radiology 2007; 243(1):148–157
4. Patronas N, Bulakbasi N, Stratakis CA, et al. Spoiled gradient recalled acquisition in the steady state technique is superior to conventional postcontrast spin echo technique for magnetic resonance imaging detection of adrenocorticotropin-secreting pituitary tumors. J Clin Endocrinol Metab 2003;88(4):1565–1569
5. Kucharczyk W, Bishop JE, Plewes DB, Keller MA, George S. Detection of pituitary microadenomas: comparison of dynamic keyhole fast spin-echo, unenhanced, and conventional contrast-enhanced MR imaging. AJR Am J Roentgenol 1994;163(3):671–679
6. Tabarin A, Laurent F, Catargi B, et al. Comparative evaluation of conventional and dynamic magnetic resonance imaging of the pituitary gland for the diagnosis of Cushing's disease. Clin Endocrinol (Oxf) 1998;49(3):293–300
7. Pierallini A, Caramia F, Falcone C, et al. Pituitary macroadenomas: preoperative evaluation of consistency with diffusion-weighted MR imaging—initial experience. Radiology 2006;239(1): 223–231
8. Stadlbauer A, Buchfelder M, Nimsky C, et al. Proton magnetic resonance spectroscopy in pituitary macroadenomas: preliminary results. J Neurosurg 2008;109(2):306–312

9. Korogi Y, Takahashi M. Current concepts of imaging in patients with pituitary/hypothalamic dysfunction. Semin Ultrasound CT MR 1995;16(4):270–278
10. Elster AD. Imaging of the sella: anatomy and pathology. Semin Ultrasound CT MR 1993;14(3):182–194
11. Symons SP, Aviv RI, Montanera WJ, Kucharczyk W. The sella turcica and parasellar region. In: Atlas SW, ed. Magnetic Resonance Imaging of the Brain and Spine, vol. 2. Lippincott Williams & Wilkins; 2008:1120–1192
12. Hagiwara A, Inoue Y, Wakasa K, Haba T, Tashiro T, Miyamoto T. Comparison of growth hormone-producing and non-growth hormone-producing pituitary adenomas: imaging characteristics and pathologic correlation. Radiology 2003;228(2):533–538
13. Ahmadi H, Larsson EM, Jinkins JR, Haba T, Tashiro T, Miyamoto T. Normal pituitary gland: coronal MR imaging of infundibular tilt. Radiology 1990;177(2):389–392
14. Tosaka M, Sato N, Hirato J, et al. Assessment of hemorrhage in pituitary macroadenoma by T2*-weighted gradient-echo MR imaging. AJNR Am J Neuroradiol 2007;28(10):2023–2029
15. Cottier JP, Destrieux C, Brunereau L, et al. Cavernous sinus invasion by pituitary adenoma: MR imaging. Radiology 2000; 215(2): 463–469
16. Tokumaru AM, Sakata I, Terada H, Kosuda S, Nawashiro H, Yoshii M. Optic nerve hyperintensity on T2-weighted images among patients with pituitary macroadenoma: correlation with visual impairment. AJNR Am J Neuroradiol 2006;27(2):250–254
17. Kim HJ, Cho WH. Optic tract hemorrhage after pituitary apoplexy. AJNR Am J Neuroradiol 2007;28(1):141–142
18. Yousem DM, Arrington JA, Zinreich SJ, Kumar AJ, Bryan RN. Pituitary adenomas: possible role of bromocriptine in intratumoral hemorrhage. Radiology 1989;170(1 Pt 1):239–243
19. Shah B, Lipper MH, Laws ER, Lopes MB, Spellman MJ Jr. Posterior pituitary astrocytoma: a rare tumor of the neurohypophysis: a case report. AJNR Am J Neuroradiol 2005;26(7):1858–1861
20. Komninos J, Vlassopoulou V, Protopapa D, et al. Tumors metastatic to the pituitary gland: case report and literature review. J Clin Endocrinol Metab 2004;89(2):574–580
21. Kaufmann TJ, Lopes MBS, Laws ER Jr, Lipper MH. Primary sellar lymphoma: radiologic and pathologic findings in two patients. AJNR Am J Neuroradiol 2002;23(3):364–367
22. Sartoretti-Schefer S, Wichmann W, Aguzzi A, Valavanis A. MR differentiation of adamantinous and squamous-papillary craniopharyngiomas. AJNR Am J Neuroradiol 1997;18(1):77–87
23. Byun WM, Kim OL, Kim D. MR imaging findings of Rathke's cleft cysts: significance of intracystic nodules. AJNR Am J Neuroradiol 2000;21(3):485–488
24. Smith AS, Benson JE, Blaser SI, Mizushima A, Tarr RW, Bellon EM. Diagnosis of ruptured intracranial dermoid cyst: value of MR over CT. AJNR Am J Neuroradiol 1991;12(1):175–180
25. Razek AAKA, Castillo M. Imaging lesions of the cavernous sinus. AJNR Am J Neuroradiol 2009;30(3):444–452
26. Kato T, Sawamura Y, Tada M, et al. Occult neurohypophyseal germinomas in patients presenting with central diabetes insipidus. Neurosurg Focus 1998;5(1):e6
27. Erdem E, Angtuaco EC, Van Hemert R, Park JS, Al-Mefty O. Comprehensive review of intracranial chordoma. Radiographics 2003;23(4):995–1009
28. Vates GE, Berger MS, Wilson CB. Diagnosis and management of pituitary abscess: a review of twenty-four cases. J Neurosurg 2001;95(2):233–241 http://dx.doi.org/10.3171/jns.2001.95.2.0233
29. Gutenberg A, Larsen J, Lupi I, Rohde V, Caturegli P. A radiologic score to distinguish autoimmune hypophysitis from nonsecreting pituitary adenoma preoperatively. AJNR Am J Neuroradiol 2009;30(9):1766–1772
30. Alvarez-Linera J, Escribano J, Benito-León J, Porta-Etessam J, Rovira A. Pituitary enlargement in patients with intracranial hypotension syndrome. Neurology 2000;55(12):1895–1897
31. Semple PL, Jane JA Jr, Laws ER Jr. Clinical relevance of precipitating factors in pituitary apoplexy. Neurosurgery 2007;61(5):956–961, discussion 961–962
32. Rogg JM, Tung GA, Anderson G, Cortez S. Pituitary apoplexy: early detection with diffusion-weighted MR imaging. AJNR Am J Neuroradiol 2002;23(7):1240–1245
33. Zagardo MT, Cail WS, Kelman SE, Rothman MI. Reversible empty sella in idiopathic intracranial hypertension: an indicator of successful therapy? AJNR Am J Neuroradiol 1996;17(10): 1953–1956

4 Medical Evaluation and Management

Mary Lee Vance

Of the many types of lesions that occur in the sella or parasellar region, a pituitary adenoma is the most common. All lesions in this area require an endocrine evaluation to determine if the lesion is a secretory pituitary adenoma and if so what type of hormone is oversecreted. Also, even if the lesion is not a pituitary adenoma, a comprehensive endocrine evaluation will assess the pituitary function and whether any hormonal replacement is required. An ophthalmologic evaluation is indicated in patients with a lesion approximating or compressing the optic apparatus (optic nerves, optic chiasm). The neuro-ophthalmologic evaluation is covered in Chapter 5.

The endocrine evaluation is accomplished with measurement of the serum hormone levels and, for the situation of possible Cushing disease, a 24-hour urine test for urine free cortisol. Additional dynamic testing may be required in patients with possible Cushing disease or acromegaly—all of which can be accomplished in the outpatient setting. The important concept is that the pituitary and the adjacent area comprise both an anatomic and a functional entity, so that a combined evaluation of the anatomy and physiology is required to determine the appropriate treatment or treatments. **Table 4.1** details the most common types of sellar and parasellar lesions that should be considered when each patient is reviewed.

Table 4.1 Types of Sellar and Parasellar Lesions

Pituitary adenoma (secretory, nonfunctioning)
Craniopharyngioma
Rathke cleft cyst
Pilocytic astrocytoma
Germinoma
Metastatic carcinoma
Infiltrative disease (giant cell granuloma, sarcoidosis, lymphocytic hypophysitis, lymphoma, plasmacytoma)
Meningioma
Chordoma
Chondrosarcoma
Infection (tuberculosis, mycosis)
Carotid-cavernous aneurysm

◆ Clinical Manifestations

A lesion in the sella often causes loss of pituitary function and/or exertion of a mass effect. Depending on the location, mass effect can cause loss of vision (eg, visual field defect, decreased visual acuity), cranial nerve dysfunction (eg, diplopia, ptosis), or headache. A lesion that causes acute visual loss requires immediate evaluation and treatment.

Hormone Deficiency

Endocrine consequences of a pituitary lesion affect the reproductive system most commonly.[1] Thus, men often have symptoms of hypogonadism—decreased libido, erectile dysfunction, and infertility. Women of reproductive age may develop irregular menses, amenorrhea, or infertility. Adolescents may experience delayed or arrested puberty. Another common pituitary deficiency is loss of growth hormone (GH) secretion, resulting in fatigue in adults and arrested or decreased growth velocity in children and adolescents. The two most important hormones are cortisol and thyroid hormone, both of which are necessary for life. Symptoms of cortisol deficiency include fatigue, headache, weight loss, diminished appetite, and in some patients hypotension and syncope. Symptoms of thyroid hormone deficiency include fatigue, cold intolerance, weight gain, constipation, difficulty concentrating, and memory problems.

Deficiency of the posterior pituitary hormone vasopressin causes polyuria (particularly nocturia), polydipsia, and potentially volume depletion if the patient does not drink an adequate amount of fluids. This condition is termed diabetes insipidus (DI), which is rare in patients with a pituitary adenoma; if there are symptoms, the possible diagnoses are a craniophyaryngioma, lymphocytic hypophysitis, sarcoidosis, or metastatic carcinoma.

Pituitary Hypersecretion

Excessive hormone secretion causes symptoms and signs associated with overproduction of prolactin, growth hormone (acromegaly), or adrenocorticotropic hormone (ACTH; Cushing disease). A prolactin-producing adenoma is the most common type of secretory pituitary adenoma. Clinical features in women of reproductive age with a prolactinoma include irregular menses, amenorrhea, or infertility; galactorrhea may or may not be present. Men with a prolactinoma develop diminished libido, erectile dysfunction, and infertility; gynecomastia and galactorrhea may also occur. Because many men and postmenopausal women seek medical attention late in the course of disease, visual loss may be the presenting feature.

Excessive GH secretion after puberty causes enlargement of the bones of the face, hands, and feet. Other clinical features of acromegaly include sleep apnea, arthralgia (particularly in the large joints), spinal stenosis, carpal tunnel syndrome, diabetes mellitus, hypertension, colon polyps, excessive sweating, oily skin, and in some patients cardiomyopathy with heart failure. Excessive GH production before puberty results in gigantism with excessive linear growth and the features described above that occur in adults.

Features of Cushing disease, which is excessive cortisol production stimulated by an ACTH-producing pituitary adenoma, include weight gain, diabetes mellitus, hypertension, osteoporosis, bone fractures, depression, and memory loss.

The least common type of secretory pituitary adenoma is the thyroid-stimulating hormone (TSH)–secreting tumor, which causes clinical or subclinical hyperthyroidism (weight loss, tachycardia, frequent bowel movements, and anxiety).

◆ Endocrine Evaluation

Table 4.2 details the necessary hormone tests to evaluate a pituitary or parasellar lesion.

Table 4.2 Endocrine Evaluation for Pituitary Hormone Deficiency and Hormone Hypersecretion

Pituitary hormone deficiency
Morning serum cortisol, ACTH (ACTH and cortisol deficiency)
Serum free T_4, TSH (TSH and thyroid hormone deficiency)
Serum LH, FSH, testosterone (men; gonadotropin deficiency)
Serum LH, FSH, estradiol (women of reproductive age)
Serum IGF-1 (growth hormone deficiency)
Pituitary hormone hypersecretion
Serum prolactin (prolactinoma)
Serum IGF-1; oral glucose test (acromegaly)
24-Hour urine free cortisol, serum ACTH (Cushing disease)
Serum TSH, free T_4 (TSH-secreting adenoma)
Serum α subunit (tumor marker)
Serum LH, FSH (tumor marker)

Abbreviations: ACTH, adrenocorticotropic hormone; FSH, follicle-stimulating hormone; IGF-1, insulin-like growth factor 1; LH, luteinizing hormone; T_4, thyroxine; TSH, thyroid-stimulating hormone.

Hormone Deficiency

The most important issue is to determine if the patient has secondary adrenal insufficiency and/or secondary hypothyroidism because these hormones are necessary for essential life functions. Low morning serum cortisol and ACTH levels may be adequate to diagnose secondary adrenal insufficiency. If there is doubt, a stimulation test such as an ACTH stimulation test or insulin-induced hypoglycemia is indicated. The insulin hypoglycemia test is the most rigorous and reliable study; this test is also the most accurate for diagnosing GH deficiency. However, the insulin hypoglycemia test must be monitored by a physician and is contraindicated in patients with coronary artery disease, a seizure disorder, or general debility.

For thyroid hormone deficiency, both the serum free thyroxine (free T_4) and TSH levels should be measured. A low serum free T_4 is the most reliable test. Patients with pituitary disease may have a "normal" serum TSH in the setting of a low free T_4 level. DI is primarily a clinical diagnosis (polyuria, polydipsia, excessive thirst, and in particular frequent nocturia—ie, urination every 30–60 minutes during the night). Serum sodium and serum osmolality are normal if the patient has intact thirst sensation and no restriction of fluid intake; serum osmolality may be normal, but the urine specific gravity should be low. Gonadotropin deficiency in men is diagnosed by clinical symptoms and by measuring the serum testosterone and luteinizing hormone (LH). In gonadotropin deficiency, the serum testosterone level will be low in the setting of a "normal" serum LH (not normal for low testosterone). In women of reproductive age, irregular menses, amenorrhea, and infertility are the best indicators of gonadal dysfunction. Serum estradiol may be low or "normal" depending on the stage of the menstrual cycle, and serum LH is usually in the "normal" range, but lack of regular menses or ovulation indicates gonadal dysfunction. GH deficiency is diagnosed by either a low serum insulin-like growth factor 1 (IGF-1) level in the setting of several pituitary hormone deficiencies or by a subnormal GH response to a stimulation test (eg, insulin-induced hypoglycemia or arginine infusion).

Pituitary Hypersecretion

Serum prolactin should be measured to determine if a pituitary lesion is a prolactinoma, because medical therapy with a dopamine agonist is the first line of treatment for a prolactinoma. The prolactin level must be correlated with the size of the pituitary or parasellar lesion. Any lesion in this region may cause a mild elevation of serum prolactin (interference with the prolactin inhibitor hormone, dopamine, through the pituitary stalk). As a general rule, in the setting of a macroadenoma (>10 mm), the serum prolactin level should be greater than 200 ng/mL for a true prolactinoma. This assessment is necessary to determine the course of treatment—medical therapy or surgery. One caution: In the setting of an elevated serum prolactin level (>200ng/mL), the serum specimen must be diluted to obtain an accurate value (prolactin >200 ng/mL is not sufficient), and the physician must request that the laboratory perform the necessary dilutions to obtain the actual value. A value of >200 ng/mL may be 2000 or 20,000 or greater. To assess the response to medical therapy, an accurate baseline prolactin value is also required.

Acromegaly is diagnosed by clinical features, an elevated serum IGF-1 level, and a serum GH level that does not decline to <1 ng/mL after oral glucose (75 or 100 g). There are important considerations about these tests. Although the IGF-1 assay is reliable and reproducible, over the past 2 years there have been false elevations of IGF-1 related to the database for the range of normal according to age. This problem is being addressed but has not yet been fully resolved. The definitive test for acromegaly is the GH response to an oral glucose challenge (oral glucose tolerance test, or OGTT). The test must be performed correctly to interpret the results. Baseline serum glucose and GH are measured, the patient drinks a glucose solution (75 or 100 g), and the serum glucose and GH levels are measured every 30 minutes for 2 hours. The current guideline for a normal response is a serum GH level of <1 ng/mL. Some patients with acromegaly may have a paradoxical increase in GH.[2]

Cushing disease is diagnosed by demonstrating a consistent overproduction of cortisol in the setting of detectable or elevated serum ACTH. Cushing disease is the most problematic of all pituitary adenoma diagnoses for several reasons, including overlap of the clinical features with those of other disorders (polycystic ovarian syndrome, obesity, depression) and the variable sensitivity and specificity of tests. Consistent overproduction of cortisol is demonstrated by three types of screening tests: elevated 24-hour urine free cortisol (preferably measured by tandem mass spectrometry), loss of circadian rhythm with elevated nighttime salivary cortisol levels, and failure of the serum cortisol to decline to <1.8 μg/dL at 8 AM after ingestion of dexamethasone at 11 PM the previous night.[3] These three types of screening tests are ~92% accurate; thus, repeated tests may be necessary to establish the diagnosis. Serum ACTH may be in the normal range or elevated. The traditional high-dose dexamethasone suppression test (8 mg overnight or 2 mg every 6 hours for 48 hours) was developed to distinguish between pituitary-dependent or ectopic ACTH syndrome. Unfortunately, these tests are not sufficiently sensitive or specific to exclude ectopic ACTH production by a tumor in the lung, pancreas, or thyroid gland. Because ~50% of patients with a pituitary adenoma causing Cushing disease have no visible lesion on magnetic resonance imaging (MRI) with a pituitary protocol and because 10% of adults with normal pituitary function have a visible lesion in the pituitary gland ("incidentaloma"), an MRI study is not sufficient to recommend pituitary surgery. The inferior petrosal sinus sampling (IPSS) study is the most precise method to determine if the source of ACTH is the pituitary gland and to exclude ectopic ACTH syndrome. This test involves comparing the central (petrosal sinus, left and right) and peripheral (inferior vena cava) ACTH levels before and after the administration of corticotropin-releasing hormone (CRH). A ratio of the basal central to the peripheral ACTH level of >2 or a CRH-stimulated ratio of >3 indicates a pituitary etiology. This invasive study should be performed only by an experienced interventional radiologist or neuroradiologist; cannulation of the inferior petrosal sinuses requires appropriate experience and expertise. This study is not without risk, including thrombosis and stroke, emphasizing the requirement that it be performed by an experienced radiologist.

An uncommon type of secretory adenoma produces excessive α subunit, which causes no specific clinical features but often causes hypogonadism. Measurement of serum α subunit serves as a tumor marker before and after surgical removal of the adenoma. Although many pituitary adenomas are gonadotrope tumors by immunohistochemical criteria, they rarely secrete excessive amounts of LH or follicle-stimulating hormone (FSH). Measurement of the serum LH and FSH serves as a tumor marker in the event the tumor produces an excessive amount of one or both hormones.

◆ Consequences of Endocrine Evaluation

A diagnosis of hormone deficiency and/or hormone hypersecretion directs treatments. As noted, a prolactin-producing adenoma is treated medically with a dopamine agonist drug. Other types of lesions are most commonly treated by resection, radiosurgery, radiation therapy, and even chemotherapy.

Replacement of cortisol and/or thyroid hormone is necessary before a therapeutic intervention. After surgery or another treatment, patients should be re-evaluated for pituitary hormone deficiency. In the case of patients with acromegaly or Cushing disease, serum GH and/or cortisol immediately after surgery is a helpful indicator of the outcome of the operation. Periodic and comprehensive re-evaluations of the endocrine status of patients should be performed to detect for tumor recurrence in the case of secretory pituitary adenomas. In addition, extended endocrine follow-up should be performed to detect hypopituitarism, which can arise months to years after intervention.[4] Delayed hypopituitarism has been observed following radiosurgery and radiation therapy for sellar and parasellar disease.[5]

◆ Conclusion

All lesions in the sellar or parasellar region require an endocrine evaluation in conjunction with ophthalmologic and surgical evaluations. A multidisciplinary approach is required for the diagnosis and treatment of lesions in this area, which is an anatomic and functional entity. Longitudinal endocrine follow-up is also required to detect and correct any endocrine abnormalities associated with intracranial disease or arising as an unintended effect of treatment.

References

1. Vance ML. Hypopituitarism. N Engl J Med 1994;330(23): 1651–1662
2. Hartman ML, Crowe BJ, Biller BM, Ho KK, Clemmons DR, Chipman JJ; HyposCCS Advisory Board; U.S. HypoCCS Study Group. Which patients do not require a GH stimulation test for the diagnosis of adult GH deficiency? J Clin Endocrinol Metab 2002;87(2):477–485
3. Arnaldi G, Angeli A, Atkinson AB, et al. Diagnosis and complications of Cushing's syndrome: a consensus statement. J Clin Endocrinol Metab 2003;88(12):5593–5602
4. Vance ML, Mauras N. Growth hormone therapy in adults and children. N Engl J Med 1999;341(16):1206–1216
5. Sheehan JP, Niranjan A, Sheehan JM, et al. Stereotactic radiosurgery for pituitary adenomas: an intermediate review of its safety, efficacy, and role in the neurosurgical treatment armamentarium. J Neurosurg 2005;102(4):678–691

5 Ophthalmologic Evaluation and Management

Steven A. Newman

◆ Core Messages

Visual signs and symptoms are extremely frequent manifestations of disease affecting the sellar and parasellar region. Medical treatment, radiation therapy, radiosurgery, and surgical intervention in and around the parasellar region may affect afferent or efferent visual function, producing problems with decreased vision, visual field defects, and double vision. Ophthalmic management of patients with skull base pathology involving the sellar region prioritizes protecting the afferent visual pathways. Rehabilitation techniques focus on patients with acuity and visual field loss, as well as double vision and ptosis.

Patients with ocular malalignment related to either direct orbital involvement or involvement of the ocular motor nerves can be treated with short-term therapy, including occlusion, botulinum toxin injection, and prisms. Long-term management includes strabismus surgery designed to maximize the field of binocular single vision.

Sensory loss to the anterior segment can compromise corneal function and needs to be addressed with appropriate intervention to open and close the lids, provide adequate tear production and corneal wetting, and deal with the potential loss of neurotrophic factors secondary to corneal denervation leading to corneal epithelial breakdown.

◆ Introduction

The sellar region represents not only the center of the skull base but also the primary ophthalmologic conjunction. Both the afferent visual pathways, represented by the two optic nerves, chiasm, and optic tract, and the efferent visual pathways, including the third, fourth, and sixth cranial nerves, course either above or lateral to the sella. It is thus not surprising that pathology affecting the sellar and parasellar region often presents with ophthalmic manifestations,[1–13] and any intervention, be it medical, surgical, or radiologic, can produce its own set of ophthalmic complications[14,15]

From an ophthalmic point of view, it is important to recognize the visual system in three parts. The afferent system can be thought of as a mapping function, taking the outside world into our consciousness. To perform this function adequately, the anterior segment of the eye needs to refract (bend and focus) light onto the photosensitive retina, which then converts the electromagnetic radiation into a series of impulses. These impulse signals are conducted via the optic nerves and visual pathways back to the cortex, where interpretation takes place. Interruption anywhere along these pathways can result in symptoms of afferent system dysfunction, including decreased vision, blurred vision, and visual field defects.

The efferent system, responsible for coordinating ocular motility, provides globe movement through the final common pathways of the six extraocular muscles. These are innervated by the third, fourth, and sixth cranial nerves, which travel through the cavernous sinus lateral to the wall of the body of the sphenoid and enter the orbit through the superior orbital fissure. Involvement of these cranial nerves can result in loss of ocular motility, manifested as double vision, blurred vision, or a sensation of spontaneous ocular motility.

Finally, the globe is supported by the orbital tissues making up the adnexal structures. These include the eyelids, responsible for maintaining and distributing an adequate tear film over the cornea, which forms the first part of the refracting surface of the eye. Adnexal tissues also include the lacrimal glands, the accessory lacrimal glands, and the structures responsible for opening and closing the eyes. Any involvement of the innervation of these structures can also result in various ophthalmic symptoms, including pain, numbness, loss of vision, problems with acuity, and double vision. Direct involvement of the orbital structures due to invasion of the orbit, either through the fissures and foramina connecting the intracranial cavities to the orbit or through the bone itself, can result in restricted motility, often producing double vision, proptosis (ie, prominence of the globe), and problems with anterior segment function. Thus, pathology affecting the sellar and parasellar region frequently results in multiple ophthalmic symptoms and signs.[16]

The autonomic nervous system has both afferent and efferent system effects. Sympathetic and parasympathetic innervation to the pupil controls the amount of light reaching the retina, and the parasympathetic innervation to the ciliary body is responsible for accommodation (ie, the ability to see close up). Sympathetic innervation to Müller's muscle helps lift the lid up, and parasympathetic supply to the lacrimal gland controls tear formation and, thus, the anterior refracting surface of the eye.

◆ History

The history of visual symptoms often provides a clue to the presence of parasellar lesions and directs decisions regarding imaging. The most common ophthalmic manifestation of pathology affecting the suprasellar region is visual loss. Compression or secondary ischemic involvement of the optic nerve, chiasm, or optic tracts often produces decreased vision or less commonly appreciated visual field defects.[14,17] The most important question is whether this is in one eye or both eyes. Loss of vision restricted to one eye implies globe, retina, or optic nerve pathology. If both eyes are involved, there still may be bilateral globe, retina, or optic nerve pathology, but chiasmal or retrochiasmal lesions are also in the differential diagnosis. The next question is that of the onset. Answers should include whether the visual loss is diffuse, central, or off to one side, and whether it is constant or intermittent. If variable, one needs to inquire as to what can make it better or worse, and whether it is progressive—either acutely, stepwise, or slowly. Any other associated neurologic or systemic complaints should also be sought. Patients should always be asked about a prior history of vascular disease (hypertension, diabetes, hypercholesterolemia, angina, myocardial infarct, irregular heart beat, cardiac valvular disease, or a documented stroke); inflammatory disease (demyelinating disease, infections including zoster, autoimmune conditions); cancer; or migraine. The patient's occupation may give a clue to exposure to toxins and agents that can affect pupil size or motility, as may a travel history. It is helpful if the patient has had prior imaging studies. History often supplies clues to "where" the pathology is, which in turn alters the differential diagnosis.

As with all complaints, rule No. 1 is essential: "Get the old records." Often, patients with complaints of visual loss will be found to have previous compromise of the visual pathways, manifested by records documenting decreased vision. Attention should be directed to identifying any source of prior ophthalmic evaluation, including the records of previous ophthalmologists and optometrists, or even the results of visual screening, such as for the Department of Motor Vehicles or military. Previous refractive correction needs to be identified, including the potential problems of nearsightedness, farsightedness, and astigmatism. If the patient wears glasses or contact lenses, these should be available and all testing done with them in place.

Bitemporal visual field defects are often unnoticed,[18] and homonymous defects are often identified incorrectly as loss of vision in the ipsilateral eye. Patients may describe objects "disappearing" off to one side while they are reading. It is important to identify which parts of words seem to be disappearing as a clue to a visual field defect.

It would be unusual for parasellar pathology to present with positive visual phenomena. Positive visual phenomena, often described as zigzag lines, lights, colors, a kaleidoscope, cracked glass, or broken images, are most commonly seen with migraine. They can uncommonly be seen with cortical pathology. Rare types of formed visual hallucinations usually occur with occipital involvement, but deafferentation anywhere along the visual pathways, including the optic nerve, chiasm, and tract, may result in release phenomena as known as the Charles Bonnet syndrome.

Distortion of vision (seeing lines as bent, warped, broken, or missing, or seeing objects as too large or too small) may represent cortical pathology but is usually due to pathology affecting the retina, more specifically the macula. This can be seen with parasellar lesions that extend to involve the orbit but would be uncommon.

Additional uncommon manifestations of pathology affecting the afferent system are visual obscurations.[19] These are brief, usually bilateral loss of vision, often associated with change in position. This is typical in patients with disc edema, and it may be seen with parasellar lesions that cause increased intracranial pressure. Transient visual loss associated with exercise may represent long-standing inflammation involving the optic nerves (Uhthoff phenomena[20]). Monocular loss of vision lasting minutes may also occur with thromboembolic phenomena (amaurosis fugax, usually related to carotid disease), or dimming or darkening of vision with ocular hypoperfusion (ocular ischemic syndrome or arteritis, particularly in the elderly). Less common symptoms include darkening of vision associated with exposure to bright lights. This can sometimes be seen in patients with carotid compromise, potentially with parasellar lesions. Less commonly, transient loss of vision may be due to ocular disease (angle closure, hyphema, dry eye) and very rarely to orbital disease (gaze-evoked amaurosis secondary to an orbital tumor).

The second most common ophthalmic complaint associated with parasellar pathology is double vision.[21] This should first be characterized as monocular or binocular, with the examiner specifically questioning whether it disappears when either eye is covered. Failure to resolve when either eye is covered indicates a monocular problem. Although this may occur as a cortical phenomenon (palinopsia), it usually represents ghost images secondary to high astigmatism due to corneal warping, surface pathology, or cataract.

Double vision that resolves by covering either eye is usually due to ocular malalignment. Attention should be directed to whether or not the double vision increases with gaze in one particular direction, specifically looking to the right or to the left, and in the four corners (up right, down right, down left, and up left). Although the natural presumption in the case of incomitant deviations (deviations that change with direction of gaze) is that they are due to a cranial nerve palsy,[22–25] it is important to recognize that alternative causes of paretic malalignment include neuromuscular transmission deficits (myasthenia gravis), and internuclear connection problems (brainstem) causing a skew deviation or internuclear ophthalmoplegia. Supranuclear palsies due to cortical or corticobulbar pathway pathology may limit motility but usually do not produce malalignment or diplopia. Limitations secondary to supranuclear processes may be overcome with infranuclear stimulation (vestibular stimulation or irrigation of the ear [calorics]).

In addition to paretic causes, incomitant ocular malalignment producing diplopia may also be due to restriction of the extraocular muscles. This requires involvement of the extraocular muscles themselves within the orbit and is most commonly seen in patients with thyroid orbitopathy. It can also be seen following trauma, with orbital inflammation, and with tumors that either extend to involve the extraocular muscles or are metastatic to the extraocular muscles or orbital tissues (particularly breast cancer). Restrictive phenomena should be suspected when there is history of orbital asymmetry, including proptosis, enophthalmos, exophthalmos, lid position abnormalities, prominent episcleral vessels, and a rushing sound in the patient's head.

Patients should be asked whether the double vision is side to side or if there is a vertical component. If the diplopia is strictly horizontal, then the problem must ultimately involve the two medial and lateral rectus muscles or their innervation. If there is a vertical component (indicating involvement of the vertical muscles [both obliques and the inferior and superior recti]), it needs to be addressed first. Patients should also be asked whether the double vision is worse at near or distance.

Not all patients with ocular malalignment will experience double vision. This may be the case if there is a history of strabismus or poor vision in one eye. Similarly, subtle abnormalities in ocular alignment, often due to mild cranial nerve palsies, may not be appreciated as double vision, but rather as "blurred" vision when the patient looks in the direction of the weakened muscle. Patients will also often adopt head posturing, including head turns or tilts, to avoid the blurred or double vision. Old records should be sought for a previous history of strabismus, including records of eye muscle surgery and problems with ocular alignment in childhood. Congenital cranial nerve palsies may decompensate, producing the onset of double vision later in life. Clues to this may be provided by old photographs showing long-standing head posturing (particularly useful in the setting of a congenital fourth nerve palsy or Duane syndrome).

Other, less common symptoms of efferent pathology include oscillopsia (a sensation of the world jumping), vertigo (a sensation of the world rotating), and tilt symptoms (a sensation of the world tilted, most commonly seen in Wallenberg lateral medullary plate syndrome owing to infarction of the posterior inferior cerebellar artery). These are usually due to pathology affecting the brainstem centers of stability and would thus be very uncommon with parasellar lesions.

Adnexal involvement can be sought with a history of numbness or pain. Pain in and around the eyes unassociated with numbness is often unrevealing. A history of numbness, however, almost always indicates significant pathology. Prominence of the globe or fullness within the orbit may indicate intraorbital pathology, potentially extending from the parasellar region. A history of lid position abnormalities, including lid retraction or ptosis, may be a clue to pathology affecting the oculomotor nerve or the orbital tissues themselves.

◆ Anatomy

Afferent System

Afferent information is carried via the optic nerves, which consist of approximately 1.2 million axons of the ganglion cells located within the inner retina. Because the fovea is located nasal to the disc, fibers from the temporal portion of the retina arc around the macula, separating fibers that are just above the temporal horizontal midline from those just below. This anatomic separation occurs within the retina and at the disc and is maintained throughout the optic nerve. Thus, any pathology that affects the optic nerve tends to produce visual field defects that are either a little bit above or a little bit below the nasal horizontal midline on visual field testing (as we see things opposite to their anatomy). This is the anatomic origin of the arcuate visual field defects that we see with any pathology affecting the optic nerve.

The fovea, which is the most sensitive portion of the retina, has the highest spatial resolution based on its relatively high (1:1 or 1:2) ganglion-to-receptor cell ratio, (in the peripheral retina, the ratio may be as low as 1:1000). In addition, the fovea, or the center of the macula, is devoid of rods and has the highest concentration of cones, responsible for color vision. Thus, color abnormalities are a common concomitant of the dysfunction of the relatively small macular fibers, which can be compromised with compressive lesions.[26] Color vision may be affected relatively early in patients with mild compression of the optic nerve. Involvement of the small fibers, which are particularly sensitive to compression, may also result in relative central scotomas. The optic nerve is approximately 1.5 mm in diameter as it exits the globe, extends less than a millimeter through the sclera, then becomes myelinated, increasing in size to approximately 3 mm. It is surrounded by the optic nerve sheath and the trabecular arachnoid, which allows cerebrospinal fluid (CSF) up to the back of the eye. This access of CSF to the back of the globe is responsible for the potential development of disc edema secondary to increased intracranial pressure.

There is redundancy in the optic nerve within the orbit, which permits the eye to move, but can be restricted if substantial proptosis ensues owing to invasion of the orbit. The central retinal artery and vein run within the optic nerve in the 8 to 10 mm just behind the globe, but outside the optic nerve posterior to this region, where the optic nerve is supplied by small branches from the optic nerve sheath. Extension of a meningioma along the optic nerve sheath can compromise the vascular supply to the optic nerve posteriorly. It also can compromise the venous outflow, resulting in the development of collaterals to the choroid circulation (optociliary shunt vessels)[27] (**Fig. 5.1**).

The optic canal measures 6 to 8 mm in length and extends superiorly and medially; it is bordered temporally by the optic strut, which separates it from the superior orbital fissure, and nasally by the sphenoid sinus. In approximately 8% of cases, there is bone dehiscence, so that the optic nerve actually may have no bony protection from pathology (or surgical exploration) within the sphenoid sinus. The exit of the optic canal takes place under a fold

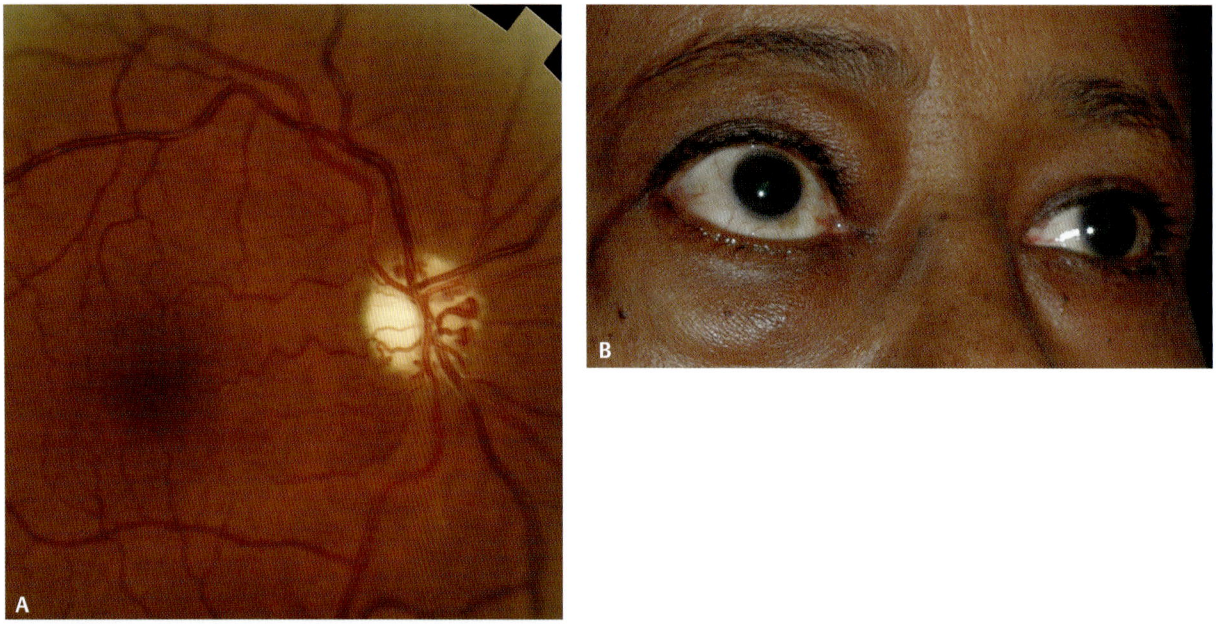

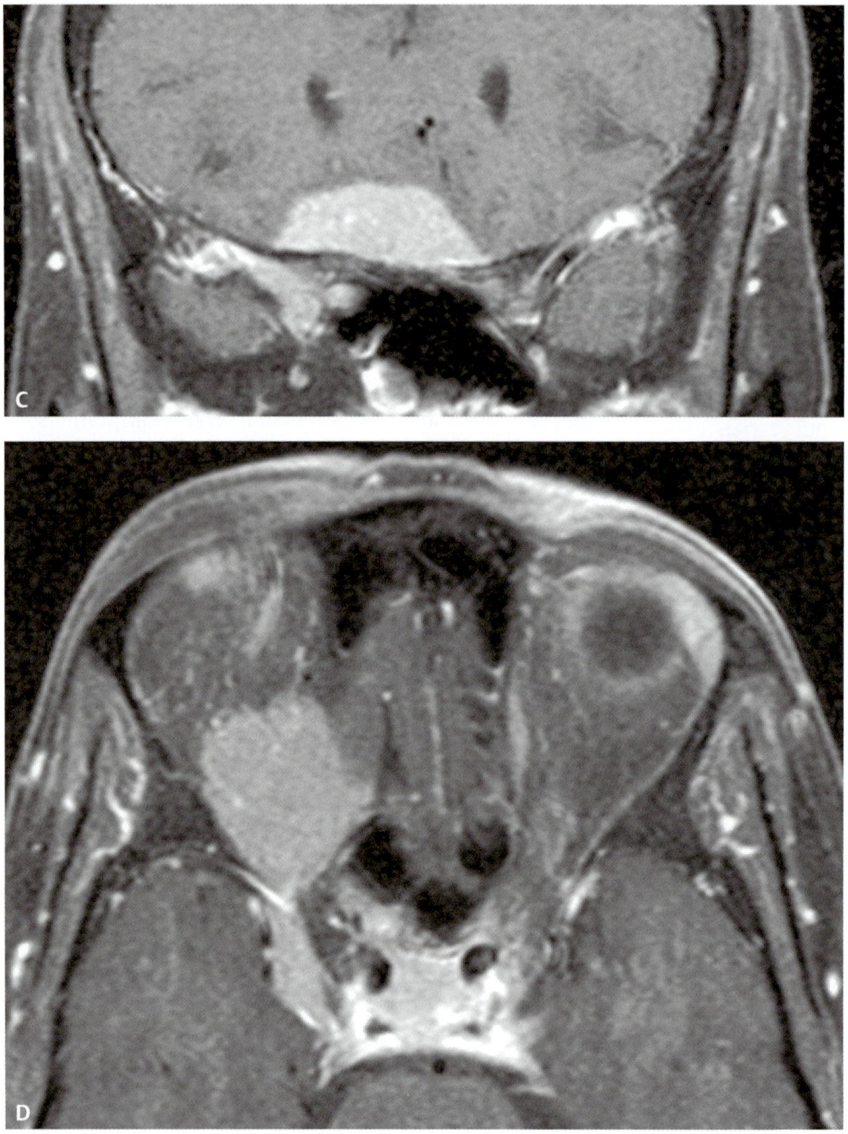

Fig. 5.1 Photo of the right fundus **(A)** of a 54-year-old woman who presented with a 7-year history of progressively decreased vision in the right eye. When evaluated, she had no light perception in the right eye and 9 mm of proptosis **(B)**. MRI reveals evidence of a skull base meningioma involving the tuberculum **(C)** and invading the orbit **(D)**, producing the optociliary shunt vessels indicated in the fundus **(A)**. Comment: Optociliary shunt vessels are pathophysiologically associated with compromise of the central retinal venous outflow. They are most commonly seen with central retinal vein occlusion but when associated with optic atrophy may be due to an optic nerve sheath meningioma or a parasellar meningioma invading the orbit.

of dura, the falciform ligament. Pathology that elevates the optic nerve can thus compress the superior portion of the nerve, resulting in an inferior visual field defect. The intracranial portion of the optic nerve (uncovered by any dural sheath) is usually approximately 10 mm. The chiasm is variably placed, so that in the case of a preplaced chiasm, there may be a much shorter distance from the exit of the canal to the beginning of the chiasm. Similarly, in a relatively postplaced chiasm, the intracranial portion of the optic nerve may be longer, such that the chiasm actually rests posterior to as well as superior to the sella. This variability is responsible for the spectrum of clinical manifestations seen in suprasellar tumor involvement. In the setting of a relatively postplaced chiasm, tumors or other mass lesions of the parasellar region often involve the optic nerve, producing central scotomas and arcuate visual field defects (**Fig. 5.2**). In the setting of a preplaced chiasm, tumors that arise from the sella can compress the optic tract, producing homonymous visual field defects.[17]

The optic nerves meet and create the chiasm, which lies variably above the level of the sella. Because more of the pupillary fibers in the anterior visual pathways cross than do not cross, pathology affecting the optic tract may produce a contralateral afferent pupillary defect[28] (**Fig. 5.3**). Damage to the tract may have a second distinguishing characteristic (not seen in cortical or optic radiation pathology) because retrograde degeneration will result in band (or bowtie) atrophy in the contralateral optic nerve head. It should be noted that this takes weeks to months to occur and will not be seen in the setting of an acute tract lesion, whereas the contralateral afferent pupillary defect develops immediately.

The chiasm is usually inclined at about a 45-degree angle, so that pathology arising from the sella most frequently affects the anterior and inferior aspects of the chiasm, first producing the characteristic superior bitemporal visual field defects seen in most patients with suprasellar pathology[29,30] (**Fig. 5.4**). The macular fibers tend to cross more posteriorly within the chiasm, and involvement of the posterior chiasm or the anterior third ventricle can result in relatively bitemporal scotomatous defects or bitemporal inferior field defects (**Fig. 5.5**).

Recent studies have suggested that the looping of the crossing fibers into the contralateral optic nerve, described in earlier anatomy texts, is an artifact of the patients who were in the original studies (following enucleation or loss of an eye).[31] Even though the so-called Wilbrand knee[32] is probably an artifact, pathology that affects the optic nerve just anterior to the chiasm often produces a central scotoma with a relative temporal defect in the opposite eye. This, therefore, remains a useful localizing sign. Rarely, a lesion may compress the optic nerve without touching the anterior chiasm. This can produce a unilateral temporal field defect, referred to as the junctional syndrome of Traquair.[33] Involvement of the posterior aspect of the chiasm is potentially seen with craniopharyngiomas or other pathology affecting the pituitary stalk, including sarcoid, histiocytosis, and germinomas. Even with posterior chiasmal compression, however, the majority of lesions are pituitary tumors because these are simply much more common.

Efferent System

The efferent visual pathways originate within the horizontal and vertical gaze centers, located within the pons and midbrain, respectively. The horizontal gaze center itself is actually within the abducens nerve nucleus, although the burst cells, which are within the paramedian pontine reticular formation, generate horizontal saccades. Pathologic involvement of the horizontal gaze center results in absence of gaze to that side. The opposite eye can still adduct owing to convergent triggering of the medial rectus in the area of the midbrain.

The vertical gaze centers are located within the dorsal rostral midbrain tegmentum. A set of three nuclei (the rostral interstitial nucleus of the medial longitudinal fasciculus [MLF], the interstitial nucleus of Cajal, and the nucleus of Darkschewitsch) are responsible for coordinating vertical gaze movements. Compression of the dorsal portion of the midbrain,[34] such as is seen with extension of lesions of the pineal gland, can result in a classic dorsal midbrain syndrome, with absent up gaze, retraction convergence nystagmus, Collier's sign of lid retraction, and light near dissociation due to involvement of the pupillary crossing fibers in the posterior commissure.[35] Seesaw nystagmus is a rare finding in patients with parasellar lesions that extend to compress the midbrain.[36] In this, one eye will elevate and intort, while the other eye depresses and extorts. This pattern then reverses.

Signals from the horizontal and vertical gaze centers travel to the extraocular muscles via the third (oculomotor), fourth (trochlear), and sixth (abducens) cranial nerves. The sixth nerve exits the pontine brainstem to run in the subarachnoid space up the clivus. It pierces the dura and enters Dorello's canal underneath the petroclinoid ligament (in conjunction with the inferior petrosal sinus), entering into the body of the cavernous sinus, where it crosses next to the carotid artery. The sympathetic fibers in the wall of the carotid artery leave the carotid within the cavernous sinus in conjunction with the sixth nerve to run more anteriorly before entering the superior orbital fissure along with branches of the first division of the fifth cranial nerve (nasociliary branch).[37] The sixth nerve enters through the superior orbital fissure within the annulus of Zinn to innervate the lateral rectus muscle approximately one-third of the way anteriorly along its medial surface.

The fourth, or trochlear, nerve nucleus is located just caudal to the third nerve nuclear complex within the tegmentum of the midbrain. Its branches run dorsally to cross in the superior medullary velum. It is the only cranial nerve that exits the brain dorsally and has the longest unprotected course in the subarachnoid space. It runs around the midbrain and travels along the edge of the tentorium anteriorly to enter the lateral wall of the cavernous sinus between the third nerve above it and the first division of the fifth nerve below it. The fourth nerve can be easily injured when the tentorium is opened (**Fig. 5.6**). The trochlear nerve is the only motor nerve that runs outside the annulus of Zinn, crossing over the optic nerve to innervate the superior oblique muscle approximately one-third along its course. Surgery to reach the optic nerve through the superior orbit can damage the trochlear nerve as it crosses in the orbital apex.

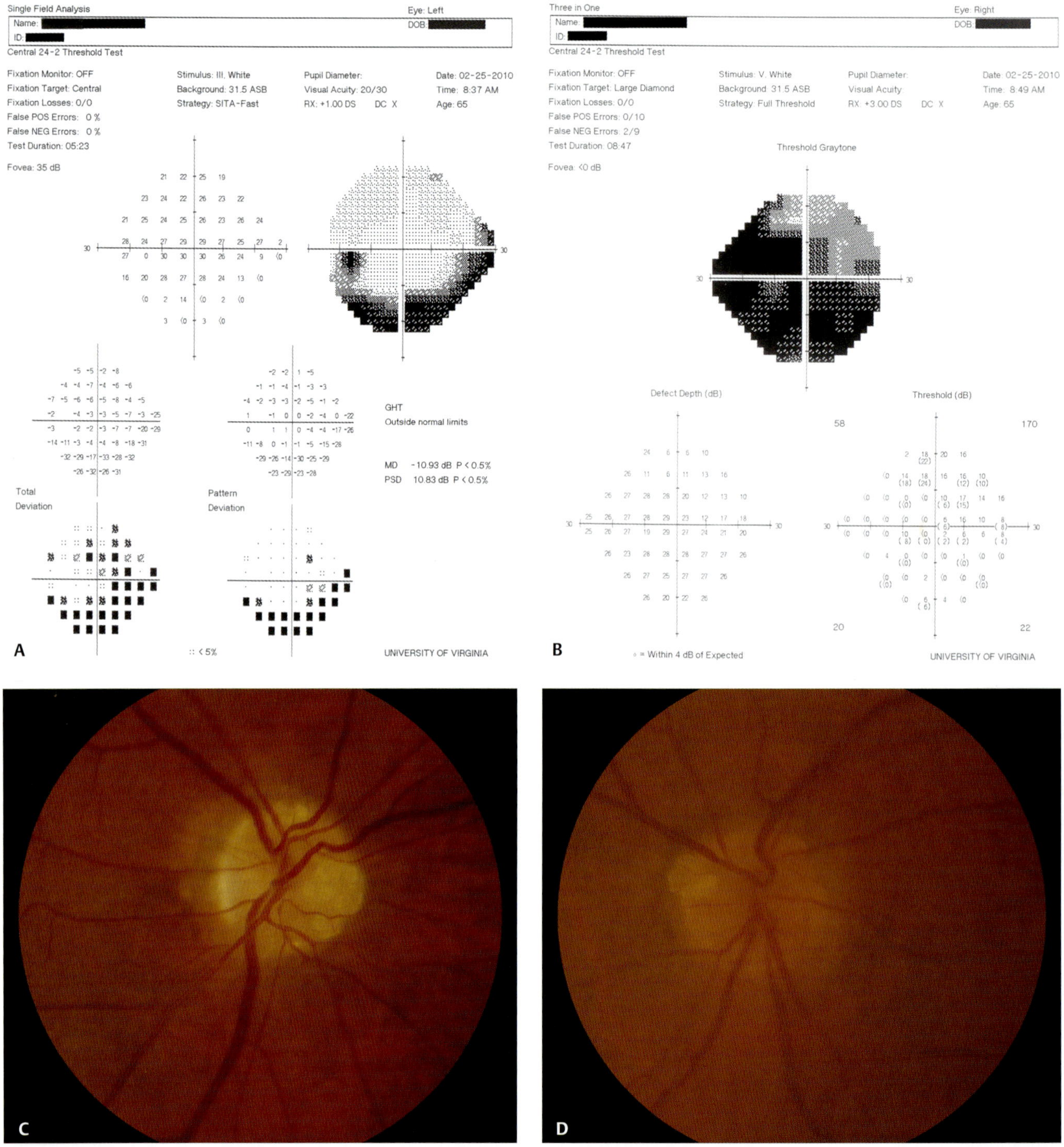

Fig. 5.2 The fields **(A,B)** of a 65-year-old woman who presented with a 1-year history of progressive visual loss in the right eye. Visual acuity was 2/200 OD and 20/30 OS with a >1.8 log unit right afferent papillary defect. The right field **(B)** demonstrates a central scotoma, and the left field **(A)** demonstrates an inferior arcuate defect. Her funduscopic examination **(C,D)** revealed evidence of drusen of the optic nerve heads bilaterally with relative optic atrophy OD > OS. The view on the right **(C)** was much better than the view on the left **(D)** because she had had her cataract on the right side removed. The arcuate changes on the left eye were compatible with the buried drusen, and the difference between the total deviation plot and the pattern deviation plot was presumably related to her cataract.

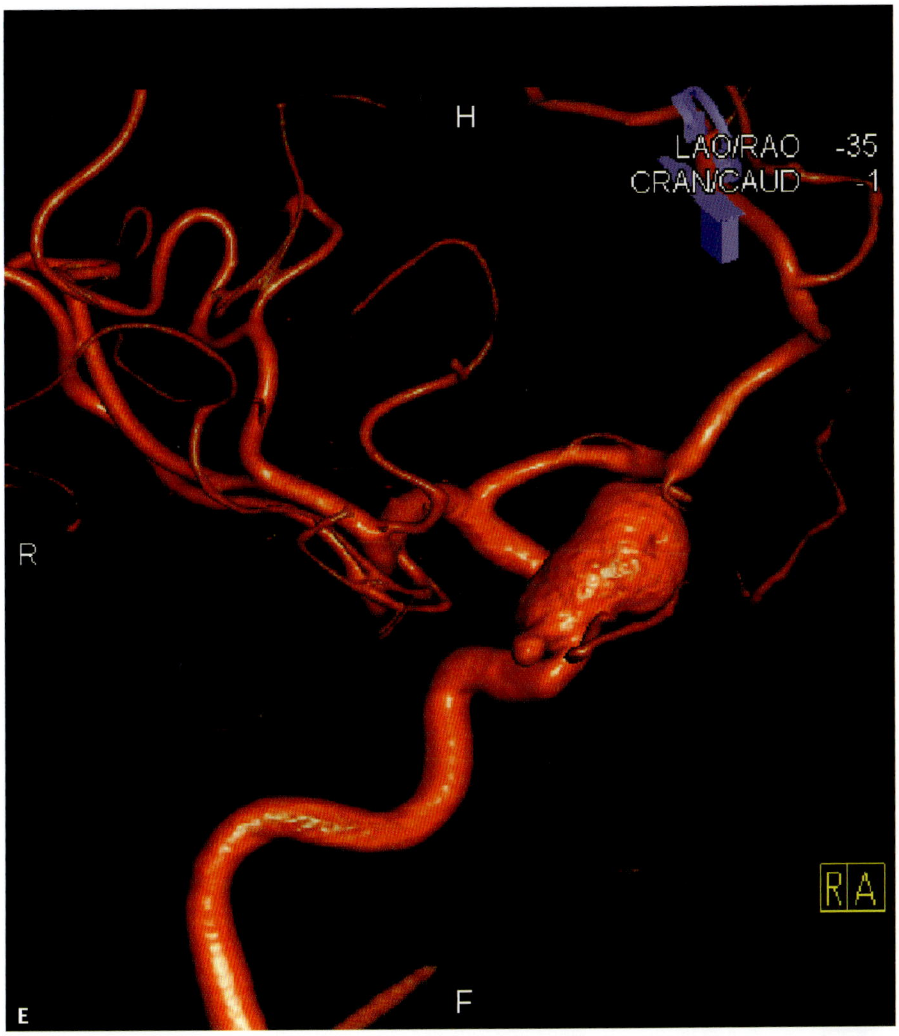

Fig. 5.2 *(Continued)* The central scotoma in the right eye, however, could not be explained by the optic nerve head drusen, and an angiogram revealed evidence of bilateral ophthalmic segment internal carotid artery aneurysms with right optic nerve compression **(E).** Evidence of bilateral optic neuropathies were confirmed on the optical coherence tomogram (OCT), which shows thinning of nerve fiber layer in both eyes **(F).** *(Continued on page 72)*

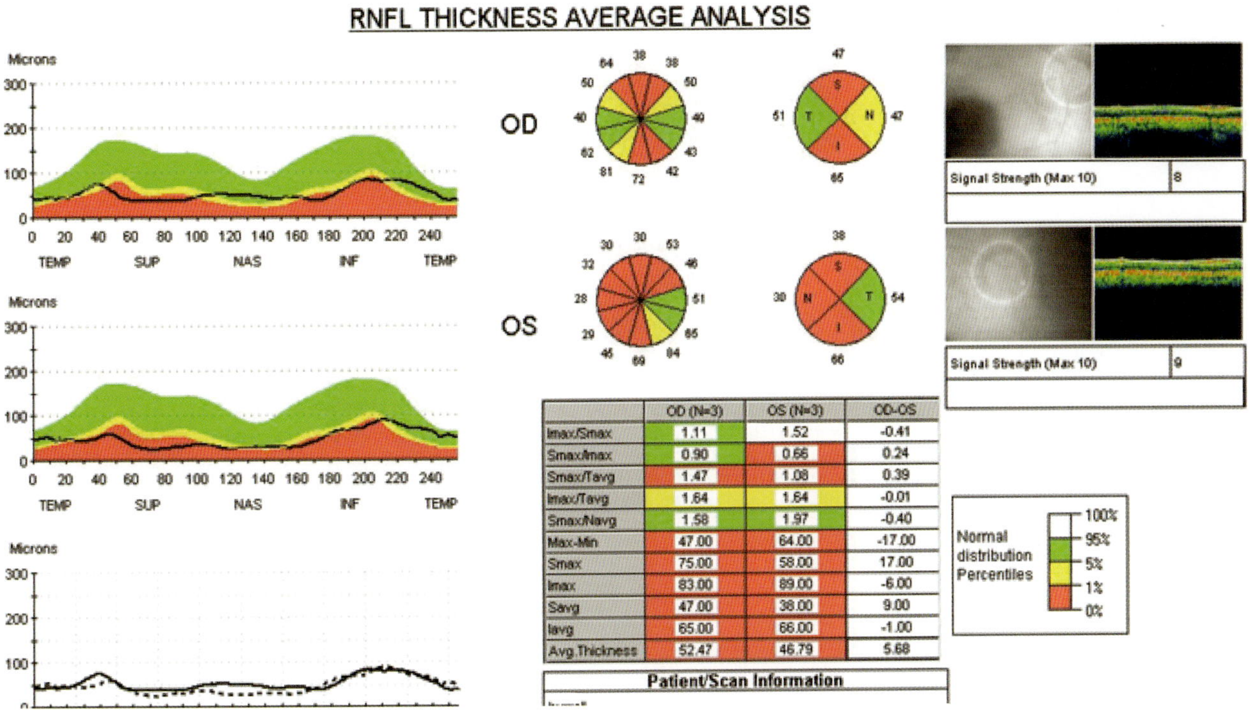

	OD (N=3)	OS (N=3)	OD-OS
Imax/Smax	1.11	1.52	-0.41
Smax/Imax	0.90	0.66	0.24
Smax/Tavg	1.47	1.08	0.39
Imax/Tavg	1.64	1.64	-0.01
Smax/Navg	1.58	1.97	-0.40
Max-Min	47.00	64.00	-17.00
Smax	75.00	58.00	17.00
Imax	83.00	89.00	-6.00
Savg	47.00	38.00	9.00
Iavg	65.00	66.00	-1.00
Avg.Thickness	52.47	46.79	5.68

F

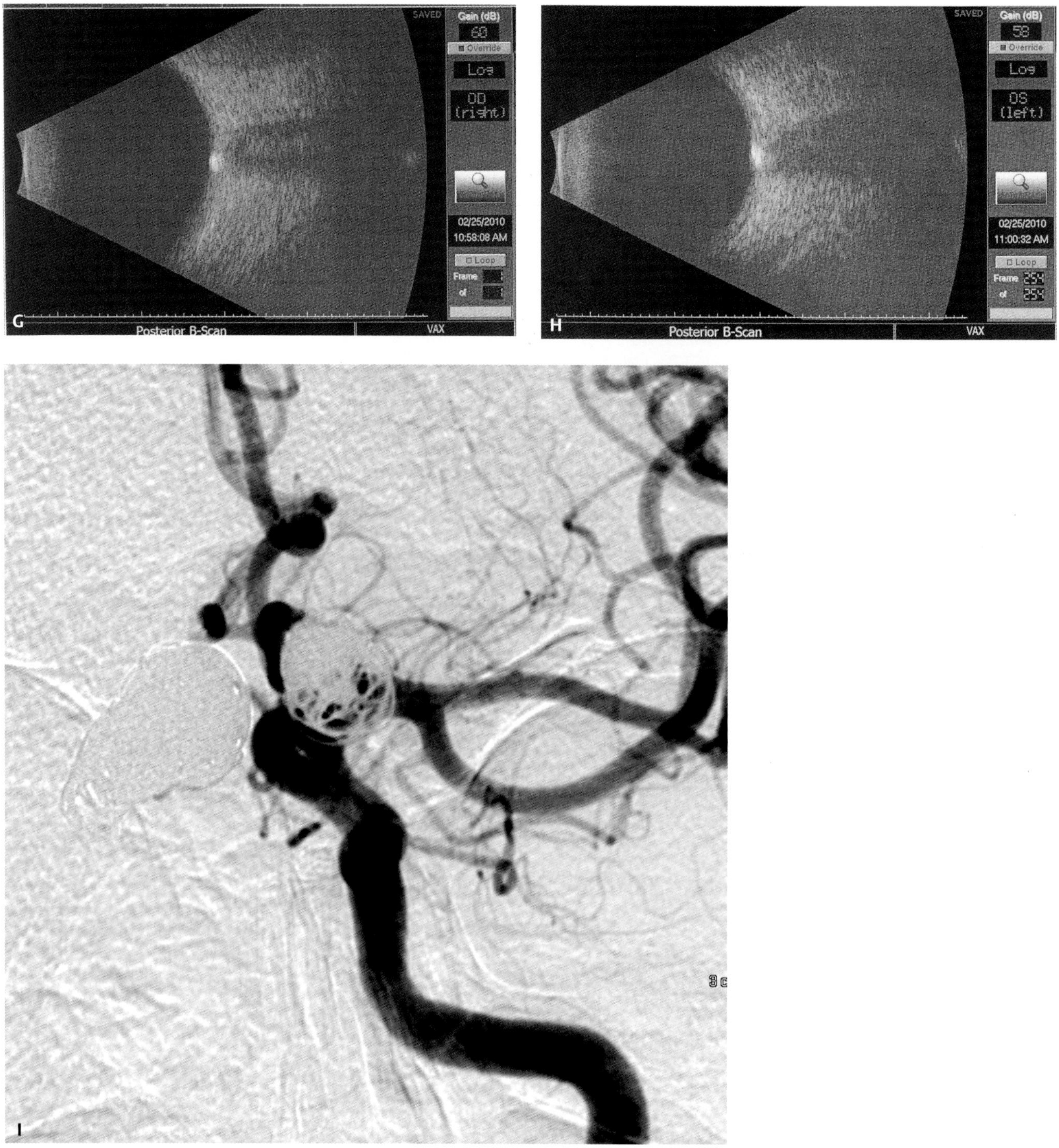

Fig. 5.2 *(Continued)* B-scan reveals hyperrefractile bodies in the optic nerve head **(G,H)**, demonstrating that this is optic nerve head drusen, not papilledema. She underwent stenting and coil embolization of both carotid aneurysms **(I)** with stabilization of her visual function. Comment: Although central scotomas are most commonly associated with macular disease, certain optic neuropathies often cause central loss of vision. Rare causes include nutritional, toxic, and hereditary (Leber) optic neuropathies. Inflammatory and compressive lesions are more common causes of visual loss. In this case, a paraclinoid aneurysm compressed the right optic nerve, producing visual loss and a central scotoma. B-scan of the optic nerve head can help distinguish papilledema (disc elevation due to increased intracranial pressure) from optic nerve head drusen.

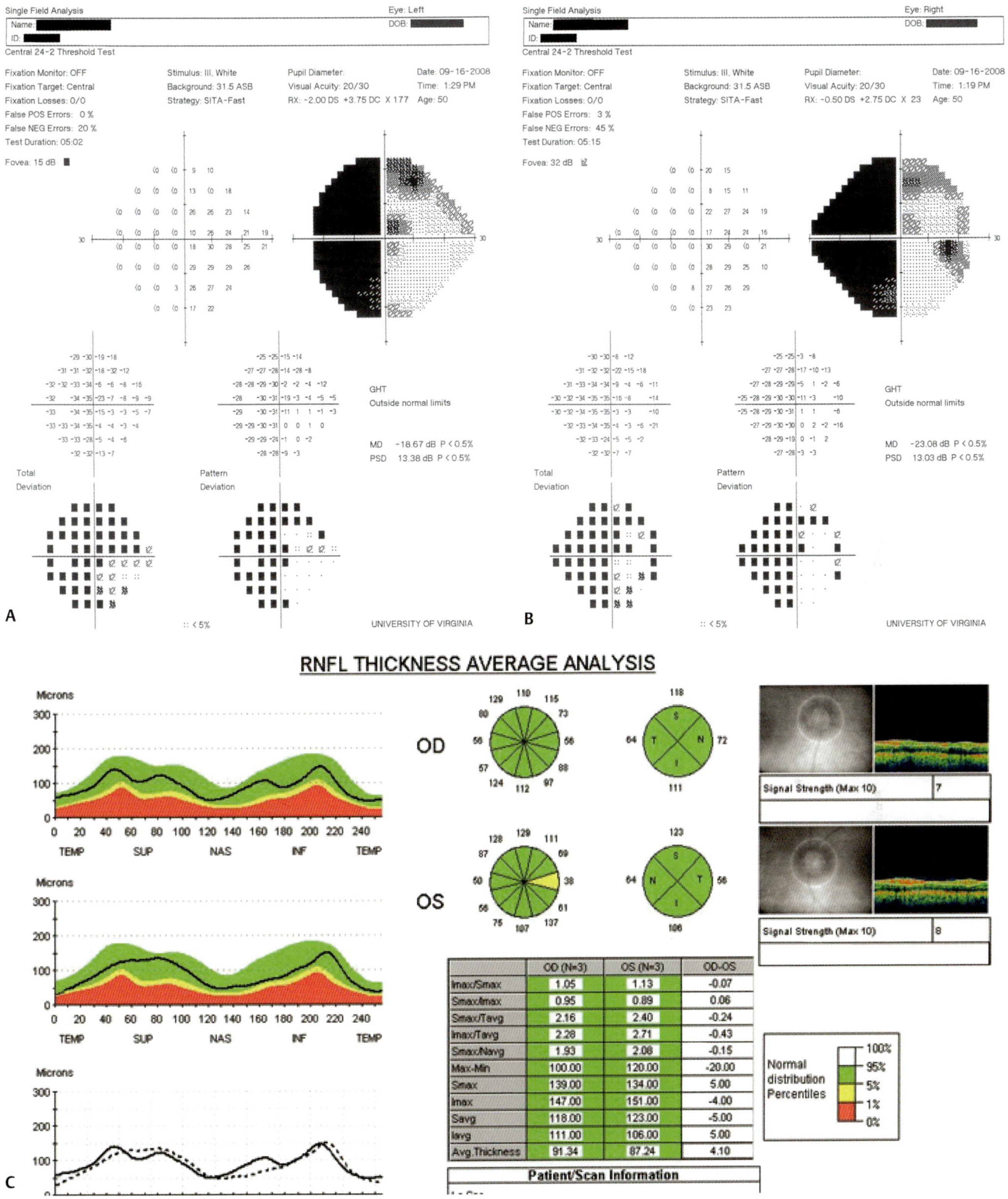

Fig. 5.3 This 50-year-old patient was referred in September of 2008. Seventeen months earlier, she had developed a "funny smell" and was seen by her local doctor, who ordered MRI. This revealed evidence of a right temporal lobe lesion, and she underwent a craniotomy in May of 2007 (16 months before her evaluation) with subtotal resection of a high-grade glioma. Three days before her referral, she had noticed increasing problems seeing to the side. Visual fields reveal a fairly dense left homonymous hemianopsia **(A,B)**. Visual acuity was preserved with 20/30 vision at distance and 4-point vision at near. She did, however, have a 0.9 log unit left afferent pupillary defect, indicating involvement of the right optic tract, which produced the left homonymous hemianopsia. Her discs at that time looked normal, and an optical coherence tomogram (OCT) of her nerve fiber layer also looked entirely normal **(C)**. *(Continued on page 74)*

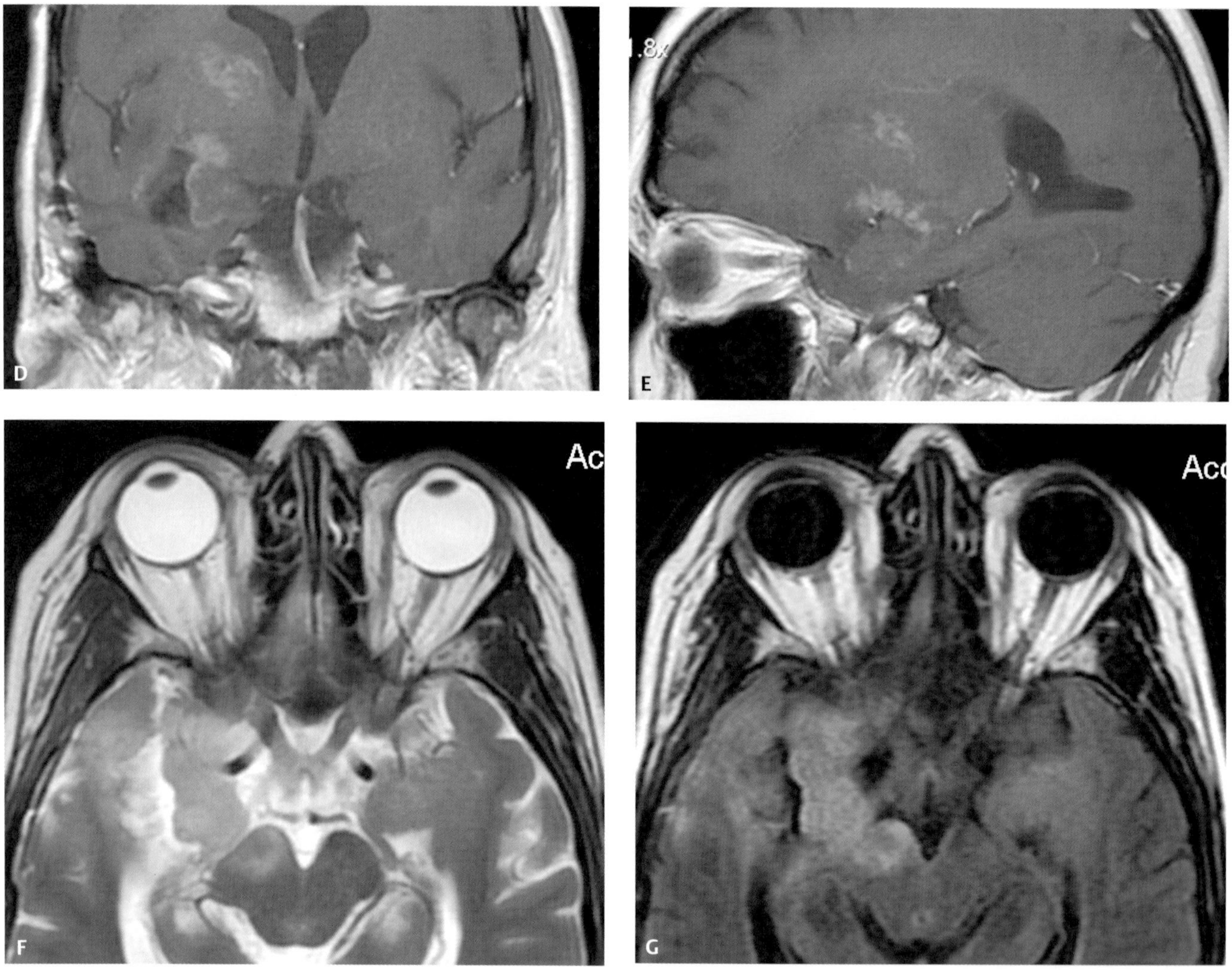

Fig. 5.3 *(Continued)* This 50-year-old patient was referred in September of 2008. Seventeen months earlier, she had developed a “funny smell” and was seen by her local doctor, who ordered MRI. This revealed evidence of a right temporal lobe lesion, and she underwent a craniotomy in May of 2007 (16 months before her evaluation) with subtotal resection of a high-grade glioma. Three days before her referral, she had noticed increasing problems seeing to the side. Repeat scan at this time revealed a lesion extending from the temporal lobe to involve the basal ganglia as well as the right optic tract **(D–G)**. Three months later, she returned with visual acuity down to 1/200 in the right eye and 20/30 in the left. She now had a dense left homonymous hemianopsia. Her afferent pupillary defect had increased to 1.8 log unit.

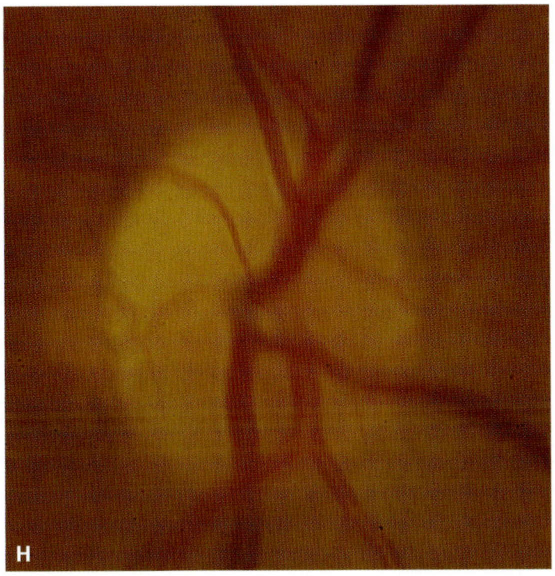

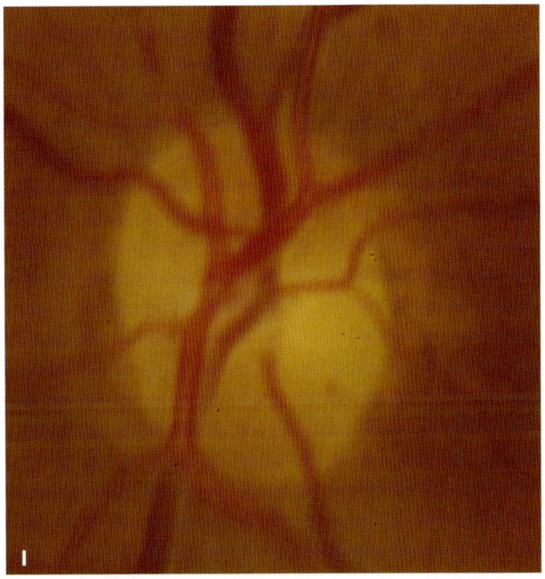

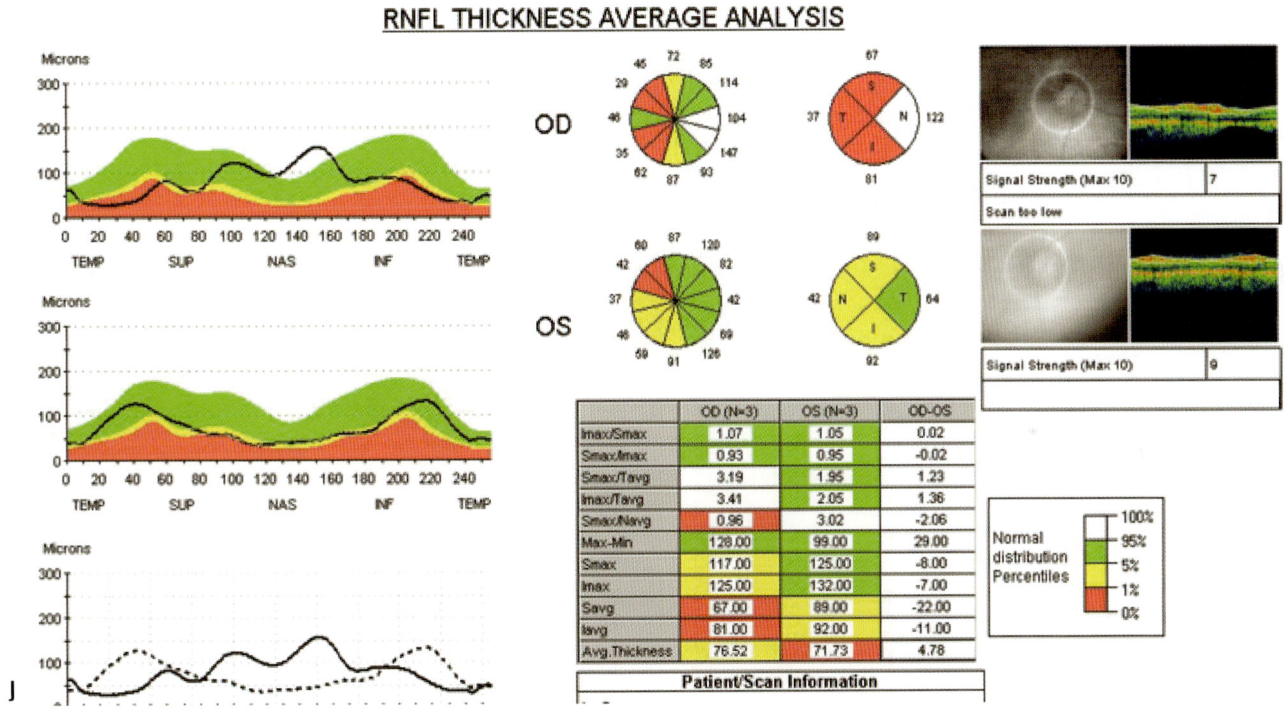

Fig. 5.3 *(Continued)* This 50-year-old patient was referred in September of 2008. Seventeen months earlier, she had developed a "funny smell" and was seen by her local doctor, who ordered MRI. This revealed evidence of a right temporal lobe lesion, and she underwent a craniotomy in May of 2007 (16 months before her evaluation) with subtotal resection of a high-grade glioma. Three days before her referral, she had noticed increasing problems seeing to the side. Three months later, she returned with visual acuity down to 1/200 in the right eye and 20/30 in the left. She now had a dense left homonymous hemianopsia. Her afferent pupillary defect had increased to 1.8 log unit. Although her optic discs did demonstrate some subtle optic atrophy, OD **(H)** greater than OS **(I)**, the progressive damage to the anterior visual pathways could be better seen in her OCT, which showed severe thinning of the nerve fiber layer on the right side and moderate thinning of the nerve fiber layer on the left **(J)**. Comment: Optic tract involvement may be suspected when there is an afferent pupillary defect on the same side as the visual defect. OCT, by giving us an in vivo biopsy, is a more quantitative way of assessing damage to the anterior afferent visual pathways. Although it is likely that when we first saw her she already had ongoing damage to the optic tract, there is a delay in the development of thinning of the nerve fiber layer and subsequent optic atrophy. The quantitation of her afferent pupillary defect also demonstrated progression, indicating involvement not only of the right optic tract but also subsequently of the right optic nerve in this patient with an aggressive glioblastoma.

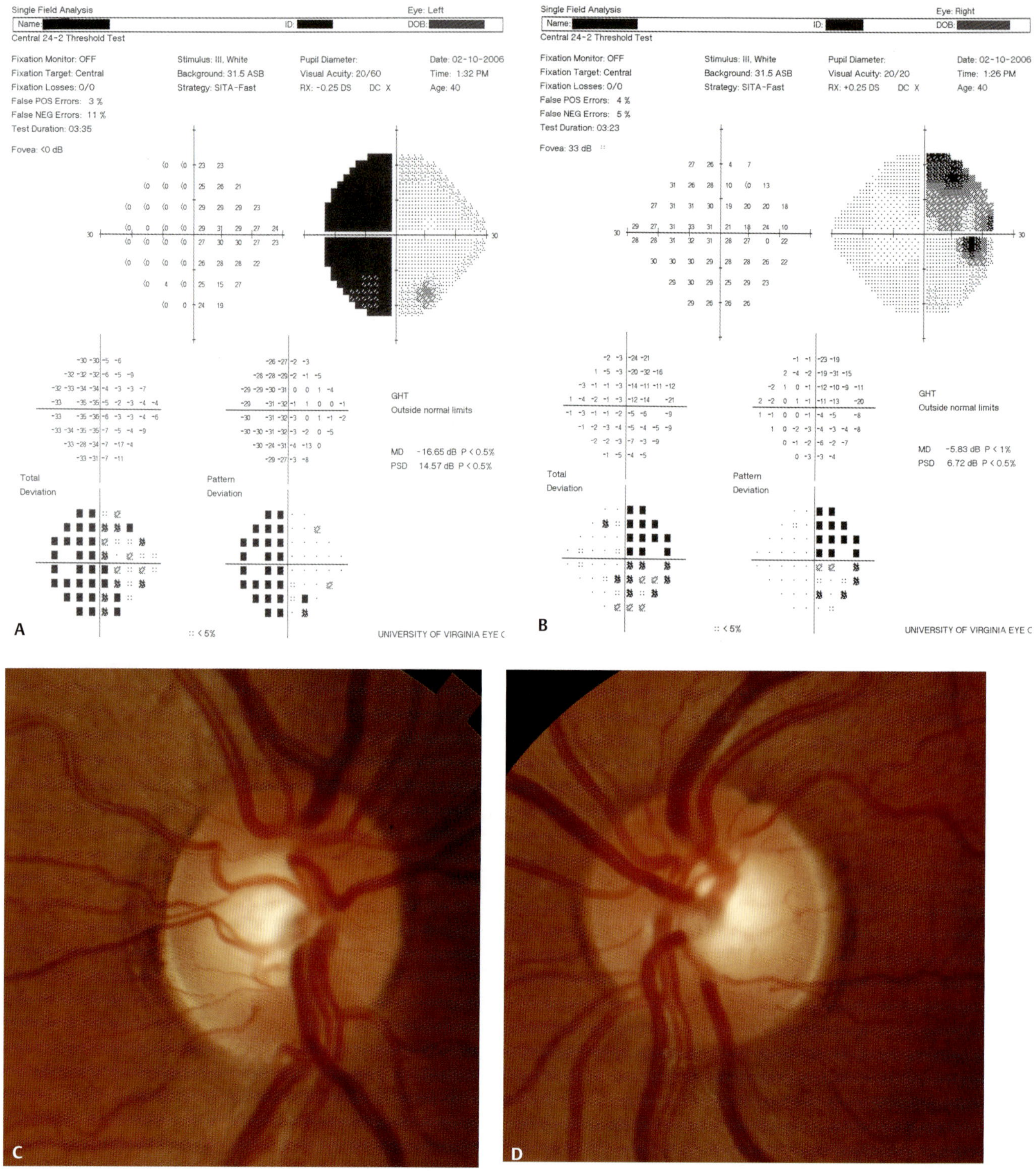

Fig. 5.4 This 40-year-old woman presented with a 3-week history of headaches and 2 weeks of blurred vision. Visual acuity was found to be 20/40 and 20/200 with near vision of 4 point and 26 point. Her visual fields revealed asymmetric bitemporal visual field defect **(A,B)**. Interestingly, her discs really did not look that abnormal **(C,D)**, and her optical coherence tomogram (OCT) showed normal nerve fiber layer thickness **(E)**.

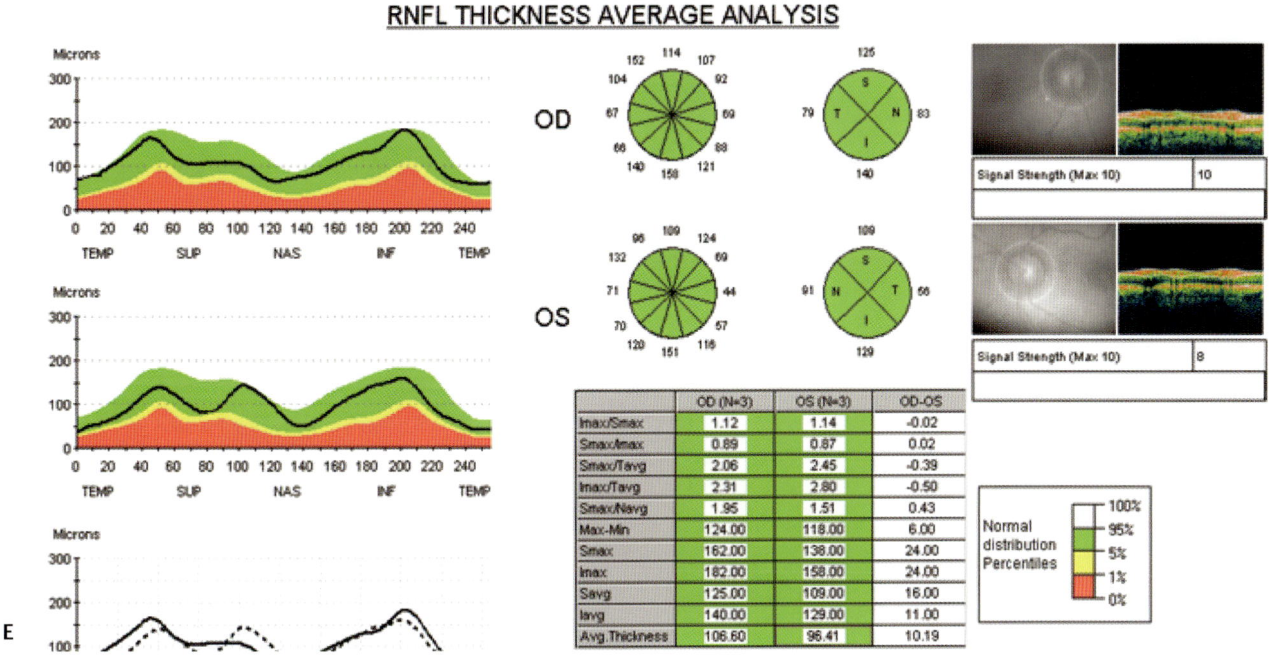

	OD (N=3)	OS (N=3)	OD-OS
Imax/Smax	1.12	1.14	-0.02
Smax/Imax	0.89	0.87	0.02
Smax/Tavg	2.06	2.45	-0.39
Imax/Tavg	2.31	2.80	-0.50
Smax/Navg	1.95	1.51	0.43
Max-Min	124.00	118.00	6.00
Smax	162.00	138.00	24.00
Imax	182.00	158.00	24.00
Savg	125.00	109.00	16.00
Iavg	140.00	129.00	11.00
Avg.Thickness	106.60	96.41	10.19

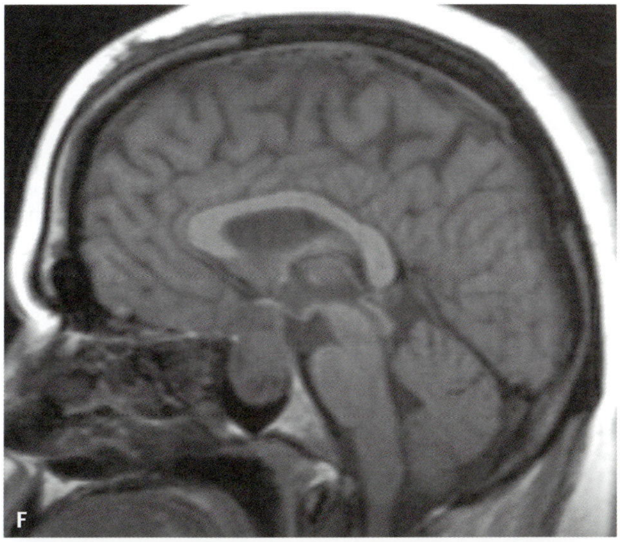

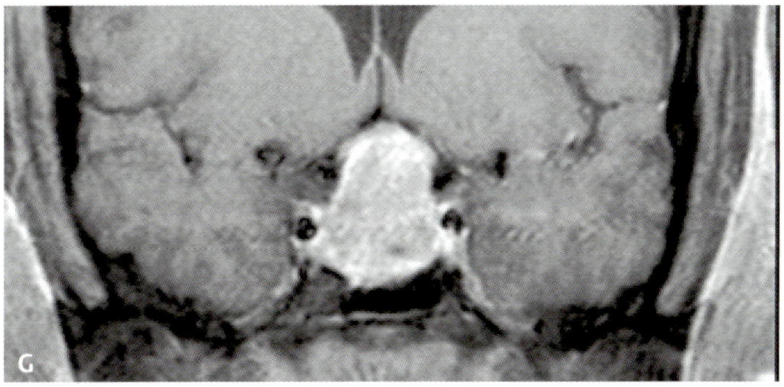

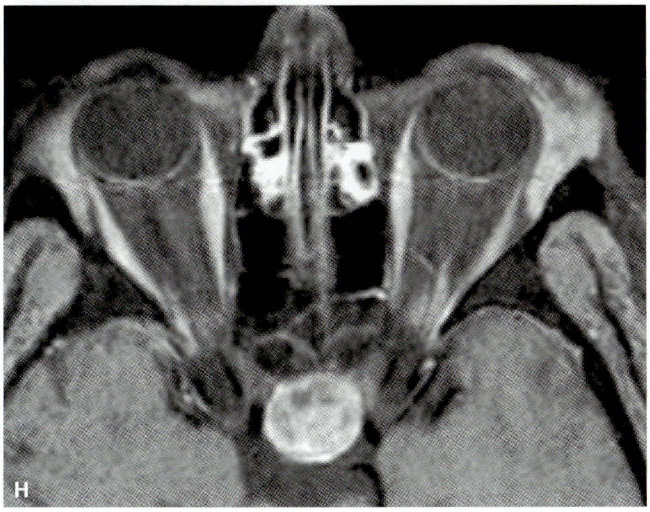

Fig. 5.4 *(Continued)* This 40-year-old woman presented with a 3-week history of headaches and 2 weeks of blurred vision. Visual acuity was found to be 20/40 and 20/200 with near vision of 4 points and 26 points. Interestingly, her discs really did not look that abnormal **(C,D)**, and her optical coherence tomogram (OCT) showed normal nerve fiber layer thickness **(E)**. Her MRI revealed a suprasellar mass lesion compressing the chiasm **(F–H)**. *(Continued on page 78)*

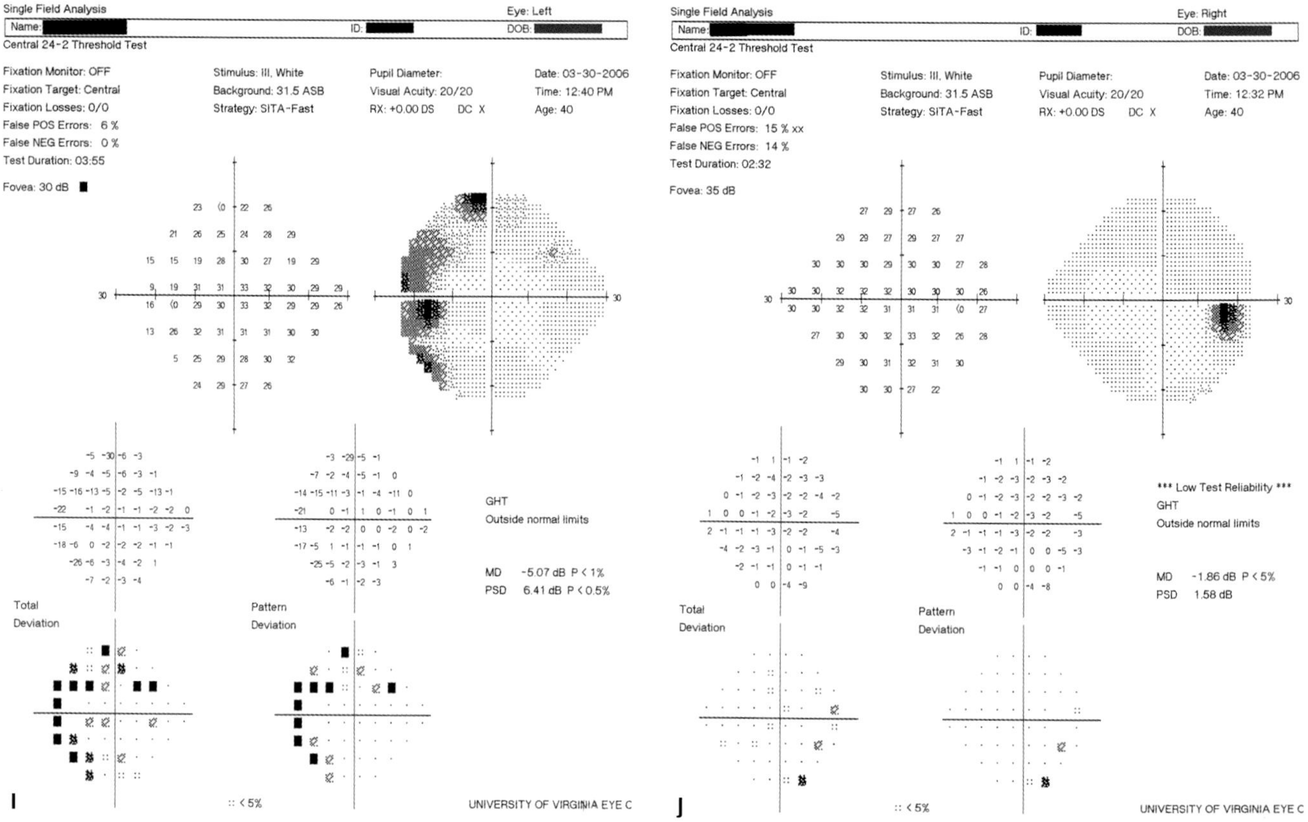

Fig. 5.4 *(Continued)* This 40-year-old woman presented with a 3-week history of headaches and 2 weeks of blurred vision. Visual acuity was found to be 20/40 and 20/200 with near vision of 4 points and 26 points. Her prolactin was elevated at 739 ng/mL. She was started on cabergoline (Dostinex) 0.5-mg tablets twice a week, and 6 weeks later she had dramatic improvement in automated static perimetry **(I,J)**. Comment: Superior bitemporal defects are the most common chiasmal syndrome due to compression of the anterior inferior chiasm by a lesion arising from the sella. Elevated prolactin indicated a prolactinoma, which responded well to medical treatment with cabergoline. Quantitative improvement in perimetry is common with medical or surgical decompression of the chiasm. The normal OCT indicated that the compression was probably not long-standing and might be a good prognostic indicator for visual recovery.

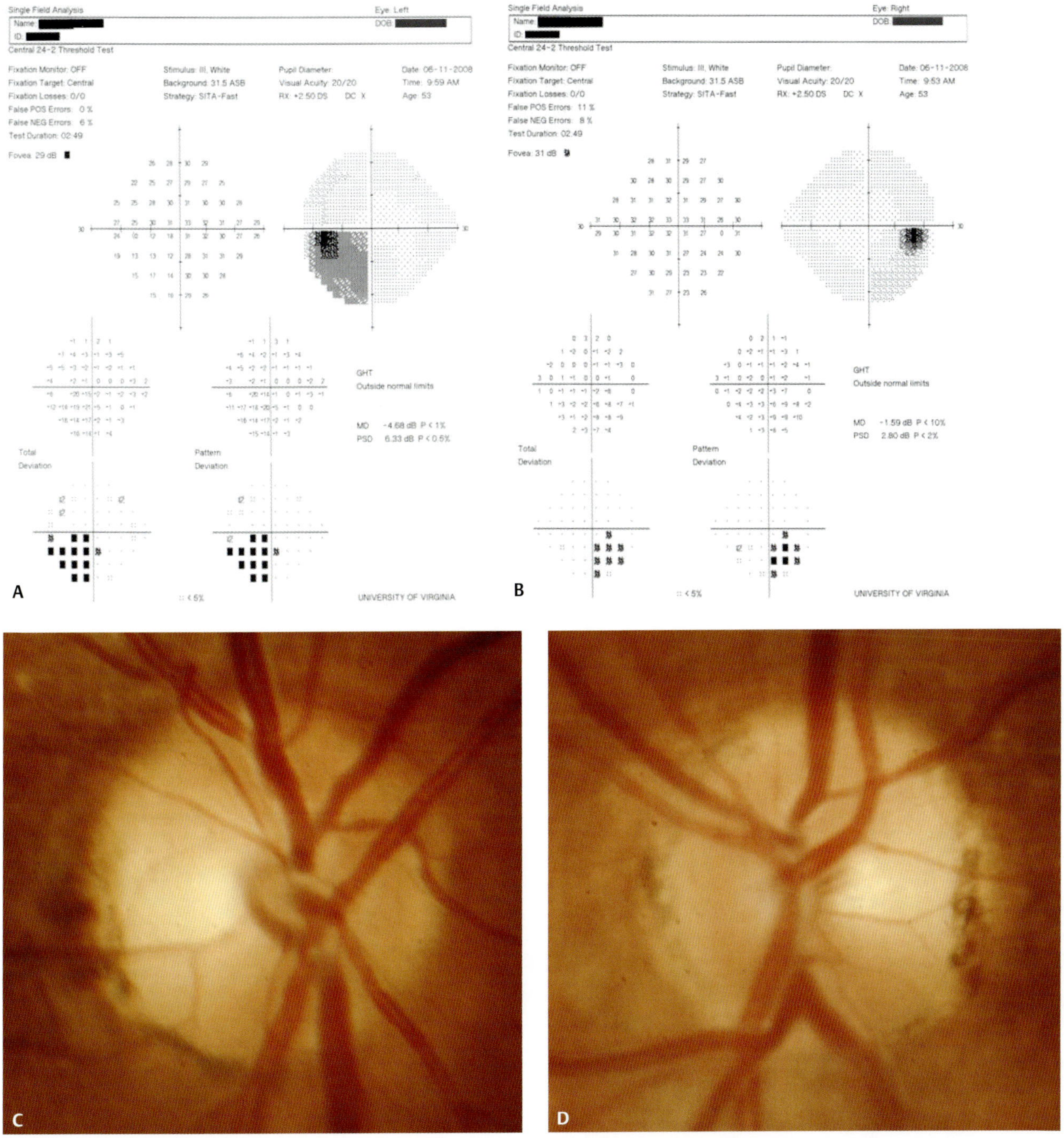

Fig. 5.5 This 53-year-old patient was referred to the neuro-ophthalmology office because of “another tumor.” Her visual fields demonstrated an inferior bitemporal visual field defect **(A,B)**, and her optic discs indicated optic atrophy **(C,D)**. *(Continued on page 80)*

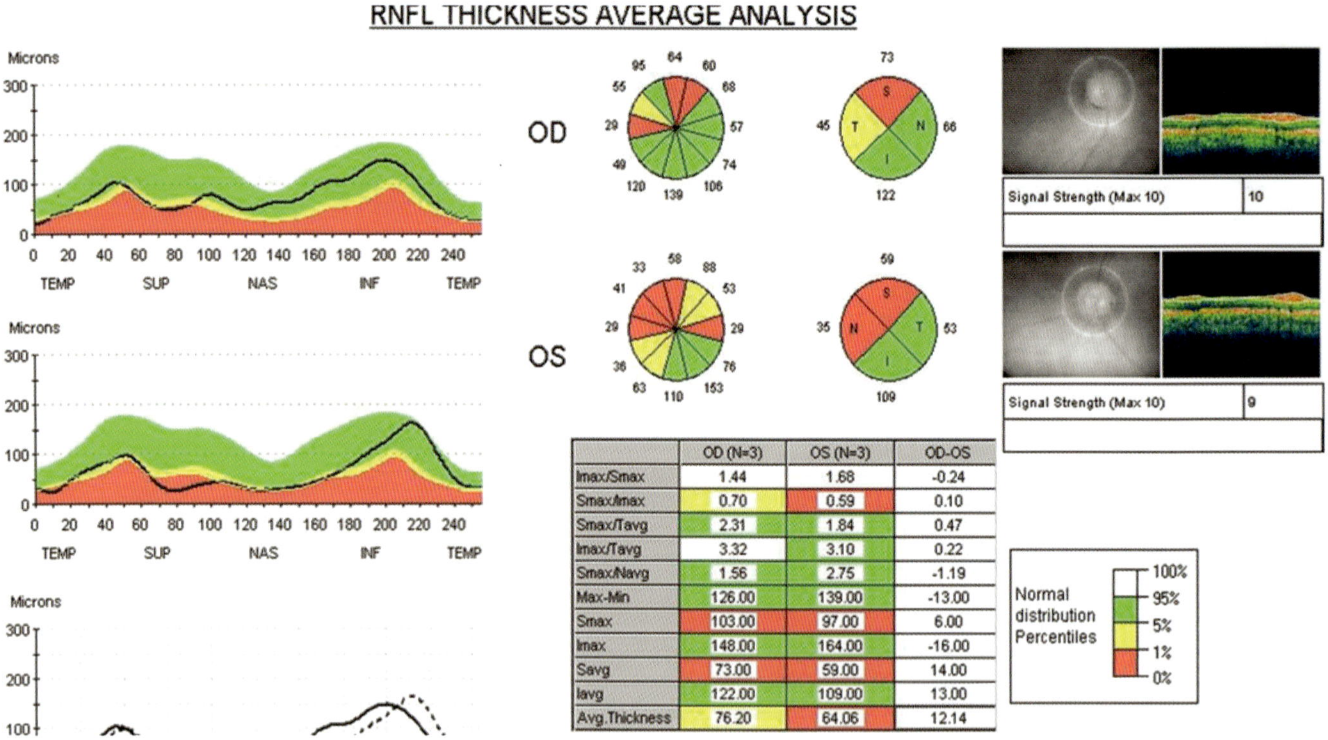

	OD (N=3)	OS (N=3)	OD-OS
Imax/Smax	1.44	1.68	-0.24
Smax/Imax	0.70	0.59	0.10
Smax/Tavg	2.31	1.84	0.47
Imax/Tavg	3.32	3.10	0.22
Smax/Navg	1.56	2.75	-1.19
Max-Min	126.00	139.00	-13.00
Smax	103.00	97.00	6.00
Imax	148.00	164.00	-16.00
Savg	73.00	59.00	14.00
Iavg	122.00	109.00	13.00
Avg.Thickness	76.20	64.06	12.14

E

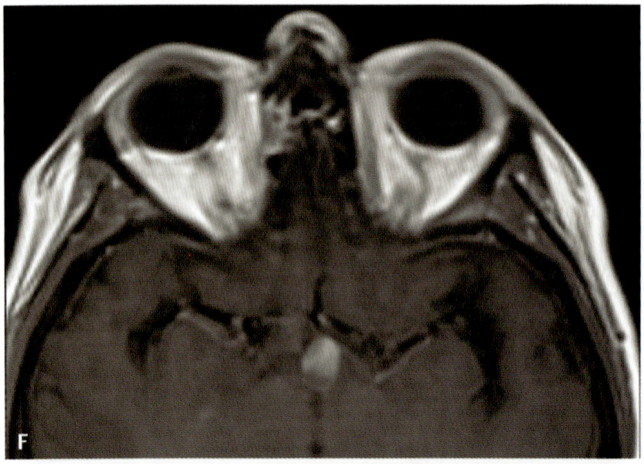

F

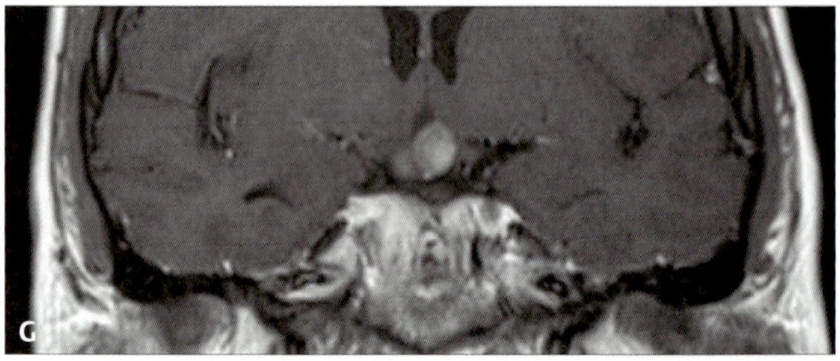

G

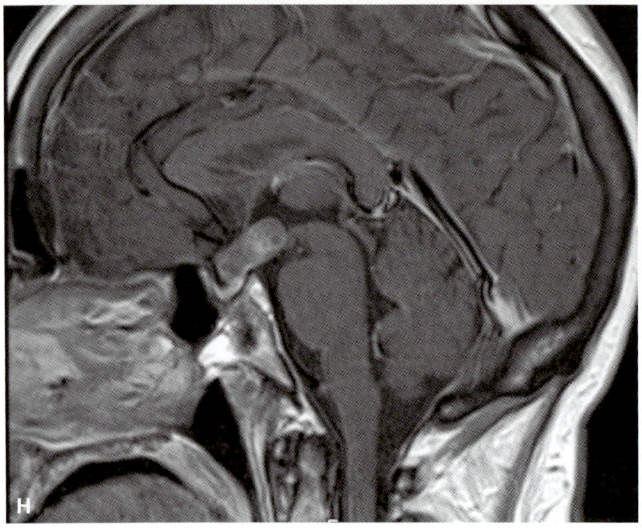

H

Fig. 5.5 *(Continued)* This 53-year-old patient was referred to the neuro-ophthalmology office because of "another tumor." Her optical coherence tomogram (OCT) confirmed the presence of bilateral optic atrophy with nerve fiber bundle dropout, more on the left than the right **(E)**. Her past medical history was remarkable for galactorrhea in 1992. She was found to have an elevated prolactin level and in June of 1995 had undergone transsphenoidal resection of a cystic nonsecretory pituitary tumor. Review of her MRI demonstrated a cystic lesion arising from the sella and compressing the posterior aspect of the chiasm **(F–H)**.

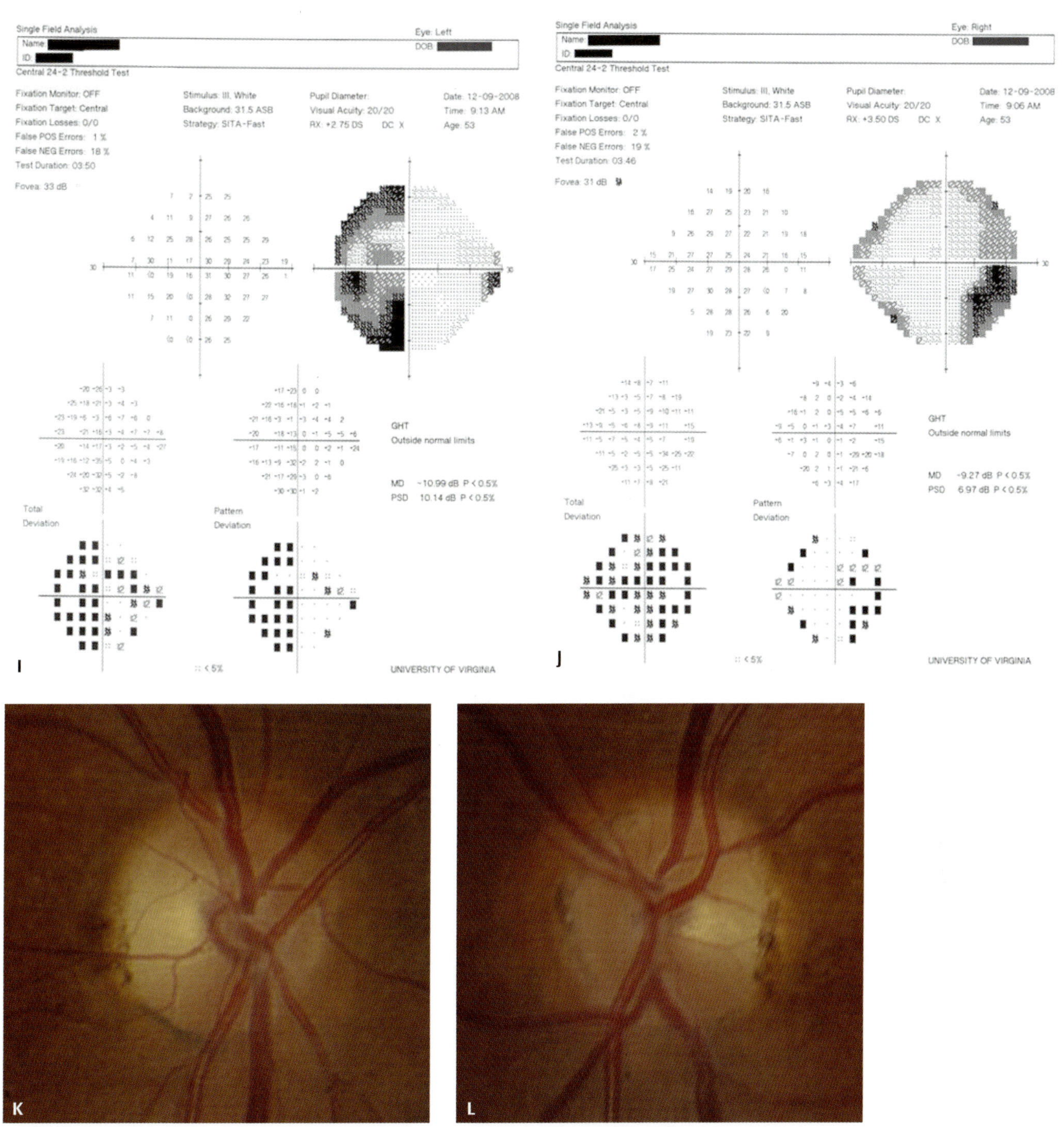

Fig. 5.5 *(Continued)* This 53-year-old patient was referred to the neuro-ophthalmology office because of "another tumor." She returned 6 months later stating that her vision had not changed, but automated static perimetry now demonstrated denser bitemporal visual field defects **(I,J)**, though her discs showed no change **(K,L)**. *(Continued on page 82)*

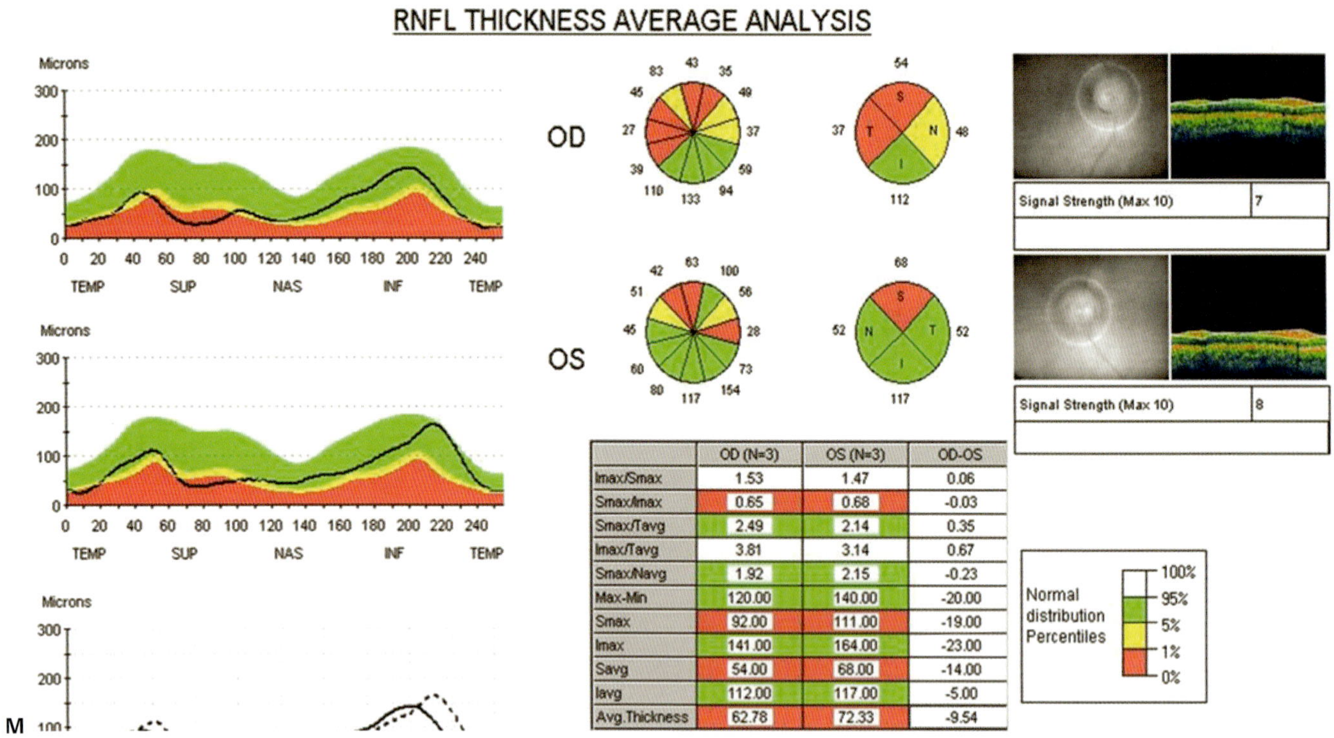

	OD (N=3)	OS (N=3)	OD-OS
Imax/Smax	1.53	1.47	0.06
Smax/Imax	0.65	0.68	-0.03
Smax/Tavg	2.49	2.14	0.35
Imax/Tavg	3.81	3.14	0.67
Smax/Navg	1.92	2.15	-0.23
Max-Min	120.00	140.00	-20.00
Smax	92.00	111.00	-19.00
Imax	141.00	164.00	-23.00
Savg	54.00	68.00	-14.00
Iavg	112.00	117.00	-5.00
Avg.Thickness	62.78	72.33	-9.54

M

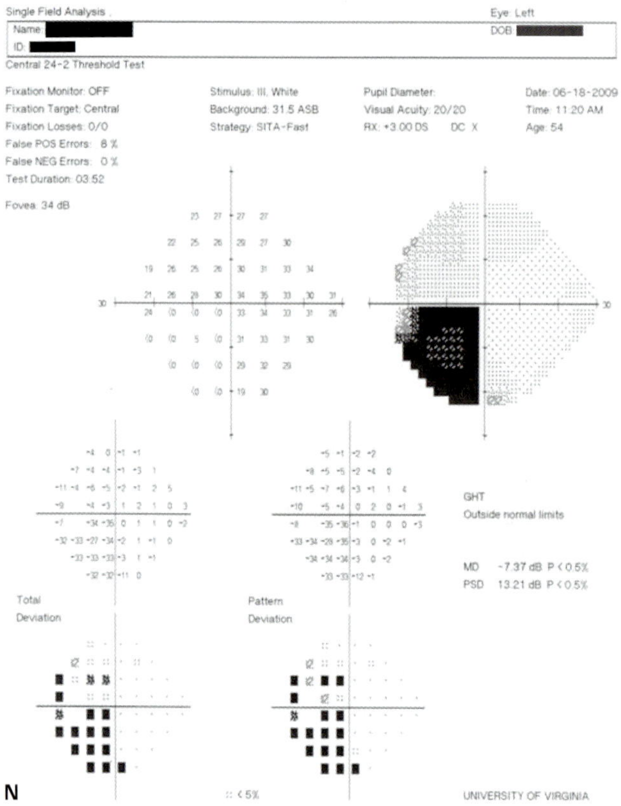

N

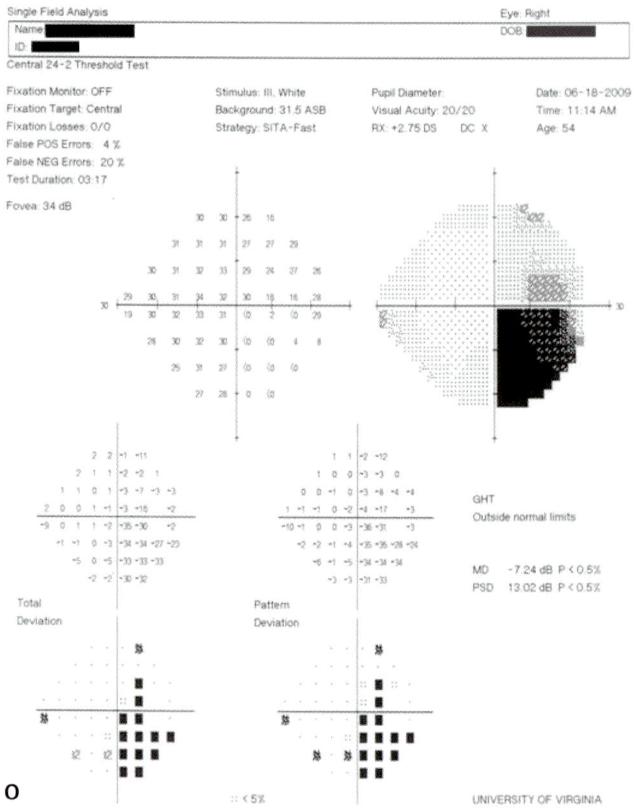

O

Fig. 5.5 *(Continued)* This 53-year-old patient was referred to the neuro-ophthalmology office because of "another tumor." OCT demonstrated further thinning of her nerve fiber layer on the right side **(M)**. She underwent decompression of what pathologically proved to be a Rathke cleft cyst. Within 6 months, her visual fields had improved, although still with a residual bitemporal defect **(N,O)**.

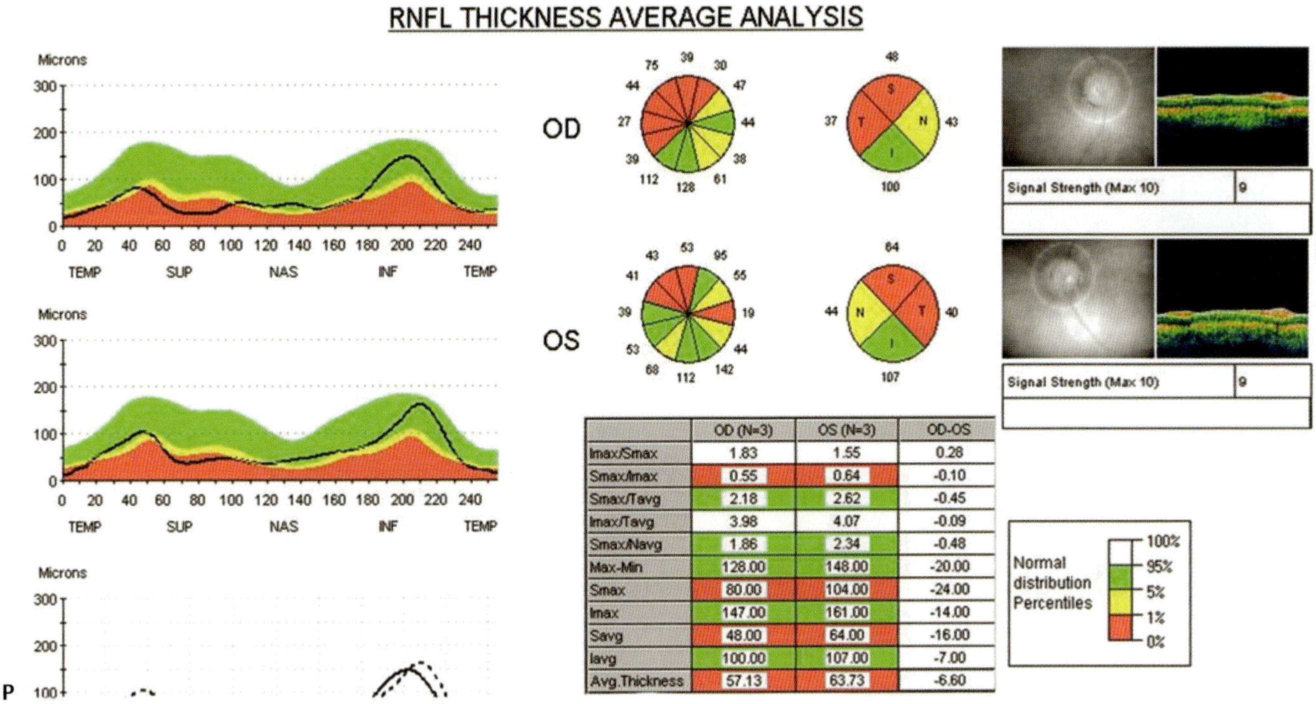

	OD (N=3)	OS (N=3)	OD-OS
Imax/Smax	1.83	1.55	0.28
Smax/Imax	0.55	0.64	-0.10
Smax/Tavg	2.18	2.62	-0.45
Imax/Tavg	3.98	4.07	-0.09
Smax/Navg	1.86	2.34	-0.48
Max-Min	128.00	148.00	-20.00
Smax	80.00	104.00	-24.00
Imax	147.00	161.00	-14.00
Savg	48.00	64.00	-16.00
Iavg	100.00	107.00	-7.00
Avg.Thickness	57.13	63.73	-6.60

Fig. 5.5 *(Continued)* This 53-year-old patient was referred to the neuro-ophthalmology office because of "another tumor." OCT showed still further thinning of her nerve fiber layer **(P)**. Comment: In the setting of a preplaced chiasm or with a posteriorly oriented suprasellar lesion, compression of the posterior aspect of the chiasm produces an inferior bitemporal defect. OCT thinning is delayed, and it is not unusual following decompression for the fields to improve but the OCT to show progressive thinning.

The oculomotor nerve originates within the tegmentum of the midbrain just rostral to the fourth nerve and just caudal to the vertical gaze centers. Several subnuclei make up the oculomotor nucleus, including a single central subnucleus for the levators of both eyes and a pair of subnuclei for the parasympathetics (Edinger-Westphal nuclei) innervating the sphincter of the iris and ciliary body. The superior rectus subnuclei send out fibers that cross over to the opposite side. The medial rectus subnucleus has been divided into several areas and probably has a subsubnucleus responsible for convergence, although this has been poorly identified.

The third nerve exits on the ventral aspect of the midbrain, having passed through the area of the red nucleus, as well as the cortical spinal pathways in the peduncle. There are multiple rootlets as the third nerve exits the brainstem, and the nerve itself passes between the superior cerebellar artery below and the posterior cerebral artery above. The nerve runs parallel to the posterior communicating artery (where it can be affected by an aneurysm) and enters the superior lateral aspect of the cavernous sinus. There is a variable sheath that makes up the inner lateral wall of the cavernous sinus. Within the lateral wall of the cavernous sinus, the third nerve usually divides into a superior and an inferior division. These both enter the superior orbital fissure within the annulus of Zinn. The superior division innervates the superior rectus and levator muscles on their inferior surfaces. The inferior division innervates the medial rectus and the inferior rectus approximately one-third of the way along their inner surfaces and the inferior oblique muscle at its midpoint, just lateral to the border of the inferior rectus. An additional branch containing the parasympathetics to the iris sphincter and ciliary muscles runs with the inferior division and synapses in the ciliary ganglion at the lateral aspect of the optic nerve in the orbital apex. The short posterior ciliary nerves then convey the parasympathetic innervation to the globe and extend anteriorly to the sphincter and ciliary muscles.

Adnexal Structures

The adnexal structures include the globe itself, which consists of a firm scleral shell composed of collagen and a specialized anterior portion, the cornea, which is optically clear. The cornea is kept clear by the action of the endo-

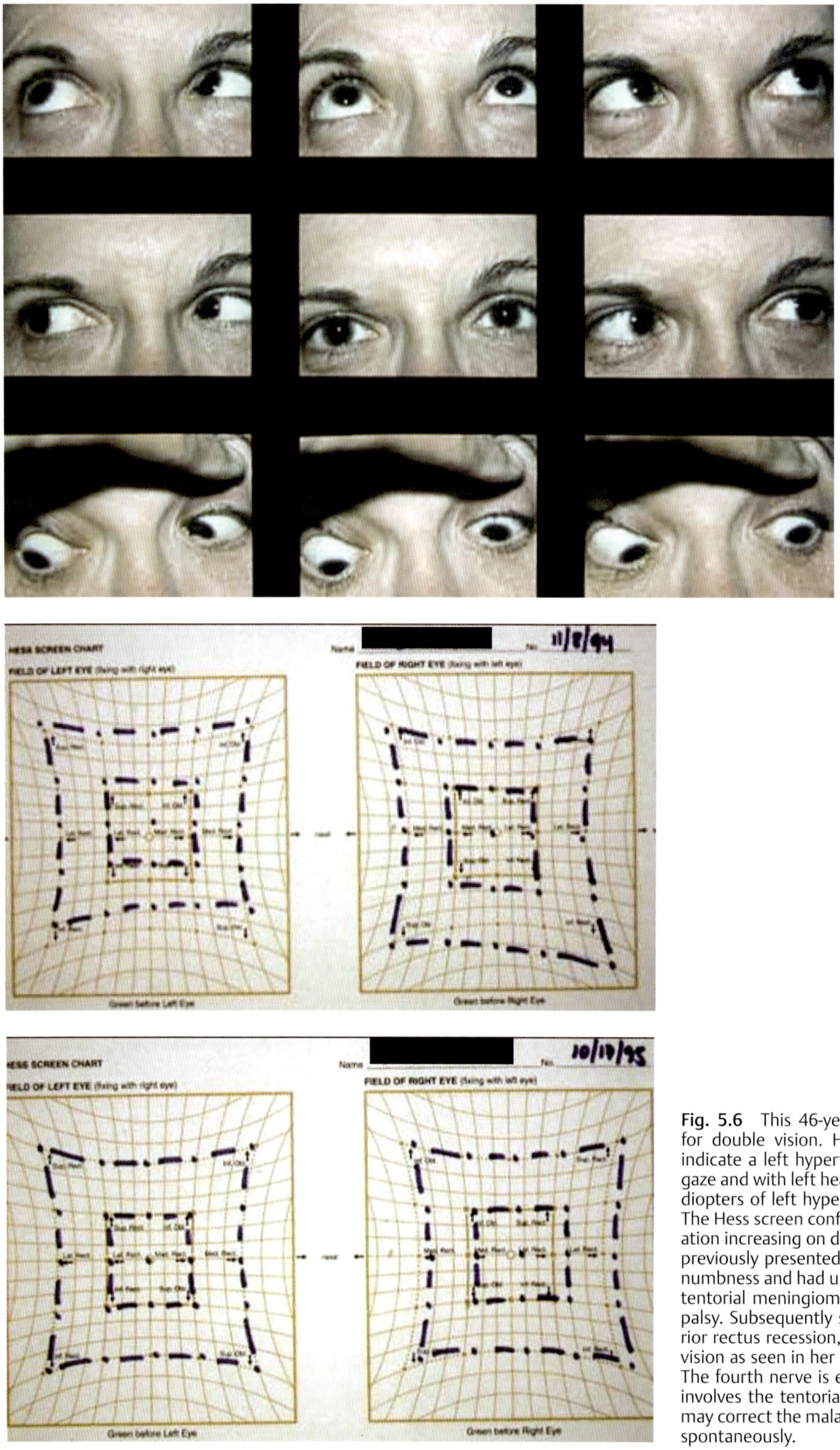

Fig. 5.6 This 46-year-old patient was referred for double vision. Her nine cardinal positions indicate a left hypertropia increasing with right gaze and with left head tilt **(A)**. She measured 16 diopters of left hypertropia in primary position. The Hess screen confirms a left hypertropia deviation increasing on down right gaze **(B)**. She had previously presented with a history of left facial numbness and had undergone resection of a left tentorial meningioma that caused her nerve IV palsy. Subsequently she underwent a right inferior rectus recession, which resolved her double vision as seen in her Hess screen **(C)**. Comment: The fourth nerve is easy to injure when surgery involves the tentorial edge. Eye muscle surgery may correct the malalignment if it does not clear spontaneously.

thelial pump, which returns interstromal fluid into the anterior chamber, relatively dehydrating the corneal stroma.

The inner surface of the globe is lined by a photosensitive layer, the retinal receptors, consisting of rods and cones. The rods line the entire retina except for the fovea. The cones are also located throughout the retina but are concentrated in the fovea. The retinal receptors send signals via the bipolar cells to the ganglion cells located in the most inner portion of the retina. The axons of the ganglion cells make up the nerve fiber layer, which then forms the optic nerve.

The inner retina is perfused through the central retinal artery, which branches into a superior and inferior arcade. The blood supply to the outer retina (the rods and cones) is through the choroid. The choroidal blood actually makes up more than 80% of the blood circulating through the eye and is supplied through the posterior ciliary arteries around the optic nerve and the anterior ciliary arteries, which run within the rectus muscles. The retinal pigment epithelium, which underlies the retinal receptors, is responsible for support and also plays an active role in the metabolic pathways that are required for the rods and cones to function.

The choroid is the posterior extent of the uveal tract. More anteriorly, the uveal tract consists of the ciliary body, which is responsible for forming aqueous (which keeps the eye inflated and supplies oxygen and nutrition to the nonvascularized lens and corneal endothelium), and the iris, which regulates the amount of light coming into the eye. Zonules, which originate from the ciliary body, support the intraocular lens. Contraction of the ciliary body releases tension on the lens, which then increases its refractive power by becoming rounder (permitting us to see objects up close).

The surface of the eye is covered by a nonkeratinized epithelial layer that is contiguous from the cornea through the conjunctiva, lining both the surface of the globe (bulbar) and the inner surface of the eyelids (tarsal). The initial refracting surface of the eye is the tear film, which is supplied by the accessory lacrimal glands lining the upper tarsus and within the cul de sac both superiorly and inferiorly. The main lacrimal gland, located supratemporally in the anterior orbit, drains into the superior cul de sac. Although the main lacrimal gland is responsible for reflex tearing, it also supplies some basic tear production. The main lacrimal gland is innervated by the parasympathetics, which originate near the salivary nucleus. These fibers leave the brainstem in the nervus intermedius and join the seventh nerve. At the geniculate ganglion, they course with the greater superficial petrosal nerve, which parallels the carotid artery within the petrous bone, to the area of the foramen lacerum, where they join the vidian nerve. They synapse in the sphenopalatine ganglion. The postganglionic fibers then run through the inferior orbital fissure before joining the lacrimal nerve to the lacrimal gland.

The eyelids are another important adnexal structure. As the outer surface of skin is keratinized, it is critical that the lids be held in an appropriate position and the keratinized surface not come in contact with the cornea. This is accomplished through the tarsus, a fibrous tissue that keeps the lids oriented. The lids are held tightly in position by the medial and lateral canthal tendons attached to the bone and are elevated by the levator and Müller's muscles superiorly. The lids are closed by the orbicularis muscle, innervated by the temporal and zygomatic branches of the seventh nerve. The pretarsal orbicularis is largely responsible for reflex blinking, whereas the remainder of the preseptal and orbital orbicularis is responsible for forced lid closure. The tarsus also contains meibomian glands, which secrete an oily film that decreases tear evaporation. Goblet cells contained within the perilimbal conjunctiva are responsible for wetting the cornea, which is otherwise hydrophobic.

The globe is moved within the orbit by six extraocular muscles: the four rectus muscles (medial, lateral, superior, and inferior) and the two oblique muscles (superior and inferior). The rectus muscles insert on the anterior aspect of the globe and will pull the eye in the direction in which they insert. The superior rectus produces elevation as well as adduction and incyclotorsion. The inferior rectus causes depression, adduction, and excyclotorsion. The oblique muscles, because they insert posterior to the equator, move the eye in the opposite direction, with the superior oblique muscle causing depression as well as incyclotortion and abduction. The inferior oblique moves the eye up and produces excyclotortion and abduction.

The eye is permitted to move because of its encasement within Tenon's capsule, which isolates the globe from the surrounding structures. The sheaths of the extraocular muscles also permit movement. These sheaths form a portion of the complicated septal anatomy within the orbit, with pockets of fat surrounding and protecting the extraocular muscles, as well as the cranial nerves and the vascular supply to the eye, muscles, optic nerve, and eyelids anteriorly. Any damage to the tissue planes often results in restricted motility and diplopia.

The orbit communicates with the intracranial space through the optic canal, which transmits the optic nerve as well as the ophthalmic artery, and the superior orbital fissure, which transmits the ocular motor cranial nerves as well as the three branches of the first division of the trigeminal nerve, the superior ophthalmic vein, and various sympathetic and parasympathetic innervation to the structures within the orbit. The orbit also communicates inferiorly with the nose, allowing drainage of the excess tears through the lacrimal sac and the nasolacrimal duct. Collateral circulation links the ophthalmic artery (branch of the internal carotid artery) to multiple branches of the external circulation via the anterior and posterior ethmoid arteries, the recurrent meningeal artery through the superior orbital fissure, and the terminal branches of the supraorbital, supratrochlear, and infratrochlear arteries with the terminal branches of the angular, transverse facial, and temporal arteries.

◆ Evaluation

Afferent System Evaluation

A basic understanding of the neuro-ophthalmic examination includes qualitative and quantitative assessment of the afferent and efferent systems. Multiple texts and chapters have addressed the neuro-ophthalmic evaluation of the afferent system.[15,33,38–44] Ophthalmic evaluations, like all examinations, can be divided into those that are qualitative, potentially localizing in nature, and those that are quantitative, providing for an assessment of the natural history of disease as well as the effects of intervention. Qualitative assessment is often adequate to confirm the presence of a lesion and to direct additional work-up. Quantitative assessment is required, however, to determine whether or not lesions are changing over time, and whether therapy has been effective.

Although qualitative acuity measurements may be listed as "normal" or "reduced," in almost all circumstances quantitative measurement of afferent visual function should be obtained. It is important to recognize that central vision as measured by Snellen or near acuity represents only macular function, and it does not assess visual perception outside the point of fixation. Macular function is traditionally recorded as the smallest Snellen optotype that can be seen, usually at the fixed distance of 20 ft. The top of the fraction recorded (eg, 20/40) indicates the testing distance and the bottom smallest optotype that can be seen. Thus, in this case, at 20 ft the patient cannot see anything smaller than the 40 optotype. The optotype is defined by the size of the letter required to subtend 5 minutes of arc at the named distance. Small improvements in distance acuity testing were introduced by Bailey and Lovie in 1976, and a modification of the chart (also called the ETDRS [Early Treatment Diabetic Retinopathy Study] chart), is often used in multicenter trials.[45] All visual function testing should be obtained with the patient's correction (glasses or contact lenses) in place. Often, acuity seems to be lost simply because the patients are not wearing their glasses. A rapid screen for the presence of refractive abnormalities, as well as corneal or surface anomalies, can be obtained with the use of a pinhole. Improvement in central visual function when the patient looks through a pinhole usually indicates that at least a component of the decreased vision is related to uncorrected refractive error, or potentially to early corneal or lens pathology.

In addition to best corrected distance acuity, near vision should be checked routinely (**Fig. 5.7**). Although this may be recorded as "equivalent," as a general rule, it should be recorded in the point system, again with the appropriate refraction for near, and with a notation of the distance at which the patient is holding the reading card. The Jaeger system, although used by ophthalmologists, does not have the universal applicability (the point system is used in all type, including computer printouts) and therefore is less useful. Lack of equivalence between distance and near measurement is another clue to the possibility of an uncorrected refractive error, but it also may occur in patients with various types of cataract formation.

An additional essential part of evaluation of the afferent system is testing extrafoveal function (visual fields).[33,41] This can be done qualitatively by confrontation testing (**Fig. 5.8**), semiqualitatively on tangent screen testing, and quantitatively by Goldmann or automated static perimetry.[46] At a minimum, all patients should be assessed for the potential presence of visual field defects that respect the vertical midline, indicating chiasmal or retrochiasmal pathology, or the nasal horizontal midline, indicating optic nerve pathology. In addition, as compressive lesions may affect the central portion of the visual field, patients should be tested for relative central visual field defects. These are common with optic nerve compression. Visual fields (like other afferent system tests) should be recorded as if you are the patient looking out. Thus, the right visual field is to the right side and the left is to the left, with the temporal fields peripherally and the nasal fields centrally.

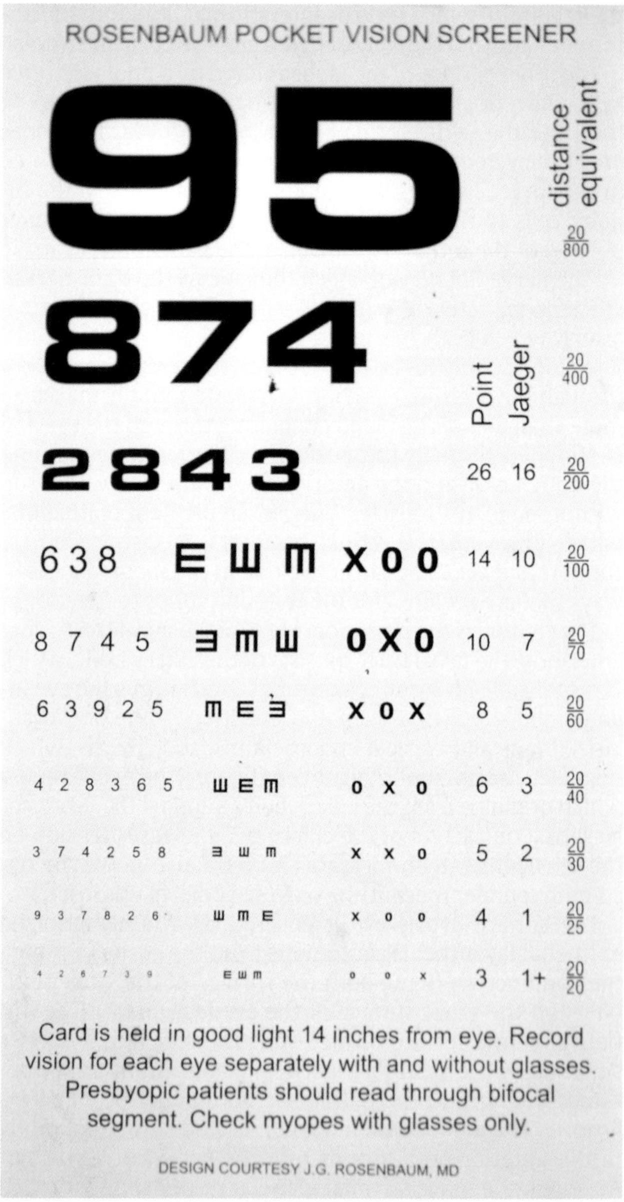

Fig. 5.7 Near card. Instructions call for this to be held at 14 in (35.6 cm). It is more important that the patient hold the card at the clearest distance and that distance be measured and recorded. Vision should be recorded in the point system. The equivalent subtended angle at distance is also given.

Visual field defects are particularly useful in localizing pathology, even without quantitative assessment. Bitemporal visual field defects, originally described clinically by McKenzie in 1835, clearly localize pathology to the area of the chiasm (**Figs. 5.4** and **5.5**). Homonymous visual field defects, in which there is a field defect to the same side in both eyes, indicates pathology affecting the post-chiasmal visual pathways (**Fig. 5.3**). Involvement of the optic nerves may produce either a central scotoma (**Fig. 5.2**) or variations of arcuate visual field defects, found on qualitative assessment by a relative step across the nasal horizontal midline. Arcuate defects are better evaluated in a more quantitative fashion either by Goldmann kinetic perimetry or automated static perimetry. In the interpretation of visual fields, the pattern deviation plot with statistical analysis

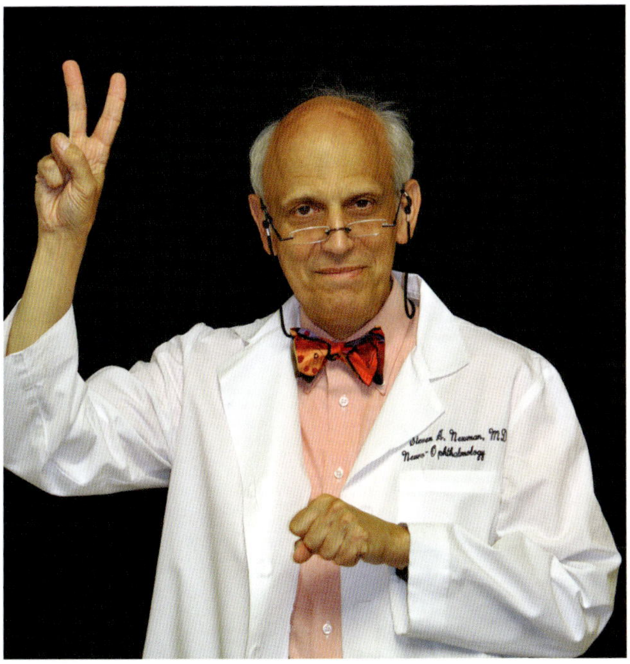

Fig. 5.8 Confrontation testing should be done by presenting one, two, or five fingers in each of the four quadrants, with each eye tested separately.

is most important in terms of recognizing and appreciating the localizing value of visual field defects. Arcuate defects indicate pathology affecting the optic nerve (less likely the retina), whereas respect for the vertical midline indicates involvement at or behind the chiasm. Central scotomas not due to macular pathology are classically seen with toxic, metabolic, or hereditary pathology, but are not uncommon with compressive or inflammatory lesions.

Evaluation of the afferent system also involves two additional studies: assessment of pupillary response and assessment of the retina and optic disc. Teleologically, the pupil is responsible for regulating the amount of light coming into the visual system.[47] When there is excess light, the pupils become smaller, and when it is relatively dark, the pupils dilate. This is under control of the sphincter muscle, innervated through the third nerve, and the dilator muscles, innervated by the sympathetics traveling with the carotid artery through the superior orbital fissure. Pupils should be examined for regularity and symmetry. Pupil size may be measured with a pupil gauge. Asymmetry is not rare, essential anisocoria, but the difference should be the same in light and dark.[48]

The presence of asymmetric optic nerve pathology produces an afferent pupillary defect; moving a bright light from one side to the other results in dilation of both pupils when the light is moved to the side where the optic nerve is involved while the patient fixes a distant accommodative target.[49] The presence of an afferent pupillary defect may be further quantitated by the placement of neutral-density filters in front of the better-functioning eye until the response is balanced[50] (**Fig. 5.9**). Although an afferent pupillary defect cannot be detected in a patient with one eye, it is possible to detect an afferent pupillary defect even when there is only one working pupil. Statements about "reverse Marcus Gunn" pupil should be avoided. No matter which pupil is being observed, the relative afferent pupillary defect indicates the side on which less light is getting into the system. The presence of an afferent pupillary defect parallels asymmetric visual fields more than central acuity and optic nerve appearance.

The eye gives us a unique ability to see in vivo into the functioning of the central nervous system. Funduscopic evaluation permits us to look at the beginning of the optic nerve, which is really the most anterior portion of the white matter tract of the brain connecting the photoreceptors via the ganglion cells to the geniculate and then the cortex. The presence of increased intracranial pressure, potentially seen in patients with parasellar lesions, can produce disc edema as it results in constipation of axonal transport (**Fig. 5.10**). Persistent disc edema due to increased intracranial pressure will eventually produce optic atrophy associated with deteriorating afferent visual function. This may be documented with photographs of the posterior pole and can be qualitatively assessed based on relative disc pallor and more recently quantitatively assessed with OCT (optical coherence tomography; **Fig. 5.5**). Papilledema is uncommonly seen with pituitary tumors unless they become large enough to obstruct the foramen of Monro. Other tumors arising in the parasellar region, however, more frequently present with increased intracranial pressures, especially meningiomas arising from the olfactory groove, from the tuberculum, or even from the anterior clinoid and medial sphenoid wing. These may present with bilateral disc edema due to increased intracranial pressure or unilateral disc edema and contralateral optic atrophy (Foster Kennedy syndrome) due to compression of one optic nerve.[51]

It should be noted that since the advent of imaging studies, the incidence of disc edema with all intracranial tumors has markedly decreased.[14] This would be particu-

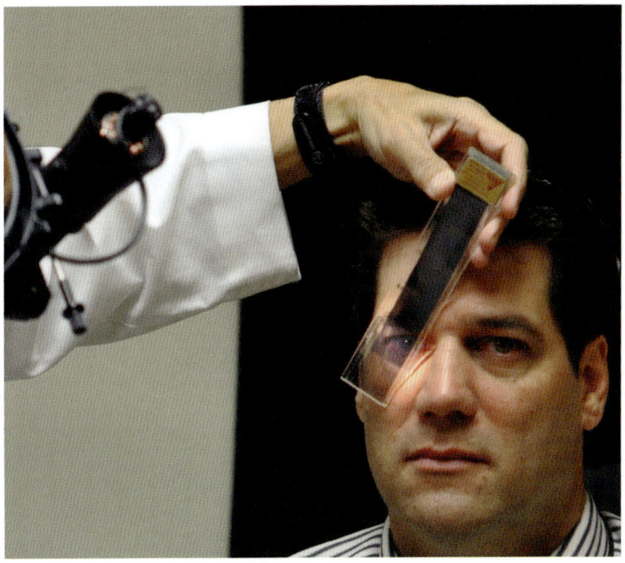

Fig. 5.9 In the presence of an afferent pupillary defect, neutral density filters may be placed in front of the better-functioning eye to quantitate the amount of asymmetry between the two eyes. It is important to use a bright light and spend equal time in the two eyes.

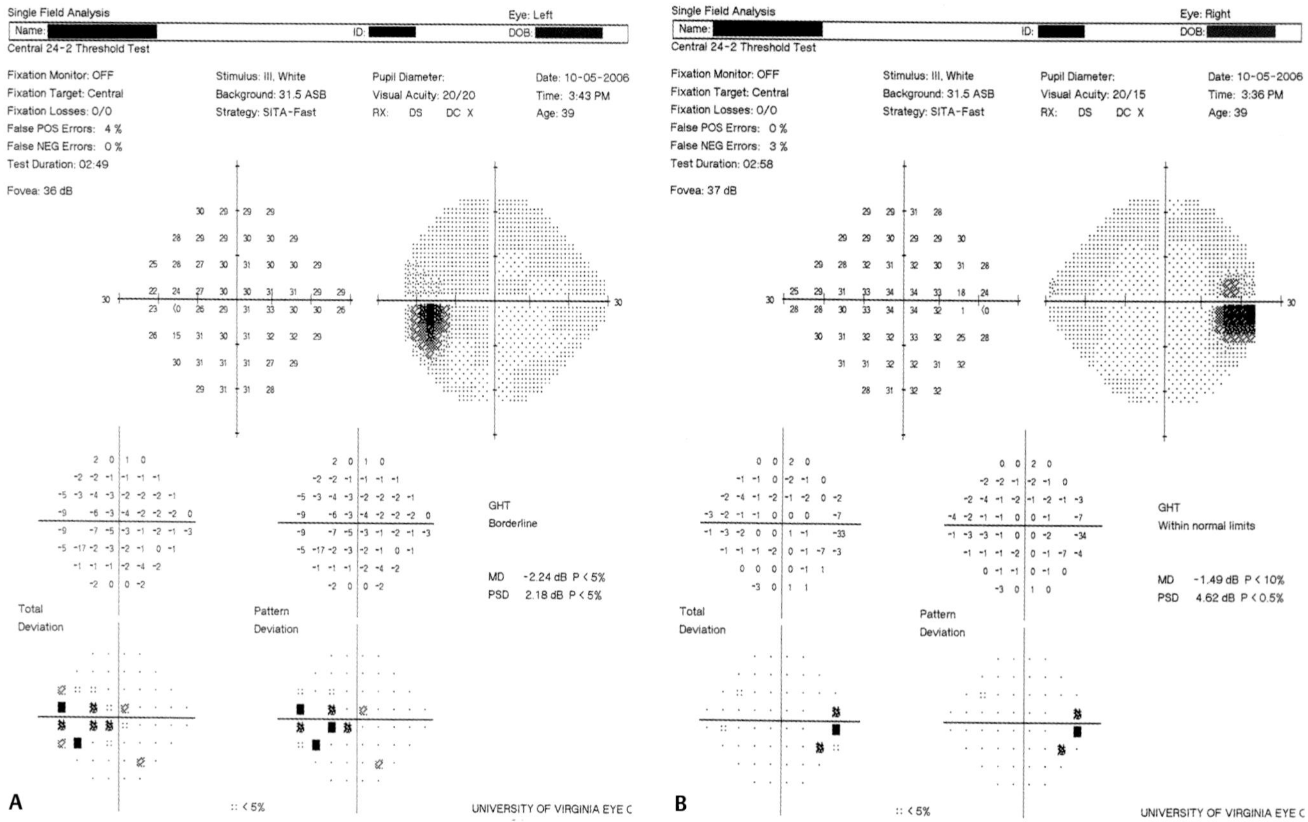

Fig. 5.10 This 39-year-old patient presented in August 2006 with a 1-month history of pounding headaches. Visual acuity was 20/20 bilaterally, but his visual fields demonstrated enlargement of the blind spot bilaterally, worse on the left **(A)** than the right **(B)**, and bilateral disc edema **(C,D)**.

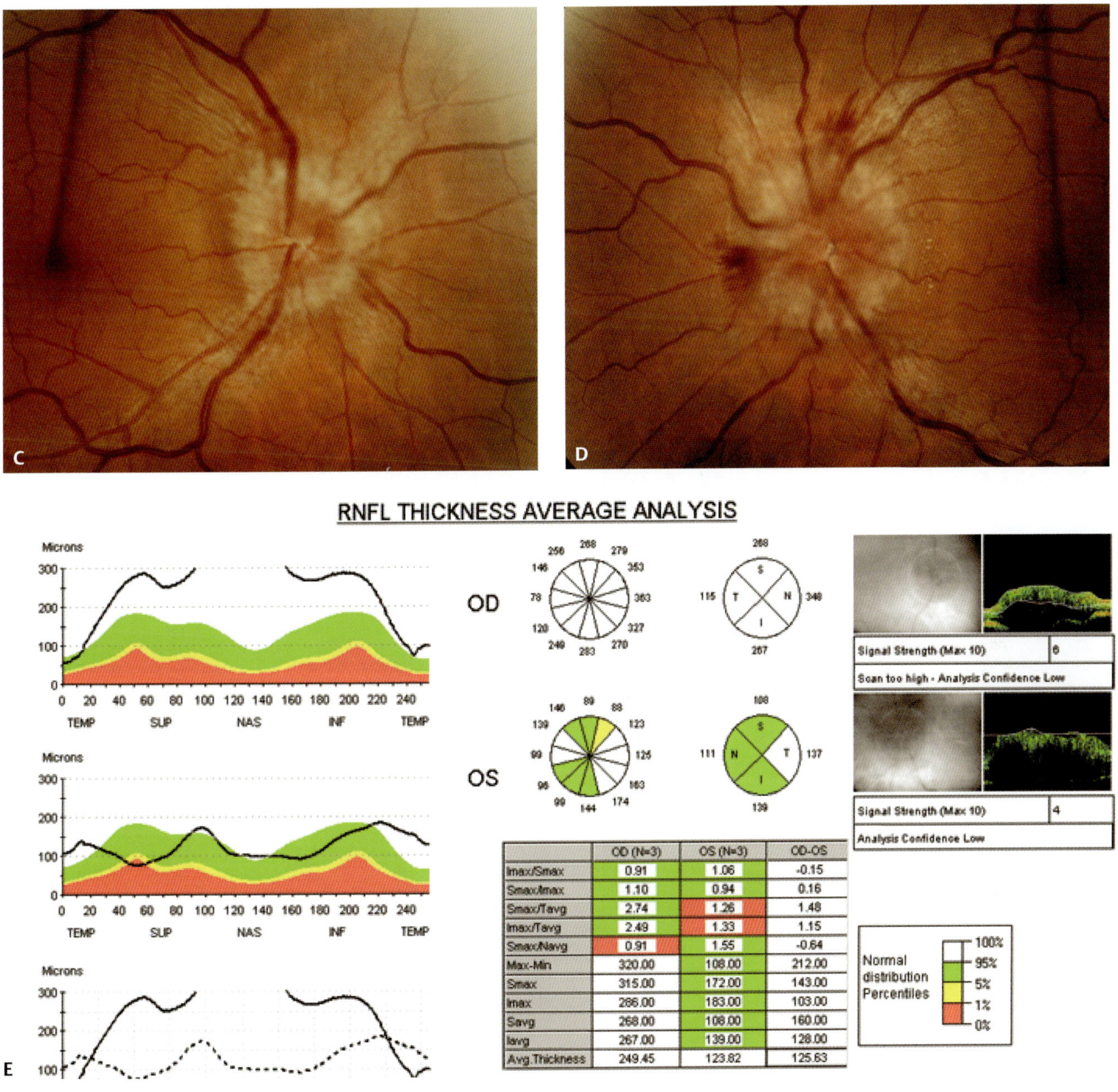

Fig. 5.10 *(Continued)* This 39-year-old patient presented in August 2006 with a 1-month history of pounding headaches. Visual acuity was 20/20 bilaterally, but his visual fields demonstrated enlargement of the blind spot bilaterally, worse on the left **(A)** than the right **(B)**, and bilateral disc edema **(C,D)**. Optical coherence tomography (OCT) confirmed the presence of marked thickening of the nerve fiber layer bilaterally, worse on the right than the left **(E)**. *(Continued on page 90)*

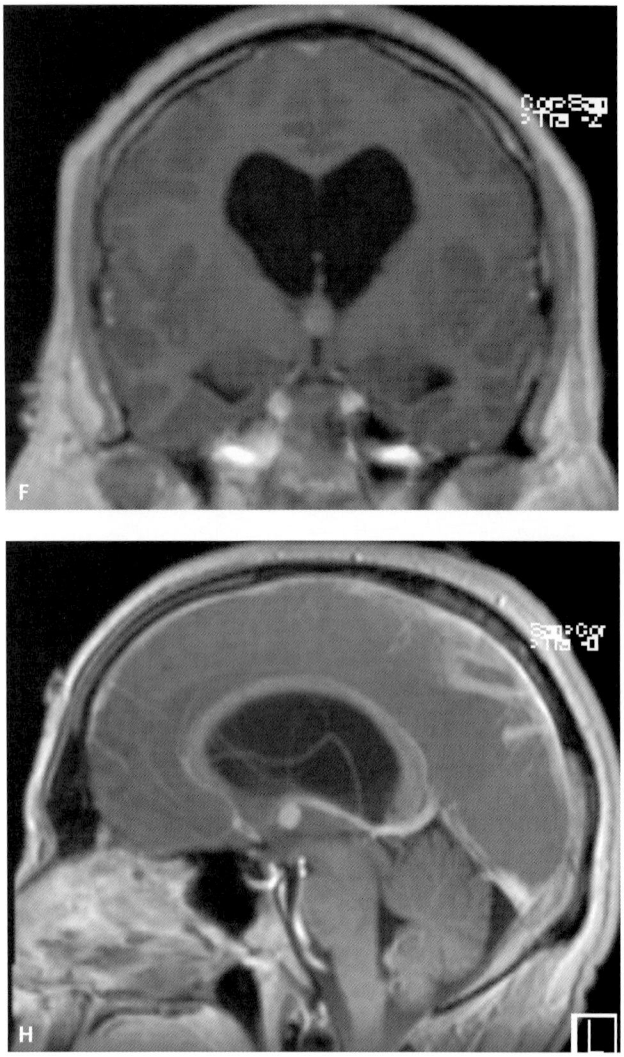

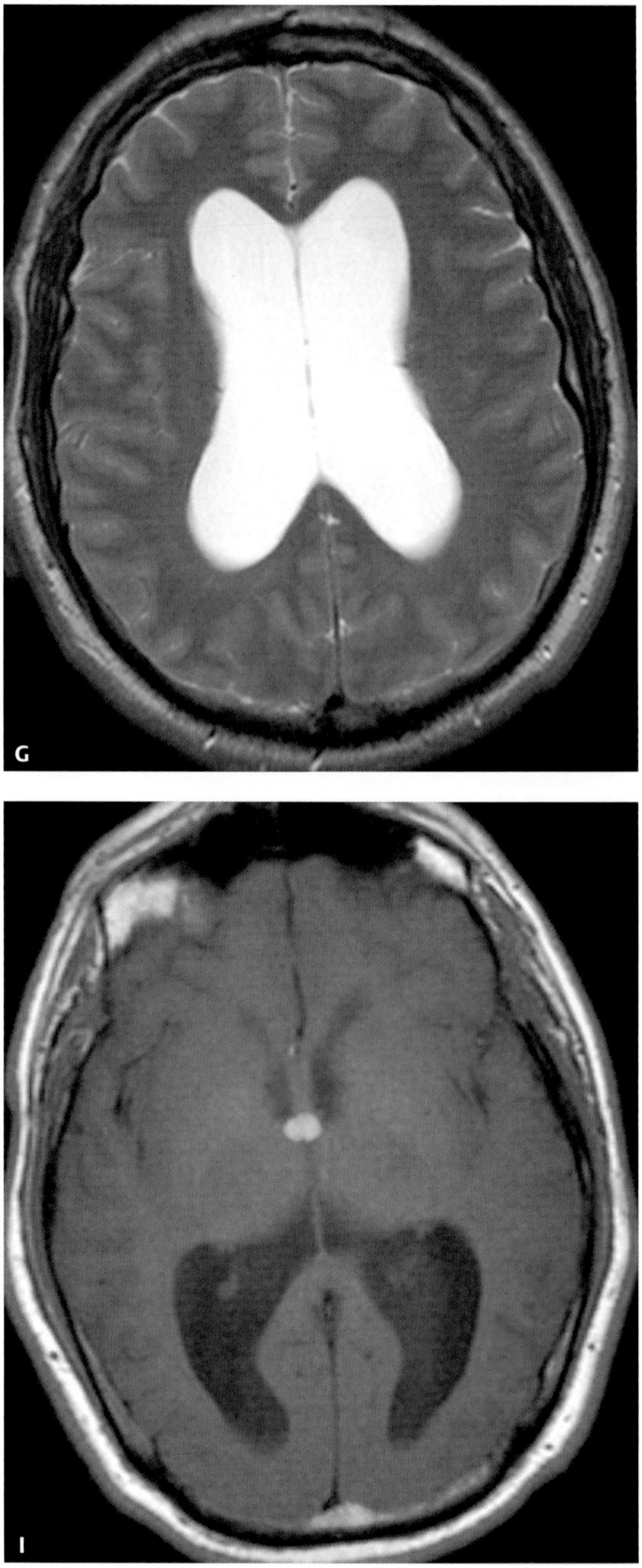

Fig. 5.10 *(Continued)* This 39-year-old patient presented in August 2006 with a 1-month history of pounding headaches. MRI revealed evidence of significant hydrocephalus, with a small colloid cyst blocking the foramen of Monro **(F–I)**.

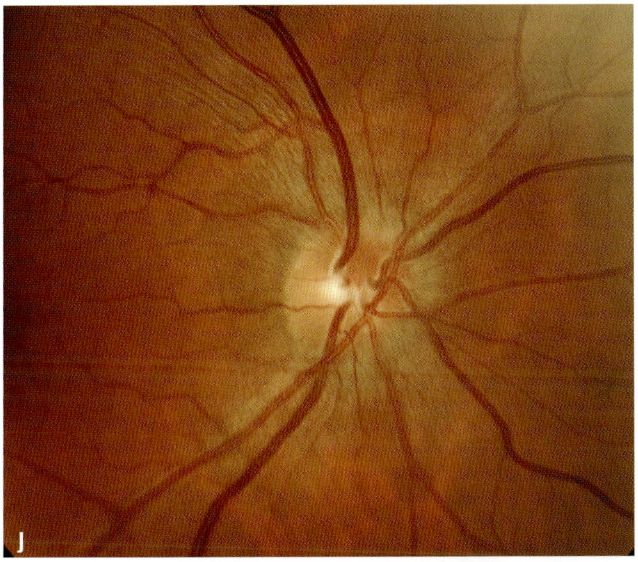

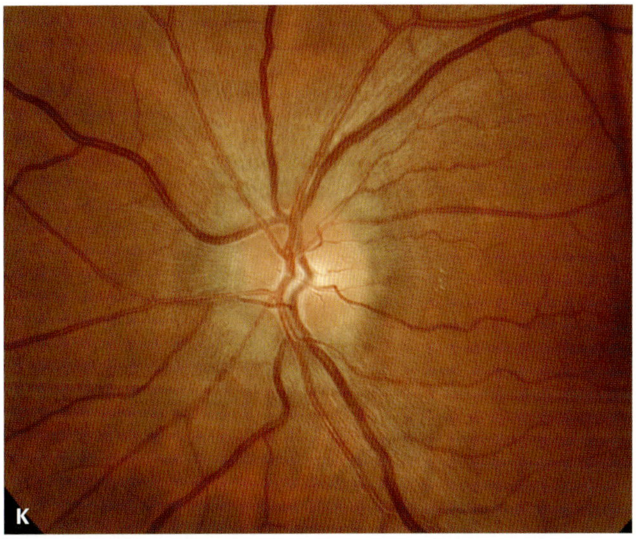

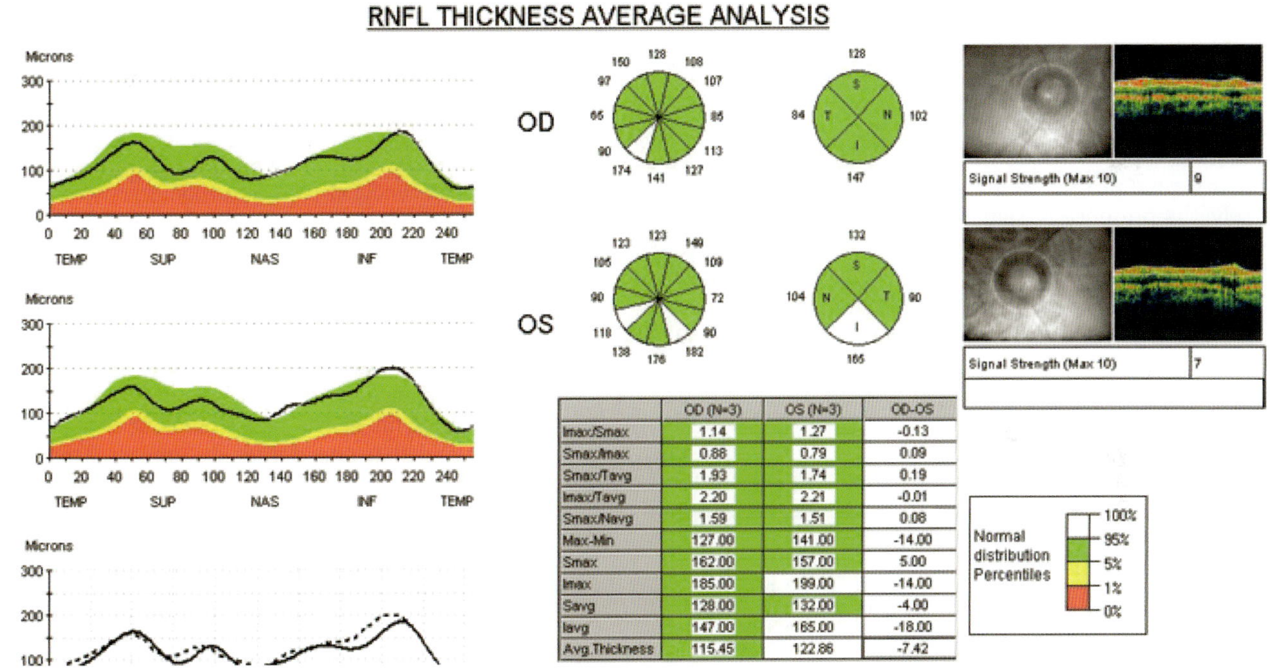

L

	OD (N=3)	OS (N=3)	OD-OS
Imax/Smax	1.14	1.27	-0.13
Smax/Imax	0.88	0.79	0.09
Smax/Tavg	1.93	1.74	0.19
Imax/Tavg	2.20	2.21	-0.01
Smax/Navg	1.59	1.51	0.08
Max-Min	127.00	141.00	-14.00
Smax	162.00	157.00	5.00
Imax	185.00	199.00	-14.00
Savg	128.00	132.00	-4.00
Iavg	147.00	165.00	-18.00
Avg.Thickness	115.45	122.86	-7.42

Fig. 5.10 *(Continued)* This 39-year-old patient presented in August 2006 with a 1-month history of pounding headaches. Following excision of the colloid cyst, the discs are seen to return to normal **(J,K)**, and the OCT shows marked thinning with return to normal **(L)**. Comment: Obstruction of ventricular flow in this case resulted in secondary increased intracranial pressure with bilateral disc edema and bilateral cecal scotomas. With restoration of the normal CSF flow, pressure was reduced, the disc edema resolved, and the thickening of the nerve fiber layer reversed (as seen on OCT).

larly true in patients with parasellar lesions, as it would be unusual for patients to be asymptomatic long enough for these lesions to reach the size that leads to papilledema.

The recent development of OCT has opened a new door to the more quantitative assessment of the optic nerve, disc, and nerve fiber layer. This can be seen to be thickened in patients with disc edema of any etiology (**Fig. 5.10**) and, more importantly, can quantitate the presence of loss of nerve fiber layer due to pathology that affects the optic nerve (paralleling optic atrophy; **Fig. 5.5**). It should be noted that there is a delay in the thinning of the nerve fiber layer for weeks, if not months, between the acute onset of optic nerve pathology and thinning seen on OCT. It is also important to note that the OCT will not thin to zero because there are support structures within the retina that will keep nerve fiber layer thickness measurements at least in the upper 30s or lower 40s range. Asymmetry between the two sides may be a useful sign of previous damage to one optic nerve. A finding of nerve fiber layer thinning may also indicate that a lesion is much more long-standing than otherwise appreciated (**Fig. 5.3**). OCT may also be prognostic in terms of visual recovery following surgical or medical decompression (**Fig. 5.4**). Just as the older literature suggested that the best prognosis was in patients with relatively brief visual loss and the absence of optic atrophy on funduscopic evaluation, the lack of OCT thinning may also be taken as a relatively good prognostic sign for potential recovery. Conversely, the presence of significant thinning of nerve fiber layer may indicate a worsened prognosis for recovery following decompression. It should be emphasized, however, that even with significant thinning, there may be substantial improvement in optic nerve function, particularly as measured by central acuity, but even by visual fields.

It is important to note that not all decreased vision is due to optic nerve or chiasmal pathology. Abnormalities in refraction and abnormalities of the cornea, lens, vitreous, or retina can also produce decreased vision. This will often require more detailed work-up. One of the tests that may be particularly suggestive of an alternative explanation for visual loss would be the absence of an afferent pupillary defect. Although an afferent may not be present if both optic nerves are involved, the presence of unilateral decreased vision but no afferent pupillary defect strongly suggests either an anterior segment or a retina problem. In photostress test a light is shined in the eye for 10 seconds, then the patient is timed until he or she can read down to one line worse than best previoiusly recorded vision. This may be a subtle way of detecting a relative macular problem as differentiated from an optic nerve problem.[52] Patients who have macular pathology will have a delay in their recovery, whereas patients with optic nerve problems will not.

The view of the back of the eye may also be very helpful. If there is an anterior segment problem, the observer often cannot see in with a direct ophthalmoscope (**Fig. 5.11**), and therefore, it is not surprising the patient cannot see out. Similarly, clear macular pathology may explain the patient's visual limitation. The appearance of the macula, unfortunately, does not always indicate its function. Additional functional tests, such as multifocal electroretinography (ERG) and autofluorescence, and anatomic tests, such OCT of the macula, may be necessary.

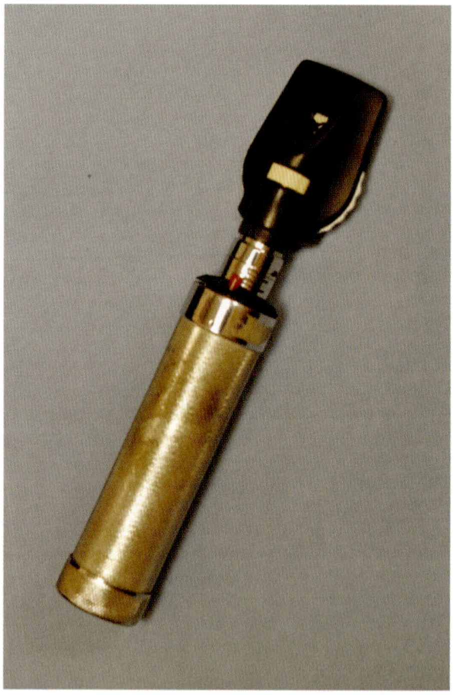

Fig. 5.11 Direct ophthalmoscope. Although a more detailed view (and in stereo) may be obtained with slit-lamp biomicroscopy or with indirect ophthalmoscopy, the direct ophthalmoscope gives a good idea of any media (cornea, lens, anterior segment) problems that may be interfering with vision. If you can see in, the patient should be able to see out.

One unusual symptom of a dense bitemporal visual field defect is the presence of postfixational blindness. When a patient converges his visual axes to look at a near target, anything beyond that near target disappears. This is not usually noticed by the patient but can be easily demonstrated on examination.

Efferent System Evaluation

Extensive literature addresses the importance of ocular motility to visual function.[21,53,54] Because we are foveate animals, to maximize our visual potential, we need to bring the eyes into alignment with the object of interest. To do that, we have developed the efferent visual system, which allows the movement of each eye. In addition, because we have overlapping visual fields, both eyes must be in alignment simultaneously. Acuity is adversely affected by movement of the eye relative to the visual environment. Thus, it is critical that the eyes be kept stable. This includes stability when the head moves and when the object of interest moves. Stability can be best judged by observing the fundus with a direct ophthalmoscope.[55] Any tendency for the eye to drift will be picked up as a movement of the observed optic disc. This can be done in primary and eccentric gaze. Gross instability may be directly observed, magnified with a Fenzel viewing system, or recorded with an eye-tracking system (electro-oculogram [EOG], infrared, coil).[56]

Each individual movement of the eyes is referred to as a duction. Ductions can be qualitatively assessed by simply looking at ocular excursion but also by looking to see if "the sclera can be buried." Ductions may also be quantitatively assessed by measurement linearly, by rotational measurements with prism, or most accurately by measuring ductions on a hemispheric bowl (Goldmann apparatus) or an arc perimeter. These measurements may be particularly helpful in following patients who are likely to develop progressive limitation in individual ocular motility, such as those with infiltration of the extraocular muscles, or in the setting of disease processes such as myasthenia gravis and progressive external ophthalmoplegia. Normally, a patient should be able to abduct and adduct approximately 50 degrees; depression is approximately 45 degrees, and elevation decreases from a maximum of 40 degrees in childhood to 15 degrees in the elderly.

Movement of the two eyes together is referred to as version. These may be movements left (levoversion), right (dextroversion), up (sursumversion), or down (deorsumversion). Vergence refers to movements of the eyes in opposite directions. Convergence is necessary to look at a near target, bringing the axes closer together, and divergence is required for looking at a distance target. Abnormalities of convergence and divergence can occur with midbrain lesions and can uncommonly be seen with parasellar lesions that enlarge to affect or involve the midbrain. Abnormal versions can lead to ocular malalignment. This, as mentioned, usually results in diplopia. Subtle abnormalities in versions can be picked up by dissociative tests such as the red glass test or, better yet, the use of a Maddox rod.[57] A white light is viewed by one eye while a Maddox rod placed over the opposite eye produces the sensation of seeing a line perpendicular to the cylinders of the Maddox rod. To assess horizontal alignment, the Maddox rod is placed so that the cylinders are aligned horizontally, thus producing the sensation of seeing a line running vertically (**Fig. 5.12A**). If the light is not seen as on the line, then there is relative horizontal malalignment of the eyes. As the patient will see the light in the opposite direction to which the eye is deviated, if the patient reports seeing the light as crossed over the line, it means that the patient has a relative exodeviation, or deviation out. Similarly, if the patient reports the light on the same side as the eye viewing, the patient has the eyes relatively crossed in, or an esodeviation. If the Maddox rod is aligned vertically, the patient will see a horizontal line (**Fig. 5.12B**). If the light is above or below the line, there is a vertical deviation. A tendency to deviate (phoria), as picked up by a Maddox rod or red glass, is common in a large percentage of the population. Most people, however, maintain alignment by the use of fusional amplitudes, which can make up for a tendency of the eyes to deviate. A breakdown of the fusional amplitudes results in a manifest deviation (tropia). Torsional abnormalities (often seen when the third or fourth nerve is involved) can be measured with double Maddox rods. Occasionally, patients are unable to perform Maddox rod or other subjective tests. Alignment may be assessed by cross-cover testing and prism measurements or, in nonresponsive patients, by judging the position of the light reflex on the cornea (Hirshberg's test). A more quantita-

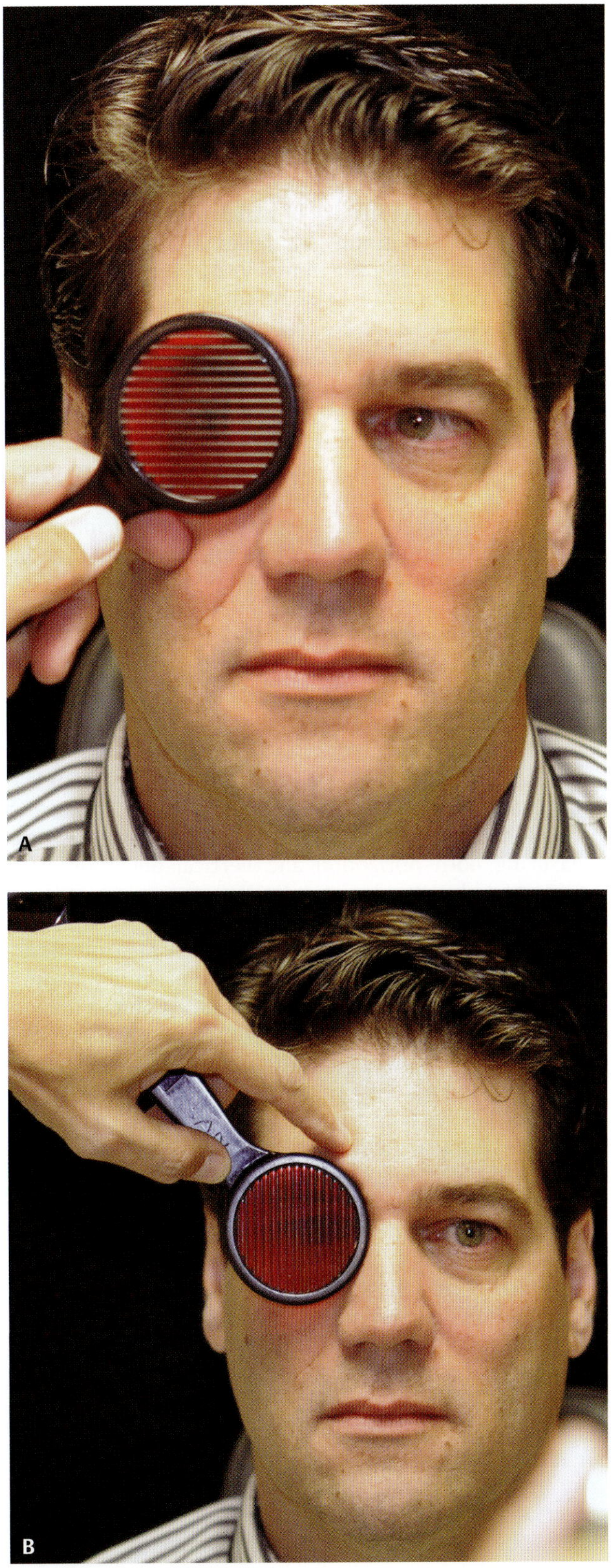

Fig. 5.12 Maddox rod. Although a red glass or cross-cover testing may also be used to check for alignment, the Maddox rod is a very quick means of assessing for any tendency to deviate (phoria) both horizontally **(A)** and vertically **(B)**. This is the quickest way to check for comitance and identify the field of maximal deviation.

tive test not requiring patient response is Krimsky's test, in which the light reflex is simultaneously centered on the cornea with the use of prisms, thus placing a number on deviation.[58]

As mentioned, not all patients who are tropic have diplopia; they may have facultative suppression, in which the brain simply ignores one image. This is usually seen in patients with a long history of malalignment, or congenital strabismus and amblyopia. Fusional amplitudes vary. They are much greater horizontally than vertically and are greater for convergence, bringing things in, than for divergence. The implications are that a patient who has a subtle problem with abduction (eg, a mild sixth nerve palsy) is more likely to be symptomatic than one with a subtle adduction problem (eg, an internuclear ophthalmoplegia). A small tendency to deviate vertically usually produces double vision because vertical fusional amplitudes are much less than horizontal, and most patients cannot fuse more than 3 or 4 diopters (1–2 degrees) of vertical malalignment. Fusional amplitudes require bilateral simultaneous vision. In the setting of a dense bitemporal defect, each eye is actually seeing half of the visual field, and any tendency to drift (a small hyperphoria that would otherwise be controlled) can result in double vision due to "hemifield slip."

Although the red glass test and Maddox rod are usually considered qualitative (assessing the presence of deviation but not quantitating it), it is possible to use them to quantitate deviation by adding a prism to balance the deviation. Quantitative assessment of ocular deviation may also be obtained by cross-cover testing in primary position, measuring both horizontal and vertical deviation with prisms and also the deviation in the other eight cardinal positions of gaze, including up, down, left, right, up right, down right, up left, and down left. Prism measurements will depend on which eye is under the prism. In incomitant deviations, when the patient fixates with the normal eye and the prisms are placed over the abnormal eye, one measures the "primary" deviation. If the prisms are then switched to the normal eye, the deviation measured when the abnormal eye is fixating is called the secondary deviation. The secondary deviation is always greater than the primary. In the setting of a comitant deviation (the same in all directions), the primary and secondary deviations are equal. In addition to the quantitative use of orthoptic or cross-cover testing with prisms, the use of a Lancaster red-green test[59,60] or a Hess screen[61] gives a semiquantitative assessment of ocular motility. This is particularly useful in following patients with ocular deviation (**Fig. 5.13**).

An additional quantitative assessment of ocular deviation can be obtained by using a Goldmann bowl and plotting the area of binocular singularity. Thus, a patient with an abduction deficit, perhaps due to a sixth nerve palsy, may be seen to have double vision when looking in the direction of the sixth nerve dysfunction but single vision when looking away. By plotting the binocular single vision fields, patients can be followed to determine whether or not sixth nerve function is improving or worsening. It should be noted that finding a deviation, either qualitatively and quantitatively, does not tell you whether the deviation is due to a paretic problem (eg, a cranial nerve palsy, a neuromuscular transmission deficit, or an inter-

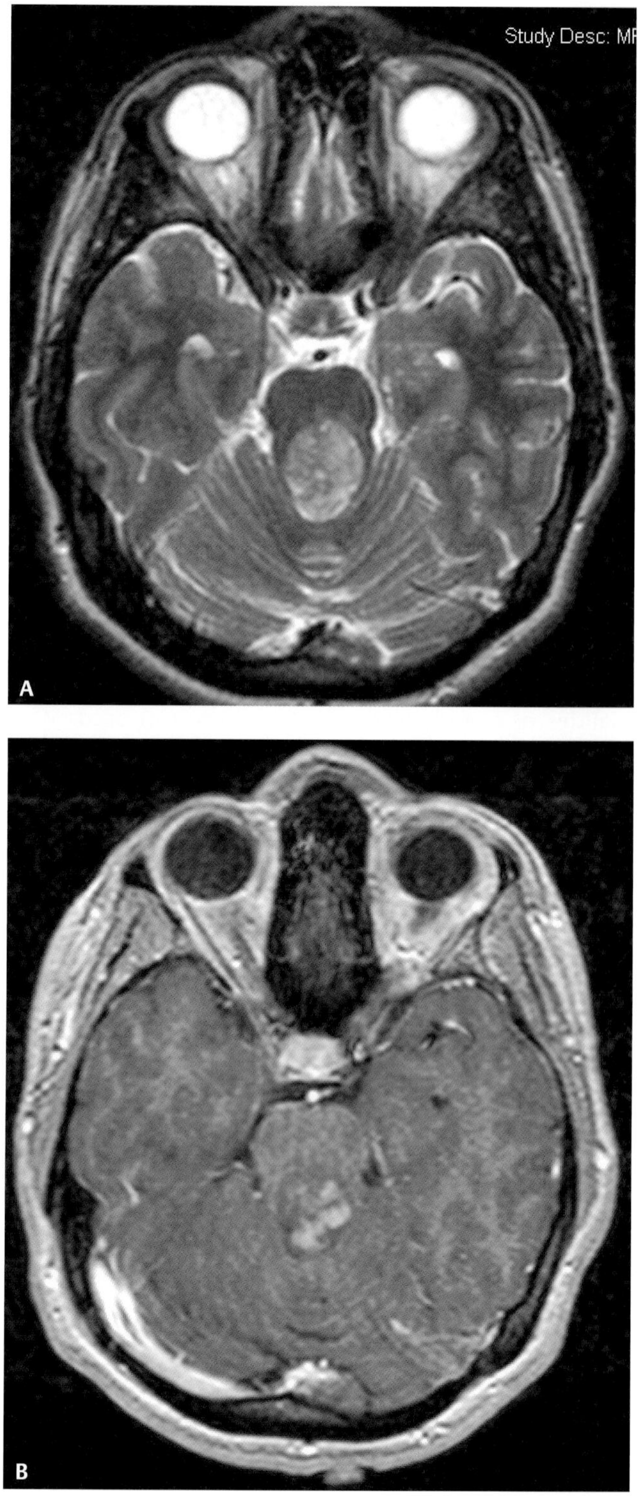

Fig. 5.13 This 24-year-old presented with a 4-month history of intermittent diplopia. Visual acuity and visual fields were normal, but she had upbeat nystagmus in primary position increasing on up gaze. MRI demonstrated a dorsal midbrain intra-axial lesion with an exophytic component **(A,B)**.

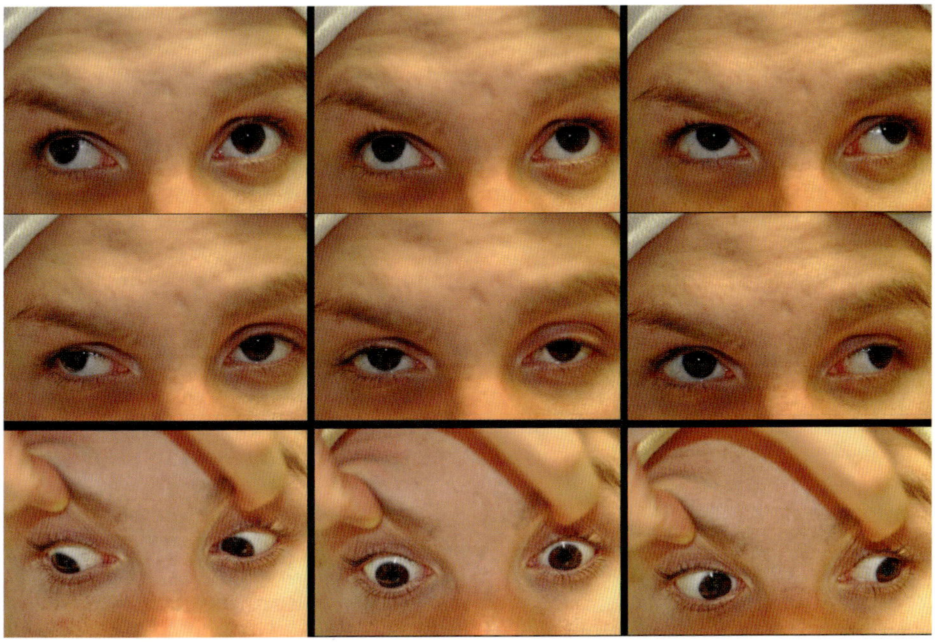

C

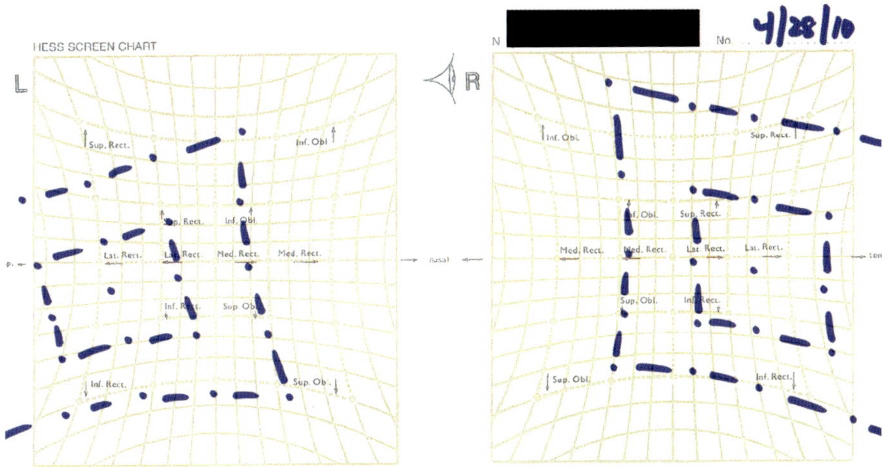

D

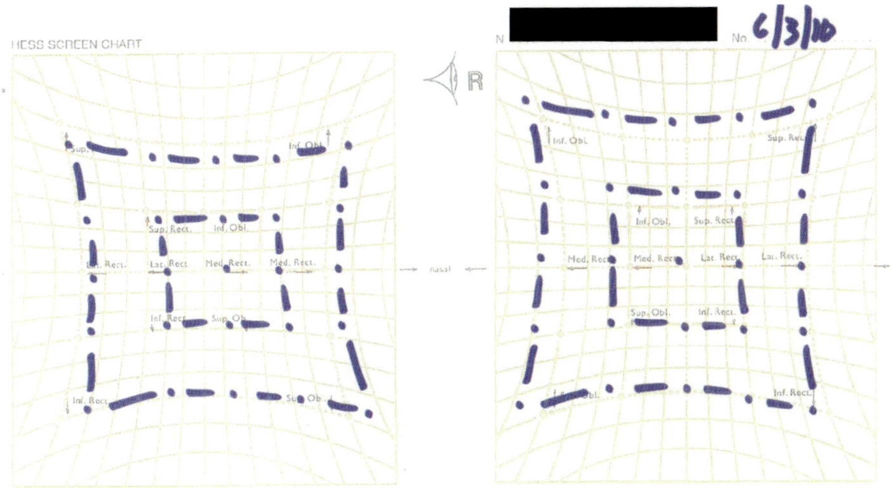

E

Fig. 5.13 *(Continued)* This 24-year-old presented with a 4-month history of intermittent diplopia. Visual acuity and visual fields were normal, but she had upbeat nystagmus in primary position increasing on up gaze. She underwent a suboccipital craniotomy and biopsy, which demonstrated a low-grade glioma. Postoperatively she had worsening of her diplopia, with an exo deviation increasing on gaze to either side **(C)** and a right hypertropia increasing on left gaze and with right head tilt. Hess screen confirmed the incomitant vertical deviation **(D).** Two months later, her double vision had significantly improved **(E).** Comment: Following craniotomy, this patient had evidence of bilateral internuclear ophthalmoplegia and a right fourth nerve palsy, which spontaneously improved. The Hess screen provides quantitative follow-up.

nuclear problem) or due to restrictive phenomena secondary to local orbital invasion. Restrictive syndromes are traditionally diagnosed by forced ductions but may also be recognized with the use of a suction cup[62] or the elevation of intraocular pressure in eccentric gaze.[63] Rarely, ocular malalignment may be due to primary overaction syndromes. Parasellar lesions that can produce overaction include ocular neuromyotonia, which often follows radiation of lesions in the parasellar region. Patients with ocular neuromyotonia can report a sensation of the eye "sticking" when they look in the direction of the affected muscle. In sixth nerve ocular neuromyotonia, when the patient looks to that side, the lateral rectus muscle will continue to fire even after the patient looks back straight, resulting in a transient exodeviation producing double vision.

Making the diagnosis of a cranial nerve palsy depends on whether or not it fits a pattern. A sixth nerve palsy should be seen as an esodeviation increasing on ipsilateral gaze and decreasing on contralateral gaze (**Fig. 5.14**). The deviation should be minimal when the patient looks away from the side of the sixth nerve. A fourth nerve palsy consists of an ipsilateral hyperdeviation that increases on contralateral gaze and ipsilateral head tilt (**Fig. 5.6**). The deviation should be minimal when the patient looks up and to the same side as the involved superior oblique. A third nerve palsy produces the pattern of an exodeviation increasing on contralateral gaze and a variable hyperdeviation with a contralateral hyperdeviation on up gaze and an ipsilateral hyperdeviation on down gaze (**Fig. 5.15**). This may be variable depending on whether or not there is divisional third nerve palsy. Two additional "fellow travelers," the eyelid position and the pupil, should be assessed. Specifically, because the third nerve innervates the levator, there is usually a concomitant ptosis, and because the third nerve also controls the sphincter muscles of the iris, the pupil on that side is often larger and does not react normally.

In the setting of a complete third nerve palsy, fourth nerve function can be determined by whether the patient has incyclotorsion while looking down. Small vessels at the limbus can be observed to see if they rotate in when the patient attempts to follow down. The finding of a concomitant fourth and third nerve palsy usually indicates cavernous sinus pathology. Multiple cranial nerve palsies may occur, particularly in the setting of cavernous sinus pathology secondary to parasellar extension.[16,64,65] However, "pieces" of a third nerve palsy, such as isolated medial rectus or isolated inferior rectus weakness, are unlikely to be related to third nerve dysfunction. Instead, they more likely indicate other causes of ocular motor problems, including myasthenia gravis, skew deviation, and restrictive pathology. The pattern of deviation is particularly easily seen on a Hess screen but also can be assessed quickly with a Maddox rod or red glass.

The acute onset of multiple cranial nerve palsies is characteristic of pituitary apoplexy.[66–68] These are often bilateral and accompanied by involvement of the afferent visual pathways, resulting in decreased vision, afferent pupillary defect, and field defects plus associated mental status changes. This event was originally felt to be an uncommon condition related to bleeding into a preexisting pituitary tumor. The advent of imaging has indicated that small bleeds into pituitary tumors are far more common than previously documented, and most patients do not have a

A

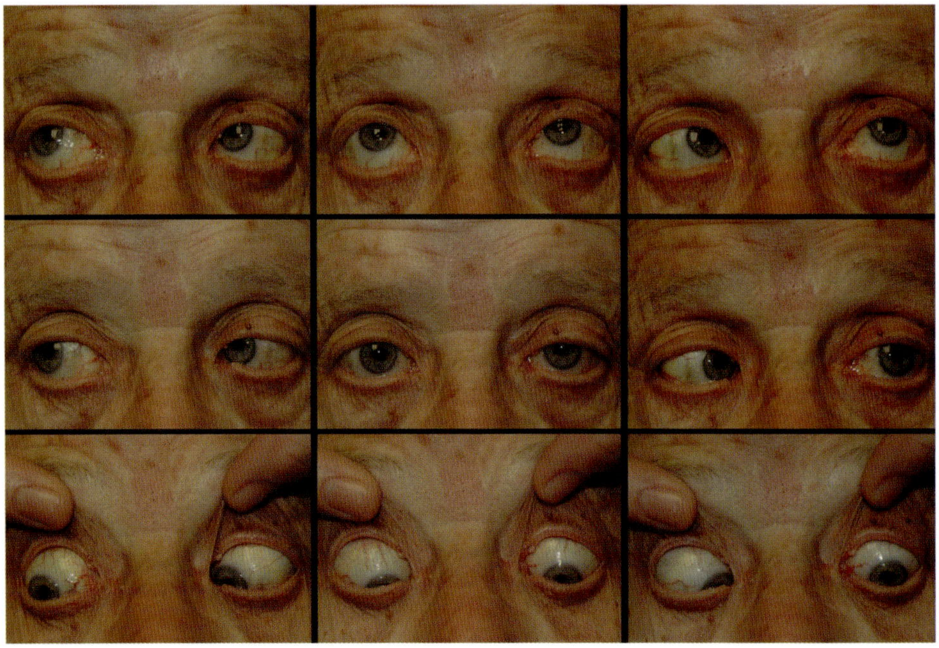

Fig. 5.14 This 78-year-old woman presented in September 2009 with double vision. Her afferent system was entirely intact, but her nine cardinal positions demonstrated an abduction deficit on the left **(A)**.

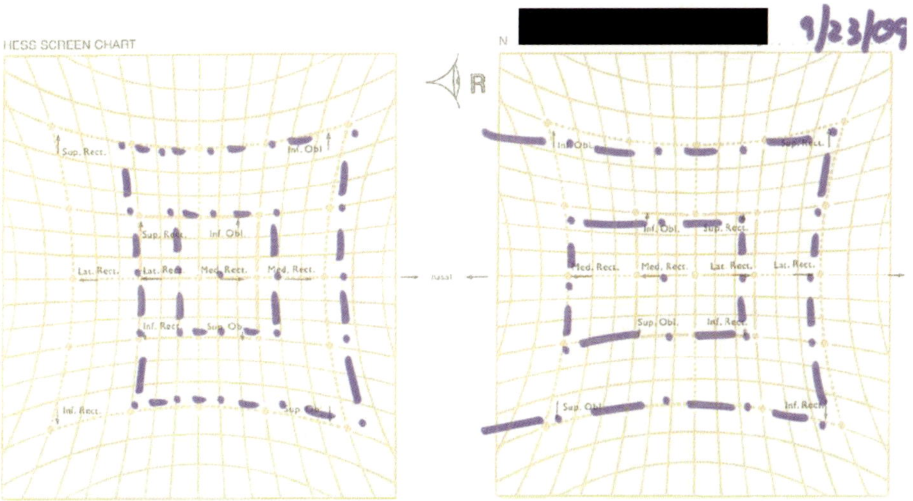

B

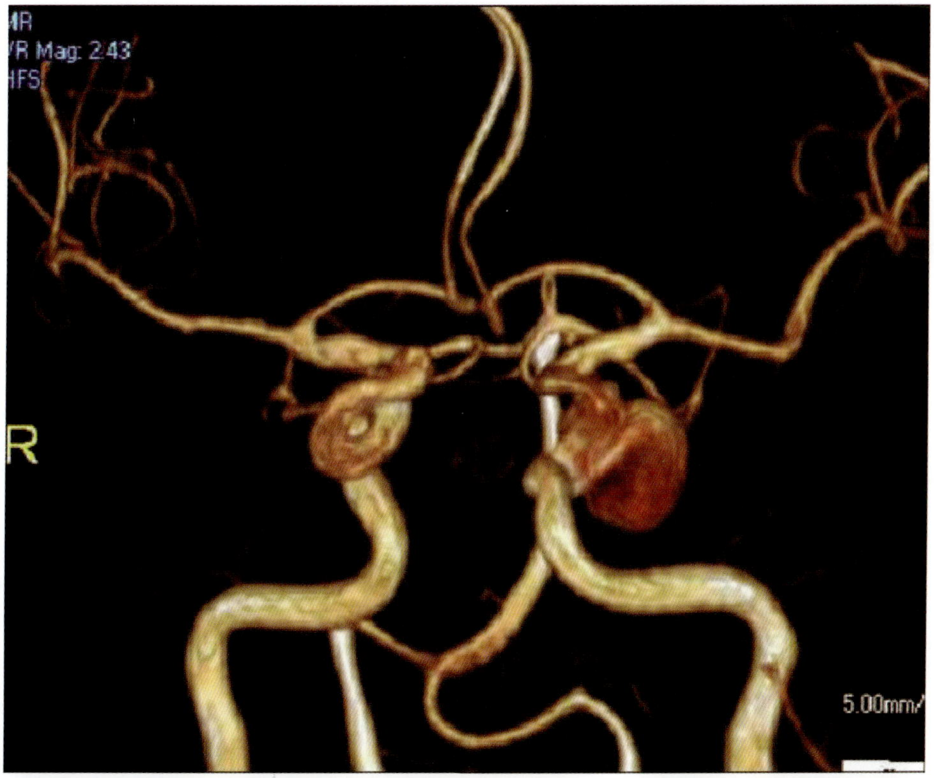

C

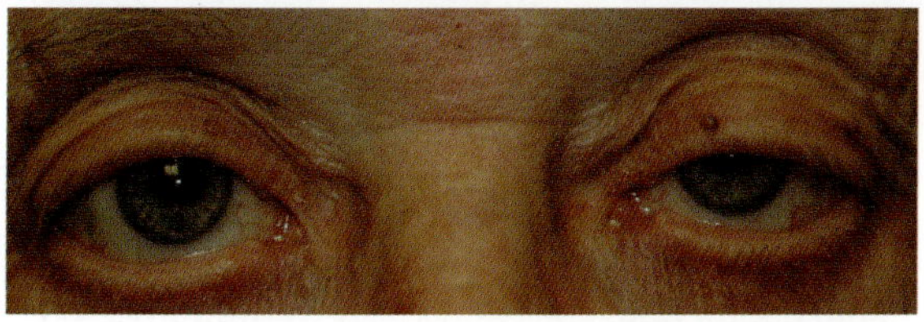

D

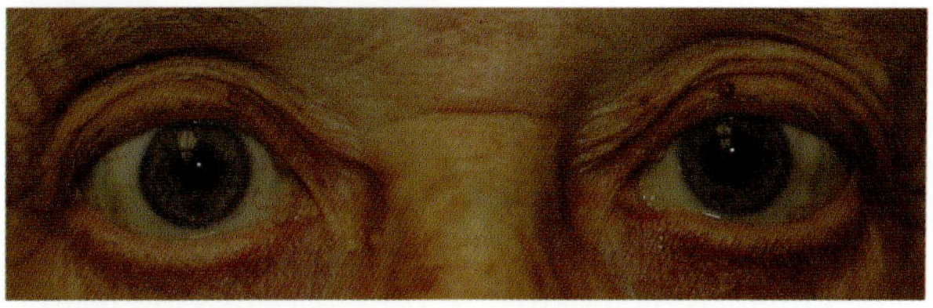

E

Fig. 5.14 *(Continued)* This 78-year-old woman presented in September 2009 with double vision. This is confirmed on her Hess screen, which shows a limitation in left abduction **(B)**. CTA revealed a left carotid cavernous aneurysm **(C)**. Her pupils were also noted to be unequal, with a miotic pupil on the left side and mild ptosis **(D)**. Following Iopidine, the smaller left pupil now is larger, indicating hypersensitivity on the left **(E)**. Comment: This is an example of a combined left sixth nerve and Horner syndrome secondary to a carotid artery aneurysm. The pattern of deviation is easily appreciated on the Hess screen.

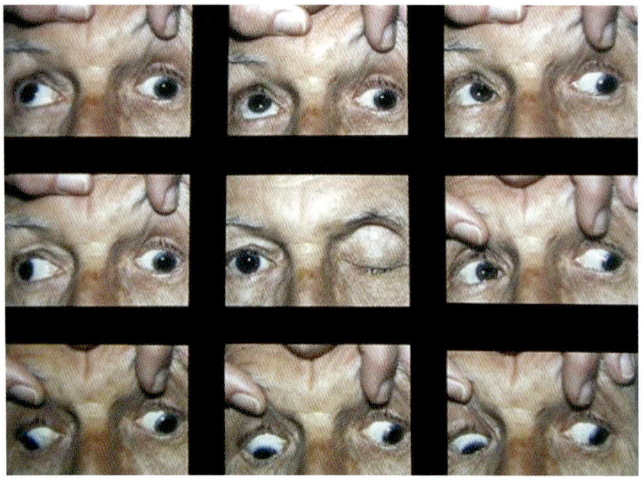

A

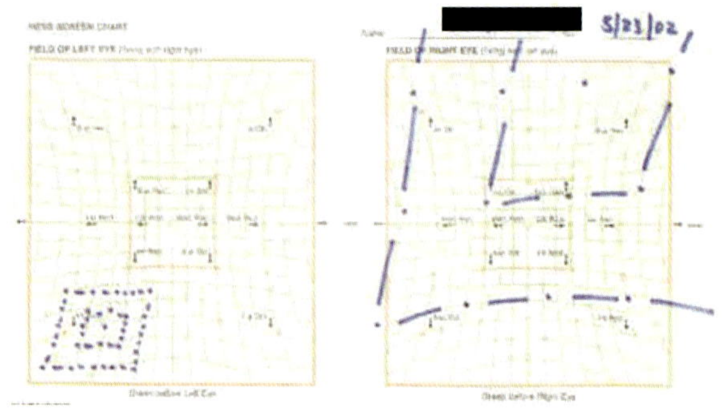

B

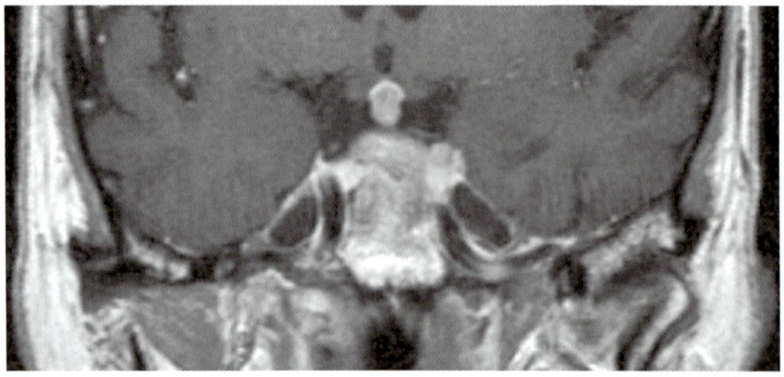

C

Fig. 5.15 This 62-year-old man presented in May of 2002 with a 3-week history of double vision. His acuity was 20/20 and 20/25 with 3-point near vision and full visual fields, but he had complete ptosis OS. Although there was no afferent pupillary defect, the pupil on the left was dilated to 5.5 mm and was nonreactive. His motility demonstrated essentially absent adduction, elevation, and depression on the left **(A)**. His motility problem was confirmed on the Hess screen **(B)**. MRI demonstrated a mass in the sella and left cavernous sinus **(C)**, which proved to be metastatic adenocarcinoma. Comment: The Hess screen demonstrates the pattern of a left third nerve palsy, with the primary deviation on the left and the secondary overaction on the right.

substantial change in their symptomatology. Nonetheless, variations of pituitary apoplexy still do occur, and the sudden onset of multiple cranial nerve palsies and afferent system dysfunction should bring that to mind.

Adnexal Assessment

Adnexal assessment is addressed by measuring the palpebral fissure opening, usually with a millimeter ruler (**Fig. 5.16**). Upper lid range gives a clue to the function of the levator muscle and Müller's muscle (**Fig. 5.17 A,B**). The presence of ptosis can be quantitated by measuring the distance between the center light reflex on the cornea and the upper lid margin. This median reflex distance (MRD; **Fig. 5.18**) decreases in patients with ptosis, or lid droop, and increases in patients with lid retraction. The presence of pathology within the orbit may be suspected by widening of the palpebral fissure, clear evidence of the eye bulging, or more quantitative evidence of relative proptosis or exophthalmos. An additional qualitative assessment may simply be obtained by looking over the patient's forehead for evidence of increased prominence of the globe. Hertel measurements are used to quantitatively assess the distance from the orbital rim to the corneal plane (**Fig. 5.19**). Although the range for normal patients has been published (varying by population), far more valuable is the symmetry expected between the two sides. More than 2 mm of difference between the two eyes usually calls for an explanation. A previous history of trauma, inflammation, or orbital tumors should be sought before it is assumed that this is related to intraorbital extension of parasellar pathology. Proptosis that varies, particularly induced by Valsalva maneuver or bending forward, usually indicates a vascular anomaly such as a venous varix. Rarely, pulsations of the eye may be seen with loss of the bony confines of the orbit. This may be related to previous surgery but can occur with congenital, neoplastic, or vascular anomalies eroding the bone. Vascular abnormalities including carotid cavernous fistulae may also cause pulsations.

One other clue to the presence of pathology involving the orbit itself may be obtained by balloting the eye. Resistance to retropulsion usually indicates pathology within the orbit. This is particularly useful when there is asymmetry between the two sides. In addition to axial displacement of the globe forward, the globe may be displaced inferiorly (dystopia) or in or out relative to the distance from the midline of the nose. This may indicate the origin of pathology affecting the globe and other adnexal structures. Displacement inferiorly usually indicates involvement of the orbit through the roof (**Fig. 5.1**). Displacement of the globe medially would indicate a more central skull base pathology, often entering the orbit through the ethmoid sinus and medial wall. Involvement of the lateral wing of the sphenoid can produce both axial proptosis and displacement of the globe medially or inferiorly. Rarely, masses may actually be palpated within the orbit.

The anterior segment, including the conjunctiva, cornea, iris, anterior chamber, and lens, is best evaluated at the slit lamp. Although a penlight may be helpful, the slit

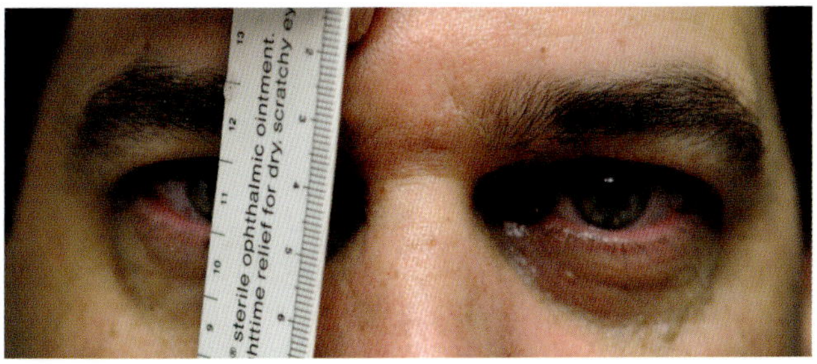

Fig. 5.16 A millimeter ruler can be used to measure the palpebral fissure opening.

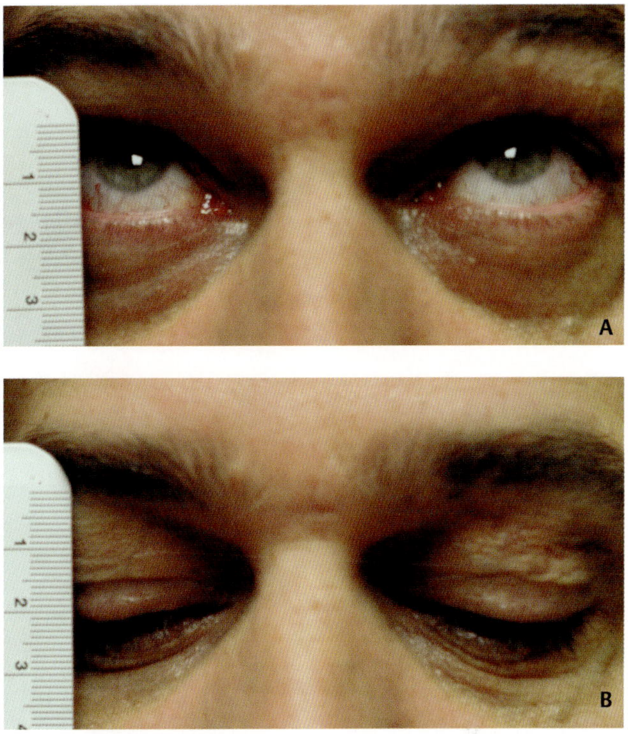

Fig. 5.17 The upper lid range is the measurement between the lid position while the patient is looking up **(A)** and its changed position when the patient is looking down **(B)**. The frontalis muscle should be splinted to more accurately measure levator function.

lamp offers binocular magnification as well as oblique and transillumination (useful for detecting old inflammation). The pupils should be examined for irregularity and symmetry. If the pupils are unequal, they should be recorded in the light and dark. If the difference is greater in light, then the larger pupil is not constricting. Assuming there are no pharmacologic (red top dilating drops), inflammatory, or traumatic causes, one must distinguish between Adie's pupil (postganglionic parasympathetic dysfunction, usually after viral infection or trauma, with vermiform iris movements, light-near dissociation, and tonic redilatation) and third nerve dysfunction, which should be associated with abnormal eye movements. If the pupillary difference is greater in the dark, then the smaller pupil is not dilating (**Fig. 5.20**). Both third nerve palsy and Horner syndrome are common symptoms of parasellar pathology affecting the cavernous sinus. A subtle dilation delay may be seen on serial photographs of the pupils taken after shutting off the lights as a sign of sympathetic dysfunction (Horner syndrome).[69] Horner syndrome may be confirmed by a lack of dilation to cocaine drops or by reversal of anisocoria following apraclonidine (Iopidine) drops (**Figs. 5.14** and **5.20**). Paredrine drops will dilate the pupil of a patient with a first- or second-order Horner syndrome (brainstem, neck, or lung apex), but not a third-order Horner syndrome (seen with parasellar disease). The larger pupil due to a third nerve palsy should react to 1% pilocarpine, whereas a pharmacologically dilated pupil will not.

Two additional critical items in adnexal assessment include evaluation of the fifth cranial nerve and lid closure. Sensation should be checked qualitatively simply by asking the patient to compare sensation in the three divisions of the distribution of the trigeminal nerve. More quantitative assessment can be obtained with an esthesiometer (**Fig. 5.21**), measuring corneal sensitivity. This may be particularly useful in potentially progressive lesions affecting the first division of the fifth nerve, resulting in corneal hypesthesia. A second critical function is that of lid closure. Although lid closure may be affected by proptosis alone, most of the time, marked problems with lid closure are secondary to weakness in the orbicularis muscle. Neuromuscular transmission deficits should always be considered, as should primary involvement of the orbicularis muscle itself (mitochondrial myopathy, as seen in patients with chronic progressive external ophthalmoplegia). Most weakness of lid closure, including decreased blinks and incomplete blinks, is related to facial nerve weakness. The presence of facial nerve paresis in the setting of suspected

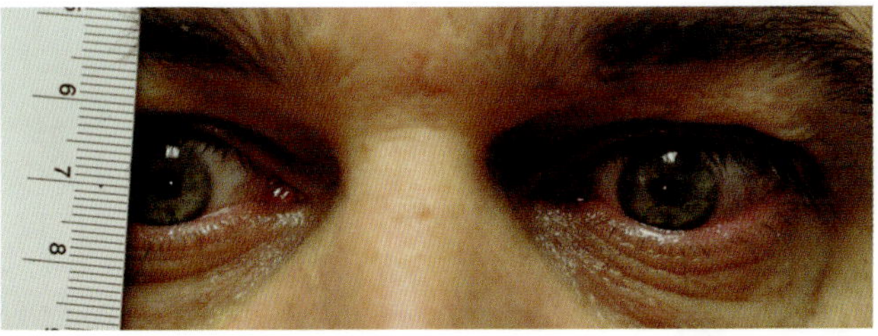

Fig. 5.18 The marginal reflex distance (MRD) is measured from the central corneal reflex to the upper lid margin. If this is less than 4 to 5 mm, there is evidence of ptosis.

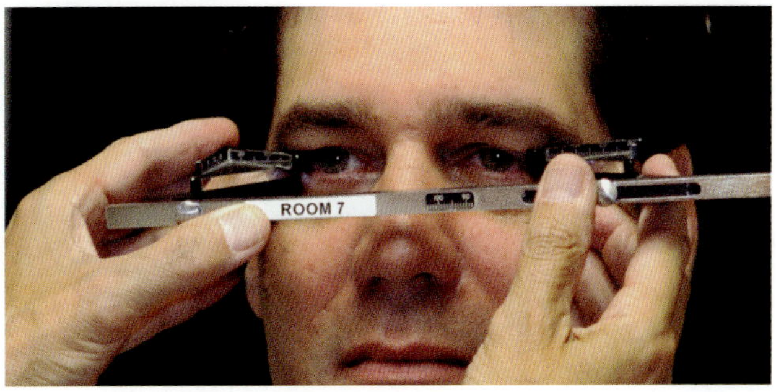

Fig. 5.19 The Hertel exophthalmometer measures the relative distance between the lateral orbital rim and the plane of the cornea. A difference of more than 2 mm suggests either proptosis (exophthalmos) on one side or enophthalmos on the other.

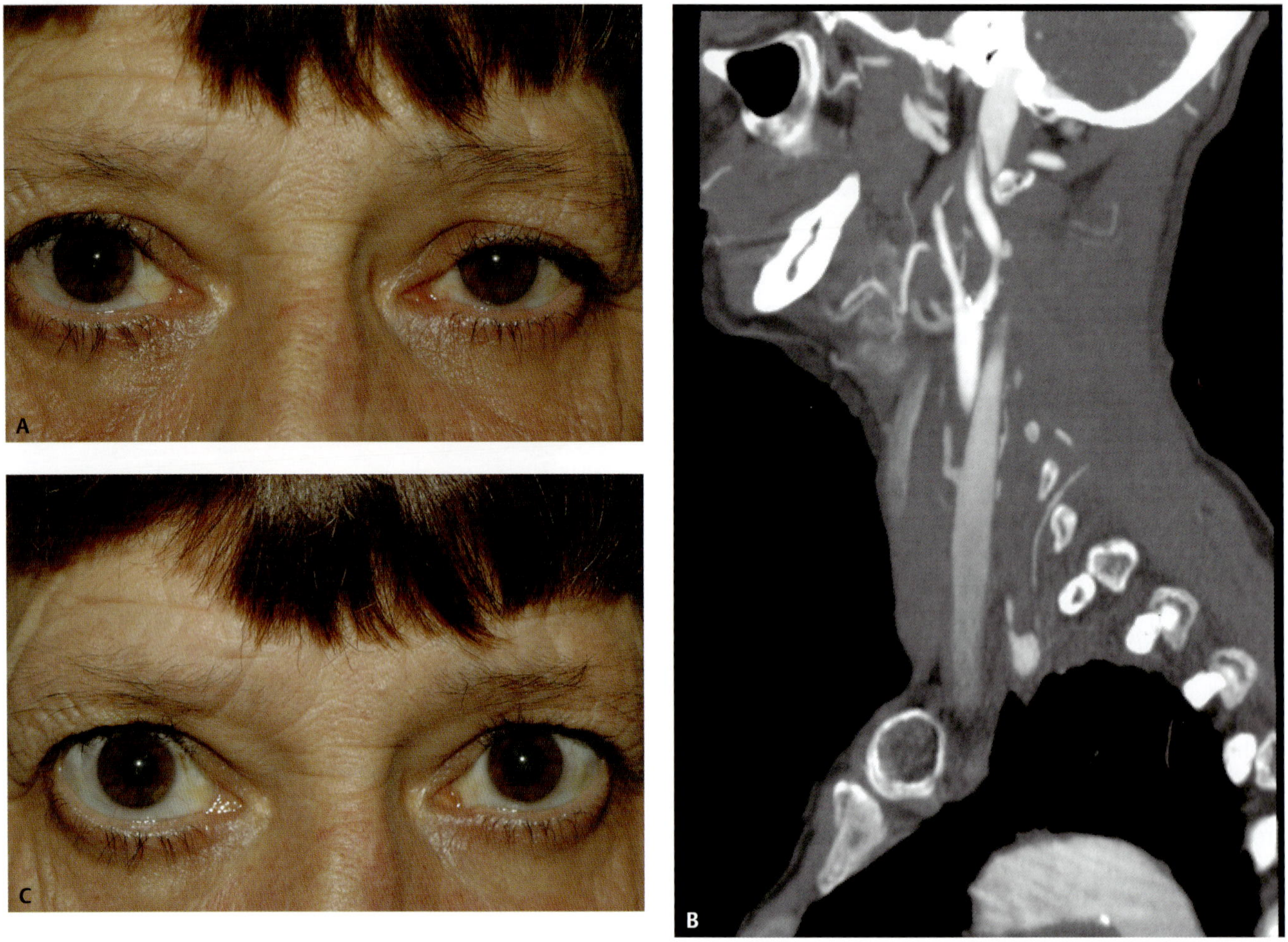

Fig. 5.20 This 50-year-old patient presented without visual complaints but was noted to have asymmetric pupils with mild ptosis on the left side. External photographs reveal mild ptosis and anisocoria with miosis OS **(A)**. Her past medical history was remarkable for a squamous cell mass involving her throat, and she had been treated 2 years earlier with 60 Gy of radiation therapy. CT of her neck revealed evidence of accelerated atherosclerosis of the left common carotid artery at the level of C6-7, undoubtedly related to her previous radiation therapy **(B)**. Iopidine drops reversed the anisocoria, with a larger pupil on the left side now indicative of hypersensitivity following sympathetic denervation **(C)**.

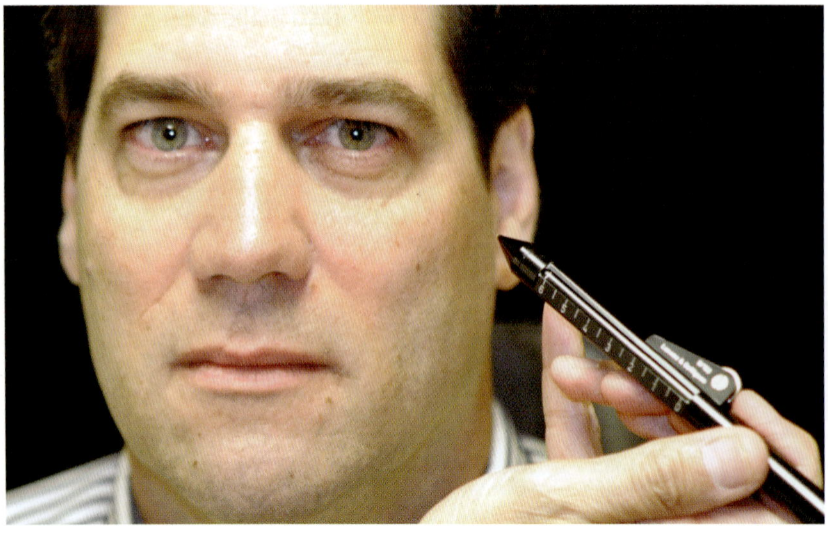

Fig. 5.21 The esthesiometer may be used to quantitatively assess corneal sensitivity.

parasellar pathology would indicate much more extensive involvement or more than a single lesion.

The presence of facial nerve weakness combined with sensory loss has a particularly worrisome implication and needs to be recognized early in the care of patients with parasellar pathology. These patients are likely to develop problems with neurotrophic keratitis, resulting in corneal epithelial breakdown and potentially corneal infection and melt. Primary loss of sensation that is progressive often indicates neurotrophic spread of a skin cancer along the trigeminal nerve. This is particularly common in patients with squamous cell carcinoma and adenoid cystic carcinoma. Extension usually goes back to the cavernous sinus, with motility problems following the loss of sensation.

Overaction of the orbicularis may occur in four settings. Most common is blepharospasm, in which increased lid closure bilaterally is often associated with other orofacial movements (Meige syndrome). Hemifacial spasm is usually unilateral and is associated with compression of the root exit zone of the facial nerve. Quivering movements of the face are seen with both facial myokymia (often due to intra-axial pathology such as multiple sclerosis) and benign facial fasciculations. Accompanying facial weakness is usually a sign of significant disease. Occasionally, the patient cannot initiate lid opening (apraxia of lid opening).

An additional adenxal problem associated with parasellar lesions is that of alteration in tear production. Baseline tear production can be assessed by measuring the wetting of a filter strip (Schirmer's test). Although most literature suggests that baseline tear secretion is unaffected by pathologic denervation of the parasympathetics to the lacrimal gland, lesions affecting the parasympathetics often result in at least mild reduction in baseline tear secretion as measured by asymmetry in Schirmer's test. Even more importantly, surgical intervention can interrupt the parasympathetic pathways, resulting in decreased baseline tear production.

Although the presence of lid retraction is most commonly seen with thyroid orbitopathy (less commonly with Collier's sign, seen with dorsal midbrain syndrome), one important type of lid retraction occurs while the patients attempt to look down and in. This is usually seen in patients with preceding third nerve palsy and indicates aberrant regeneration of the third nerve (**Fig. 5.22**). Fibers that used to go to the medial rectus and inferior rectus are now misdirected to the levator. Other signs of aberrant regeneration include pupillary miosis on up and down gaze, persistent co-contraction of the superior and inferior recti (leading to restricted vertical movement), and adduction with elevation and depression. The lid elevation with depression and adduction is the most classic and obvious sign of aberrant regeneration. In rare cases, a slowly expanding parasellar lesion, such as a giant cavernous carotid aneurysm or meningioma, may produce aberrant regeneration without a history of an acute third nerve palsy. This form of "primary aberrant regeneration" is very suggestive of a slowly expanding parasellar lesion.[70,71]

Relative enophthalmos is most commonly due to previous trauma, including blowout fractures of the orbit or previous hemorrhage resulting in orbital fat atrophy. Chronic inflammation of the maxillary sinus can result in enlargement of the orbit and enophthalmos (so-called silent sinus syndrome). Metastatic breast carcinoma often can produce shrinkage of the fat, resulting in a combination of enophthalmos and restricted motility.

Enlargement of the greater wing of the sphenoid, frequently related to meningioma, often presents with proptosis. However, involvement of the orbit from any direction, including through the superior orbital fissure, from and through the roof with hyperostosis, and from the sphenoid sinus and posterior ethmoids, can result in axial displacement (proptosis) as well as dystopia, with the globe displaced inferior or laterally, and less commonly medially or superiorly.

◆ Rehabilitation

Rehabilitation of Afferent System Dysfunction

Ability to improve compromised optic nerve function is limited. Unlike goldfish, which can regrow their optic nerves, at this point we have limited options to influence the recovery of optic nerve function. It should be pointed out that visual fields often will continue to improve for periods of up to a year or more following surgical decompression of optic nerve or chiasmal compression (**Fig. 5.23**). This can be seen with gradual improvement in visual field function in patients with pituitary tumors following surgery.[72,73] It is likely that this functional improvement is separate from anatomic improvement because OCT thinning and optic atrophy tend to remain (**Fig. 5.23**). It is important to note that psychophysical functioning, electrophysiologic studies, and anatomic studies such as OCT and disc appearance, although paralleling each other, may not always be exactly linked. This is particularly obvious in patients with optic neuritis, whose central acuity and even visual fields may return to normal despite clear evidence of residual optic atrophy, OCT thinning, and electrophysiologic abnormalities, including prolonged latency on visual evoked potential. Thus, it is important to recognize that each of these assessments of afferent visual system does not replace the others.

Patients with visual impairment can be helped with various low-vision aids. These may be low-tech, including simple high-plus magnifiers that allow patients to see small objects by holding them closer, or fairly sophisticated magnification systems, including computer-driven closed circuit TV monitors. Although substantial work is being done on bionic replacement for dysfunctional afferent visual pathways, at present this is strictly theoretic and research-driven. Low-vision aids, however, can be very useful if patients can define the exact function they would like to improve. Although it is often impossible to resupply visual acuity for some of the activities of daily living, such as driving, reading can be helped, as can functioning at particular defined distances.

Visual field defects also represent a substantial challenge. Although there have been attempts at encourag-

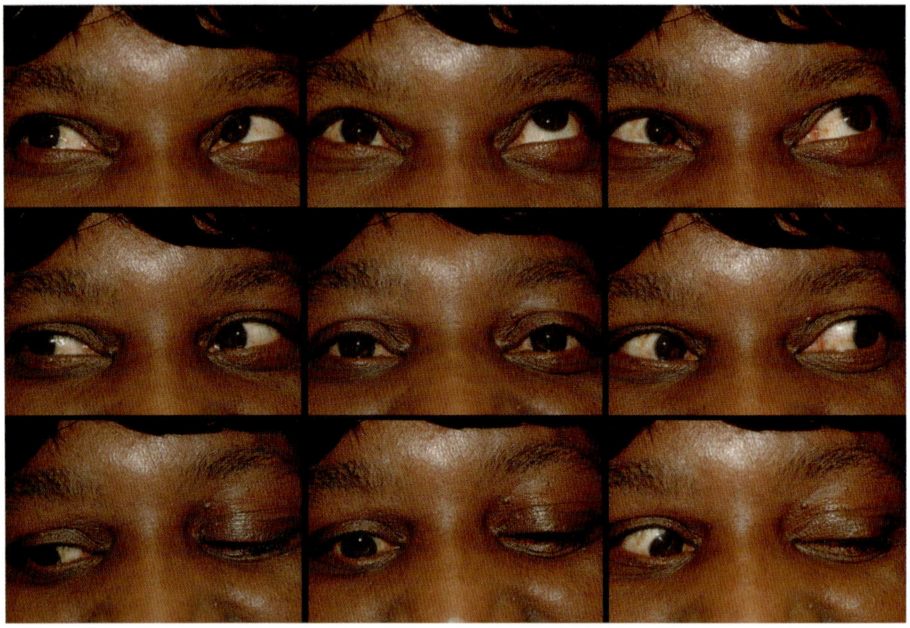

A

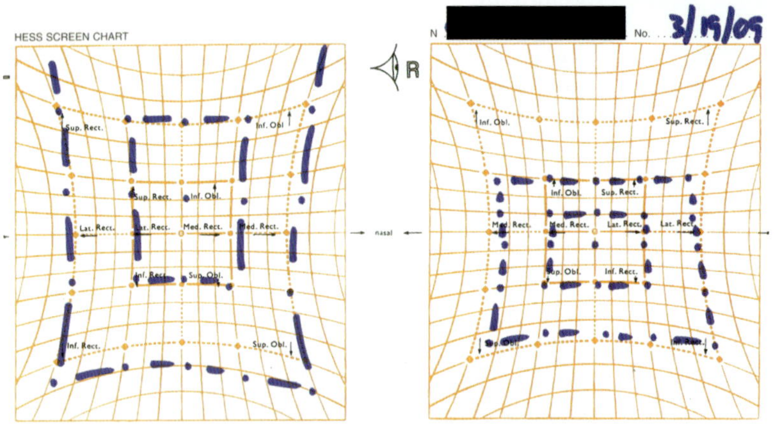

B

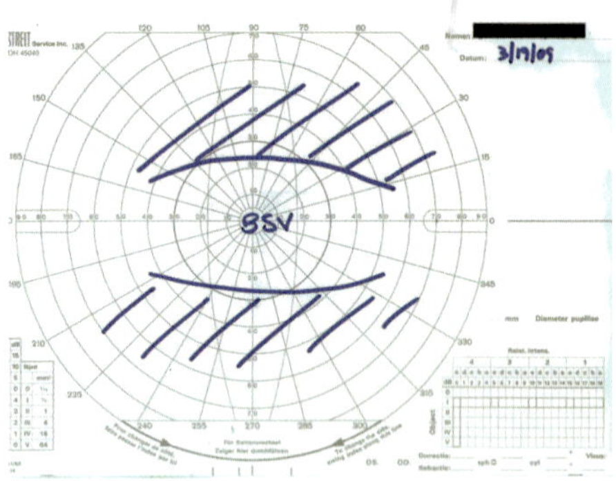

C

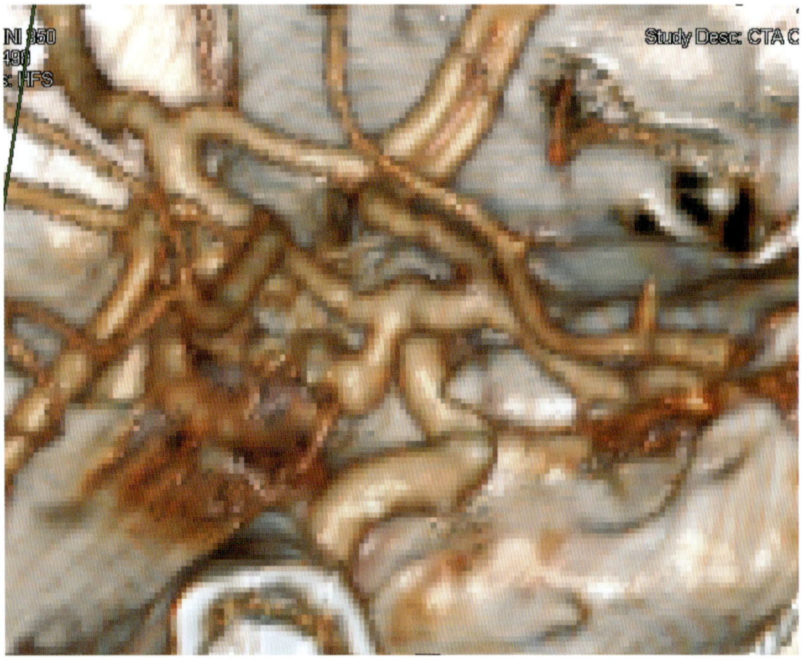

D

Fig. 5.22 This 54-year-old woman was seen in March of 2009 with mild persistent double vision. On examination, she could see 20/20 bilaterally with 4-point and 3-point vision. Her visual fields were full. She did, however, have limitation in vertical gaze on the right and 1.5 mm of right ptosis, and when she looked down and to the left, her right eyelid was elevated **(A)**. Hess screen confirmed limitation in vertical (particularly up) gaze **(B)**. Binocular single vision fields demonstrated single vision when she looked straight ahead but double when she looked up or down **(C)**. Eight months earlier, she had acutely developed a severe headache. CT revealed evidence of subarachnoid hemorrhage, and CTA demonstrated a right posterior communicating artery aneurysm **(D)**.

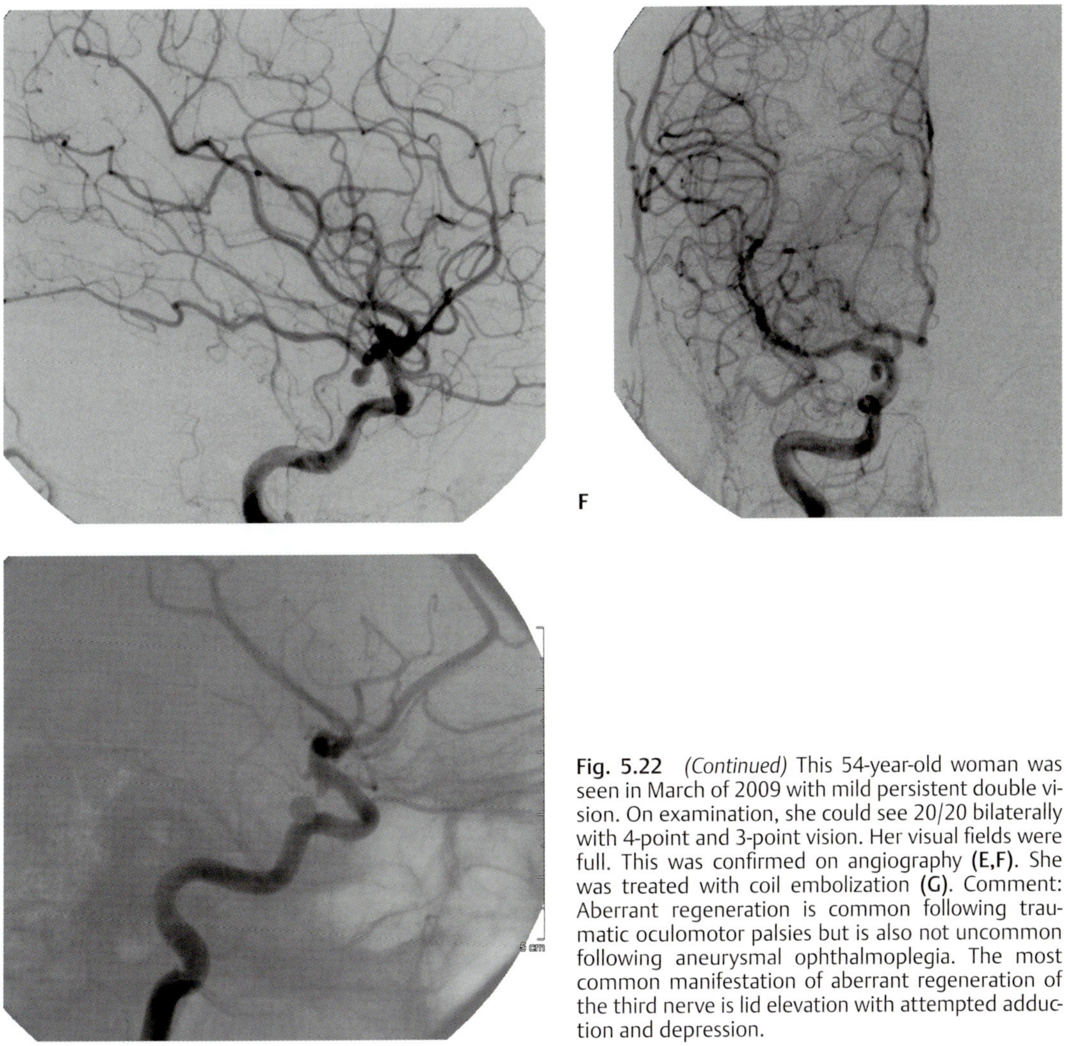

E

F

G

Fig. 5.22 *(Continued)* This 54-year-old woman was seen in March of 2009 with mild persistent double vision. On examination, she could see 20/20 bilaterally with 4-point and 3-point vision. Her visual fields were full. This was confirmed on angiography **(E,F)**. She was treated with coil embolization **(G)**. Comment: Aberrant regeneration is common following traumatic oculomotor palsies but is also not uncommon following aneurysmal ophthalmoplegia. The most common manifestation of aberrant regeneration of the third nerve is lid elevation with attempted adduction and depression.

ing visual plasticity, it is unlikely that major field defects can be bypassed. Practice with visual field defects, however, can markedly improve the ability to read. Simple techniques such as orienting letters vertically, in the case of patients with homonymous visual field defects, can sometimes improve the ability to read,[74,75] and the use of simple tricks, such as leading the eye proprioceptively with a finger or a ruler to find the next line, can be helpful in the rehabilitation of patients with marked visual field abnormalities. High-power prisms have been used to try to bring objects into a seeing field from a nonseeing field. This has limited applicability, however, and it certainly should not be promised as a way of restoring the ability to drive to patients with dense homonymous visual field defects. They may occasionally be useful to alert patients to events in their nonseeing field.

Efferent System Rehabilitation

It is usually not possible to restore normal ductions. In the setting of restrictive strabismus, particularly after involvement of the orbit by a tumor or by a surgical approach, restrictive strabismus can be released by recessing the affected fibrotic muscle. This, unfortunately, does not usually improve ductions overall. In the setting of marked limitation of ductions, something that may occur following prolonged complete involvement of the third cranial nerve or more likely the sixth cranial nerve, in which the eye may gradually drift into abduction or adduction, the eye can be recentered with eye muscle surgery. This should be undertaken only once there is stability. A more common challenge is the problem of double vision, seen in patients with ocular malalignment. The most likely short-term solution is simply to occlude one eye. Although this sometimes

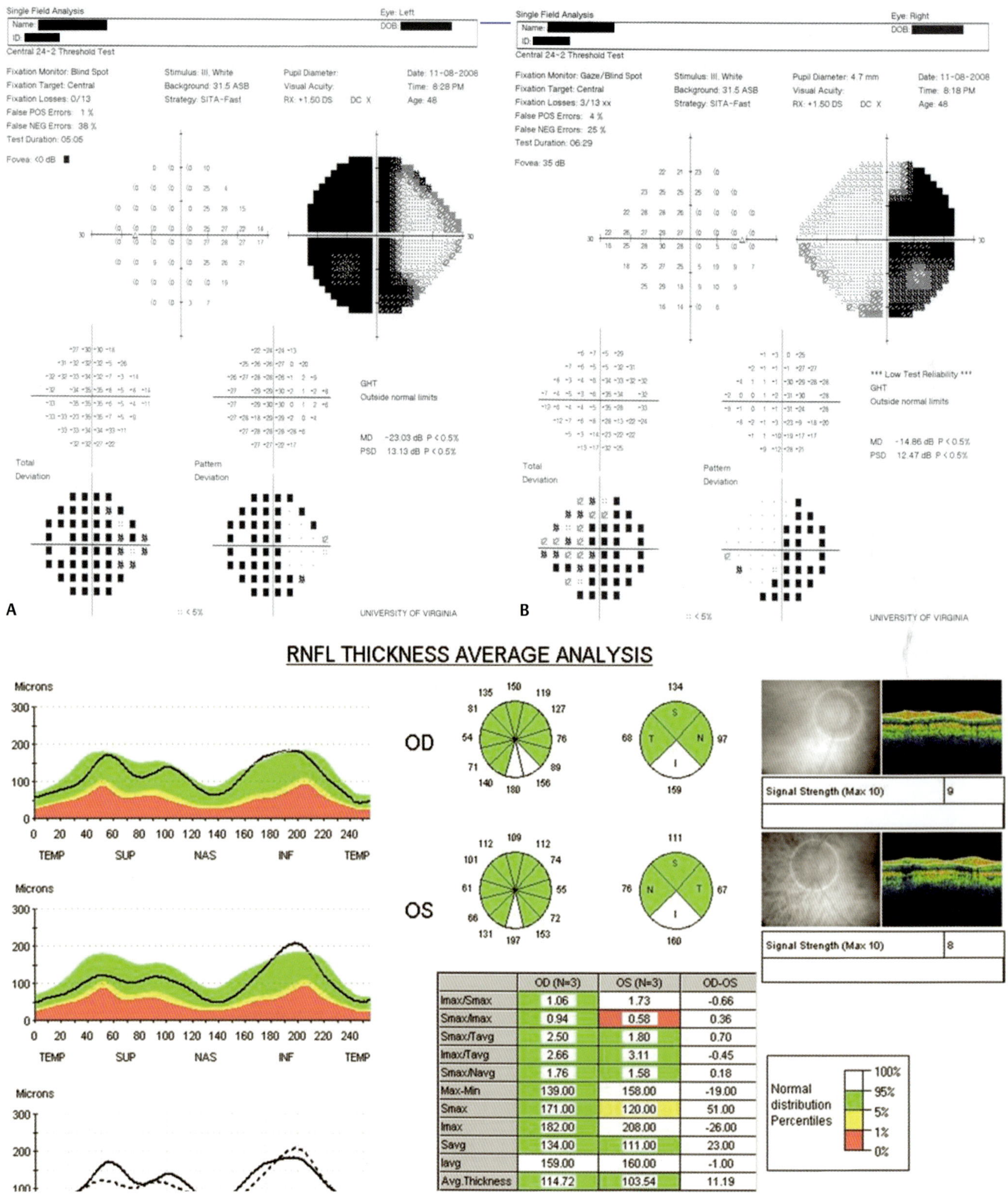

Fig. 5.23 These are the visual fields **(A,B)** of a 48-year-old woman who was referred with a 1-month history of decreasing vision. Visual acuity when evaluated was 20/30 on the right and 8/200 on the left, with a 0.3 log unit afferent pupillary defect. Her funduscopic examination was unremarkable, and optical coherence tomography (OCT) demonstrated a normal nerve fiber layer **(C)**.

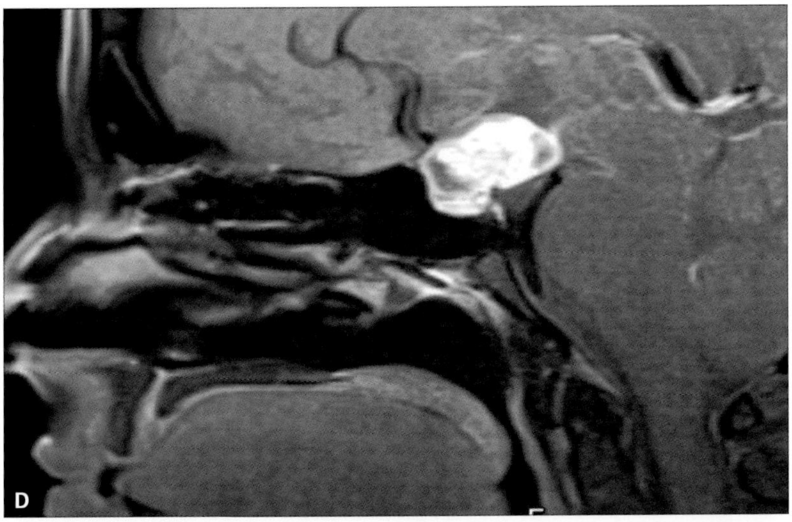

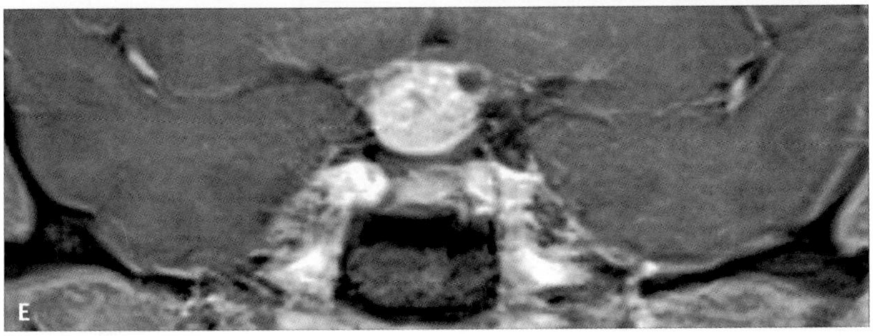

Fig. 5.23 *(Continued)* MRI, however, revealed a suprasellar lesion compressing the chiasm and impacting both optic nerves **(D,E)**. Her past medical history was remarkable for a 10-month history of polydipsia and polyuria, a 7-month history of amenorrhea, and a 1-month history of severe headaches, nausea, and vomiting. Transsphenoidal surgery demonstrated a craniopharyngioma, which was endoscopically decompressed. Follow-up visual fields 2 months later revealed dramatic improvement in the bitemporal defect **(F,G)**, with visual acuity improving to 20/25 and 20/20. *(Continued on page 106)*

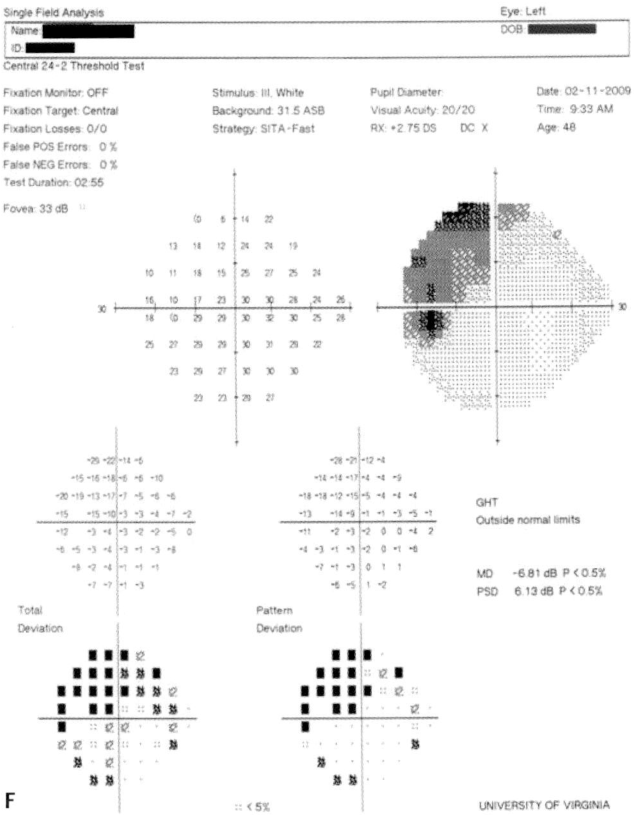

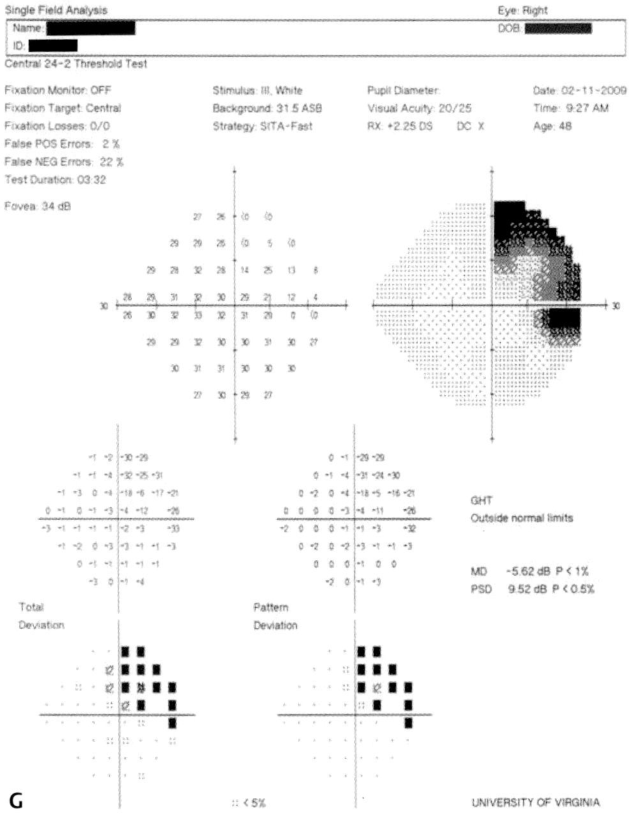

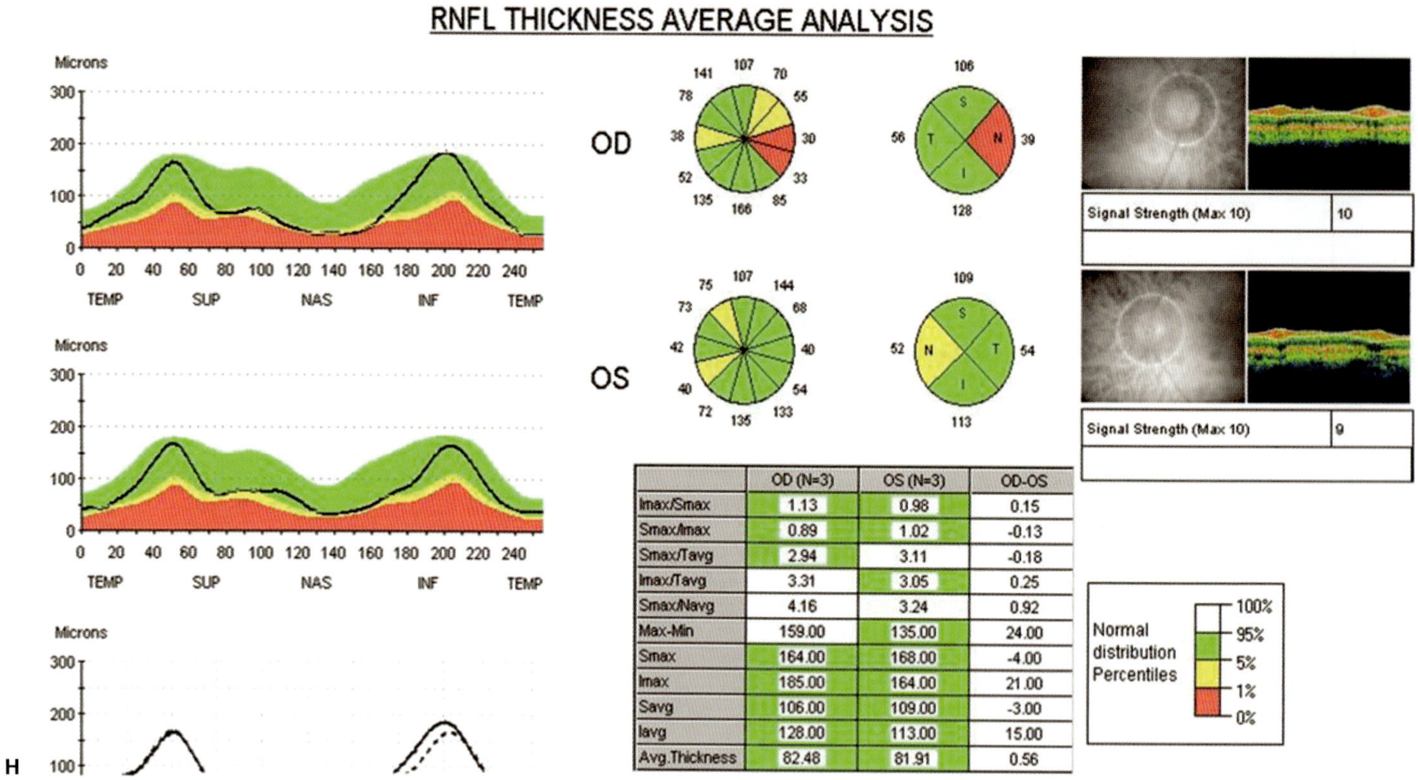

	OD (N=3)	OS (N=3)	OD-OS
Imax/Smax	1.13	0.98	0.15
Smax/Imax	0.89	1.02	-0.13
Smax/Tavg	2.94	3.11	-0.18
Imax/Tavg	3.31	3.05	0.25
Smax/Navg	4.16	3.24	0.92
Max-Min	159.00	135.00	24.00
Smax	164.00	168.00	-4.00
Imax	185.00	164.00	21.00
Savg	106.00	109.00	-3.00
Iavg	128.00	113.00	15.00
Avg.Thickness	82.48	81.91	0.56

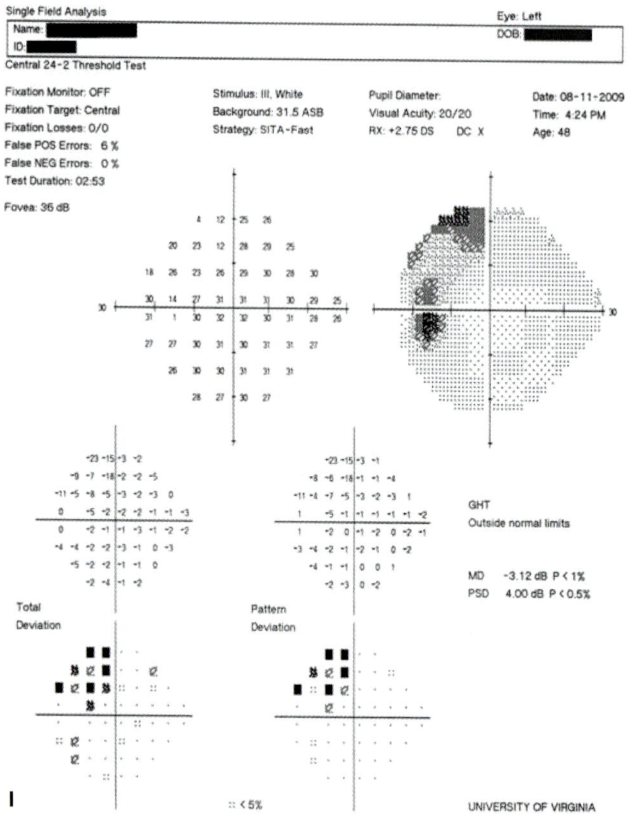

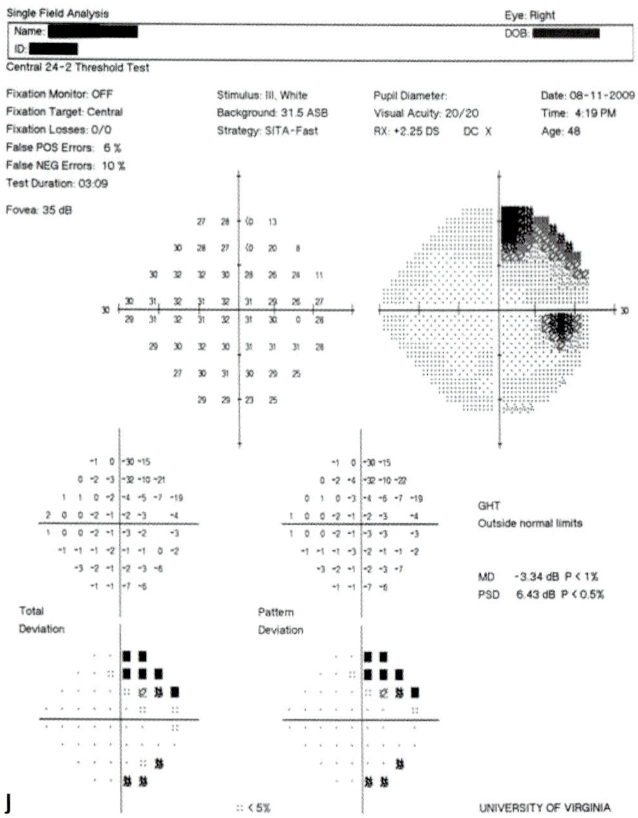

Fig. 5.23 *(Continued)* Despite the improvement in her fields, her OCT demonstrated thinning of the nerve fiber layer nasally in both eyes **(H)**. Follow-up 6 months after that revealed further improvement in the bitemporal visual field defects **(I,J)**, but with some residual optic atrophy **(K,L)** and further thinning of the nerve fiber layer, worse on the left than the right **(M)**.

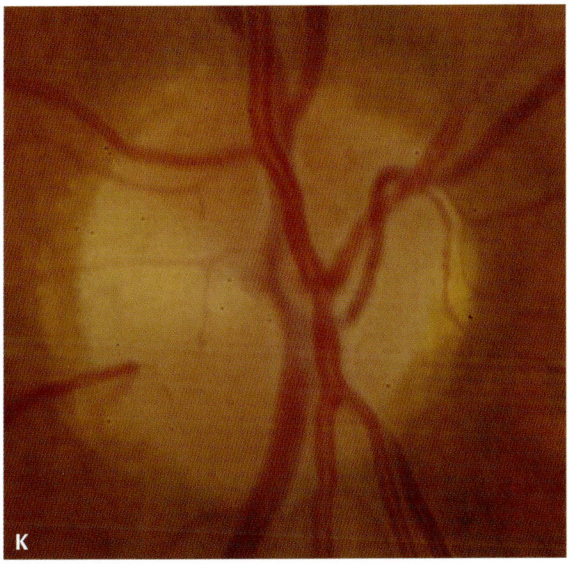

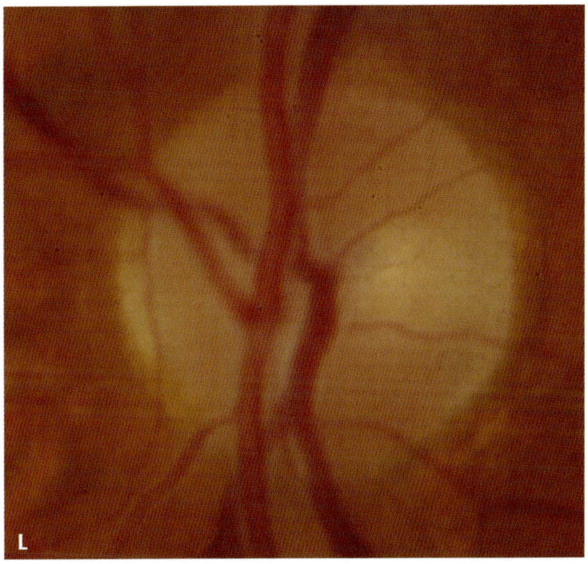

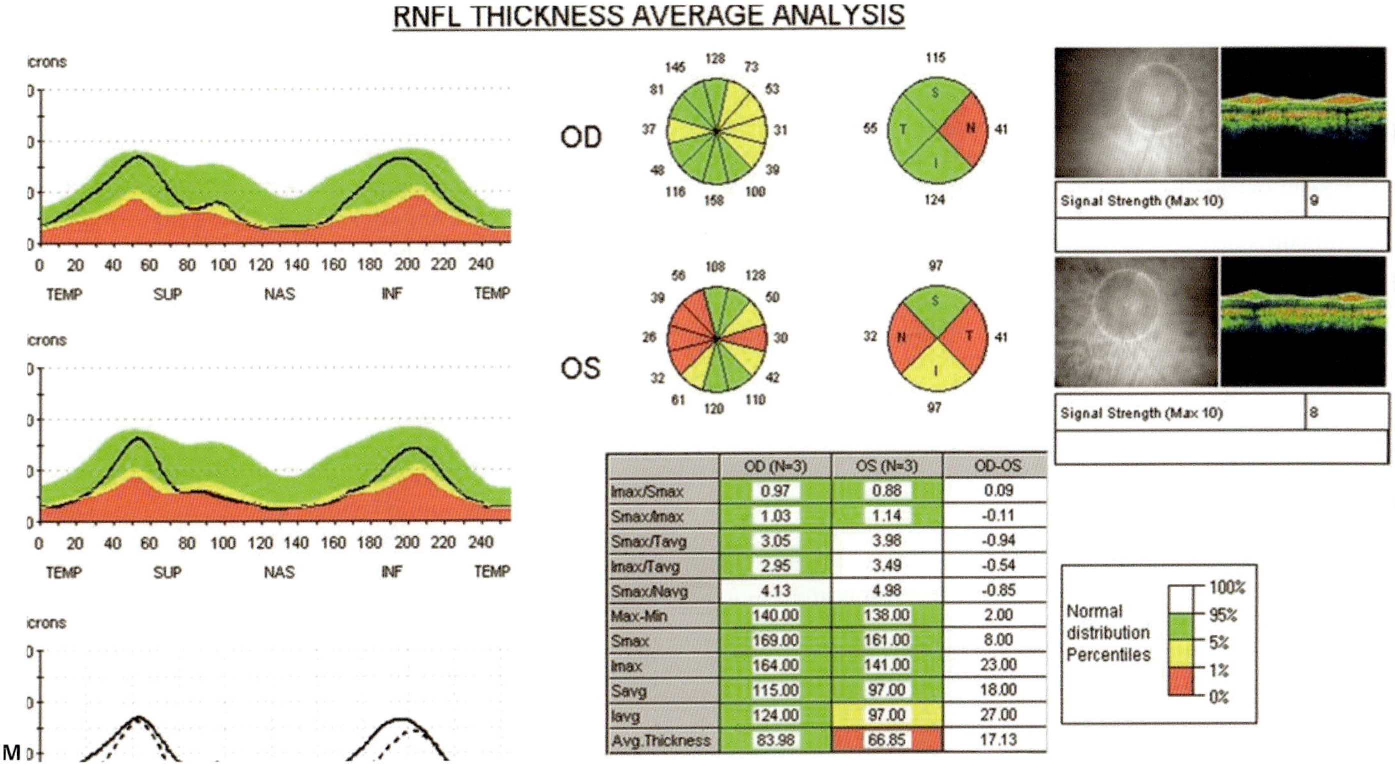

	OD (N=3)	OS (N=3)	OD-OS
Imax/Smax	0.97	0.88	0.09
Smax/Imax	1.03	1.14	-0.11
Smax/Tavg	3.05	3.98	-0.94
Imax/Tavg	2.95	3.49	-0.54
Smax/Navg	4.13	4.98	-0.85
Max-Min	140.00	138.00	2.00
Smax	169.00	161.00	8.00
Imax	164.00	141.00	23.00
Savg	115.00	97.00	18.00
Iavg	124.00	97.00	27.00
Avg.Thickness	83.98	66.85	17.13

Fig. 5.23 *(Continued)* Follow-up 6 months after that revealed further improvement in the bitemporal visual field defects **(I,J)**, but with some residual optic atrophy **(K,L)** and further thinning of the nerve fiber layer, worse on the left than the right **(M)**. Comment: The presence of a normal nerve fiber layer when the patient was first evaluated suggested that the compression of the chiasm was relatively acute. Recent studies suggest that this may be a good prognostic sign for improvement in both acuity and visual fields, as was the case here. Although acuity often improves immediately following decompression, visual fields may take months or more to show improvement. Despite the field improvement, however, she was left with residual optic atrophy and nerve fiber layer thinning.

takes some getting used to, patients can function perfectly well and can engage in most activities of daily living, including driving, with a single eye. The chief challenge early on is that of reaching for near objects because it is difficult to judge near distances. The loss of stereopsis, however, is usually not important for any distance substantially beyond arm's length. Even for objects close up, over time patients learn to use monocular clues to more accurately judge distances. Although botulinum toxin (Botox) injections into the muscle opposite to the involved muscle can result in decreased contracture, it is unlikely that the patient will achieve substantial functional realignment because the effects tend to be variable, and injection of the extraocular muscles often results in inadvertent development of vertical movement problems. Prisms are seldom useful in the acute setting because most deviations secondary to ocular motor nerve palsies are markedly incomitant, meaning the deviation varies depending on where the patient is looking. Sometimes, however, realignment is possible, at least in primary position, and a second prism power in down reading gaze may allow them to use both eyes together.

Over time, if the deviation does not clear or if we have been unable to improve things, there is a natural tendency for any residual deviation to become increasingly comitant. This so-called spread of comitance is due to the unequal innervation of the yoke muscles (violation of Hering's law). This change makes it easier to correct any residual deviation with the use of prisms, or possibly with extraocular muscle surgery. It is imperative that patients remain stable before any sort of surgical intervention is considered. A minimum of 6 to 9 months is required before eye muscle surgery can be entertained. As mentioned, Botox injection to the extraocular muscles is sometimes useful, particularly to avoid contracture of shortening muscles due to unopposed action. This is particularly true in patients with complete sixth nerve palsies who develop progressive esodeviation that can be at least partially relieved or tempered by injecting the medial rectus muscle. This can be accomplished under direct electromyographic control; small doses of Botox can weaken the overacting medial rectus, at least over the short run, and reduce or mitigate further contracture. As mentioned, it is important to undertake a quantitative assessment of ocular motility, including quantitative use of a Maddox rod or cross-cover testing with prisms or, better yet, use of the Hess screen and binocular single vision fields to demonstrate stability, before eye muscle surgery is considered.

Once the eye is stable, eye muscle surgery can be planned, particularly with use of the Hess screen. It is usually impossible to improve the ductions of a limited eye secondary to persistent residual cranial nerve palsy. This is particularly true in patients who develop aberrant regeneration of the third nerve. In this, persistent co-contraction of the superior and inferior rectus muscles limits vertical excursion. As it is impossible to rewire the eye, the only way of increasing binocularity is to limit the movement of the better-moving eye. Although this takes some explaining to the patient and family, it is possible to increase the area of binocularity and reduce diplopia. This is best accomplished through the use of posterior fixation sutures (Faden procedure), in which a combination of recessing the muscle and adding sutures placed well posteriorly limits the overall excursion of the better-moving eye (**Fig. 5.24**). Again, it is essential to make sure the eye is stable before this sort of intervention is considered.

In the setting of a complete sixth nerve palsy, to provide a tonic abducting force, a transposition procedure can be accomplished, moving the superior and inferior rectus muscles to the insertion of the lateral (**Fig. 5.25**). This may be done as a full-thickness transposition or as a partial-thickness transposition, which may potentially spare some of the circulation to the anterior segment. The presence of pulleys controlling the position of the muscles[76] limits the extent of transposition, and an important recent modification of this technique involves the use of posterior fixation sutures along the area of the globe equator. This moves the effectiveness of the transposition more posteriorly and results in a greater abducting effect than does a simple transposition procedure alone. This so-called Foster modification is part of the routine in moving the eye out following a complete sixth nerve palsy. A similar procedure may be used in the absence of elevation (double elevator palsy), in which the medial and lateral rectus muscles are moved superiorly to act as elevators. The pulley system controlling the extraocular muscles again limits the amount of transposition possible. Decisions about the type of extraocular muscle surgery usually depend on whether or not the defect is complete. In the setting of a complete sixth nerve palsy, the usual sequence would be to perform a transposition procedure to give some tonic abduction to the eye, followed by limiting procedures on the opposite yoke muscle (the medial rectus in the opposite eye). In the setting of an incomplete sixth nerve palsy, weakening of the medial rectus in the opposite eye, which would include a recession procedure and Faden operation, would be the primary surgical intervention. This can later be fine-tuned by a recession and resection of the various muscles on the involved side to move the eye into better alignment. It is also important to recognize that any subtle residual defect can be managed with prism in glasses, although ground-in prism is limited to approximately 6 degrees of malalignment (12 diopters of ground-in prism). Although larger Fresnel prisms may be applied to the glasses, these usually degrade acuity by blurring visual function. They are often not tolerated for lengths of time but can be tried as a temporary measure.

Adnexal Rehabilitation

Probably the most important aspect of adnexal rehabilitation is to provide for adequate lid function. In the setting of a seventh nerve palsy, it is critical to ensure lid closure to avoid neuroparalytic keratitis. Short-term measures include aggressive lubrication, including ointment at nighttime, and potentially taping the eye at night. During the day, adequate lubrication without blurring of the vision can be obtained with semiviscous solutions such as Refresh Liquigel and GenTeal Gel. Partial tarsorrhaphies or even central tarsorrhaphies can protect the globe in the short term if the patient has epithelial breakdown, particularly in the setting of combined facial nerve palsy and trigemi-

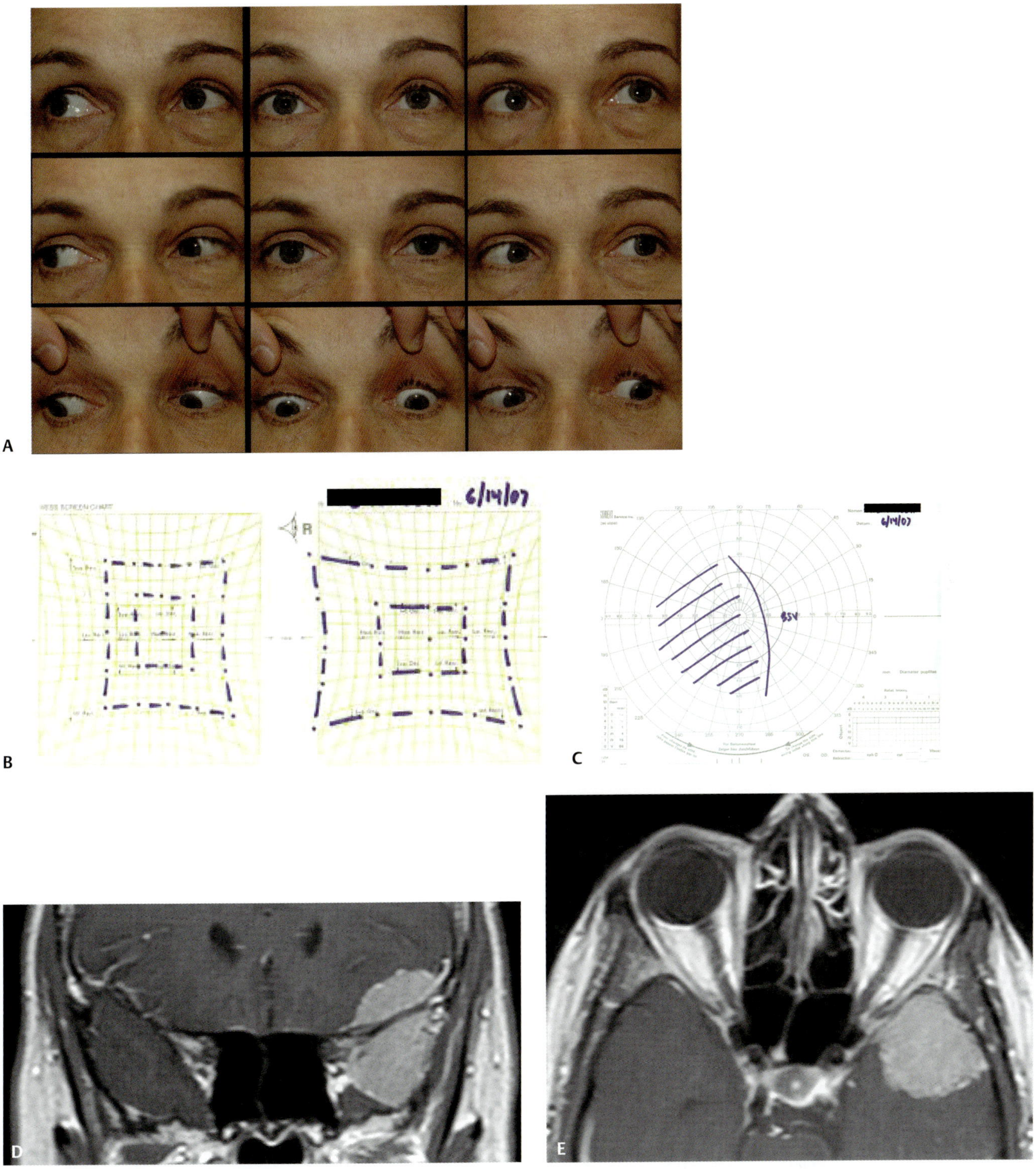

Fig. 5.24 In June of 2007 a 50-year-old woman was referred for diplopia. Her acuity and visual fields were normal, but she had evidence of an abduction deficit on the left side **(A)** with an esotropia increasing on left gaze **(B)**. Binocular single vision fields **(C)** confirmed diplopia on left gaze. Seven months earlier, she had begun to have episodes of "voices in my head." EEG demonstrated an epileptogenic focus, and MRI in April had revealed a sphenoid wing meningioma **(D,E)**. *(Continued on page 110)*

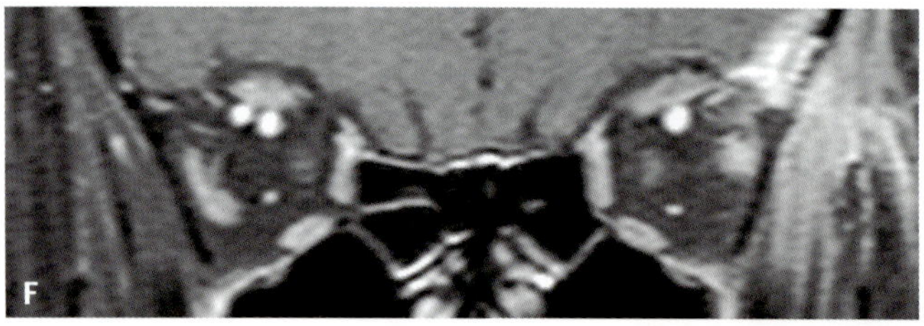

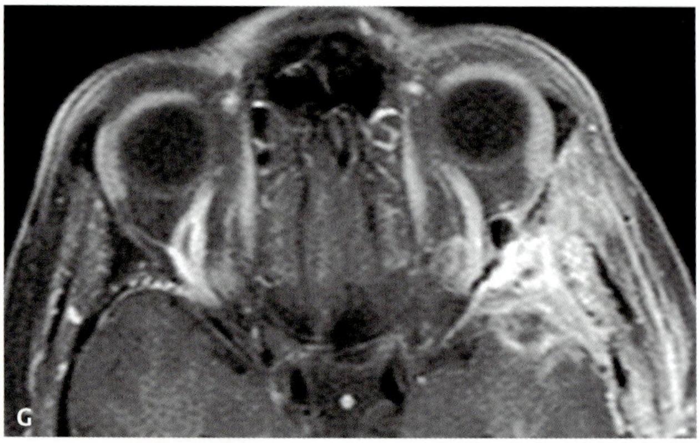

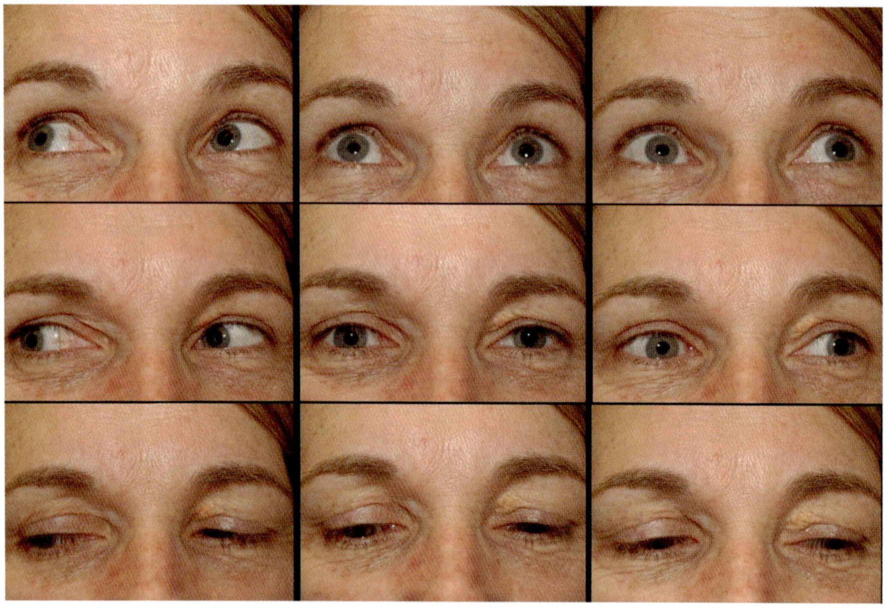

H

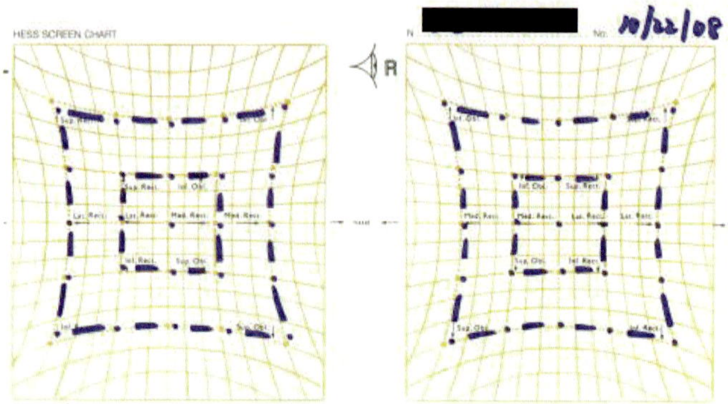

I

Fig. 5.24 *(Continued)* In June of 2007 a 50-year-old woman was referred for diplopia. One month later, she had undergone pterional craniotomy and tumor resection. Repeat MRI demonstrated damage to the left lateral rectus muscle **(F,G)**. One year later, when her motility failed to improve spontaneously, she underwent a right medial rectus recession and Faden procedure. This limited the adduction on the right to match the limited abduction on the left **(H)** and completely eliminated her double vision **(I)**. Comment: With both paretic and restrictive causes of limitation in motility, it is often impossible to improve ductions. Although the eye can be straightened in primary position to maximize binocularity, surgery on the contralateral eye may be advisable.

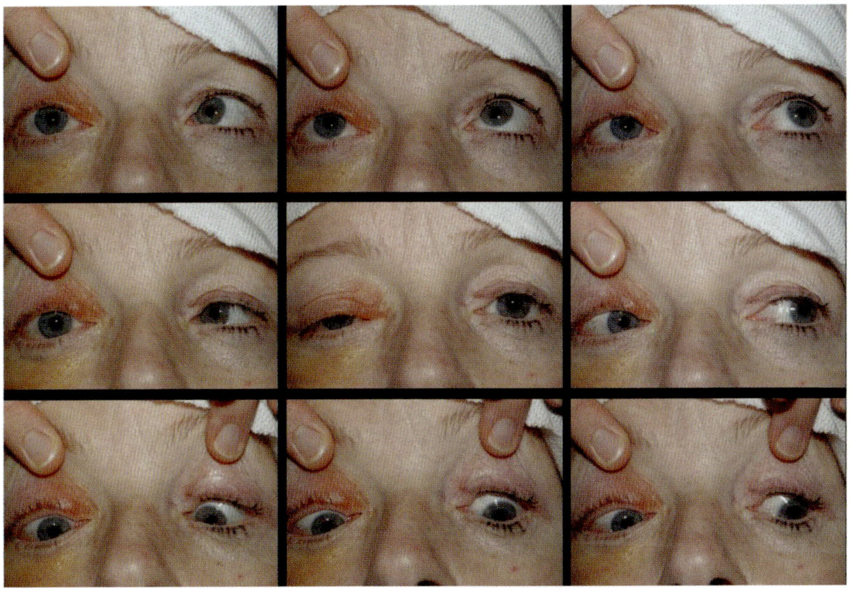

A

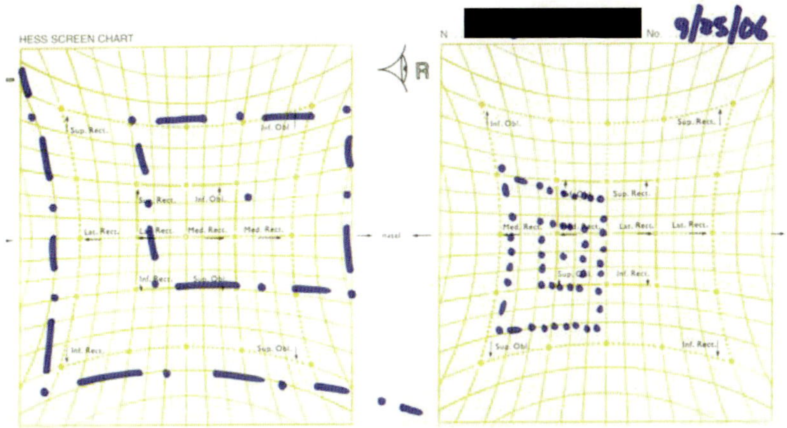

B

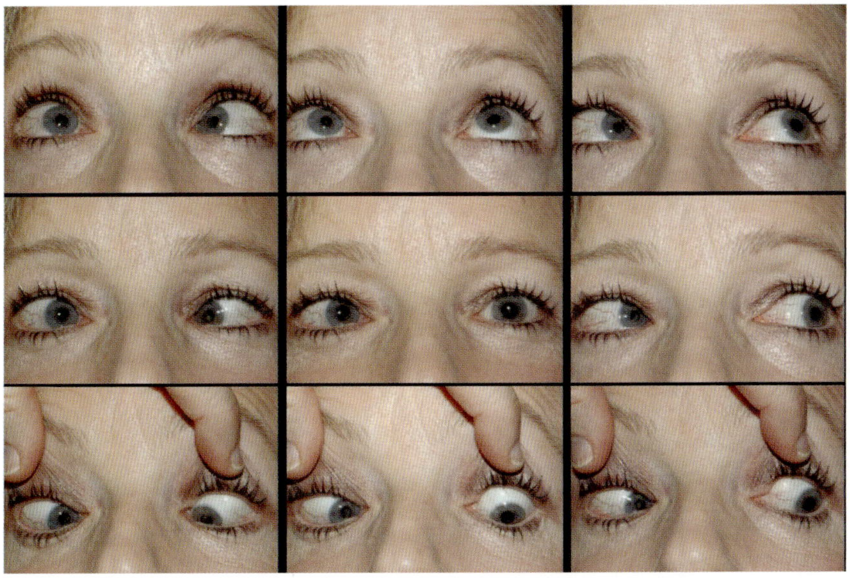

C

Fig. 5.25 This 48-year-old patient noted some ringing in her ears, and MRI demonstrated a parasellar right cavernous meningioma. She underwent pterional craniotomy and resection, which left her with a right IV, V, and VI cranial nerve palsy. Immediately following surgery, the abduction deficit could be seen on her nine cardinal positions **(A)**, and the Hess screen **(B)** confirmed a problem with abduction. There was no recovery of nerve VI, and by 4 months following surgery she had developed 50 diopters of right esotropia **(C)**. She was treated with injection of 5 units of Botox into the right medial rectus muscle, which resulted in a decrease in adduction on the right **(D)** as well as some inadvertent problems with down gaze on the right side, but her right eye did not deviate out at all, indicating that her nerve VI was still complete. *(Continued on page 112)*

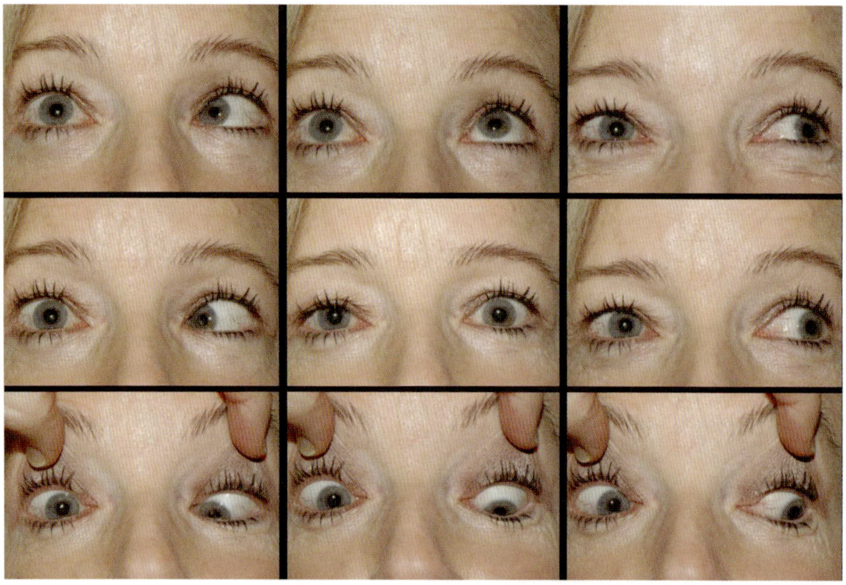

D

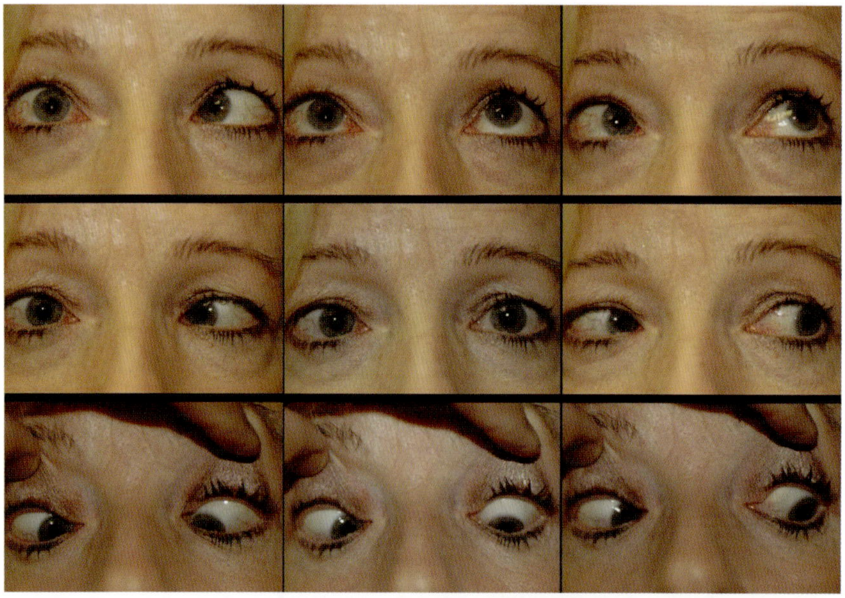

E

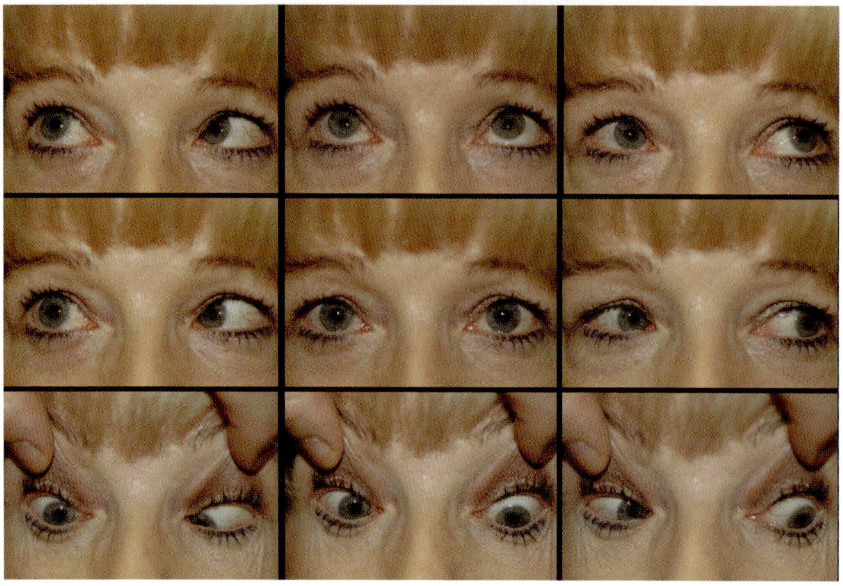

F

Fig. 5.25 *(Continued)* This 48-year-old patient noted some ringing in her ears, and MRI demonstrated a parasellar right cavernous meningioma. She underwent pterional craniotomy and resection, which left her with a right IV, V, and VI cranial nerve palsy. As the Botox began to wear off, the right eye began to drift back in **(E)**. Botox was reinjected into the right medial rectus muscle, and the patient underwent a full tendon transfer of the right superior and right inferior rectus muscles to the origin of the lateral rectus along with a posterior fixation suture (Foster modification), which substantially straightened her eye **(F)**. Seven months later, she had an area of binocularity centrally, although she still had double vision when she looked down, left, or right **(G,H)**.

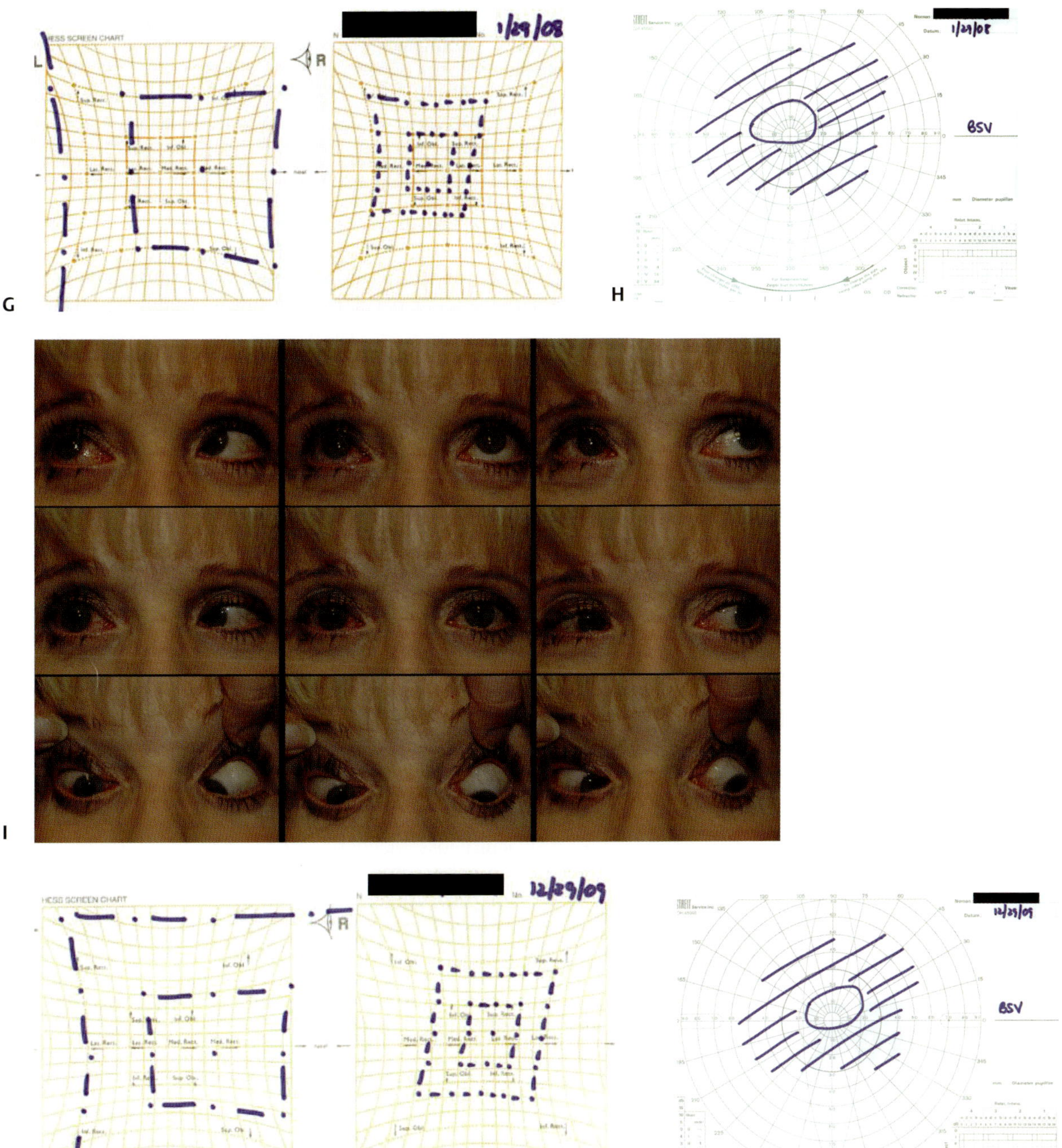

Fig. 5.25 *(Continued)* This 48-year-old patient noted some ringing in her ears, and MRI demonstrated a parasellar right cavernous meningioma. She underwent pterional craniotomy and resection, which left her with a right IV, V, and VI cranial nerve palsy. Seven months later, she had an area of binocularity centrally, although she still had double vision when she looked down, left, or right **(G,H)**. This has remained stable **(I)**, and when seen 30 months following her strabismus surgery, she still had an area of binocularity centrally and was pleased with her ability to function **(J,K)**. She was noted to have some redness in the right eye due to neurotrophic changes because of the loss of normal sensation. Comment: The patient was made functional here by muscle transposition surgery. She remains at risk because of the lack of fifth nerve innervation and therefore can easily develop epithelial breakdown. It is imperative that these patients be followed carefully.

nal nerve palsy. Failure of seventh nerve function to recover usually requires surgical intervention to help close the lid. Although it is still possible to implant an elastic band (Arion sling) or springs, the easiest way to help lid closure is with gravity assist by implantation of a gold or platinum weight. Although some weights can be applied externally, most of these are usually implanted in a pretarsal or, less commonly, preseptal location. Although the preseptal implants are less obvious cosmetically, they tend not to be as effective. Some surgeons will use a single-size weight, but it is usually advisable to tailor the gold weight to the particular status of the patient. I prefer to implant the heaviest weight that the patient can easily lift up, producing a minimal amount of ptosis. The heavier the weight, the more likely are good lid closure and eye protection. It is imperative to note that patients who are otherwise compromised and therefore supine in bed should never have a gold weight implanted because they cannot sit up to allow gravity to have an appropriate effect. In that setting, it is often better to simply perform a tarsorrhaphy to protect the eye.

◆ Exacerbation of Ophthalmic Findings Following Surgical Intervention

Because of the proximity of both the afferent and efferent visual pathways to lesions in the parasellar region, surgical intervention, whether transsphenoidal or transcranial, carries substantial risks for exacerbating existing or causing new neuro-ophthalmic findings. It is often critical to have a baseline examination before intervention because unrecognized previous compromise related to the presence of tumors can put patients at increased risk. Medicolegally, it is also nice to know what is preexistent. As mentioned above, quantitative assessment of both the afferent and efferent visual pathways is paramount. The presence of OCT thinning or optic atrophy may indicate previous optic nerve compromise, even when central visual function and visual fields appear normal. Subtle comitant deviations, including eso-, exo-, and hyperdeviations, may be left over from previous cranial nerve palsies. Fusional amplitudes may mask these. Preexisting motility problems may also be unrecognized if the patients have poor central vision or a previous history of strabismus, amblyopia, or facultative suppression.

Transsphenoidal surgery has the potential for injuring the optic nerve in its path through the lateral wall of the sphenoid bone, or the chiasm and tract in their suprasellar location. Additionally, injury to the carotid artery may produce secondary ischemic effects that may cause central peripheral visual field defects or even a chiasmal syndrome. Blood liberated into the subarachnoid space can result in secondary vasospasm and related ischemic changes. Following transsphenoidal surgery, infectious or inflammatory conditions can affect the optic nerve and chiasm. Overpacking the sphenoid sinus and sella can actually compress and elevate the optic nerves and chiasm, producing additional or new visual field defects. Later herniation of the chiasm into an empty sella may also produce delayed problems with visual exacerbation.

Worsening of extraocular motility following transsphenoidal surgery usually implies involvement of the cavernous sinus. As the ocular motor nerves run lateral to the carotid artery, it is unusual to produce cavernous sinus syndrome unless there is aggressive manipulation, hemorrhage, vasospasm, or vascular compromise. It is even less likely that the orbital structures themselves may be injured during transsphenoidal surgery, although the orbit may be entered if the surgeon becomes disoriented laterally.

The potential for injury of the afferent and efferent visual pathways with transcranial surgery depends on the approach. A transfrontal approach can result in injury to the optic nerves and chiasm and frequently cause problems with the olfactory nerve. A pterional approach can injure the optic nerve, particularly during a takedown of the anterior clinoid (especially if this is done extradurally). Aggressive surgery in the area of the cavernous sinus, of course, can result in compromise of the third, fourth, and sixth cranial nerves, but also the fifth nerve, producing neurotrophic problems (**Fig. 5.25**). Aggressive retraction of the scalp flap can injure branches of the seventh nerve, and although this usually causes brow ptosis alone, it can theoretically compromise lid closure. The burr hole placed at the pterion can be misdirected into the orbit, producing damage to the superior rectus and levator muscles (resulting in ptosis and diplopia), or to the lateral rectus (**Fig. 5.24**). Overly aggressive retraction of the temporal lobe during a pterional approach can produce secondary ischemia and infarction, compromising the visual pathways within the temporal lobe and resulting in homonymous hemianopsia, usually superior and incongruous, secondary to involvement of Meyer's loop.

Radiation therapy can result in delayed radiation optic neuropathy, usually appearing 6 months to 2 years following fractionated radiation therapy. This often presents with the sudden onset of altitudinal visual field loss followed by central acuity loss. Magnetic resonance imaging (MRI) findings include enhancement of the optic nerve extending to the chiasm. Radiosurgery with the gamma knife, Cyber Knife, or modified linear accelerators (LINAC) may result in acute necrosis, which can involve the optic nerve, chiasm, or optic radiations in the temporal lobe.[77] Stereotactic radiosurgery that encompasses the cavernous sinus has a small but not insignificant incidence of worsening of ocular motor palsies.

◆ Conclusion

The neuro-ophthalmic evaluation is an essential part of the assessment of any patient suspected of having a parasellar lesion. Although there is a tendency to believe that the clinical evaluation has been replaced by imaging, it is usually the examination that leads to appropriate imaging, and it clearly is quantitative assessment in the evaluation that will determine whether or not lesions are changing (natural history), even when the imaging studies remain the same. This can be an important indicator for intervention and may also be used to follow patients after intervention to determine whether that intervention, be it medical treatment, surgery, or radiation, has been effective. The psychophysical testing of the neuro-ophthalmic evaluation is far better attuned to what our patients experience than any of the radiologic or anatomic studies that may indicate disease. As such, determining what our patients see and how their eyes move and function is a critical part at all stages in following those with parasellar pathology.

◆ Appendix I: The Neuro-ophthalmic Examination for the Neurosurgeon

Assessment of the Afferent System

Snellen Acuity

Requirements: Snellen chart, good lighting, patient's refractive correction for distance, pinhole if no refractive correction is available. If a refractionist is available, this should be used in the absence of glasses.

Testing points: Test each eye separately, making sure that the opposite eye is occluded. Encourage patients to guess. Ensure adequate lighting. Watch out for the ability to read only the last letters because this may indicate a visual field defect. Use a 200 E (**Fig. 5.26**) to quantitate acuity less than 20/400, reporting the distance at which the patient can see the direction in which the E is pointed. Patients should be allowed to hold the E in any position they like (make sure the opposite eye is covered) to avoid visual field defects. Test patients who cannot see the 200 E at any distance for "hand motion"; determine the direction in which the tester's hand is moving. If hand motion is not present, determine if the patient can perceive light ("light perception") and its direction ("with projection").

Near Vision

Requirements: Use of a near chart (**Fig. 5.7**), near refractive correction (or add), measurement of distance at which the card is held.

Testing points: Make sure each eye is tested separately. Make sure the patient is wearing appropriate near correction. Allow patients to hold the reading material at the distance at which they see most clearly. Measure the distance to the near chart. Record the near acuity in the point system. If no correction is available, have a plus lens (usually +2.50 to +3.50) to put in front of the patient's eye to ensure that the patient is adequately corrected for near.

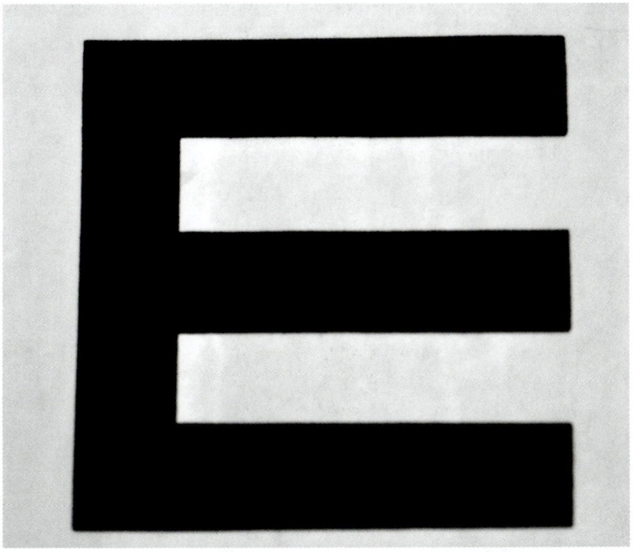

Fig. 5.26 A 200 optotype E (9 cm in size) can be held at the farthest distance at which the patient can identify the direction in which the E is pointed. Ideally, patients will hold the card themselves. This permits quantitative assessment of acuity of less than 20/400, and is more quantitative and reproducible than "count fingers."

Adjunctive Macular Function Tests

Color Vision

Requirements: Commercially available (Ishihara AO pseudoisochromatic plates) color vision plates are designed to test for congenital red-green color blindness (8% of the male population). Subtle reduction in color vision can be determined with quantitative color testing by using the American Optical Hardy-Rand-Ritter (AO-HRR) plates, the 100 hue test, or the desaturated D-15 test. Other color tests are available.

Testing points: Subtle washout of colors can be recorded as a substitute if formal color vision testing is not available by comparing colored (usually red) test objects (**Fig. 5.27**).

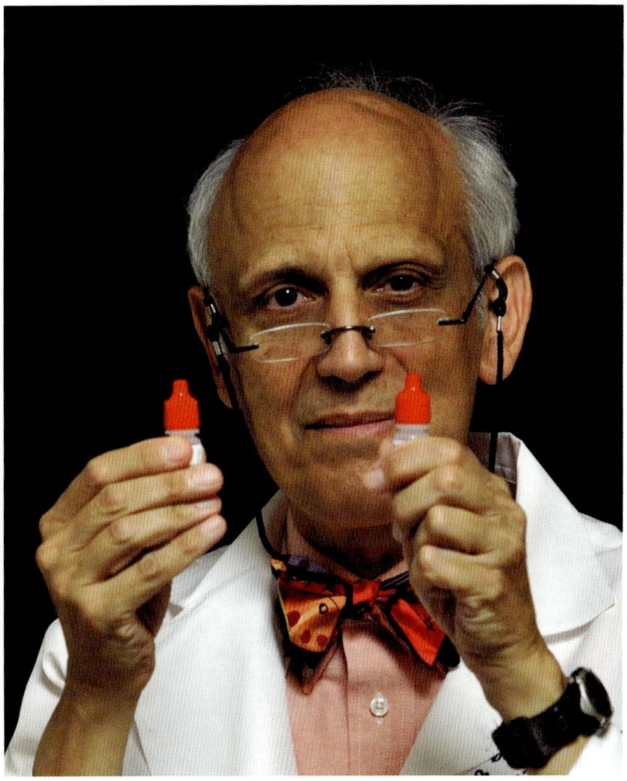

Fig. 5.27 Subtle optic nerve dysfunction may be appreciated as dimming or desaturation of a red test object. This is particularly useful for comparing the two eyes and may also be used to pick up subtle visual field defects by comparing red test objects across the vertical midline.

Contrast Sensitivity

Requirements: Special contrast sensitivity testing, including the Vistech system, sinusoidal gradings, and Pelli-Robson charts. Adequate lighting and appropriate refractive correction are critical.[78]

Testing points: Subtle abnormalities in contrast sensitivity may be detected following previous damage to the optic nerves even when Snellen acuity is normal.

Stereo Acuity

Requirements: Stereo testing can be done with the Titmus test and Randot test; usually, polarized glasses are used (**Fig. 5.28**). Fusion and fusional amplitudes can be measured with an amblyoscope.

Testing points: The presence of normal stereopsis indicates that both maculae are working well. This is a triple check on the previous Snellen vision and near vision.[79]

Visual Field Testing

Requirements: Central scotomas in particular can be picked up on Amsler grid testing (**Fig. 5.29**), in which patients are given a grid and asked to look at the center dot and describe whether parts of the grid are missing. A response of distortion of the lines is particularly seen in patients with macular disease. Qualitative perimetry may include Amsler grid testing and confrontation testing (**Fig. 5.28**), in which fingers are counted (one, two, or five) at an equal distance from the patient, allowing the observer to compare his or her own field with the patient's field.[80] This should be done monocularly. A moving or waving target can also be used to pick up dense defects. The visual fields of patients who are confined to bed may be tested by projecting a target with a laser pointer on the ceiling. This can be presented statically (on/off) or kinetically (moving from periphery to the center). Semiquantitative testing may be obtained by using a tangent screen on which variously sized test objects are moved from nonseeing to seeing kinetically or presented statically by flipping them over. Comparison testing across the vertical midline, particularly of red test objects, may pick up subtle desaturation. This can also be used across the nasal horizontal midline. Simultaneous appearance in both hemifields can pick up subtle neglect due to higher cortical dysfunction. Quantitative visual field testing usually involves dedicated apparatus, either kinetic (Goldmann bowl perimeter) or static (Humphrey, Octopus automated static perimetry). Because of longer time and duration, static perimetry in particular is often concentrated centrally, although peripheral testing is possible when indicated.

Testing points: Visual field testing is required to assess extrafoveal function. Three anatomic correlates of visual fields emphasize the importance of testing centrally across the nasal horizontal midline and across the vertical midline.

1. The small fibers responsible for central vision are partially sensitive to macular disease and certain optic neuropathies, particularly metabolic, hereditary, toxic, compressive, or inflammatory etiologies. Thus, these lesions (including compressive lesions) tend to cause central scotomas. Most central scotomas are related to macular disease.
2. The disc is located nasal to the fovea (arcuate visual field defects are an indicator of optic nerve pathology).[81]
3. The visual pathways segregate left and right information at the chiasm (visual field defects that respect the vertical midline indicate chiasmal and retrochiasmal involvement).

Therefore, all visual field tests should be designed to detect central scotomas, field defects that respect the nasal hori-

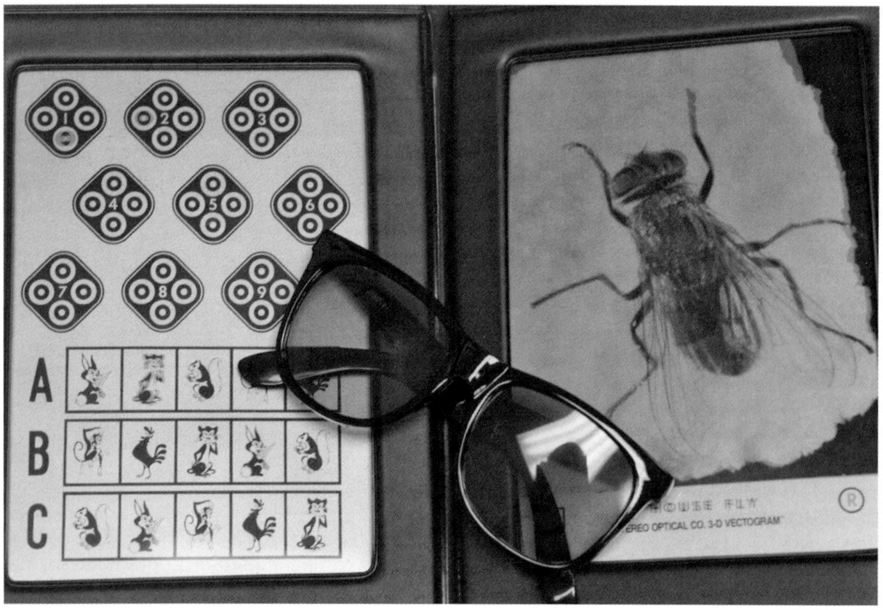

Fig. 5.28 The Titmus test can be used to detect stereoacuity. Normal stereopsis requires bilaterally good acuity. Stereoacuity may be absent in the setting of amblyopia, strabismus, or monofixation syndrome.

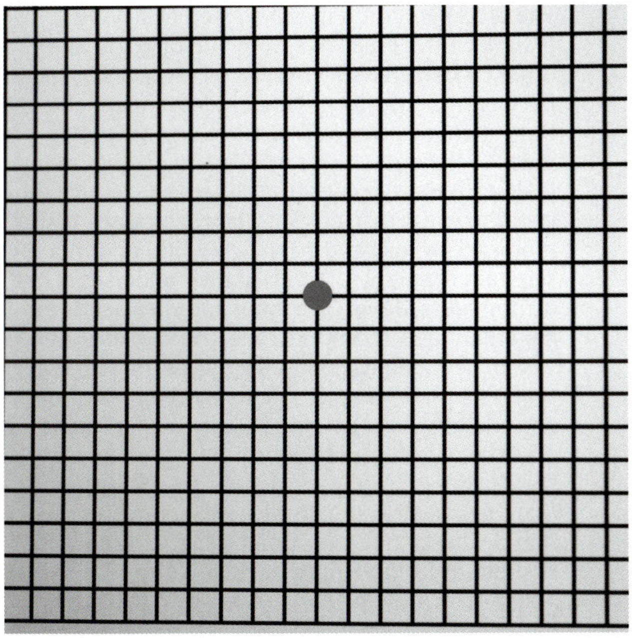

Fig. 5.29 An Amsler grid is very useful for picking up subtle distortion, which may be seen with macular disease, but it may also detect early visual field abnormalities, particularly if the patient is asked to compare parts of the grid across the vertical and nasal horizontal midline.

zontal midline, and field defects that respect the vertical midline. Visual field testing should be thought of as qualitative (looking to detect the presence of an abnormality in the visual field) versus quantitative (looking for how much of a visual field defect there is). Field testing is divided into kinetic perimetry, in which a fixed-intensity target is moved from areas of nonseeing to areas of seeing, and static, in which a fixed location is tested with an increasingly intense stimulus.

Assessment of the Pupil

Requirements: Fixation target so that accommodation does not change (patient should be instructed to fixate on a distant target, not just a light or "my nose"). An external camera can document pupil size in varying illumination. A bright light (not enough to produce an aversive response but bright enough to ensure adequate pupillary reactivity), such as a muscle light or indirect ophthalmoscope, should be used. A pupil gauge or ruler can quantitatively measure pupil size. A neutral-density filter bar can be placed in front of the better-functioning eye to grade an afferent pupillary defect (**Fig. 5.9**).

Testing points:

1. Pupils should be examined in both light and dark with a pupil gauge or millimeter ruler; the examiner should look for subtle asymmetry in pupil size. Subtle asymmetry is common (essential anisocoria may occur in >50% of the population when a 0.2- to 0.3-mm difference is looked for).
2. Anisocoria that increases in the dark usually indicates that the smaller pupil is not dilating and may be an indicator to check locally for inflammation, and also for Horner syndrome.[69] Anisocoria that increases in the light suggests that the larger pupil is not constricting and usually is an indicator to check both locally for evidence of inflammation, synechiae (best seen by slit lamp), a history of the use of eye drops, and also the possibility of motility disturbance that would parallel a third nerve palsy. Vermiform movements of the iris (best seen at the slit lamp) may indicate an old Adie syndrome due to involvement of the ciliary ganglion.
3. In a test for an afferent pupillary defect, patients should fixate an accommodative distance target. The examiner should move the bright test light quickly from one eye to the opposite eye, looking for initial contraction and release. Any asymmetry can be quantitated further by placing neutral-density filters in front of the better-reacting pupil.[50] Important point: An afferent pupillary defect may be detected even when only one pupil is working.
4. Pupils that do not react to light should be tested for response to a near target accommodation. Light-near dissociation may be seen in patients with any of the following: previous laser treatment of the eye, Adie syndrome (due to pathology affecting the ciliary ganglion), complete optic neuropathies in which they still retain pupillary response when given a proprioceptive near target, or dorsal midbrain pathology.

Assessment of the Efferent System

Ocular Motor Stability

Requirements: A direct ophthalmoscope (**Fig. 5.11**) is a very sensitive means of assessing stability of the eyes in primary and eccentric gaze.[55] More quantitative analysis of eye stability, as well as spontaneous and voluntary movements, can be obtained with infrared tracking, video monitoring, EOG, or electromagnetic coil recording.[56]

Testing points:

1. Eyes should be examined for stability in primary position. Spontaneous eye movements may indicate underlying pathology affecting the ocular motor pathways. Small conjugate refixation movements are normal (square wave jerks). An increase in their amplitude (better seen on funduscopic examination with a direct ophthalmoscope) may indicate cerebellar pathology. Tendencies for the eyes to spontaneously drift in a conjugate direction may be a sign of congenital nystagmus but also may develop following asymmetric vestibular pathology. Stability in primary position but drift back to the center when the patient looks eccentrically usually indicates pathology affecting the neural integrator (gaze paretic nystagmus). This can be best seen during subtle movement of the eye following dilation by

using a direct ophthalmoscope but is often picked up easily simply by direct observation. Neural integrator pathology may be seen with intoxication, antiseizure medications, sedatives, and metabolic abnormalities.
2. Quantitative assessment may be obtained with ocular motor recordings that use infrared tracking, EOG, or ocular search coil technology.

Assessment of Ocular Motor Systems

Requirements: Observation is usually adequate for qualitative assessment. Ocular motor recording with video, infrared tracking, EOG, or search coil technology will permit more quantitative analysis.

Testing points:

1. The vestibular ocular reflex may be tested by viewing the disc while rotating the patient in the dark. If the disc moves off fixation, the vestibular ocular reflex gain has been affected. Subtle abnormalities in vestibular ocular reserve may be detected by having patients shake their head from side to side in the dark and open their eyes while the examiner observes the disc for a drift to one side. Drift induced by head shaking suggests asymmetric vestibular reserve, often seen in patients with old vestibular pathology (eg, acoustic neurinoma).

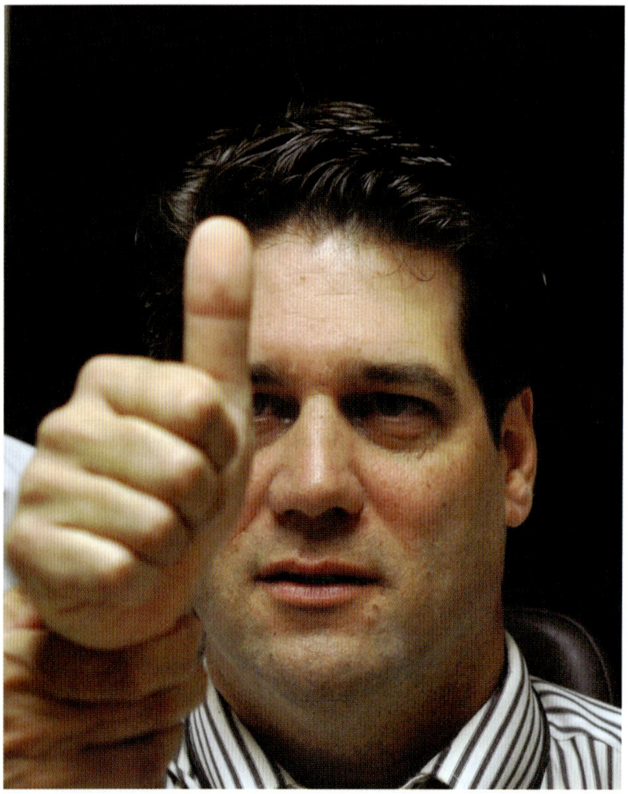

Fig. 5.30 Subtle abnormalities in the pursuit system may be detected by rotating patients while observing their ability to maintain fixation on their thumb.

2. The saccadic system may be tested by having patients move their eyes from one target to another.[82] Characteristics of normal saccades include latency (usually 250 milliseconds between when the patient is instructed to move and the movement), velocity (which can be estimated by simply looking at the saccades [the larger the saccade, the faster the peak velocity] or quantitatively by ocular motor recording), and accuracy (whether or not the saccades reach their target). If they undershoot and drift in (glissade) or overshoot and then achieve alignment by a second saccade, the saccades are said to be dysmetric. Saccadic dysmetria suggests cerebellar pathology. Problems with initiation of saccades can be seen congenitally (ocular motor apraxia) or with frontal lobe pathology. Slowing of saccades is usually a sign of burst cell pathology (paraneoplastic) but may also be seen with primary muscle disease (chronic progressive external ophthalmoplegia, mitochondrial myopathy).
3. The pursuit system can be tested by having the patient fixate a small accommodative target that moves (should not be any faster than about 30 degrees per second). Another subtle means of testing pursuit is to have patients fixate a thumb while rotating in a chair (**Fig. 5.30**). As the vestibular system would normally move their eyes in the opposite direction to which they are rotated, keeping their eyes on the thumb indicates that the vestibular reflex can be canceled. This usually indicates an intact pursuit system. Interruption by saccades ("cogwheel pursuit") suggests pathology affecting the pursuit system somewhere between the middle temporal gyrus and the pontine nuclei.
4. The convergence system can be tested by having the patient look between a distant and a near accommodative target. Failure of convergence may be seen by the development of an exodeviation at near. Lack of effort or cooperation may be suspected if there is failure of miosis, which should accompany convergence.

Assessment of Ocular Malalignment

Requirements: Qualitative malalignment[21] may be directly observed, noted by asymmetry of the corneal light reflex (Hirshberg), or identified by dissociative testing (red glass, Maddox rod; **Fig. 5.12**). Quantitative measurements may be made with prisms or on an amblyoscope. Dissociative tests such as the Maddox rod can be quantitated by adding prisms. The Hess screen[61] and binocular single vision assessed with a Goldmann bowl can further quantitate relative movements of the two eyes. Malalignment due to restrictive pathology may be separated from paretic problems by forced duction testing (anesthetic, forceps, suction cup[62,83]) or measurement of intraocular pressure in eccentric gaze (pneumotonometer, Tonopen).

Testing points: Ductions can be assessed qualitatively by determining whether the eye crosses midline and whether it reaches appropriate eccentric gaze. The easiest clue to an abnormality in ductions is provided by asymmetric movement of the eyes. Ductions can be further quantitated with a linear ruler measurement, prisms, or most quantitatively with a Goldmann bowl. Versions are movements of the eyes relative to each other. They can be qualitatively noticed if there is adducting or abducting delay or if one eye reaches the desired position more quickly than the opposite eye. This will also be seen as malalignment. Malalignment may be measured qualitatively by using a red glass or a Maddox rod test,[57] or quantitatively by using a Hess screen[61] and cross-cover testing with prisms. Maddox rod permits easy demonstration of incomitant deviations (does not distinguish between paretic and restrictive causes) and allows critical identification of the direction of maximal deviation and also of minimal deviation.

Adnexal Evaluation

Basic Adnexal Evaluation

Requirements: A ruler is critical for measurements of the palpebral fissures (**Fig. 5.16**), upper lid range (**Fig. 5.17**), and orbital symmetry. External photographs are very useful for documenting adnexal anatomy. A Hertel apparatus can be used to determine proptosis (**Fig. 5.19**). Sensation can be qualitatively evaluated with a cotton tip or quantitatively with an esthesiometer (**Fig. 5.21**). Sophisticated orbital evaluation can be done with an ultrasound (**Fig. 5.2**).

Testing points:

1. The patient's face should be examined for symmetry. Often, one eye is slightly higher than the other, and this should be recorded.
2. The distance between the upper and lower lids should be recorded bilaterally as the palpebral fissure opening.
3. The distance from a light reflex in the center of the pupil to the upper lid should be recorded as the marginal reflex distance (**Fig. 5.18**).
4. Excess skin on the upper lid may be recognized as dermatochalasis, which can become clinically significant if it droops over the lid margin.
5. Normally, the lids will cross the limbus both superiorly and inferiorly. Being able to see the sclera between the limbus of the cornea and the lid indicates lid retraction. This can be both superior and inferior.
6. Levator function is recorded by splinting the frontalis muscle and having the patient look way up and way down.
7. Relative proptosis can be seen qualitatively by looking over the patient's forehead and quantitated by using a Hertel apparatus.
8. Facial sensation should always be checked, with the examiner looking for symmetry.
9. Blinks should be assessed for both frequency and completeness. Patients who have incomplete blinks should be examined for their ability to close completely. Failure to close completely (lagophthalmos) is often associated with corneal exposure problems.
10. Orbicularis strength can be qualitatively assessed and the two sides compared.
11. Spontaneous movement of the face (blepharospasm, hemifacial spasm, facial myokymia, benign facial fasciculations) may also be recorded.

Adjunctive Adnexal Assessment

Requirements: High-tech equipment for examining the orbit and adnexal structures include a slit lamp, ultrasound, OCT unit (for both anterior and posterior segment evaluation), and fundus cameras.

Testing points:

1. Patients with pathology within the orbit may have abnormal resistance to retropulsion. This is tested by ballottement.
2. Auscultation of the orbit may also be obtained and can demonstrate a bruit in the setting of a carotid cavernous fistula.
3. The anterior segment may be assessed, ideally with a slit lamp providing illumination from the side so that the various levels of the globe can be evaluated. A pen light examination can reveal abnormalities in the cornea, anterior chamber, iris, and lens.
4. Funduscopic examinations should concentrate on the disc, macula, and posterior pole structures. The disc should be evaluated for size and symmetry, cupping, abnormal blood vessels, elevation or hyperemia, hemorrhage, exudate, and the possible presence of optic atrophy. The macula should be evaluated for thickening, hemorrhage, and exudate. Vessels should be inspected for narrowing or dilatation as well as tortuosity, anomalies, crossing changes (where the artery crosses the vein), and irregularities in the wall. Other posterior pole pathology includes new vessels (neovascularization) and obstruction of vessels, including Hollenhorst plaques, loss of nerve fiber layer, inflammatory infectious pathology, and various degrees of hemorrhage. Hemorrhage may be under the retina, in the retina (flame-shaped or dot-blot), in front of the retina (preretinal, subhyaloid), or in the vitreous (**Fig. 5.31**). The retina may be elevated by traction (following trauma or related to diabetes) or underlying fluid (rhegametogenous—due to a hole or related to exudate). Mass lesions (inflammatory or neoplastic) may be located in the choroid (subretinal) or retina, or may extend into the vitreous. Funduscopic evaluation can be greatly improved by dilating the patient's pupils. A nonmydriatic fundus camera may also be a useful way of seeing the posterior globe better.
5. Ultrasound may record the size of the extraocular muscles and the possible presence of intraorbital mass lesions.

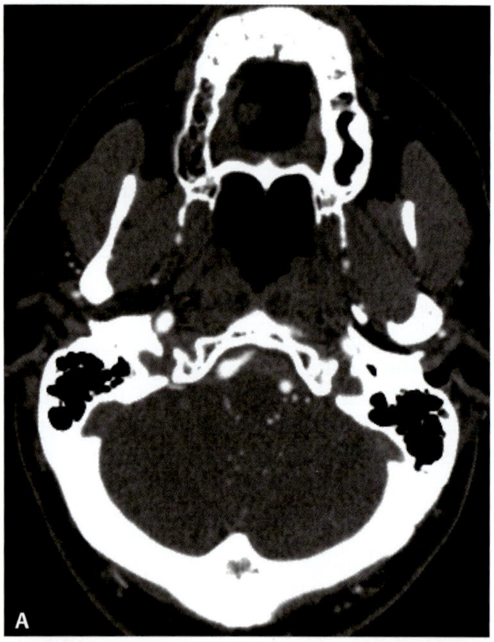

Fig. 5.31 This 52-year-old man presented with the acute onset of the "worst headache of his life" and severe blurred vision. CT showed evidence of an aneurysm at the skull base **(A)** in the distal vertebral artery with a dissection extending into the basilar artery and subarachnoid hemorrhage. Funduscopic examination revealed evidence of bilateral preretinal, interretinal, and subretinal hemorrhage related to an acute increase in intracranial pressure **(B,C)**. The patient's Terson syndrome resolved over 6 months, with a return in visual acuity from the 20/400 when he was first seen to 20/30 and 20/40. Comment: Terson syndrome is vitreous hemorrhage associated with a subarachnoid hemorrhage. Most cases occur in the setting of a ruptured intracranial aneurysm. The hemorrhage may often clear spontaneously over weeks to months. Those that fail to clear may be treated with vitrectomy.

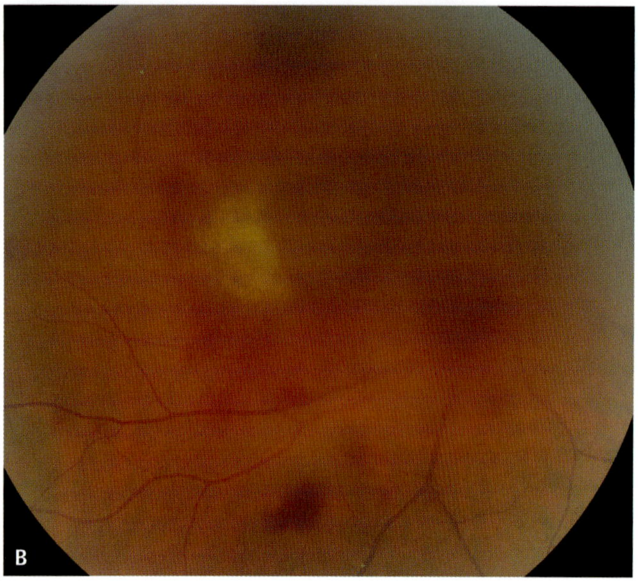

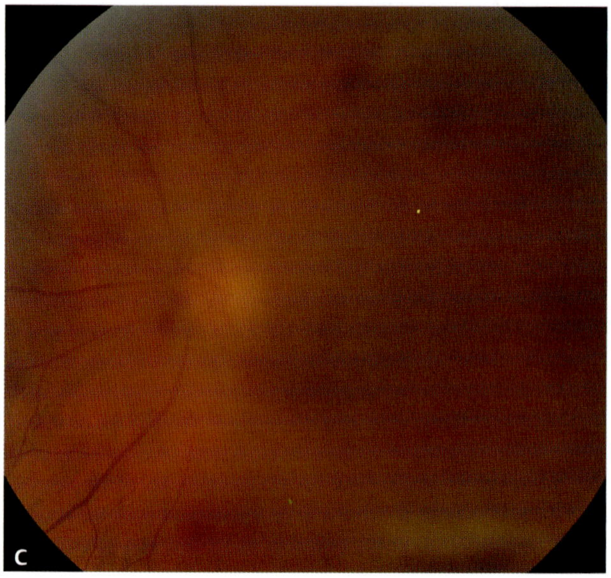

◆ Appendix II

Basics in Your Pocket

Direct ophthalmoscope (light, plus lenses)
Near card (can use as near accommodative target)
200 E
+3.00 lens
Pinhole
Ruler
Amsler grid
Red top dilating drops (tropicamide)
Maddox rod

Patient Supplies

Their glasses
Name of their eye doctor for old records

Your Neuro-ophthalmologist

Hertel
Optokinetic nystagmus (OKN) strip or drum
Neutral-density filter for quantitating an APD
External camera
Indirect ophthalmoscope
Portable slit lamp
Pressure measure (applanation tonometer, Tonopen)
Titmus test
Schirmer strips
Stethoscope for auscultation (carotid, orbit)

In the Clinic

Slit lamp with biomicroscopic lenses
Gonioprism
Color tests (AO-HRR plates, D-15, 100 hue)
Contrast tests (Pelli-Robson, Vistech)

High Tech

Automated static perimetry
OCT
Fluorescein angiography
Visual evoked potential (latency increase suggests inflammation, not compression)
Multifocal ERG (abnormality suggests maculopathy)
Hess screen
Goldmann bowl
Ultrasound
Video recording
Infrared tracking
Scleral search coil

References

1. Cushing H. The chiasmal syndrome: of primary optic atrophy and bitemporal visual field defects in adults with a normal sella turcica. Arch Ophthalmol 1930;3:505–551
2. Cushing H, Walker CB. Distortion of the visual fields in cases of brain tumor. Brain 1915;37:341–400
3. Godfredsen E. Eye and nerve symptoms in connection with cranial chordomas. Acta Ophthalmol (Copenh) 1944;21:224–236
4. Berson EL, Freeman MI, Gay AJ. Visual field defects in giant suprasellar aneurysms of internal carotid. Report of three cases. Arch Ophthalmol 1966;76(1):52–58
5. Jefferson G. On compression and invasion of the optic nerves and chiasma by neighboring gliomas. Trans Ophthalmol Soc U K 1945;65:262–304
6. Finn JE, Mount LA. Meningiomas of the tuberculum sellae and planum sphenoidale. A review of 83 cases. Arch Ophthalmol 1974;92(1):23–27
7. Kirkham TH. The ocular symptomatology of pituitary tumours. Proc R Soc Med 1972;65(6):517–518
8. Walsh FB. The ocular signs of tumors involving the anterior visual pathways. Am J Ophthalmol 1956;42(3):347–377
9. Hollenhorst RW, Younge BR. Ocular manifestations produced by adenomas of the pituitary gland: analysis of 1000 cases. In: Kohler PO, Ross GT, eds. Diagnosis and Treatment of Pituitary Tumors. Excerpta Medica; 1973:53–68
10. Neetens A, Selosse P. Oculomotor anomalies in sellar and parasellar pathology. Ophthalmologica 1977;175(2):80–104
11. Sharpe JA. Visual dysfunction with basal skull tumours. Can J Neurol Sci 1985;12(4):332–335
12. Snyder H, Robinson K, Shah D, Brennan R, Handrigan M. Signs and symptoms of patients with brain tumors presenting to the emergency department. J Emerg Med 1993;11(3):253–258
13. Trobe JD, Tao AH, Schuster JJ. Perichiasmal tumors: diagnostic and prognostic features. Neurosurgery 1984;15(3):391–399
14. Huber A. Eye Signs and Symptoms in Brain Tumors. 3rd ed. CV Mosby; 1976
15. Levin LA. Topical diagnosis of chiasmal and retrochiasmal disorders. In: Miller NR, Newman NJ, Biousse V, Kerrison JB, eds. Walsh

& Hoyt's Clinical Neuro-Ophthalmology. 6th ed. Lippincott Williams & Wilkins; 2005:503–573

16. Jefferson G. The Bowman Lecture. Concerning injuries, aneurysms and tumors involving the cavernous sinus. Trans Ophthalmol Soc U K 1953;73:117–152
17. Newman SA, Miller NR. Optic tract syndrome. Neuro-ophthalmologic considerations. Arch Ophthalmol 1983;101(8):1241–1250
18. Fujimoto N, Saeki N, Miyauchi O, Adachi-Usami E. Criteria for early detection of temporal hemianopia in asymptomatic pituitary tumor. Eye (Lond) 2002;16(6):731–738
19. Sadun AA, Currie JN, Lessell S. Transient visual obscurations with elevated optic discs. Ann Neurol 1984;16(4):489–494
20. Uhthoff W. Die Augenveräderungen be idem Erkrankungen des Gehirnes. In: Graefe-Saemisch Handbuch der gesamten Augenheilkunde, vol. 11. Wilhelm Engelmann; 1915:1143
21. Borchert MS. Principles and techniques of the examination of ocular motility and alignment. In: Miller NR, Newman NJ, Biousse V, Kerrison JB, eds. Walsh & Hoyt's Clinical Neuro-Ophthalmology. 6th ed. Lippincott Williams & Wilkins; 2005:887–905
22. Schoepf D, Zangemeister WH, Vines FS, et al. Correlation of ocular motor reading strategies to the status of adaptation in patients with hemianopic visual field defects. Ann N Y Acad Sci 1993;682:404–408
23. Currie J, Lubin JH, Lessell S. Chronic isolated abducens paresis from tumors at the base of the brain. Arch Neurol 1983;40(4):226–229
24. Savino PJ, Hilliker JK, Casell GH, Schatz NJ. Chronic sixth nerve palsies. Are they really harbingers of serious intracranial disease? Arch Ophthalmol 1982;100(9):1442–1444
25. Volpe NJ, Lessell S. Remitting sixth nerve palsy in skull base tumors. Arch Ophthalmol 1993;111(10):1391–1395
26. Hart WM Jr. Acquired dyschromatopsias. Surv Ophthalmol 1987;32(1):10–31
27. Frisèn L, Royt WF, Tengroth BM. Optociliary veins, disc pallor and visual loss. A triad of signs indicating spheno-orbital meningioma. Acta Ophthalmol (Copenh) 1973;51(2):241–249
28. Bell RA, Thompson HS. Relative afferent pupillary defect in optic tract hemianopias. Am J Ophthalmol 1978;85(4):538–540
29. Adler FH, Austin G, Grant FC. Localizing value of visual fields in patients with early chiasmal lesions. Arch Ophthalmol 1948;40:579–600
30. Hoyt WF. Correlative functional anatomy of the optic chiasm. 1969. Clin Neurosurg 1970;17:189–208
31. Horton JC. Wilbrand's knee of the primate optic chiasm is an artefact of monocular enucleation. Trans Am Ophthalmol Soc 1997;95:579–609
32. Wilbrand HL. Schema des verlaus der Schnervenfasern durch das Chiasma. Z Augenheilkd 1926;59:135–144
33. Traquair HM. An Introduction to Clinical Perimetry. CV Mosby; 1927
34. Posner M, Horrax G. Eye signs in pineal tumors. J Neurosurg 1946;3:15–24
35. Seybold ME, Yoss RE, Hollenhorst RW, Moyer NJ. Pupillary abnormalities associated with tumors of the pineal region. Neurology 1971;21(3):232–237
36. Daroff RB. See-saw nystagmus. Neurol (Tokyo) 1965;15:875–877
37. Parkinson D, Johnston J, Chaudhuri A. Sympathetic connections to the fifth and sixth cranial nerves. Anat Rec 1978;191(2):221–226
38. Kestenbaum A. Clinical Methods of Neuro-Ophthalmological Examination. 2nd ed. Grune & Stratton; 1961
39. Enoksson P. Perimetry in neuro-ophthalmological diagnosis. Acta Ophthalmol (Copenh) 1965;82(suppl):82, 1–54
40. Frisén L. Visual acuity. In: Clinical Tests of Vision. Raven Press; 1990:24–39
41. Frisén L. The foundations of visual field testing. In: Clinical Tests of Vision. Raven Press; 1990:55–77
42. Burde RM, Savino PJ, Trobe JD. Clinical Decisions in Neuro-Ophthalmology. 3rd ed. CV Mosby; 2002
43. Wall M, Johnson CA. Principles and techniques of the examination of the visual sensory system. In: Miller NR, Newman NJ, Biousse V, Kerrison JB, eds. Walsh & Hoyt's Clinical Neuro-Ophthalmology. 6th ed. Lippincott Williams & Wilkins; 2005:83–149
44. Biousse V, Newman NJ. Neuro-Ophthalmology Illustrated. Thieme; 2009
45. Bailey IL, Lovie JE. New design principles for visual acuity letter charts. Am J Optom Physiol Opt 1976;53(11):740–745
46. Katz J, Tielsch JM, Quigley HA, Sommer A. Automated perimetry detects visual field loss before manual Goldmann perimetry. Ophthalmology 1995;102(1):21–26
47. Lowenfeld IE. The Pupil. Butterworth; 1999
48. Lam BL, Thompson HS, Corbett JJ. The prevalence of simple anisocoria. Am J Ophthalmol 1987;104:69–73
49. Levatin P. Pupillary escape in disease of the retina or optic nerve. Arch Ophthalmol 1959;62:768–779
50. Thompson HS, Corbett JJ, Cox TA. How to measure the relative afferent pupillary defect. Surv Ophthalmol 1981;26(1):39–42
51. Kennedy RF. Retrobulbar neuritis as an exact diagnostic sign of certain tumors and abscesses in the frontal lobes. Am J Med Sci 1911;142:355–368
52. Glaser JS, Savino PJ, Sumers KD, McDonald SA, Knighton RW. The photostress recovery test in the clinical assessment of visual function. Am J Ophthalmol 1977;83(2):255–260
53. Roper-Hall G. Methods and theories of testing extraocular movements. Int Ophthalmol Clin 1978;18(1):1–18
54. Leigh RJ, Zee DS. The Neurology of Eye Movements. 3rd ed. FA Davis; 1999
55. Zee DS. Ophthalmoscopy in examination of patients with vestibular disorders. Ann Neurol 1978;3(4):373–374
56. Bechert K, Koenig EA. A search coil system with automatic field stabilization, calibration, and geometric processing for eye movement recordings in humans. Neuroophthalmology 1996;16: 163–170
57. Maddox EE. A new test for heterophoria. Ophthalmol Rev 1890;9:129–133
58. Choi RY, Kushner BJ. The accuracy of experienced strabismologists using the Hirschberg and Krimsky tests. Ophthalmology 1998;105(7):1301–1306
59. Lancaster WB. Detecting, measuring, plotting and interpreting ocular deviations. Arch Ophthal 1939;22(5):867–880
60. Zee DS, Chu FC, Optican LM, Carl JR, Reingold D. Graphic analysis of paralytic strabismus with the Lancaster red-green test. Am J Ophthalmol 1984;97(5):587–592
61. Hess WR. Ein einfaches messendes Verfahren zur Motilitätsprufung der Augen. Z Augenheilkd 1916;35:201–219
62. Knox DL. Suction cup forced duction. Am J Ophthalmol 1974;77(5):762–763
63. Zappia RJ, Winkelman JZ, Gay AJ. Intraocular pressure changes in normal subjects and the adhesive muscle syndrome. Am J Ophthalmol 1971;71(4):880–883
64. Trobe JD, Glaser JS, Post JD. Meningiomas and aneurysms of the cavernous sinus. Neuro-ophthalmologic features. Arch Ophthalmol 1978;96(3):457–467
65. Detry-Morel M. [The eye and cavernous sinus disorders (author's transl)]. J Fr Ophtalmol 1981;4(8-9):603–618
66. Cardoso ER, Peterson EW. Pituitary apoplexy: a review. Neurosurgery 1984;14(3):363–373
67. Wakai S, Fukushima T, Teramoto A, Sano K. Pituitary apoplexy: its incidence and clinical significance. J Neurosurg 1981;55(2):187–193
68. McFadzean RM, Doyle D, Rampling R, Teasdale E, Teasdale G. Pituitary apoplexy and its effect on vision. Neurosurgery 1991;29(5):669–675
69. Pilley SF, Thompson HS. Pupillary "dilatation lag" in Horner's syndrome. Br J Ophthalmol 1975;59(12):731–735
70. Savino PJ, Hilliker JK, Casell GH, Schatz NJ. Chronic sixth nerve palsies. Are they really harbingers of serious intracranial disease? Arch Ophthalmol 1982;100(9):1442–1444
71. Cox TA, Wurster JB, Godfrey WA. Primary aberrant oculomotor regeneration due to intracranial aneurysm. Arch Neurol 1979;36(9):570–571
72. Falconer MA, Stafford-Bell MA. Visual failure from pituitary and parasellar tumours occurring with favourable outcome in pregnant women. J Neurol Neurosurg Psychiatry 1975;38(9):919–930
73. Jakobsson KE, Petruson B, Lindblom B. Dynamics of visual improvement following chiasmal decompression. Quantitative pre- and postoperative observations. Acta Ophthalmol Scand 2002;80(5):512–516

74. Pameijer JK. Reading problems in hemianopia. Ophthalmologica 1970;160(5):322–325
75. Schoepf D, Zangemeister WH. Correlation of ocular motor reading strategies to the status of adaptation in patients with hemianopic visual field defects. Ann N Y Acad Sci 1993;682:404–408
76. Demer JL, Miller JM, Poukens V, Vinters HV, Glasgow BJ. Evidence for fibromuscular pulleys of the recti extraocular muscles. Invest Ophthalmol Vis Sci 1995;36(6):1125–1136
77. Stafford SL, Pollock BE, Leavitt JA, et al. A study on the radiation tolerance of the optic nerves and chiasm after stereotactic radiosurgery. Int J Radiat Oncol Biol Phys 2003;55(5):1177–1181
78. Moseley MJ, Hill AR. Contrast sensitivity testing in clinical practice. Br J Ophthalmol 1994;78(10):795–797
79. Donzis PB, Rappazzo JA, Burde RM, Gordon M. Effect of binocular variations of Snellen's visual acuity on Titmus stereoacuity. Arch Ophthalmol 1983;101(6):930–932
80. Trobe JD, Acosta PC, Krischer JP, Trick GL. Confrontation visual field techniques in the detection of anterior visual pathway lesions. Ann Neurol 1981;10(1):28–34
81. Kearns TP, Rucker CW. Arcuate defects in the visual fields due to chromophobe adenoma of the pituitary gland. I. Clinics in perimetry. Am J Ophthalmol 1958;45(4 Part 1):505–507
82. Baloh RW, Sills AW, Kumley WE, Honrubia V. Quantitative measurement of saccade amplitude, duration, and velocity. Neurology 1975;25(11):1065–1070
83. Chamberlain W. Restriction in upward gaze with advancing age. Am J Ophthalmol 1971;71(1 Pt 2):341–346

6 Surgical Treatment of Pituitary Adenomas

Soriya Motivala, Yakov Gologorsky, Joshua Bederson, and Kalmon D. Post

Pituitary adenomas are epithelial tumors arising from the adenohypophysis that can manifest with neurologic symptoms resulting from local mass effects or as a variety of clinical entities depending on the type of hormone secreted. Pituitary adenomas comprise 10 to 15% of intracranial tumors, although the incidence has been noted to be as high as 24% in autopsy series. They are most common in the third and fourth decades of life and overall affect both sexes equally. There are, however, differences in frequency between the sexes for certain subtypes, such as Cushing disease, which is more frequent in women; prolactin-secreting adenomas, which are more common in young women; and null cell adenomas, oncocytomas, and gonadotropin-secreting adenomas, which are more common in men.

The classification of pituitary neoplasms has undergone a variety of modifications over time, but they are now commonly stratified based on the hormone they secrete. Endocrinologically, they are considered either active or inactive and are classified as active only if the amount of hormone secreted leads to excessive levels in the blood and clinically evident symptomatology. Inactive adenomas contain the secretory and cellular components necessary for hormone production, but they are not associated with clinical and biochemical evidence of hormone excess. This functional classification is now being further modified to incorporate recent advances in molecular and immunohistochemical staining in pituitary research.

The variability of pituitary neoplasms has engendered the need for multiple algorithms of treatment dependent upon the behavior of the classes of tumors themselves. In this chapter, we discuss the indications for surgical treatment as well as the surgical techniques available for the major classifications of pituitary adenomas.

◆ Surgical Management of Cushing Disease

Cushing disease is a life-shortening illness caused by hypercortisolism secondary to an adrenocorticotropic hormone (ACTH)–secreting pituitary adenoma. Pituitary surgery is considered the treatment of choice in these cases, providing the greatest likelihood for remission of symptoms, although results thus far have been less than perfect. Recent advances in surgical strategy, endocrinologic assessment, and adjuvant therapies have improved the ability to treat this devastating disease.

The large majority of these tumors (89%)[1] are microadenomas (<1 cm in diameter) and can be difficult to localize on imaging. In 25 to 45% of cases, magnetic resonance imaging (MRI) does not demonstrate an identifiable neurosurgical target despite biochemical confirmation of pituitary-driven Cushing syndrome.[2] In cases in which preoperative imaging is nondiagnostic, preoperative bilateral inferior petrosal sinus sampling (IPSS) with corticotropin-releasing hormone (CRH) stimulation may help to identify the pituitary as the site of pathology. In experienced hands, IPSS preceded by CRH stimulation can correctly lateralize a tumor in 83% of cases in which there is an ACTH gradient of more than 1.4 pg/mL between the two sides.[3]

In cases in which the lesion is not identifiable on MRI or at the time of microsurgical exploration, the operating surgeon may, depending on the severity of the patient's symptomatology and expressed desires, opt for hemihypophysectomy in a small percentage of patients or, rarely, complete hypophysectomy with the knowledge that such measures can result in lifelong hypopituitarism requiring hormone replacement and still may not result in remission. Hemihypophysectomy in these cases is usually guided by the results of preoperative IPSS, whereas complete hypophysectomy is usually reserved for patients in whom resolution of the hypercortisolemic state is an absolute necessity.

Some surgeons recommend the use of an intraoperative ultrasound device to aid in localization of the adenoma. This author has not found it to be beneficial in our practice.[2]

We prefer the term *remission* to *cure*. In the setting of Cushing disease, remission is defined as resolution of clinical symptoms secondary to hypercortisolemia, biochemical confirmation of normal diurnal cortisol secretion levels, and resumption of normal hypothalamic-pituitary-adrenal function. Initial remission rates following surgery range from 78 to 87% in experienced hands. However, relapse rates of 7 to 11% have been reported following surgery. (Long-term remission rates following surgery have been reported as 42–86%.[4])

Owing to the relatively high rate of recurrence, much attention in the literature has focused on immediate postoperative factors, which may predict long-term outcomes. In some cases, ACTH and cortisol levels remain unchanged or even may be seen to be elevated in the immediate 24-hour period after surgery. This is most likely attributable to the stress of surgery or anesthesia. However, with a few exceptions in which "late" remission has been documented, levels that remain elevated beyond postoperative day 1 often indicate surgical failure.[5]

Cortisol levels that decrease to less than 2 to 3 μg/dL within 24 to 72 hours after surgery usually indicate a biochemical remission.[6] Simmons et al reported that a comparison of serum cortisol levels measured preoperatively at midnight and ~30 hours after the operation offer the most sensitive indication of long-term remission. With these two measurements, a lower postoperative level offers 95% sensitivity and a 95% positive predictive value for remission up to 2 years following surgery.[5] They stress that the administration of exogenous steroids in the immediate postoperative period is unnecessary except in a small percentage of patients with laboratory-documented hypocortisolemia accompanied by symptoms of steroid withdrawal. In fact, routine administration of postoperative steroids often only delays accurate biochemical assessment in the remaining majority of patients.

It is also this author's practice not to routinely prescribe perioperative steroids. Our algorithm requires that patients be closely monitored for signs of addisonian symptoms for 2 days in the hospital, during which time serum cortisol and ACTH levels are sent daily. Patients are subsequently discharged on replacement therapy until the postoperative results become available. If a patient exhibits signs of hypocortisolemia while in the hospital, serum levels are immediately drawn and replacement therapy is initiated without delay.

Although they may be dramatically decreased from preoperative values, 1-week postoperative serum cortisol levels within the normal range are not predictive of remission. This finding in fact often signifies trauma to the abnormal ACTH-producing tissue that may eventually lead to divergent outcomes of further necrosis and remission or resumption of secretory activity. In one study of patients with normal serum cortisol levels in the immediate postoperative period, 29% went on to demonstrate long-term remission, whereas 71% demonstrated recurrence from 2 to 4 years following surgery.[7] Another indication of viable tumor cells in the immediate postoperative period is a measurable response of serum ACTH level to CRH stimulation. In a series of 82 patients, a normal or exaggerated response predicted recurrence in 18% and 43%, respectively, whereas an absent response can be a predictor of long-term remission at 2-year follow-up.[7]

Macroadenomas are easier to identify on preoperative imaging and localize intraoperatively. However, they portend a worse prognosis and higher surgical failure rate than microadenomas. In a series of 137 patients with microadenomas at Massachusetts General Hospital, 123 (90%) were cured with transsphenoidal surgery with or without adjuvant therapy. This contrasts with a surgical cure rate in 11 of 17 (65%) patients from the same series who harbored macroadenomas. The 5-year cure rates in this series for patients with microadenomas versus macroadenomas were 96% and 91%, respectively, whereas the 10-year cure rates were 93% and 55%.[1]

Outcomes have not been found to correlate with the presence of a lesion on preoperative imaging. Remission rates after the initial surgical resection were found to be 79.3% in patients with a normal or inconclusive preoperative MRI, compared with 82.3% of patients with MRI-identifiable adenomas ($P = 1.0$) in a retrospective review of 248 consecutive patients identified with Cushing disease.[8]

In many cases, histologically identifiable ACTH-secreting adenomatous tissue is not seen postoperatively. Over the years, there has been much debate as to the significance of this finding. A recent study demonstrated that among patients who underwent transsphenoidal resection for Cushing disease, rates of remission for those with no histologically identifiable tissue were 50%, compared with an 88% remission rate ($P < 0.001$) for those with identifiable pathologic tissue. This is likely due to incomplete extirpation and may necessitate more close observation and follow-up of this particular subset of patients.[9]

Given the current data, coupled with our own experience, our philosophy has been to rely on the 24-hour urinary free cortisol levels as well as the midnight salivary cortisol levels. If those have been found to be abnormal, confirming Cushing syndrome, then MRI with high-resolution thin cuts through the pituitary sella is performed. If an adenoma is identifiable on MRI, then we proceed to transsphenoidal resection of the tumor. If an ACTH-immunostaining tumor is not found and cortisol and ACTH values remain elevated, an IPSS study with CRH stimulation is done to confirm the diagnosis of Cushing disease. Conversely, if no lesion is seen on the initial MRI, then IPSS studies are done to confirm that the pituitary is the cause of the Cushing disease, as well as to suggest laterality in the gland to help locate the adenoma. We request a 24-hour urinary free cortisol level the day before the IPSS study to ensure that the patient is not eucortisolemic at the time of the IPSS study.

The indication for bilateral IPSS (BIPSS) in the preoperative work-up of Cushing disease is controversial. Whereas some centers perform BIPSS in all patients with presumed Cushing disease before transsphenoidal surgery, others do not. We studied this issue, and in our series BIPSS was performed only in patients without a clear adenoma on MRI or if biochemical testing was not fully consistent with Cushing disease. The study, which was a retrospective analysis of 187 adult patients (153 women, 34 men; mean age, 41 ± 13.8 years; range, 18–74 years) with presumed Cushing disease, addressed whether the selective indication for BIPSS in the preoperative work-up of Cushing disease might have affected the early postoperative remission. Early postoperative remission required fasting serum cortisol levels of less than 5 μg/dL and/or urine free cortisol excretion of less than 50 μg/24h. One hundred patients (53.5%) underwent BIPSS before transsphenoidal surgery. Ninety-one of these had either a normal or an inconclusive MRI, and only 9 of the 87 patients with an adenoma on MRI had a BIPSS. Of all patients, 175 (93.6%) showed an early postoperative remission. Of the 100 patients with a preoperative BIPSS,

94 (94%), and of the 87 patients without a BIPSS, 81 (93.1%) had a postoperative remission. All patients without BIPSS and no early remission had an ACTH-positive adenoma on pathology, and therefore we suggested that the performance of a BIPSS would not have changed the management of these patients. In summary, 93.6% of all patients had an early postoperative remission. The selective indication for BIPSS in the preoperative work-up of Cushing disease did not negatively affect the outcome and thus should be considered more broadly.[8]

Repeat Surgery

Patients who demonstrate elevated postoperative ACTH and cortisol levels are candidates for attempted surgical re-exploration. In addition, some authors advocate repeat surgery in the immediate postoperative period when cortisol levels are within the normal range, given the high rate of recurrence. They argue that in early re-exploration, the lack of scar formation and the surgeon's acquaintance with the surgical target facilitate access and resection. In all cases of repeat surgery, the biochemical and radiologic work-up must be rescrutinized and possibly repeated to verify a pituitary origin of disease. Mandatory testing in this setting includes IPSS for ACTH with CRH stimulation if not previously performed. A small percentage of patients may in fact harbor an ectopic source of abnormal ACTH-secreting cells, such as within the cavernous sinus, that would not be amenable to repeat surgery.[10] Notwithstanding such cases, if no discrete adenoma is found at the time of repeat exploration, the surgeon may opt for hemihypophysectomy or complete hypophysectomy, as previously discussed. Remission rates following repeat surgery for residual or recurrent disease range from 30 to 53%.[1,11] Hypopituitarism, as well as complications including infection and cerebrospinal fluid (CSF) leaks, are more common following repeat surgery, most likely because of the tendency to perform more aggressive procedures.

Surgical Technique

This author uses a wide transnasal transsphenoidal exposure, opening from carotid canal to carotid canal (cavernous sinus to cavernous sinus) with either a microscope or endoscope technique. If the lesion was visible on the MRI, then we proceed to the area of the adenoma. If there was no visible lesion on the MRI, then we start on the side with the higher ACTH values on IPSS. Exploration begins between the gland and the dura. If no tumor is visible between the gland and dura, we then incise into the gland vertically on the suspected lateral wing of the gland (**Fig. 6.1**). If tumor is found, it is removed gently with the ring curettes and microdissectors. At this point, if the adenoma is still not visible, a vertical incision is made into the opposite lateral wing vertically. If adenoma is not identified, then a horizontal incision is made across the lower third of the anterior surface of the gland and the depth of the gland is explored. If no tumor has been seen and the IPSS study shows strong laterality, a hemihypophysectomy is done on that side. If remission is not achieved after the first exploration and testing is definitive for a pituitary etiology, a second exploration is performed more vigorously, with the understanding that hypopituitarism may develop. If two surgical procedures fail to yield remission, adjunctive therapy such as stereotactic radiosurgery and/or medical therapy with ketoconazole is recommended (**Figs. 6.2** and **6.3**).

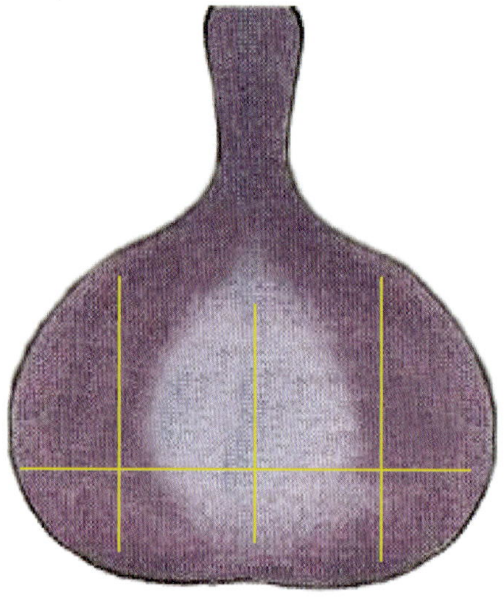

Fig. 6.1 Diagram of the incisions made into the pituitary gland during an exploration for Cushing disease with a normal MRI.

◆ Surgical Management of Acromegaly

Acromegaly is a disease of chronic overproduction of growth hormone (GH). In the child and preadolescent, excess GH leads to abnormally increased height and gigantism as well as organomegaly. Once the epiphyseal plates have closed, the manifestations are those of acromegaly. The consequences of GH hypersecretion are numerous. Bone and soft-tissue overgrowth is almost always present, resulting in changes in shoe size and ring size and a coarsening of the facial features, with enlargement of the lips, macroglossia, a prominent brow, prognathism, and increased spaces between the teeth. A low voice is a product of laryngeal hypertrophy. Patients often go on to develop skeletal abnormalities secondary to new bone growth, including vertebral body osteophyte formation leading to spinal stenosis and bowing of the long bones. Overgrowth contributes to a significant increase in weight and stress on the joints, cartilaginous erosion, and severe osteoarthritis. More seriously, acromegaly causes numerous cardiovascular complications, such as cardiomyopathy, arrhythmias, and coronary artery disease. GH elevation contributes to markedly increased rates of diabetes and hypertension.

Mortality is significantly increased in patients with untreated or uncured acromegaly. The goals of treatment are control of GH and insulin-like growth factor 1 (IGF-1)

Potential causes of failed surgery in patients with Cushing disease.

Incorrect preoperative diagnosis

- Syndrome of ectopic ACTH hypersecretion
- Ectopic pituitary adenoma (cavernous sinus, suprasellar, stalk)
- Corticotroph hyperplasia
- Pseudo-Cushing syndrome

Incomplete or failed tumor resection

- Inexperienced neurosurgeon
- Invasive disease
- Abnormal MRI, but not an adenoma

Fig. 6.2 Potential causes of failed surgery in patients with Cushing disease.

A logical approach to the postoperative evaluation of patients with suspected residual or recurrent Cushing disease.

Confirm presence pathologic ACTH hypersecretion exists after surgery
- Elevated urine free cortisol on 2-3 occasions
- Abnormal diurnal variation in serum or salivary cortisol levels

Confirm preoperative diagnosis of ACTH-dependent hypercortisolism
- Review data to determine if pathologic hypercortisolism was indeed present prior to surgery
- Review preoperative MRI studies to determine if pituitary tumor was present

Review histopathology for evidence of ACTH-producing pituitary tumor
- ACTH-immunopositive lesion?
- Crooke's hyaline change present?

Consider differential diagnosis
- MRI to evaluate for pituitary tumor
- Inferior petrosal sinus sampling with CRH stimulation if surgical pathology was negative

Fig. 6.3 A logical approach to the postoperative evaluation of patients with suspected residual or recurrent Cushing disease.

levels, such that GH levels are less than 1 µg/L after an oral glucose load and IGF-1 levels are normal, adjusted for age and sex. The tumor mass needs to be removed or significantly reduced, such that the optic nerves are free of compression or impending threat of such.[12] It is common for patients with acromegaly to require multimodality therapy.[13]

Transsphenoidal microsurgery is the preferred primary treatment for acromegaly, although rarely craniotomy may be necessary in the case of certain tumors that have a significant extrasellar or suprasellar component.[14] Surgical resection of the adenoma provides the greatest hope for cure and is generally safe, with acceptable morbidity.[15]

As one would expect, tumor size has clearly been shown to influence the likelihood of remission. The success rate for modern microadenoma resection alone ranges from 72 to 88% in this author's series. Success rates for operating on macroadenomas are expectedly lower than those for smaller tumors. Macrodenomas that are noninvasive have modestly lower remission rates of 50 to 56%.[14] Those tumors found to be invading the cavernous sinus or surrounding structures have a further reduced rate of remission. Major decreases in remission exist when the tumor is invasive and larger than 20 mm. GH levels may be predictive of the likelihood of success. According to Shimon et al, whereas patients with preoperative GH levels of less than 20 µg/L and 20 to 50 µg/L had cure rates of 90 and 79%, respectively, those with GH levels of more than 50 µg/L were cured at a rate of 16%.[16] Similar data by Freda et al found 90 and 80% cure rates for microadenomas and macroadenomas, respectively, when the preoperative GH level was less than 10 µg/L; these fell to 55% for patients with GH levels of of 30 to 50 µg/L. No patients were cured who had a preoperative GH level of more than 200 µg/L.[17] Because GH levels rapidly fall following resection, while IGF-1 can take a longer time to normalize, GH levels are routinely the test of choice in the immediate postoperative period. Early GH levels can be predictive of success or failure. There is not a clear cutoff in the early postoperative laboratory results to define cure, but GH levels of less than 2 µg/L on the first postoperative day have been found to correlate with surgical success in 99% of patients.[18] Accordingly, only 1 of 65 patients with a GH level of more than 2 µg/L on postoperative day 1 was later determined to have biochemical cure.[18] Dural invasion and extrasellar extension of tumors have been shown to be associated with persistent disease.

Patients with acromegaly usually present because of their endocrinologic disturbances. Some patients, however, present with visual disturbances. The majority of patients recover some degree of visual function following transsphenoidal surgery. The recovery of visual function relates to the duration of optic nerve compression and the ability to adequately decompress the nerves in the operating room. As patients with acromegaly largely have other symptoms as well, they are more likely to be diagnosed at an earlier point in their disease. Nonetheless, some patients do present with significant nerve compression and/or pituitary apoplexy leading to acute visual deterioration. In one study of patients with acromegaly and optic nerve compression at the time of surgery, 75% had an improved visual examination following transsphenoidal decompression.[15]

There is a small subset of patients who will not present until their elderly years. As many as 3 to 5% of patients with acromegaly do not present until they are older than 65 years of age.[19] Many clinicians are tempted to steer these patients away from surgical resection because of the belief that they are unable to handle the stresses of surgery. Minniti et al, in a series of 22 patients with acromegaly past the age of 65, reported no significant perioperative morbidity and no mortality due to transsphenoidal resection. Sixty-eight percent of patients were reported cured based on biochemical criteria and significant improvement in cardiovascular function and glucose tolerance.[19]

Transsphenoidal surgery for GH-secreting tumors is very safe. In general, the morbidity associated with surgical resection of tumors in patients with acromegaly mirrors that of surgery in patients with other tumors via the same method. Anesthetic considerations may be somewhat different if there is significant airway compromise. The soft-tissue, cartilaginous, and bony overgrowth associated with the disease may contribute to a narrowed surgical corridor, especially when a transnasal route is employed, making instrument manipulation even more challenging. Another consideration for surgical planning in these patients is the significant narrowing of the inner borders of the carotid sinus giving rise to a reduced intercarotid distance, which, if neglected, may result in an increase in vascular injury.[20] In experienced hands, major complications such as visual impairment, severe meningitis, and death have been reported in fewer than 2% of cases. CSF leaks, hypopituitarism, and diabetes insipidus have been reported in roughly 5% of postoperative patients. The risks of transsphenoidal surgery as well as the likely rates of cure reported in this chapter are predicated on the procedure being done by an experienced surgeon.[21–24]

Reoperation for acromegaly is a controversial subject. Rates of surgical success in these patients have been historically quite poor. Recent experience by dedicated pituitary surgeons has been quoted as 44 to 76%.[25] This can most likely be attributed to extensive tumor involvement, given that at the time of surgery 70 to 80% of tumors are macroadenomas, which are less amenable to complete surgical resection.[26] The postoperative patient with persistent disease is a complex clinical entity. There is much controversy surrounding the ideal course of treatment after surgical failure. Goals of therapy are fourfold: to gain biochemical control, reverse medical comorbidities and risk for mortality, relieve signs and symptoms of the disease, and limit local tumor mass effects.[27] Some patients need reoperation for progressive visual deterioration. In general, surgical re-exploration is reserved for those who on follow-up demonstrate persistent compression of the optic pathway or in whom residual tumor may have become more surgically accessible over time. It has been noted that patients undergoing reoperation for impairment do not generally seem to garner as much visual improvement as those undergoing a primary operation with the same complaint.

What defines recurrence of active acromegaly is a confusing issue. As testing becomes more sensitive, more patients are noted to have subtle signs of endocrinologic laboratory abnormality. Some patients now considered to have recurrence may just have had mild GH dysfunction that was not detected by earlier, less accurate tests. We have previously reported on a subset of patients with postoperative IGF-1 levels that normalized but failed to be suppressed to less than 1 µg/L. Five of these 14 patients later developed evidence of elevated IGF-1.[28] This suggests a group of patients with subtle endocrinologic dysfunction who, although they have normal IGF-1 levels and hence are technically in remission, probably still have some latent disease. Although no intervention is considered necessary provided the IGF-1 remains under control, this group may benefit from closer monitoring.

The current treatment paradigm for acromegaly involves a multidisciplinary approach (**Fig. 6.4**). It is incumbent on the patient's primary care doctor to notice the signs and symptoms of the disease early and refer the patient for definitive treatment. Success correlates with pretreatment GH levels. To reduce the patient's risk for mortality to baseline levels, the IGF-1 level must be normalized and the GH level suppressed to less than 1 µg/L following an oral glucose tolerance test. Surgery offers the best possible

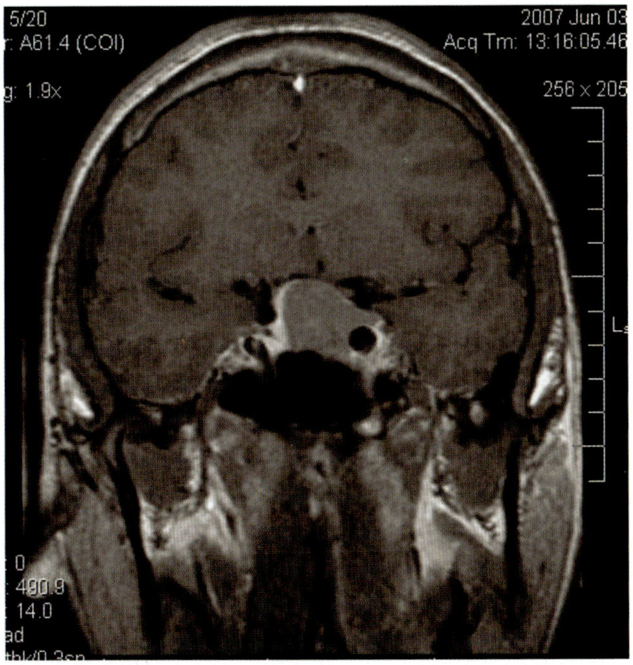

Fig. 6.4 Coronal gadolinium-enhanced T1 MRI of a patient with acromegaly. Even though adenoma may invade the left cavernous sinus, transsphenoidal surgery would be the first treatment option. Preoperative treatment with a somatostain analogue could be offered but might not change the surgical outcome.

opportunity for cure. In experienced hands, cure rates for patients with a microadenoma approach 90%; those with larger and/or invasive tumors do not fare quite so well. Patients who do not have full normalization of their IGF-1 level postoperatively should be considered for further therapy or reoperation. Reoperation can be considered, but rates of cure are significantly lower than in the primary surgical group. Medical therapy is successful in lowering GH and IGF-1 levels and may be employed both presurgically and postsurgically, but its effects are sustained only during the course of administration. New, long-acting depot forms of somatostatin analogues are available that offer equal efficacy and longer dosing intervals. The newer GH antagonist holds further promise in the medical armamentarium, but patients' GH levels can no longer be followed. Radiation is a good treatment option for patients with uncured acromegaly following surgery. The cure is slow to develop, but more than 50% of patients may achieve normalized IGF-1 levels this way. Both radiation therapy and stereotactic radiosurgery carry significant risks of panhypopituitarism necessitating hormone therapy. Similar to the prolonged time to cure, patients have a gradual onset of pituitary hormone dysfunction, should it develop.

Surgical Technique

The incidence of difficult intubation in patients with acromegaly has been reported to vary from 10 to 30%.[29–31] Airway difficulty has been attributed to morphologic changes produced by excess GH. These changes include prognathism, macroglossia, and thickening of the pharyngeal and laryngeal soft tissue. Thickening of the vocal cords, recurrent laryngeal nerve paralysis, narrowing of the cricoid arch, and hypertrophy of aryepiglottic and ventricular folds have also been cited as causes of difficult intubation in patients with acromegaly.[32] Of our patients with acromegaly and a preoperative evaluation of a difficult airway, 61% proved to be difficult intraoperatively. Conversely, 91% of patients with GH-secreting tumors who required three or more attempts at intubation were felt to have a "difficult" airway preoperatively. Our 17.3% rate of difficult intubation is well within the range of difficult airway in acromegaly of 10 to 30% reported in the literature. Patients with acromegaly were 4.4 times more difficult to intubate than were patients with non–GH-secreting/non–ACTH-secreting tumors. Although considered the gold standard, fiberscopic intubation was only 85% successful in securing the airway (**Fig. 6.5**).

Surgical techniques, whether via a microscopic or endoscopic venue, are the same as for other pituitary adenomas. There is no need to explore the gland, as is necessary with Cushing disease, because no patient whom we operate on has a normal MRI. Because of the potentially narrowed distance between the carotid arteries, a micro Doppler probe is often used before the dura is incised.

◆ Surgical Management of Prolactinomas

Prolactinomas are the most commonly diagnosed pituitary adenomas, representing ~30% of cases.[33] Rarely life-threatening, they cause symptoms primarily as a result of hyperprolactinemia, which in turn results in alterations in reproductive and sexual function and may also cause symptoms related to mass effect. This is the pituitary tumor for which a reliably effective medical treatment is most often available and that in most cases is the favored

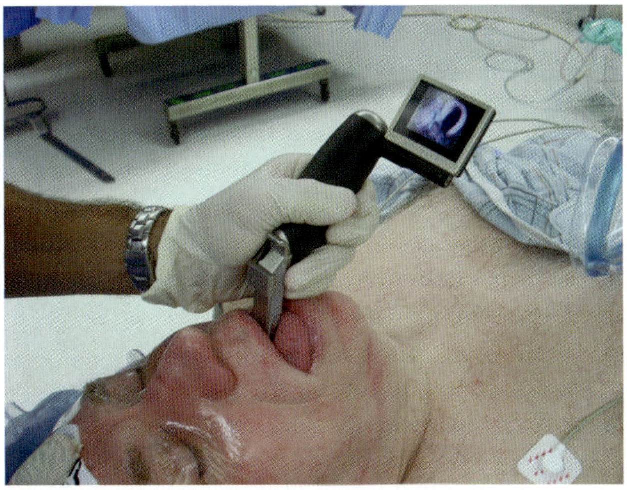

Fig. 6.5 A patient with acromegaly being intubated with the McGrath Series 5 video laryngoscope (Aircraft Medical, Edinburgh, Scotland).

primary therapy. Surgical treatment, however, has proved to provide similar results as in other endocrine-secreting adenomas and is applicable as the appropriate intervention for prolactinomas in certain cases.

The treatment options available to a patient with a prolactinoma include observation, medical therapy, surgical therapy, and radiotherapy. The best treatment depends on tumor size, prolactin level, clinical manifestations, tolerance of medical therapy, and the desire for fertility. Studies have demonstrated that the vast majority of microprolactinomas (<10 mm) do not increase in size. Additionally, autopsy series have found the frequent occurrence of incidental microprolactinomas. Based on this, if patients have only mildly elevated prolactin, normal pituitary function, no clinical symptoms, and no desire for pregnancy, observation with serial radiographic and endocrine evaluation is reasonable.

Lactotropes are controlled by a negative dopaminergic effect from the hypothalamus, and based on this, dopamine agonists have become the standard medical therapy. Dopamine agonists have been remarkably effective in both reducing the size of the tumor and normalizing serum prolactin levels below the accepted remission level of 20 ng/mL. Bromocriptine was the first of these medications, but more recently others, such as cabergoline, quinagolide, lisuride, pergolide mesylate, and terguride, are also used. Dopamine agonists have been shown to have a high response rate, with reports of normalization of prolactin in 70 to 80%, tumor shrinkage in 80 to 90%, and restoration of ovulation in 80 to 90%.[34] Based on these results, some would argue that medical treatment should be used in all patients except the few with significant side effects from medical treatment. In addition, in an important study, it has been shown that a majority of patients who respond to cabergoline with normalization of prolactin levels and a reduction in tumor size may experience remission of hyperprolactinemia following discontinuation of the drug.[33] This study suggests the potential for a curative treatment with medical therapy in a selected group of patients.

Dopamine agonists do have some significant disadvantages that may temper their use in all patients. The effects on the tumor are reversible, making the therapy lifelong in most cases and thus requiring significant compliance. Additionally, there can be significant side effects, including nausea, vomiting, postural hypotension, headaches, depression, and anxiety, that can make long-term compliance even more difficult in some patients. In cases of pituitary apoplexy and in tumors with large cystic components, dopamine agonists are not effective in effecting shrinkage. A group of bromocriptine-resistant prolactinomas with increased aggressiveness and increased incidence in male patients has been recently described.[35] There have been recent reports of an association between valvular heart disease and dopamine agonists in patients being treated for Parkinson disease. However, these patients with Parkinson disease were receiving doses approximately seven times higher than the maximal dose used for the treatment of prolactinomas.[12] In a review of the current literature on the subject, Valassi et al reported that most published articles on the subject do not show an association between the use of dopamine agonists and valvulopathy; however, they recommend using the lowest dose possible and that the physician address the use of echocardiographic monitoring on a case-by-case basis.[36]

The role of surgery in the treatment of prolactinomas has been under discussion. Some argue that surgery should be the initial treatment of microprolactinoma, with medical therapy as an adjunct only in cases without remission.[37] The rate of long-term remission varies significantly, however, depending on the size of the tumor and preoperative prolactin levels. The most favorable results have been demonstrated in patients with microadenomas and levels below 200 ng/mL, with remission rates ranging from 50 to 84% in long-term follow-up.[34,37,38] The remission rate drops with macroadenomas and with prolactin levels from 200 to 500 ng/mL, even though these tumors are amenable to surgical resection. Surgery has not been shown to be useful alone in patients with giant adenomas or tumors with prolactin levels higher than 500 ng/mL, in whom the remission rate decreases to zero. These lesions are better treated with medical therapy, possibly in conjunction with surgery and radiation. Overall, a lower prolactin level portends a greater chance of long-term remission.

Based on the most current literature, surgical removal can be recommended for most patients with a macroadenoma and a prolactin level of less than 200 ng/mL, with anticipation of a high remission rate. Patients with tumors larger than 2 cm and/or a prolactin level below 500 ng/mL should first treated with a dopamine agonist to reduce the tumor volume and then undergo surgical resection. Any residual tumor can then be treated medically. For patients with very large or invasive tumors or tumors with a prolactin level above 500 ng/mL, medical therapy should be the primary treatment modality.

Another consideration in the management of these patients is the incidence of spontaneous CSF leak after the medical treatment of macroprolactinomas, which is a well-known phenomenon. A recent study of a small series of patients found that those subjects with adenomas invading the sphenoid sinus were at the highest risk for spontaneous CSF leaks after medical treatment that required neurosurgical repair.[39]

The subgroup requiring specific discussion comprises patients who are pregnant and harbor prolactinomas. If the patient becomes symptomatic, a dopamine agonist can be administered. The data regarding the effects of continuous dopamine agonist therapy on the fetus are limited but suggest no ill effect. During pregnancy, surgery should be undertaken only if the tumor does not respond to medical treatment and if there are progressive neurologic symptoms. Patients with macroadenomas who desire pregnancy should undergo a transsphenoidal resection before conception or remain on bromocriptine during the pregnancy.

◆ Surgical Management of Adenomas Secreting Thyroid-Stimulating Hormone

Adenomas secreting thyroid-stimulating hormone (TSH) are the least common of the pituitary tumors, representing only 1 to 2% of cases.

Patients can present with constitutional problems consistent with long-standing thyroid dysfunction, such as heat intolerance, diarrhea, weight loss, fatigue, and exophthalmos, or manifestations of local mass effect, such as headaches, visual changes, and symptoms of hypopituitarism. There is often a delay in the diagnosis of these tumors because they are commonly misdiagnosed as Graves disease and are detected only when already large and invasive. They can be difficult to cure.

Before any surgical intervention, the hyperthyroidism should be controlled to minimize the risk for cardiac arrhythmias that may occur during induction of anesthesia or intraoperatively. This is commonly done with a preoperative β blocker. If the surgery is nonemergent, an antithyroid drug (propylthiouracil or methimazole) can be added. Transsphenoidal surgery is the primary treatment but is associated with cure rates of only ~35 to 62% when performed alone and 55 to 81% when performed in conjunction with medical treatment and radiotherapy.[40–42] The criteria for cure in TSH-secreting adenomas have not yet been well defined. Radiosurgery or radiation therapy can be used if clinical remission is not obtained with surgery alone. However, radiosurgery and radiotherapy are not typically used as a primary treatment modality.

◆ Surgical Management of Nonsecreting Pituitary Adenomas

Approximately one-third of pituitary tumors are considered nonsecreting (also called nonfunctioning) adenomas. They are generally associated with older age, with a peak in the fifth decade. Patients usually present with signs and symptoms of hypopituitarism, and commonly with associated visual field defects and other ophthalmologic problems. Despite their similar clinical presentation, endocrine-inactive tumors are a heterogeneous group. Ultrastructural studies have demonstrated that these tumors actually contain secretory granules and that a majority of them synthesize follicle-stimulating hormone (FSH), luteinizing hormone (LH), and the α subunit, with a smaller subset producing other anterior pituitary hormones that do not have clinical manifestations.[43] No clear and consistent difference in treatment or prognosis has emerged among the various subtypes, however.

Because endocrine-inactive tumors do not cause hypersecretory syndromes, patients usually present with symptoms associated with mass effect. Patients usually describe headaches, visual changes, and symptoms of pituitary insufficiency. In a majority of cases, the tumor is a macroadenoma at the time of diagnosis.

Surgery remains the primary treatment of patients with inactive adenomas. The goals are to relieve the mass effect, restore pituitary function, and obtain a tissue diagnosis. As with other pituitary adenomas, the preferred approach is transsphenoidal, but cases with significant eccentric extension outside the sella may require a transcranial approach. The results of surgery for endocrine-inactive tumors are not as clearly described as those of surgery for other adenomas because there are no clear criteria for cure. Studies have consistently demonstrated that 70 to 80% of patients experience significant improvement in visual function. In addition, nearly 100% of patients report resolution of headaches, and there is an improvement in pituitary function ranging from 15 to 57%, depending on the series and the criteria for hypopituitarism.[44]

Clinical improvement is not suggestive of complete tumor removal. Postoperative imaging a few months after surgery is required to assess the extent of tumor resection. Early imaging may not be as helpful or accurate because of confounding edema, postoperative hemorrhage, and hemostatic material. This study then acts as a baseline for future comparison. We do not discuss adjunctive therapy for residual tumor in this chapter. Rather, it is discussed in other chapters in this book.

◆ Surgical Technique for Pituitary Adenomas

The historical development of transsphenoidal surgery is a complex tale of innovative leaps in ideology coupled with periods of extensive surgical experimentation and even complete rejection of the technique. Summaries of the historical movements that have resulted in its adoption as the preferred approach to tumors of the hypophysis have already been well documented. However, within this history there exist some significant revolutions in technique and technology that have further advanced the utility of this operation and merit further study. The first of these revolutions was in surgical technique, with the introduction of sublabial and transnasal approaches to the pituitary. Then, with the introduction of intraoperative image intensification by Gerard Guiot in 1958 and the surgical microscope by Jules Hardy in 1967, many of the technical difficulties faced by pioneers such as Harvey Cushing could be circumvented. This laid the foundation for the advances that now shape modern transsphenoidal surgery, including the use of endoscopy, intraoperative imaging, frameless guidance, and radioimmunoassay. Currently, the transsphenoidal approach is the preferred approach for more than 90% of pituitary tumors. Occasionally, a transcranial approach becomes necessary for those very large or asymmetric tumors with minimal sellar content.

The transsphenoidal procedure is reasonably similar whether a microscopic or endoscopic technique is used. The microscope gives a clear three-dimensional view, whereas the endoscope gives a far more extended view (**Figs. 6.6, 6.7, 6.8,** and **6.9**). With a microscope, the average exposure of the sella is ~12 mm in width and from the tuberculum to the clivus in the vertical plain. Generally, the carotid canals can be visualized. In the sphenoid sinus, the endoscope allows visualization of the entire inner surface of the sphenoid sinus, which is far more important in the extended transsphenoidal operation for tumors other than adenomas, such as meningiomas and craniopharyngiomas. Within the sella, the endoscope allows more lateral inspection of the cavernous sinus walls as well as the suprasellar region, provided that the arachnoid membrane and diaphragma sellae have not completely descended into the sella with tumor decompression. We have used both approaches and often add the endoscope as an adjunct

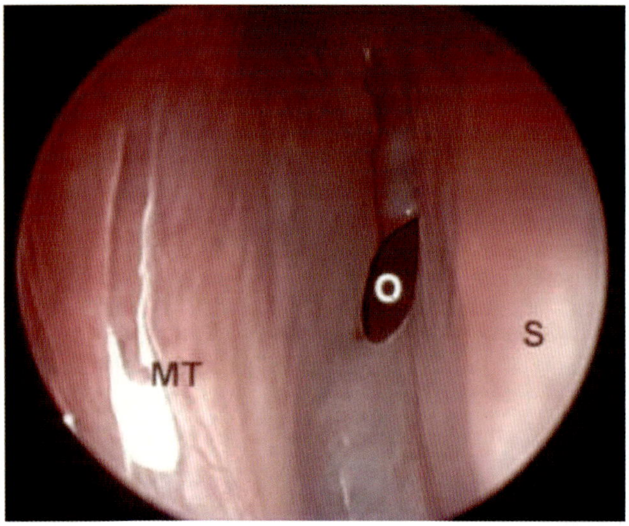

Fig. 6.6 An endoscopic view through the right naris of the ostium into the sphenoid sinus.

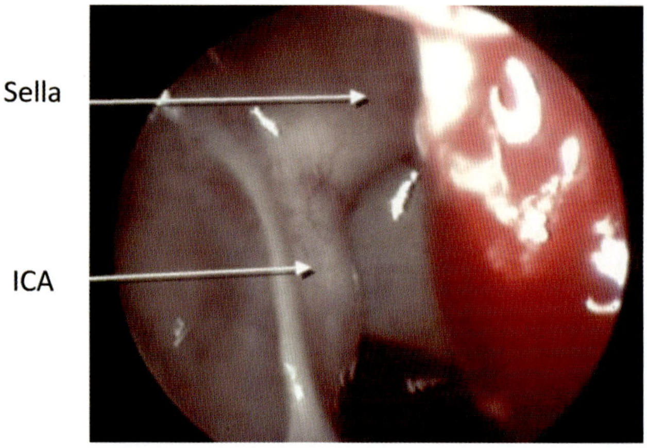

Fig. 6.7 Endoscopic view of the sellar floor and lateral carotid canal.

when we use the microscope. During an endoscopic procedure, a speculum may be inserted so that the microscope can be added as an adjunct. Clearly, both techniques are excellent, and the surgeon may have both available and should be adept with both.

For anatomic localization and direction to the sella, fluoroscopy was the mainstay but offered only one plane, lateral, and entailed the problem of radiation exposure. Newer techniques with MRI- or CT-directed BrainLab/Stealth equipment may make fluoroscopy unnecessary. These techniques offer the advantage of multiplane views as well as lower or no radiation exposure. There are numerous studies showing that in practiced hands, these techniques do not add substantially to the operative time and may reduce complications, such as carotid artery injury, of migrating from the midline approach. A small error in the angle toward the sella during exposure can lead directly to the carotid canals.

We operate with the patient in the supine position and the head just slightly flexed and tilted toward the left because the surgeon is generally on the patient's right side. With an endoscopic approach, the head may be kept straighter because a four-handed technique with one surgeon on either side of the patient may be advantageous. The right lower corner of the abdomen is also prepared in case there is need of a fat graft to seal an exposure of the CSF space. Either the fluoroscope or BrainLab equipment is positioned for localization and direction.

A transnasal submucosal exposure of the front of the sphenoid sinus is created with use of the vomer to ensure the midline if fluoroscopy is used. The orifices into the sphenoid are enlarged, allowing exposure of the back wall of the sphenoid sinus and anterior sella wall. If the sella is dramatically enlarged, or if it is anticipated that a large opening into the CSF space will be created, such as with an extended procedure, a pedicled mucosal flap along the midline is created and tucked aside in the nasal cavity for closure at the end of the procedure. We lean more toward a microscopic approach and therefore insert a bivalved microspeculum through the nares with one blade on either side of the vomer beneath the mucosal flaps. In the past, when a sublabial exposure was done with a larger speculum, care was taken to avoid putting the blade of the

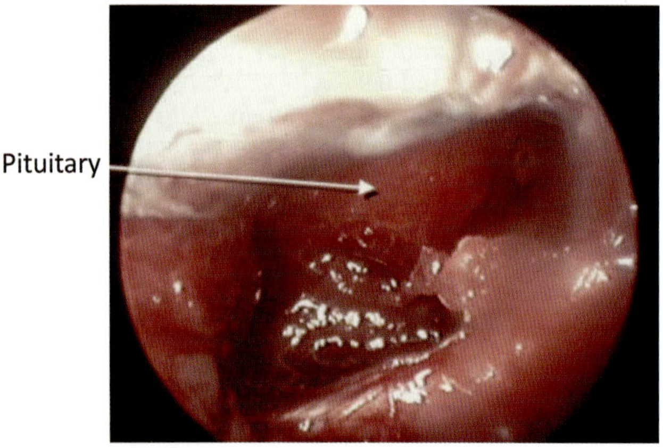

Fig. 6.8 Endoscopic view of the pituitary.

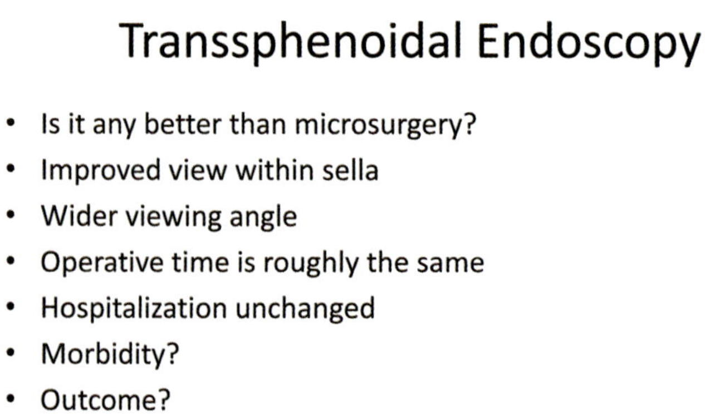

Fig. 6.9 Transsphenoidal endoscopic surgery.

speculum into the sphenoid sinus for fear of fracturing the medial walls of the orbits. With a transnasal approach and a microspeculum, we tend to place the speculum just inside the sphenoid sinus wall and open it gently to avoid fractures. This gives better exposure and keeps the speculum from rotating out of the vertical position. With an endoscopic technique, a speculum may be unnecessary.

Once the anterior sellar wall is exposed, it may be opened with a microdissector if it is thin or with a drill or osteotome if it is thick. It must be opened to the medial wall of cavernous sinus on both sides. This can be confirmed with BrainLab or visually by a change in direction of the dura as well as a color change. A micro Doppler probe may be helpful in confirming that the exposure is not too far lateral, exposing the carotid artery to injury. The dura can be opened sharply in an X fashion or with excision of a large rectangle anteriorly. If tumor is clearly invading through the dura, the latter opening is used to excise the invaded dura. A vertical cross-opening yields less exposure of the gland.

Tumor dissection varies with the size of the adenoma. With macroadenomas, the tumor is usually evident upon opening the dura. With microadenomas, dissection is guided by the preoperative imaging studies. With both microadenomas and macroadenomas, a clear plane can be found between the adenoma and the normal gland. This is the plane we follow to completely excise the tumor. We advise removing the tumor that is central, inferior, and lateral before approaching the suprasellar portion. If the superior tumor is removed first, the diaphragma sellae and arachnoid may herniate into the sella, significantly obscuring the field. At this point, the endoscope may be of great value to inspect the medial walls of the cavernous sinuses as well as the suprasellar walls to be as certain as possible that no further tumor exists. A wider view with an angled endoscope is an advantage.

After the adenoma has been resected, closure is somewhat dependent upon whether CSF has been seen. We ask anesthesia to perform a Valsalva maneuver to raise the intracranial pressure to see if CSF leakage is present. If CSF is not seen at any time during the procedure, we do not routinely use fat or other substances to fill the sella. If the sella has been markedly eroded, with a large expanse of arachnoid seen in the sella, then fat may be placed in the sella regardless of whether CSF was seen. The sella floor is closed with a piece of vomer bone that was removed during the exposure. If an adequate piece of bone is not available, then a biodegradeable plate is used instead. The bone or plate is wedged under the edges of the opened sellar wall. If the erosion of the sellar wall has been so extensive that no edges exist, this cannot be done. If there has been CSF leakage during surgery, the back of the sphenoid sinus is packed with fat harvested from the abdomen. We rarely place a spinal drain for CSF diversion either before or after surgery.

Once the speculum is removed, the mucosa is reapproximated to the midline and a Mercilene sponge is placed in the nares for 48 hours. Patients are hospitalized for 2 days on our service and are generally back at full activity within 1 week.

◆ Conclusion

Pituitary adenomas are relatively common tumors within the sellar and parasellar region. Surgical resection represents an important part of the treatment paradigm for patients with hypersecretory adenomas and nonsecretory adenomas exerting mass effect. Radiologic and endocrine results after pituitary adenoma surgery are favorable. Long-term follow up of these patients is required to detect recurrence. Reoperation generally affords less favorable results than the initial surgery.

References

1. Swearingen B, Biller BM, Barker FG II, et al. Long-term mortality after transsphenoidal surgery for Cushing disease. Ann Intern Med 1999;130(10):821–824
2. Watson JC, Shawker TH, Nieman LK, DeVroom HL, Doppman JL, Oldfield EH. Localization of pituitary adenomas by using intraoperative ultrasound in patients with Cushing's disease and no demonstrable pituitary tumor on magnetic resonance imaging. J Neurosurg 1998;89(6):927–932
3. Kaltsas GA, Giannulis MG, Newell-Price JD, et al. A critical analysis of the value of simultaneous inferior petrosal sinus sampling in Cushing's disease and the occult ectopic adrenocorticotropin syndrome. J Clin Endocrinol Metab 1999;84(2):487–492
4. Atkinson AB, Kennedy A, Wiggam MI, McCance DR, Sheridan B. Long-term remission rates after pituitary surgery for Cushing's disease: the need for long-term surveillance. Clin Endocrinol (Oxf) 2005;63(5):549–559
5. Simmons NE, Alden TD, Thorner MO, Laws ER Jr. Serum cortisol response to transsphenoidal surgery for Cushing disease. J Neurosurg 2001;95(1):1–8
6. Findling JW, Raff H. Cushing's syndrome: important issues in diagnosis and management. J Clin Endocrinol Metab 2006;91(10):3746–3753
7. Nishizawa S, Oki Y, Ohta S, Yokota N, Yokoyama T, Uemura K. What can predict postoperative "endocrinological cure" in Cushing's disease? Neurosurgery 1999;45(2):239–244
8. Jehle S, Walsh JE, Freda PU, Post KD. Selective use of bilateral inferior petrosal sinus sampling in patients with adrenocorticotropin-dependent Cushing's syndrome prior to transsphenoidal surgery. J Clin Endocrinol Metab 2008;93(12):4624–4632
9. Pouratian N, Prevedello DM, Jagannathan J, Lopes MB, Vance ML, Laws ER Jr. Outcomes and management of patients with Cushing's disease without pathological confirmation of tumor resection after transsphenoidal surgery. J Clin Endocrinol Metab 2007;92(9):3383–3388
10. Ohnishi T, Arita N, Yoshimine T, Mori S. Intracavernous sinus ectopic adrenocorticotropin-secreting tumours causing therapeutic failure in transsphenoidal surgery for Cushing's disease. Acta Neurochir (Wien) 2000;142(8):855–864
11. Chee GH, Mathias DB, James RA, Kendall-Taylor P. Transsphenoidal pituitary surgery in Cushing's disease: can we predict outcome? Clin Endocrinol (Oxf) 2001;54(5):617–626
12. Melmed S. Update in pituitary disease. J Clin Endocrinol Metab 2008;93(2):331–338
13. Trepp R, Stettler C, Zwahlen M, Seiler R, Diem P, Christ ER. Treatment outcomes and mortality of 94 patients with acromegaly. Acta Neurochir (Wien) 2005;147(3):243–251, discussion 250–251
14. Buchfelder M, Schlaffer S. Surgical treatment of pituitary tumours. Best Pract Res Clin Endocrinol Metab 2009;23(5):677–692
15. Kreutzer J, Vance ML, Lopes MB, Laws ER Jr. Surgical management of GH-secreting pituitary adenomas: an outcome study using modern remission criteria. J Clin Endocrinol Metab 2001;86(9):4072–4077
16. Shimon I, Cohen ZR, Ram Z, Hadani M. Transsphenoidal surgery for acromegaly: endocrinological follow-up of 98 patients. Neurosurgery 2001;48(6):1239–1243, discussion 1244–1245
17. Freda PU, Wardlaw SL, Post KD. Long-term endocrinological follow-up evaluation in 115 patients who underwent transsphenoidal surgery for acromegaly. J Neurosurg 1998;89(3):353–358

18. Krieger MD, Couldwell WT, Weiss MH. Assessment of long-term remission of acromegaly following surgery. J Neurosurg 2003;98(4):719–724
19. Minniti G, Jaffrain-Rea ML, Esposito V, et al. Surgical treatment and clinical outcome of GH-secreting adenomas in elderly patients. Acta Neurochir (Wien) 2001;143(12):1205–1211
20. Ebner FH, Kuerschner V, Dietz K, Bueltmann E, Naegele T, Honegger J. Reduced intercarotid artery distance in acromegaly: pathophysiologic considerations and implications for transsphenoidal surgery. Surg Neurol 2009;72(5):456–460, discussion 460
21. Ahmed S, Elsheikh M, Stratton IM, Page RC, Adams CB, Wass JA. Outcome of transsphenoidal surgery for acromegaly and its relationship to surgical experience. Clin Endocrinol (Oxf) 1999; 50(5):561–567
22. Bates PR, Carson MN, Trainer PJ, Wass JA; UK National Acromegaly Register Study Group (UKAR-2). Wide variation in surgical outcomes for acromegaly in the UK. Clin Endocrinol (Oxf) 2008;68(1):136–142
23. De P, Rees DA, Davies N, et al. Transsphenoidal surgery for acromegaly in Wales: results based on stringent criteria of remission. J Clin Endocrinol Metab 2003;88(8):3567–3572
24. Lissett CA, Peacey SR, Laing I, Tetlow L, Davis JR, Shalet SM. The outcome of surgery for acromegaly: the need for a specialist pituitary surgeon for all types of growth hormone (GH) secreting adenoma. Clin Endocrinol (Oxf) 1998;49(5):653–657
25. Scacchi M, Cavagnini F. Acromegaly. Pituitary 2006;9(4):297–303
26. Sheppard MC. Primary medical therapy for acromegaly. Clin Endocrinol (Oxf) 2003;58(4):387–399
27. Katznelson L. Approach to the patient with persistent acromegaly after pituitary surgery. J Clin Endocrinol Metab 2010;95(9): 4114–4123
28. Freda PU, Nuruzzaman AT, Reyes CM, Sundeen RE, Post KD. Significance of "abnormal" nadir growth hormone levels after oral glucose in postoperative patients with acromegaly in remission with normal insulin-like growth factor-I levels. J Clin Endocrinol Metab 2004;89(2):495–500
29. Nemergut EC, Zuo Z. Airway management in patients with pituitary disease: a review of 746 patients. J Neurosurg Anesthesiol 2006;18(1):73–77
30. Messick JM Jr, Cucchiara RF, Faust RJ. Airway management in patients with acromegaly. Anesthesiology 1982;56(2):157
31. Schmitt H, Buchfelder M, Radespiel-Tröger M, Fahlbusch R. Difficult intubation in acromegalic patients: incidence and predictability. Anesthesiology 2000;93(1):110–114
32. Nemergut EC, Dumont AS, Barry UT, Laws ER. Perioperative management of patients undergoing transsphenoidal pituitary surgery. Anesth Analg 2005;101(4):1170–1181
33. Colao A, Di Sarno A, Cappabianca P, Di Somma C, Pivonello R, Lombardi G. Withdrawal of long-term cabergoline therapy for tumoral and nontumoral hyperprolactinemia. N Engl J Med 2003;349(21):2023–2033
34. Molitch ME. Disorders of prolactin secretion. Endocrinol Metab Clin North Am 2001;30(3):585–610
35. Delgrange E, Sassolas G, Perrin G, Jan M, Trouillas J. Clinical and histological correlations in prolactinomas, with special reference to bromocriptine resistance. Acta Neurochir (Wien) 2005;147(7): 751–757, discussion 757–758
36. Valassi E, Klibanski A, Biller BM. Clinical Review: Potential cardiac valve effects of dopamine agonists in hyperprolactinemia. J Clin Endocrinol Metab 2010;95(3):1025–1033
37. Tyrrell JB, Lamborn KR, Hannegan LT, Applebury CB, Wilson CB. Transsphenoidal microsurgical therapy of prolactinomas: initial outcomes and long-term results. Neurosurgery 1999;44(2):254–261, discussion 261–263
38. Couldwell WT, Rovit RL, Weiss MH. Role of surgery in the treatment of microprolactinomas. Neurosurg Clin N Am 2003;14(1):89–92
39. de Lacy P, Benjamin S, Dixon R, Stephens JW, Redfern R, Price DE. Is surgical intervention frequently required for medically managed macroprolactinomas? A study of spontaneous cerebrospinal fluid rhinorrhea. Surg Neurol 2009;72(5):461–463, discussion 463
40. Brucker-Davis F, Oldfield EH, Skarulis MC, Doppman JL, Weintraub BD. Thyrotropin-secreting pituitary tumors: diagnostic criteria, thyroid hormone sensitivity, and treatment outcome in 25 patients followed at the National Institutes of Health. J Clin Endocrinol Metab 1999;84(2):476–486
41. Losa M, Giovanelli M, Persani L, Mortini P, Faglia G, Beck-Peccoz P. Criteria of cure and follow-up of central hyperthyroidism due to thyrotropin-secreting pituitary adenomas. J Clin Endocrinol Metab 1996;81(8):3084–3090
42. Sanno N, Teramoto A, Osamura RY. Long-term surgical outcome in 16 patients with thyrotropin pituitary adenoma. J Neurosurg 2000;93(2):194–200
43. Black PM, Hsu DW, Klibanski A, et al. Hormone production in clinically nonfunctioning pituitary adenomas. J Neurosurg 1987;66(2):244–250
44. Losa M, Mortini P, Barzaghi R, Franzin A, Giovanelli M. Endocrine inactive and gonadotroph adenomas: diagnosis and management. J Neurooncol 2001;54(2):167–177

7 Surgical Treatment of Meningiomas

Ossama Al-Mefty and Ian F. Dunn

The surgeon approaching tumors in the parasellar region must contend with a highly congested neurovascular anatomy surrounding the pituitary gland and stalk. In particular, the optic chiasm and nerves, carotid artery and branches, and upper cranial nerves merit meticulous attention, especially when meningiomas of unforgiving consistency are handled.

Accumulated experience with meningiomas and other parasellar tumors has established surgery as a technically feasible and clinically durable method of managing them in patients in whom tumor control by total removal is desired and in whom transsphenoidal access is ill advised. Below, we review the clinical presentation, radiographic features, and surgical treatment principles of meningiomas of the parasellar region, focusing on surgical management of tumors of the tuberculum sellae, diaphragma sellae, cavernous sinus, and anterior clinoid. Such approaches used for meningiomas are generally applicable to other parasellar and sellar tumors. We review the two primary surgical approaches adopted for tumor resection in this region—the supraorbital and the cranio-orbitozygomatic—and discuss the tumors attacked with each technique.

◆ Surgical Approaches

Although each tumor type warrants individual consideration, the authors use two primary surgical approaches to the parasellar region: the supraorbital and the cranio-orbitozygomatic (COZ).[1] The supraorbital approach minimizes frontal lobe retraction while providing unobstructed access to the floor of the anterior fossa from planum to the sella. The COZ approach affords wide exposure of the entire cavernous sinus and the proximal and distal carotid artery with minimal cerebral retraction. We usually use the supraorbital approach for tuberculum sellae and diaphragma sellae meningiomas. We use the COZ frequently for cavernous sinus and clinoidal meningiomas, which often encase the carotid artery and require arterial control. Below, we review the technical features of each approach and the tumor types commonly resected with their application.

◆ Supraorbital Approach: Technique

We perform this approach based on that originally described by Jane et al.[2] For the supraorbital approach, the patient is placed supine and the head and trunk elevated 20 degrees so the head is above the heart. The head is moderately extended to allow the frontal lobes to fall backward and kept straight to facilitate anatomic orientation. We monitor somatosensory evoked and brainstem auditory evoked potentials.

For patients with small to medium-sized tumors, a spinal drain is inserted so that spinal fluid may be released in a controlled fashion for brain relaxation. The scalp incision is begun 1 cm anterior to the tragus and is continued in curvilinear fashion behind the hairline to the level of the superior temporal line on the opposite side (**Fig. 7.1A**). The superficial temporal artery is behind the incision, and the facial nerve branches are in front of the incision. A large pericranial flap based on the supraorbital and frontal vessels beginning well behind the skin incision and extending from one superior temporal line to the other is raised and reflected over the scalp flap anteriorly and dissected off the superior and lateral orbital walls. The supraorbital nerve is freed from its notch or freed with a high-speed drill from its foramen.

The superior aspect of the temporalis muscle is the only part that needs to be mobilized. To do this, a subfascial dissection of the temporalis fascia is performed by incising both layers of temporalis fascia to expose the temporalis muscle, beginning at the keyhole and proceeding behind the course of the facial nerve to approximately the level of the sylvian fissure. The fascial layers are reflected forward, and the temporalis muscle, dissected free from its overlying fascia, is released from its insertion at the superior temporal line and along the superior and lateral orbit and reflected inferiorly. The junction of the zygomatic, sphenoidal, and frontal bones is thus exposed. The bone flap is usually a unilateral supraorbital bone flap, although large tumors may be approached with a bifrontal supraorbital flap. The unilateral flap begins with placement of a burr hole at the anatomic keyhole ~1 cm behind the frontozygomatic suture (**Fig. 7.1B**). When drilled correctly, the

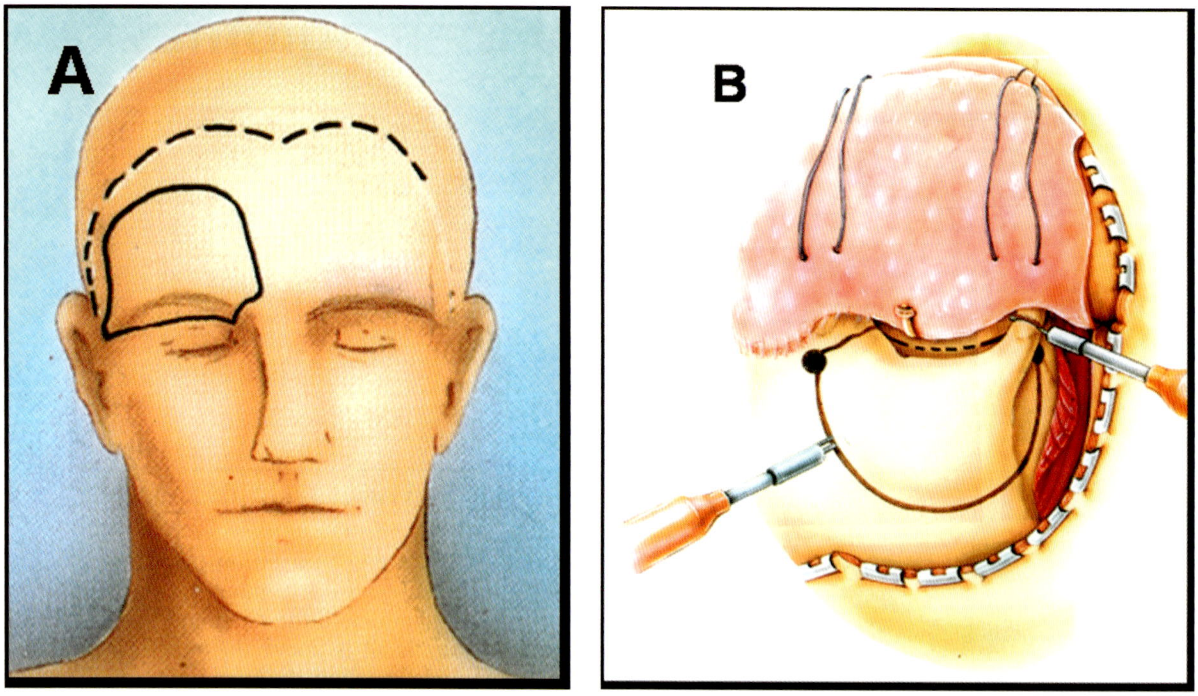

Fig. 7.1 (A) Schematic showing the incision (*hatched line*) and its relationship to the planned frontal craniotomy, which includes the superior orbital rim. **(B)** The superior aspect of the temporalis muscle is detached and the supraorbital nerve is released; the frontal burr hole is optional, but the keyhole site is essential to the supraorbital flap. (Part A from Al-Mefty O. Operative Atlas of Meningiomas. Lippincott–Raven Publishers; 1998. Part B from Al-Mefty O, Ayoubi S. Clinoidal meningiomas. Acta Neurochir Suppl (Wien) 1991;53:92–97. Reprinted with permission.)

superior half exposes the frontal lobe dura, and the lower half exposes the periorbita, with the orbital roof in the center of the burr hole separating the frontal lobe and orbit. A more posterior burr hole on the superior temporal line may also be made. The frontal aspect of the keyhole burr hole and the posterior superior temporal burr hole are connected with the craniotome, and the craniotomy continues into the frontal bone ~4 cm above the superior orbital rim and is curved medial to the supraorbital notch to avoid the frontal sinus. An additional cut is made in the lateral orbital rim and continued to the keyhole.

Finally, the flap is completed with a superior orbital roof osteotomy by placing a chisel straddling the lateral aspect of the superior orbit exposed in the keyhole and completing the osteotomy. If the frontal sinus is entered during the exposure, the sinus is exenterated and its posterior wall removed. A small piece of fat or temporalis muscle is used to pack the sinus and thereby obliterate the frontonasal duct. In **Fig. 7.2A**, the craniotomy flap has been removed, but the dura is intact.

After tack-up stitches are placed, the dura is opened transversely and reflected over the orbit. In a bilateral approach, the sagittal sinus is ligated and the falx cut anteriorly.

Because the superior orbital rim is removed, frontal lobe retraction is minimal (**Fig. 7.2B**). The frontal lobe is gently elevated and the olfactory nerve preserved by dissecting it off the inferior frontal lobe; a drop of fibrin glue can help decrease the risk for avulsion. Tumor feeders in tuberculum sellae tumors—typically arising inferiorly from the internal maxillary or posterior ethmoidal arteries—are cauterized medially, avoiding optic nerve injury laterally. The tumor is then debulked with a combination of ultrasonic aspiration and bipolar cautery.

Once the tumor is debulked, the remainder of the tumor is carefully dissected from the optic nerves, often starting near the chiasm and carefully preserving arterial supply to the optic apparatus. Although the tumor often appears adherent to the nerve, a plane of dissection can usually be established. Tuberculum sellae tumors usually extend into at least one optic canal, so one or both may need opening; cavernous sinus extension is managed as explained previously in this chapter. The ophthalmic artery and its branches should be preserved when tumor inside the optic canal is removed. The carotid is dissected from the tumor, as are its branches, with careful attention paid to the A1 segments because they may be stretched and susceptible to tearing. The pituitary stalk is distinct in its color and vascular arborization (**Fig. 7.3**). Tuberculum sellae meningiomas usually displace the stalk posteriorly and rarely will engulf the stalk, requiring careful microdissection. Hypophyseal branches off the carotid are spared.

The involved dura of the tuberculum and planum is resected and any hyperostotic bone drilled with a high-speed diamond burr. Paranasal sinus entry is handled by exenterating the sinus mucosa and packing the spaces with fat. A piece of free pericranium or fascia lata is then placed intradurally and secured to the native dura over the resected dura, and after the dural closure, the pericranial flap is turned over the orbit and frontal bone and spread over any defect in the anterior fossa floor.

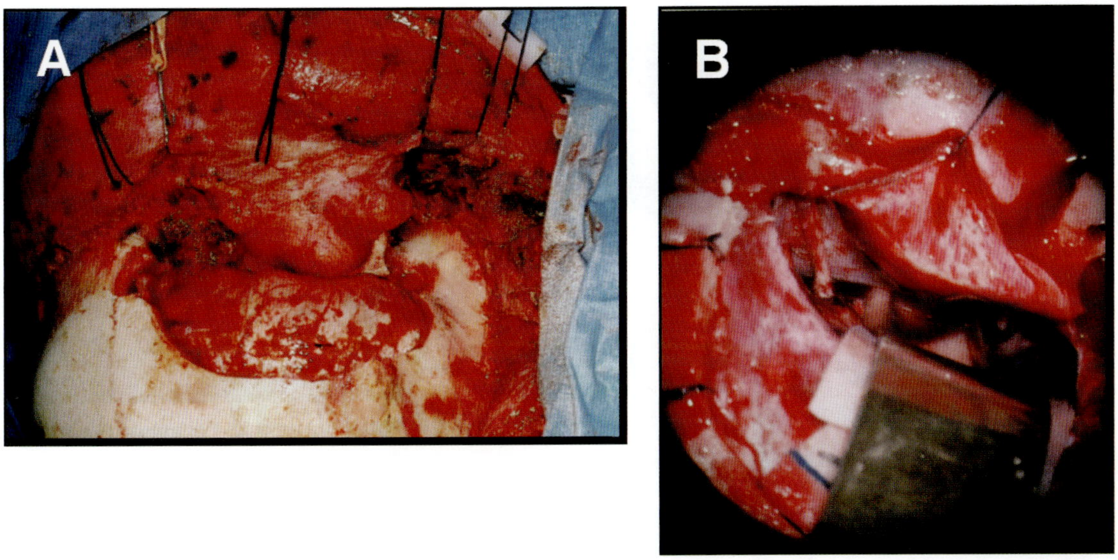

Fig. 7.2 (A) The surgical view after the supraorbital flap has been removed. (B) The view through the surgical microscope achieved through the supraorbital approach. The dura has been incised transversely and reflected over the orbit. The olfactory tract is dissected and preserved, and the optic nerve is clearly seen. (From Al-Mefty O, Ayoubi S. Clinoidal meningiomas. Acta Neurochir Suppl (Wien) 1991;53:92–97. Reprinted with permission.)

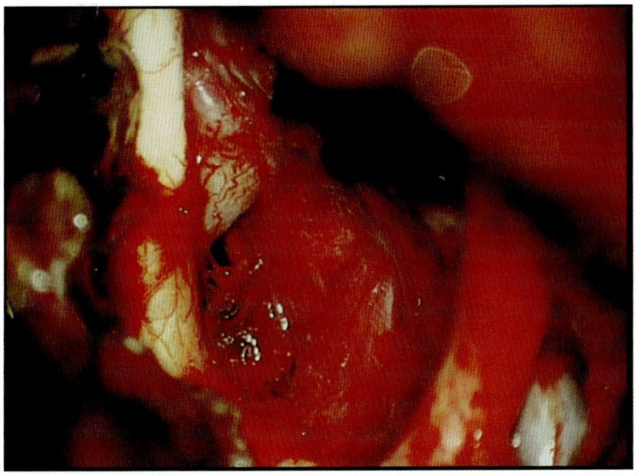

Fig. 7.3 The distinct vascularity of the pituitary stalk, shown between and below the optic nerves, is seen here after resection of a tuberculum sellae meningioma. (From Al-Mefty O, Ayoubi S. Clinoidal meningiomas. Acta Neurochir Suppl (Wien) 1991;53:92–97. Reprinted with permission.)

◆ Supraorbital Approach: Applications to Parasellar Tumors

Tuberculum Sellae Meningiomas

These tumors, originating in front of the sella and arising from the tuberculum, chiasmatic sulcus, and limbus sphenoidale, account for 5 to 10% of meningiomas in the series of Cushing and Eisenhardt.[3] They often invade the floor of the anterior fossa, causing hyperostosis commonly in front of the sella (**Fig. 7.4A**). As they enlarge, they displace the optic nerves laterally and chiasm superiorly (**Fig. 7.4B**). They also impinge on the pituitary stalk posteriorly, as well as the basilar artery, and can extend to the interpeduncular space. Although preoperative pituitary dysfunction is uncommon in these tumors, a preoperative endocrine evaluation is still recommended. The blood supply is typically inferior from the posterior ethmoidal arteries, and meticulous attention must be paid to the anterior cerebral artery complex, which, depending on the size, may be encased or displaced superiorly. Careful attention must be paid to small medial lenticulostriates.

The relationship of these tumors to the visual apparatus confers their dominant clinical presentation. The classic clinical manifestation, the chiasmal syndrome, denotes a primary optic atrophy with a bitemporal field defect.[4] Visual field defects are typically incongruous and asymmetric. In the senior author's most recent series, quadrantanopsia and a unilateral temporal defect were the most common visual findings.[5] More than 50% of patients reported failing vision in one eye. A markedly asymmetric visual field examination has been found to be highly indicative of optic canal involvement, which has specific surgical implications.[6] A full visual field and acuity examination is warranted before surgery.

Specific Surgical Principles

We favor the unilateral or bilateral supraorbital approach as originally described by Jane et al,[2] as previously stated. The main principles of the approach as it pertains to tuberculum sellae tumors are the low frontobasal exposure, which facilitates access to the tumor without undue frontal retraction and yet access to both optic canals. Removing the supraorbital rim as part of the frontal craniotomy flap affords access to the base of the anterior fossa without frontal lobe retraction; further relaxation is achieved by

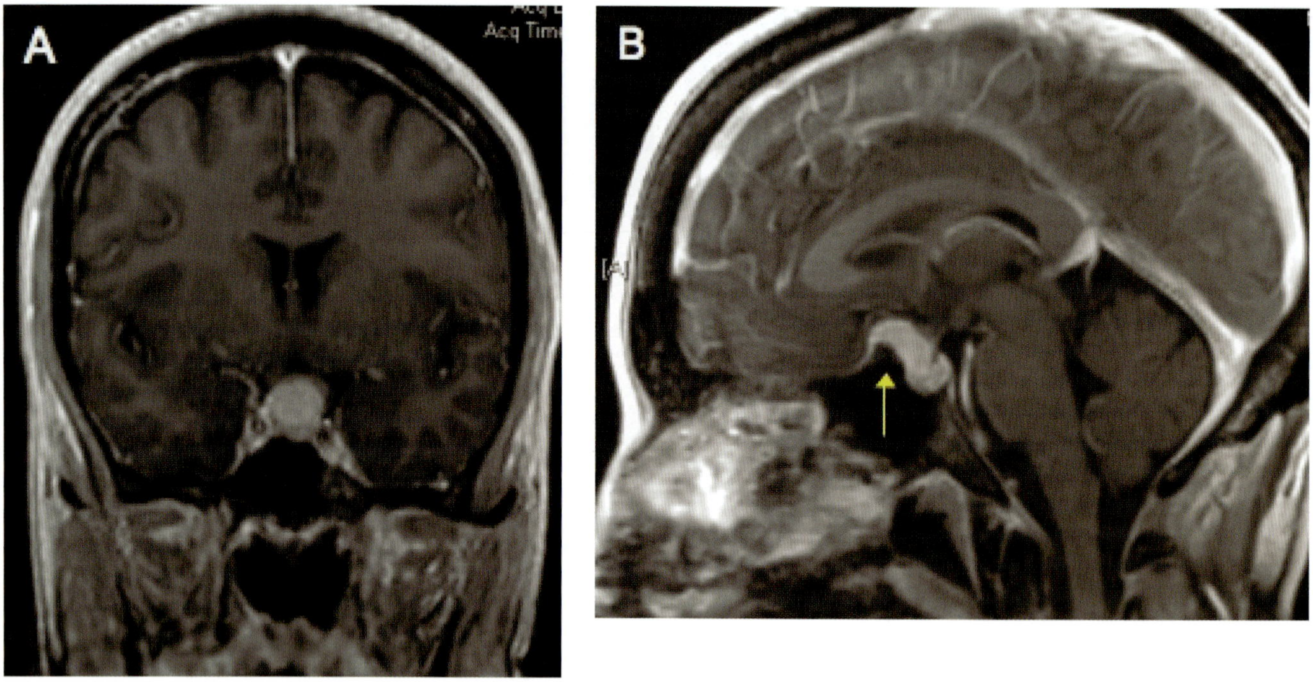

Fig. 7.4 (A,B) This tuberculum sellae meningioma, shown on coronal T1 axial postcontrast imaging, is displacing the optic nerves (A) superiorly and laterally and is associated with hyperostosis as seen on (B) sagittal views (*arrow*).

spinal drainage. When the tumor is encountered, its basal posterior ethmoidal arterial feeders are coagulated to devascularize the tumor, after which central debulking may be undertaken by ultrasonic aspiration or other means. The optic chiasm is usually displaced superiorly and the optic nerves superiorly and laterally. Should the nerves be engulfed in tumor, dissection should begin at the chiasm and proceed proximally. The arterial supply to the optic chiasm and nerves is preserved. All associated dura is resected, and any hyperostotic bone at the tuberculum and planum is drilled away with a high-speed diamond burr.

Decompression of the visual apparatus is not complete until the optic canals are unroofed; in a recent series, 67% of tuberculum sellae tumors were associated with tumor extension into one (40%) or both (60%) optic canals.[4] Moreover, tumor left inside the optic canal may be the source of recurrence or of mitigated visual improvement after surgery.[7] One optic canal or both are exposed and unroofed with a high-speed drill under constant irrigation to avoid thermal injury to the optic nerve. The falciform ligament and optic sheath are opened sharply. Optic nerve decompression should proceed as far anteriorly toward the globe as is needed to ensure that all optic extension of the tumor has been extirpated. Although the clinical presentation may suggest extension of the tumor into only one optic canal, one should be prepared to decompress both canals based on intraoperative findings. Even the slightest suggestion of canalicular extension should prompt at minimum opening of the falciform ligament.

Visual improvement was noted in 74% of patients who presented with visual deterioration in the senior author's series. Pituitary dysfunction is rare after surgery, and if present, it is usually transient in the early postoperative period.

Diaphragma Sellae Meningiomas

Although the entity was first reported in 1954,[8] diaphragma sellae meningiomas were not formally classified until more recently[9]; they are probably considered along the spectrum of tuberculum tumors in most series. Diaphragma sellae meningiomas may be considered distinct clinical entities separable into three types according to their relationship to the pituitary stalk and their specific diaphragmatic origins (**Fig. 7.5**). Each subtype is also associated with particular clinical symptoms related to proximity to the optic apparatus, pituitary, hypothalamus, and limbic system. Surgically, types A and B are approached similarly to tuberculum tumors, whereas type C tumors may be approached transsphenoidally.

Type A tumors originate from the upper leaf of the diaphragma sellae anterior to the pituitary stalk. In this way, these tumors resemble tuberculum sellae tumors and do present with visual field disturbances, but they are more likely than tuberculum tumors to present with manifestations of pituitary compromise, such as diabetes insipidus. Headache is also a common presenting symptom. On imaging, the tumors are supradiaphragmatic and may be difficult to differentiate from tuberculum sellae tumors.

Type B tumors also originate from the upper leaf of the diaphragma and are supradiaphragmatic, but unlike type A tumors, they are located posterior to the stalk and feature a greater incidence of pituitary disturbance preoperatively. Common presenting symptoms include headache, unilateral and bilateral visual disturbances in 50% of patients, and pituitary dysfunction in 38% of patients. These are also supradiaphragmatic on imaging, with a normal sella.

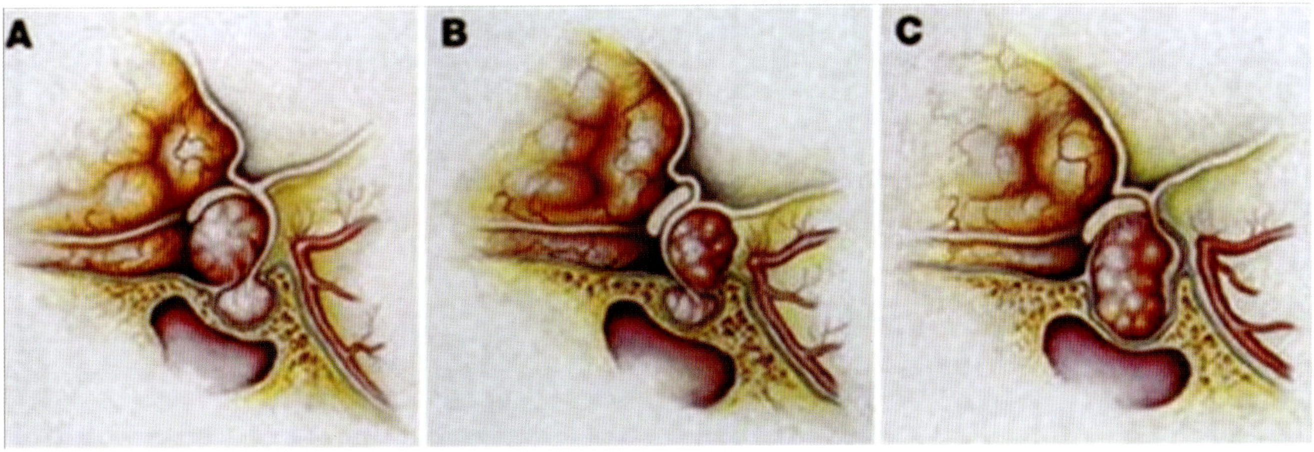

Fig. 7.5 Three types of diaphragma sellae meningiomas. (A) Type A tumor originates from the upper leaf of the diaphragma sellae anterior to the pituitary stalk. (B) Type B tumor originates from the upper leaf of the diaphragma sellae posterior to the pituitary stalk. (C) Type C tumor originates from the inferior leaf of the diaphragma sellae. (From Busch E, Mahneke A. A case of meningioma from the diaphragm of the sella turcica. Zentralbl Neurochir 1954;14(1–2):25–28. Reprinted with permission.)

Unlike type A and B tumors, **type C** tumors arise from the inferior leaf of the diaphragma and are thus infradiaphragmatic. Symptoms are similar to those produced by nonfunctioning pituitary adenomas. Half of patients presented with bitemporal hemianopsia, and 40% presented with hypopituitarism. Distinct from types A and B tumors, enlarged sellar and intrasellar tumors are demonstrated on imaging.

Diagnostically, it may be difficult to distinguish types A and B tumors from tuberculum sellae meningiomas, and type C tumors from pituitary adenomas, although the latter distinction may be aided by the more avid enhancement in type C tumors and smaller sella in comparison with pituitary adenomas.[10]

In the senior author's original description, patients with type A tumors had excellent outcomes; those with type B or C tumors had higher rates of transient pituitary dysfunction postoperatively. Although transsphenoidal approaches may be attempted in type C tumors, the supraorbital approach offers excellent access to types A and B tumors.

◆ Cranio-orbitozygomatic Approach: Technique

The COZ approach adds an anterolateral skull base approach to the supraorbital approach, rendering it ideal for accessing tumors that may engulf or displace structures superiorly and laterally in the parasellar region.

A lumbar drain is placed for cerebrospinal fluid (CSF) drainage, and the patient is positioned supine with the upper body slightly elevated and the head rotated 30 degrees to the opposite side. Leads to monitor somatosensory evoked potentials, brainstem auditory evoked potentials, and cranial nerves V and VII are placed at this time, with those to monitor nerves III, IV, and VI placed later. The ipsilateral part of the neck is prepared should more proximal carotid control be required, and the abdomen is prepared for fat graft harvest.

The skin incision for the COZ approach starts at the zygomatic root and is carried behind the hairline toward the contralateral superior temporal line (**Fig. 7.6A**). The superficial temporal artery is identified and carefully protected, and a large pericranial flap is raised by undermining the scalp posterior to the incision and dissecting sharply against the scalp flap anteriorly. A subfascial dissection of the temporalis fascia is performed to preserve the frontal branches of the facial nerve. The zygomatic arch and superior and lateral orbital margins are exposed by subperiosteal dissection, after which the zygoma is divided at either end and displaced inferiorly on its masseteric pedicle. The temporalis muscle is then elevated in subperiosteal fashion, beginning low on the temporal squama and proceeding superiorly to detach the muscle at the superior temporal line. The entire temporalis muscle is then reflected inferiorly with the freed zygoma.

The superior and lateral orbital rims are dissected free from the periorbita, with the supraorbital nerve and vessels preserved (**Fig. 7.6B**). A burr hole is placed in the keyhole to gain simultaneous entrance into the cranium and orbit. Burr holes are then placed anteriorly and posteriorly, adjacent to the temporal floor. A cut is made from the medial aspect of the lateral orbital wall to its lateral aspect and is continued to the keyhole. The keyhole is then connected to the posterior burr hole by cutting through the temporal fossa. A cut starting at this burr hole is brought superiorly to the frontal bone, then anteriorly through the supraorbital rim, with care taken to protect the orbital contents during any cuts involving the bony orbit. Care must be taken to ensure that the posterior wall of the frontal sinus is cut if the sinus has been entered. A cut is made from the first burr hole through the orbit, again with care taken to protect the orbital contents. A notched osteotome is used to incise the orbital roof from the second burr hole toward the nasion, while the orbital contents are protected during this cut. The bone flap is now elevated. Remaining portions of the orbital roof, lateral orbital wall, and sphe-

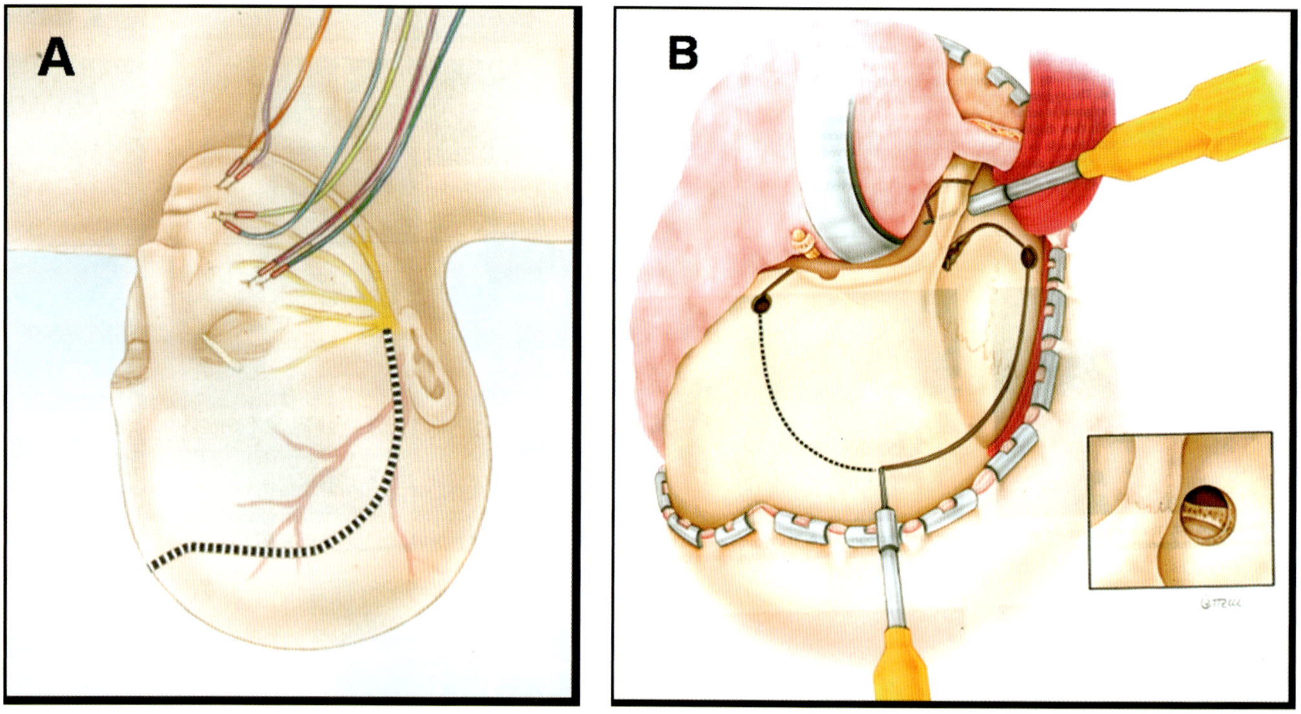

Fig.7.6 (A) Proposed scalp incision and monitoring electrode placement. (B) For the cranio-orbital flap, burr holes are placed in the keyhole (inset) and posteroinferiorly in the temporal squama. A cut is made across the lateral orbital wall, then brought up to the keyhole. The keyhole is connected posteriorly to the posterior burr hole. The cut is then continued up to the frontal bone and through the supraorbital bar. Orbital contents must be protected when the bony orbit is drilled. A V-chisel is then used to cut the orbital roof from the keyhole (right inset) to the medial cut behind the supraorbital bar. (From Al-Mefty O, Ayoubi S. Clinoidal meningiomas. Acta Neurochir Suppl (Wien) 1991;53:92–97. Reprinted with permission.)

noid wing can be removed with the craniotome for later reconstruction. With the orbit now exposed, electromyographic electrodes may be directly placed into the superior oblique, superior rectus, and lateral rectus muscles to monitor cranial nerves III, IV, and VI.

Proximal control of the carotid artery is the next objective. The middle fossa dura is elevated in a posterior-to-anterior direction. The greater superficial petrosal nerve (GSPN) emerges from the facial hiatus and should be dissected free of the dura. Traction of the GSPN is avoided to alleviate transmission to the geniculate ganglion, which can lead to facial palsy. The middle meningeal artery is identified, thoroughly electrocoagulated, and divided. Continued dural elevation reveals nerve V_3 and the foramen ovale. The apices of Glasscock's triangle are now exposed: the facial hiatus, the anterior aspect of the foramen ovale, and the intersection of the GSPN and the lateral aspect of V_3. This triangle overlies the carotid artery, and drilling here with a diamond bit and constant irrigation exposes the carotid artery. This may be sufficient for proximal control of the artery or to allow drilling posterolaterally from the known location of the artery. Proximal control may be obtained by sufficient exposure for placement of a temporary clip on the petrous carotid artery, if necessary. Alternatively, a Fogarty catheter may be inserted into the carotid canal. Should vascular control be required, the catheter balloon can be inflated to occlude the carotid artery in the carotid canal.[11]

Medial exposure of the cavernous sinus and exposure of the paraclinoid carotid artery are obtained by drilling out the remainder of the orbital roof, the superior orbital fissure, the anterior clinoid process, and the optic strut. Drilling adjacent to the orbital apex and optic canal mandates a diamond burr and copious irrigation to dissipate the heat of drilling. The anterior clinoid process is cored out with the drill and then disarticulated by drilling out the optic strut. The clinoid is subperiosteally dissected and resected. The superior orbital fissure is opened by drilling along the lesser sphenoid wing. This procedure exposes the subclinoid portion of the carotid artery, which is both extradural and extracavernous, and provides distal control of the carotid artery.

Entrance into the cavernous sinus has been described in relationship to the intervals between the neurovascular structures of the cavernous sinus. These intervals have been annotated as 10 triangles distributed among the parasellar, middle fossa, and paraclival locations.[12] The actual approach taken depends on the anatomy of the lesion in relationship to the cavernous sinus structures and must be individualized for each patient. In general, there are two approaches for entry into the cavernous sinus: a superior approach and a lateral approach. The superior approach is particularly suited to those lesions adjacent to the anterior loop of the carotid artery, and those that are superior and/or medial to the cavernous carotid artery. The lateral approach lends itself well to exposing those lesions lateral and/or inferior to the carotid artery and those that are posteriorly located within the cavernous sinus. Frequently, these approaches are combined for lesions widely involving the sinus.

Superior Entry

After the superior surface of the cavernous sinus has been exposed (**Fig. 7.7A**), the dura overlying the optic nerve is divided over the length of the optic canal to free the optic nerve. The distal carotid ring is now divided. The dura is then incised toward the oculomotor nerve, providing initial entry into the cavernous sinus. Exposure can be increased by dissecting along the length of the carotid artery. Further exposure can be obtained by subperiosteal dissection of the posterior clinoid process and drilling off the process, the dorsum sellae, and the superior clivus. These maneuvers allow increased exposure of the posterior fossa.

For tumors with medial extension, the planum sphenoidale can be drilled away. This allows exposure of the sphenoid sinus. Dissection and incision of the diaphragma sellae allow visualization of the pituitary gland. Great care must be taken during closure to obliterate any communication between the cavernous sinus and sphenoid sinus to prevent CSF leakage.

Lateral Entry

Lateral entry into the cavernous sinus can be intradural or extradural. Extradural entry begins by incising the dura propria overlying V_3. The dura propria is peeled away from the trigeminal branches and ganglion with superiorly directed traction. This will initially expose the third division and lateral ganglion, followed by the second division and most of the remainder of the ganglion. Drilling bone here will also free the trigeminal branches and will, in turn, allow greater mobility of these branches and the ganglion. A mass beginning to enter the posterior fossa can be further exposed by drilling the petrous apex. This drilling also allows greater exposure around and under the trigeminal ganglion.

For lesions requiring intradural exposure, intradural entry into the cavernous sinus is achieved through Parkinson's triangle (**Fig. 7.7B**). Cranial nerves III and IV are identified over the tentorial edge. An incision beneath the anticipated position of the fourth nerve is fashioned and extended ~8 mm anteriorly and 8 mm inferiorly. The external dural layer is peeled away from the thin inner dural layer in which nerves III, IV, and V are found. The dural flap can be further dissected from the trigeminal ganglion to expose the Meckel cave. Exposure can be increased posteriorly and into the posterior fossa by drilling the petrous apex.

The inner dural layer between the fourth nerve and the ophthalmic division can be incised to expose the lateral space of the cavernous sinus, the posterior bend and the horizontal segment of the intracavernous carotid artery, and the lateral cavernous and meningohypophyseal arteries. The abducens nerve is the only cranial nerve coursing inside the cavernous sinus proper, often appearing in fascicles of two to five nerves, and should be carefully located and protected. Frequently, meningiomas necessitate the combination of extradural and intradural cavernous sinus dissection with a combination of superior and lateral entry.

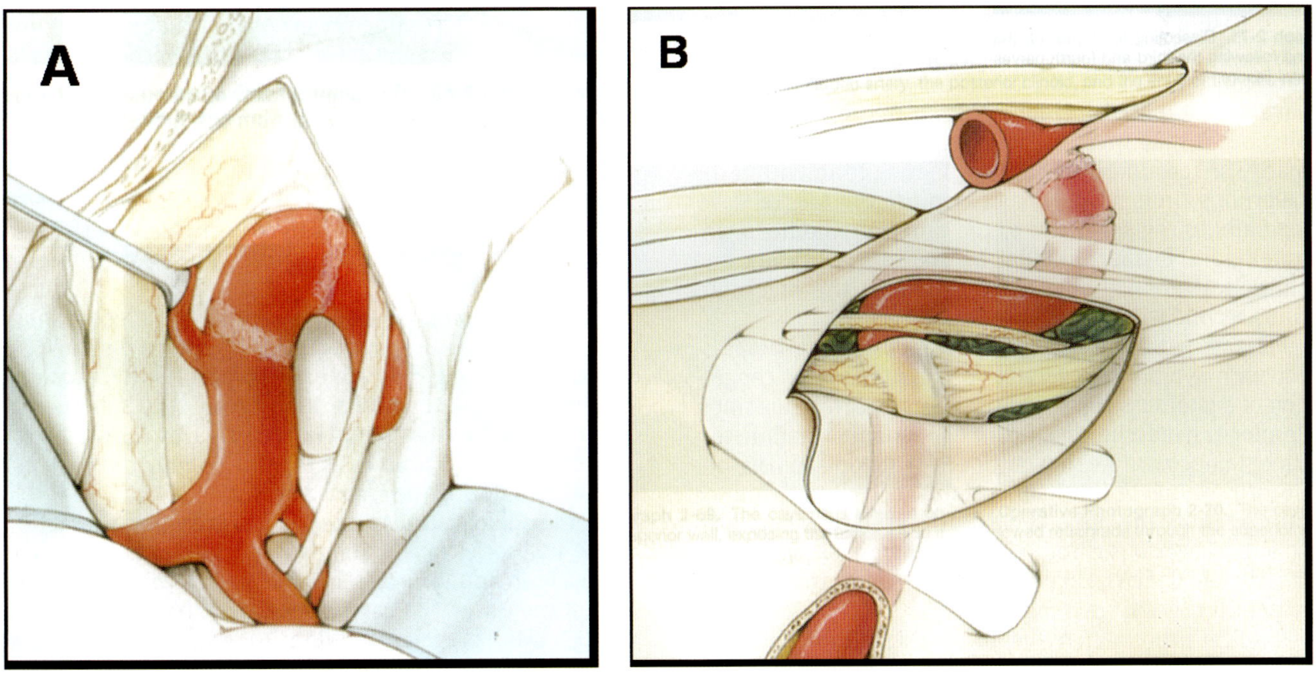

Fig. 7.7 **(A)** Superior entry into the cavernous sinus. Superior exposure obtained after the anterior clinoid is removed and the dura over the optic nerve and medial cavernous sinus is incised. **(B)** Operative anatomy of a lateral approach to the cavernous sinus with the lateral wall opened; the superior aspect of the opening is just beneath cranial nerve IV. (From Al-Mefty O, Ayoubi S. Clinoidal meningiomas. Acta Neurochir Suppl (Wien) 1991;53:92–97. Reprinted with permission.)

Reconstruction after the COZ approach begins with attention directed toward preventing CSF leaks by searching for and obliterating any feature of the dissection that may result in a CSF leak. Any entrance into the paranasal sinuses or the eustachian tube should be obliterated with fat and fascia. Any tenuous or incomplete dural closures should be reinforced with tissue—preferably autologous—such as fascia, muscle, or fat. Fibrin glue can be used for further reinforcement. The thick pericranial flap is now brought down under the frontal lobe, over the orbit, and over any sinus entries in the middle fossa or petrous apex. The orbital roof is reconstructed to prevent late enophthalmos. Dural tack-up sutures are placed circumferentially, including in the subtemporal region, to obliterate dead space and prevent postoperative development of epidural hematomas. If the frontal sinus has been entered, the mucosa should be exenterated and the cavity packed with fat or tissue to prevent mucocele formation and CSF leakage. The cranio-orbital flap is secured in place with titanium miniplates. Bony defects can be obliterated with titanium plates or mesh, or any of several cranioplastic materials, such as hydroxyapatite cement. The temporalis muscle is sutured to the superior temporal line. The zygoma is plated into position with titanium miniplates. The scalp is closed in layers, and a craniotomy head wrap is applied to decrease postoperative fluid collection under the flap.

◆ Cranio-orbitozygomatic Approach: Applications to Parasellar Tumors

Cavernous Sinus Meningiomas

The development, refinement, and careful application of skull base approaches, in particular the COZ approach, has made obsolete the notion of the cavernous sinus as a surgical "no man's land." Cavernous sinus meningiomas have an estimated incidence of 0.5 per 100,000.[13] Meningiomas may involve the cavernous sinus either primarily or secondarily. Those originating from within the cavernous sinus proper may extend to the Meckel cave, medially to the sella, and to the anterior, middle, or infratemporal fossae. Clinoidal, medial sphenoid wing, and petroclival meningiomas may extend to the cavernous sinus secondarily.

Patients with tumors in the cavernous sinus may present with symptoms referable to compression or congestion of anatomic structures in or near the cavernous sinus. Proptosis, headache, facial pain or numbness, and disturbances of ocular function or motility (diplopia, ptosis, anisocoria, complete ophthalmoplegia) are common. Tumors can compress the optic nerve, with resultant visual field deficits. Cavernous carotid artery compression may result in ischemic deficits. Less commonly, patients may present with pituitary dysfunction.

Physical examination should include a thorough neurologic examination, with particular attention paid to the function of cranial nerves II through VI, including a formal visual field assessment. An endocrine evaluation should be performed because tumors may displace the stalk and gland. Examination of coordination and motor, sensory, and cerebellar functions assists the assessment of any tumor extension into the posterior fossa with brainstem compression.

The outcome of any treatment for cavernous sinus meningiomas must be weighed against the natural history of these tumors. Asymptomatic patients or minimally symptomatic patients with cranial nerve involvement may be managed conservatively.

Specific Surgical Principles

Technical advances in skull base surgery have established the cavernous sinus as an approachable space whose contents may be navigated successfully during meningioma surgery. Core principles of these approaches include maximal bone removal for exposure; the avoidance of brain retraction; and control of the carotid artery in its petrous, cavernous, and/or clinoid segments. Two primary surgical approaches to the cavernous sinus are used by the authors: the COZ approach and the zygomatic approach.[14] The COZ approach affords wide exposure of the entire cavernous sinus and the proximal and distal carotid artery with minimal cerebral retraction. The zygomatic approach is used for tumors in the posterior cavernous sinus and petrous apex. This approach is more limited, does not offer readily obtainable distal carotid control, and does not expose the medial or superior cavernous sinus as easily as does the COZ approach. During tumor resection, arachnoid planes facilitate tumor removal, but these planes become scarred and obliterated after initial resection or irradiation, emphasizing the importance of extensive resection during an initial operation. If necessary, when no plane is encountered, small remnants of adherent tumor are left on the carotid artery. The same philosophy is true regarding the cranial nerves. As mentioned, once the cavernous sinus is entered, the abducens nerve should be located and preserved. Any cranial nerve that is frankly severed should be directly repaired. If a tension-free direct repair is not possible, an interposition graft should be performed. Injury to the carotid artery can be addressed in several ways. Temporary clipping and direct repair of tears can be performed with 8–0 suture; more severe carotid injury can be treated by vein graft repair.

Attempts should be made to remove all affected dura, and any affected dura that cannot be resected should be electrocoagulated, if possible. All involved or hyperostotic underlying bone should be drilled away. Any submucosal tumor spread within the paranasal sinuses should be removed. Sphenoid sinus defects must be repaired with extreme care during the reconstruction.

In the senior author's experience, gross total resection (GTR) in a series of 41 patients was achieved in 76% of patients, with an 11% recurrence rate in cases of GTR. A more recent review of 163 cases operated on by the senior author (OAM) has shown a GTR rate of 44%, with 7% of these patients experiencing recurrence.

Stroke is a significant concern during cavernous sinus meningioma surgery, and fortunately reported rates of ischemic complications; in the senior author's series, 7 of 188 patients (3.7%) experienced ischemic stroke.

Cranial nerve morbidity is a central issue in cavernous sinus meningioma surgery. The preponderance of evidence shows that existing preoperative cranial nerve deficits infrequently improve, and that few new permanent cranial nerve deficits appear postoperatively. Most series of aggressive surgical resection have reported that the majority of preoperative cranial neuropathies remain the same. In a recent re-evaluation of the cases operated on by the senior author (OAM), 21 of 163 patients (12.8%) experienced new cranial nerve deficits, 14 of 163 operated patients (8.5%) experienced worsening of a preoperative deficit, and 11 of 163 patients (6.7%) experienced both a new cranial nerve deficit and a deterioration of existing deficits. The majority of neuropathies remained stable.

Clinoidal Meningiomas

Cushing and Eisenhardt recognized this entity in their original treatise, noting that there exist meningiomas arising from "the deep or clinoidal third."[15] Although they were historically grouped in discussions of medial sphenoid wing meningiomas, an increasing recognition of clinoidal meningiomas[16,17] has culminated in an anatomic description of these meningiomas in three distinct subgroups (types I, II, and III) with specific surgical implications[18,19] (**Fig. 7.8**).

In group I tumors, the tumor originates proximal to the end of the carotid cistern, typically from the undersurface of the anterior clinoid process. In this manner, the tumor may encase the carotid adventitia without an intervening arachnoidal layer. The tumor thus grows along the vessel wall to the carotid bifurcation and beyond, "pushing" a sleeve of arachnoid with it. The absence of an arachnoidal layer between tumor and vessel greatly complicates the dissection. However, the optic chiasm and nerves are invested by the arachnoid of the chiasmatic cistern and should be able to be freed from tumor.

Group II tumors originate from the superior or lateral aspect of the anterior clinoid process above the carotid and are invested by cisternal arachnoid. In these cases, a layer of arachnoid separates tumor from vessel from the carotid to the bifurcation and into the sylvian fissure. Microdissection of meningioma from the carotid and its branches is thus rendered feasible by the investing layer of arachnoid, which separates tumor from vascular adventitia. As with group I tumors, the optic apparatus is sheathed in arachnoid and can be dissected from tumor.

In group III, the tumor originates on the medial aspect of the anterior clinoid process at the optic foramen. These tumors are usually small because they present early with visual compromise. The arachnoidal layer may be present between tumor and carotid but may be absent between tumor and optic nerve.

Clinoidal meningiomas commonly present with initial unilateral visual loss, frequently associated with optic atrophy; the contralateral eye may be affected, depending on chiasmal involvement. Cranial nerve involvement and exophthalmos may occur as the tumor involves the superior orbital fissure and cavernous sinus. Preoperative endocrine disturbance is rare.

Specific Surgical Principles

Preoperative imaging should include fine-cut computed tomograms through the skull base to assess hyperostosis in the region of the anterior clinoid process, optic strut, and superior orbital fissure. Standard magnetic resonance (MR) imaging sequences should be paired with vascular imaging (eg, MR arteriography and MR venography) because the carotid may be narrowed owing to tumor encasement.

The COZ approach allows a shorter working distance to the tumor; minimizes brain retraction; and permits subfrontal, transsylvian, and subtemporal routes of attack. The anterior clinoid process should be removed to resect involved bone, intercept middle meningeal artery feeders, and facilitate internal carotid artery exposure. We typically do this extradurally. Once the dura is opened, CSF drainage is accomplished by splitting the sylvian fissure and facilitating partial CSF egress through a lumbar catheter.

Tumor dissection should begin with a sylvian fissure split, during which tumor may be encountered. Dissection should continue along the middle cerebral artery to the

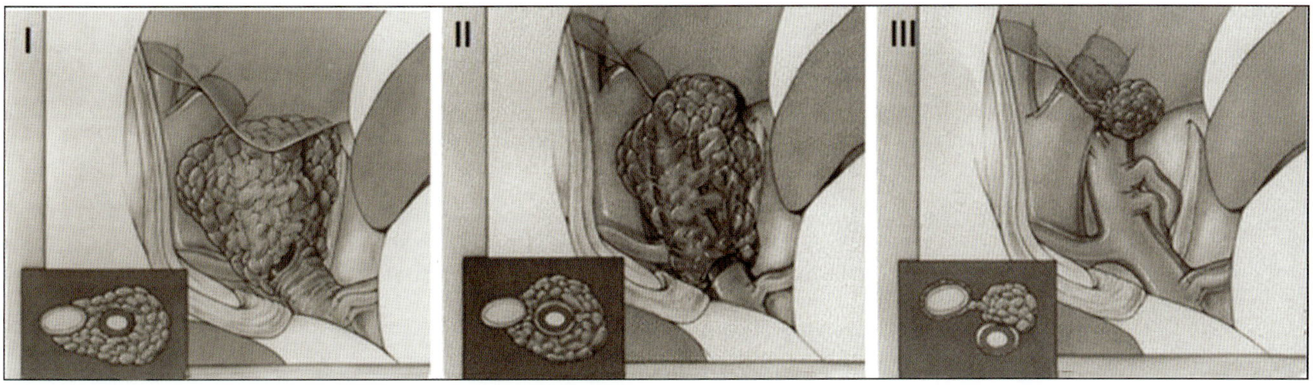

Fig. 7.8 Three types of anterior clinoidal meningiomas. Group I tumors arise proximal to the carotid cistern and adhere directly to the carotid adventitia (*inset*). Group II tumors may be dissected off the carotid and its branches owing to the presence of an arachnoid plane between vessel and tumor. Group III tumors originate at the optic foramen and extend into the optic canal. (From Ojemann R. Meningiomas: clinical features and surgical management. In: Wilkins R, Rengachary S, eds. Neurosurgery. McGraw-Hill; 1985:635–654. Reprinted with permission.)

carotid and to the anterior cerebral artery and Heubner's artery, respecting the medial and lateral lenticulostriates. Laterally, the posterior communicating and anterior choroidal arteries reside in a separate cisternal compartment, facilitating this dissection. Posteriorly, Liliequist's membrane is usually intact, facilitating removal from the interpeduncular fossa. The optic nerve may be elevated, depressed, or engulfed in tumor—it is often easiest to find the nerve at the chiasm and dissect toward the optic canal, with care taken to preserve the vascular supply of the nerve. If tumor extends into the optic canal, the falciform ligament should be opened and the optic canal unroofed, followed by optic sheath sectioning.

The pituitary stalk is recognized by its reddish color and vascular arborization; it is usually pushed back and to the opposite side. Any extension into the cavernous sinus is dealt with as with cavernous sinus meningiomas.

The complete resection of groups I and III tumors depends on the adherence of tumor to the carotid and optic nerve, respectively; an intervening arachnoid layer may be absent. Group II meningiomas in the senior author's series could be completely resected.

◆ Conclusion

Parasellar meningiomas and other tumors of this area are challenging lesions whose proximity to cranial nerves, the carotid artery, the brainstem, and the pituitary gland mandates meticulous microsurgical technique. With the exception of type C diaphragma sellae meningiomas, parasellar tumors are usually managed with such skull base approaches as the COZ or supraorbital technique. A thorough understanding of the patient's history, physical examination findings, and radiographic findings and the results of other evaluations is crucial. Although pituitary dysfunction is uncommon, preoperative and postoperative endocrine evaluation is nevertheless essential because the gland and stalk are often displaced and manipulated during surgery.

References

1. Al-Mefty O. Operative Atlas of Meningiomas. Lippincott-Raven Publishers; 1998
2. Jane JA, Park TS, Pobereskin LH, Winn HR, Butler AB. The supraorbital approach: technical note. Neurosurgery 1982;11(4):537–542
3. Cushing H, Eisenhardt L. Suprasellar meningiomas. In: Meningiomas: Their Classification, Regional Behavior, Life History, and Surgical End Results. Charles C Thomas; 1938:224–249
4. Cushing H. The chiasmal syndrome of primary optic atrophy and bi-temporal field defects in adults with a normal sella turcica. Arch Ophthalmol 1930;3(5):505–551
5. Mahmoud M, Nader R, Al-Mefty O. Optic canal involvement in tuberculum sellae meningiomas: influence on approach, recurrence, and visual recovery. Neurosurgery 2010;67(3, Suppl Operative):ons108–ons118, discussion ons118–ons119
6. Pamir MN, Ozduman K, Belirgen M, Kilic T, Ozek MM. Outcome determinants of pterional surgery for tuberculum sellae meningiomas. Acta Neurochir (Wien) 2005;147(11):1121–1130, discussion 1130
7. Schick U, Hassler W. Surgical management of tuberculum sellae meningiomas: involvement of the optic canal and visual outcome. J Neurol Neurosurg Psychiatry 2005;76(7):977–983
8. Busch E, Mahneke A. A case of meningioma from the diaphragm of the sella turcica. Zentralbl Neurochir 1954;14(1–2):25–28
9. Kinjo T, al-Mefty O, Ciric I. Diaphragma sellae meningiomas. Neurosurgery 1995;36(6):1082–1092
10. Cappabianca P, Cirillo S, Alfieri A, et al. Pituitary macroadenoma and diaphragma sellae meningioma: differential diagnosis on MRI. Neuroradiology 1999;41(1):22–26
11. Wascher TM, Spetzler RF, Zabramski JM. Improved transdural exposure and temporary occlusion of the petrous internal carotid artery for cavernous sinus surgery. Technical note [see comment]. J Neurosurg 1993;78(5):834–837
12. Borba LAB, Al-Mefty O. Normal anatomy of the cavernous sinus. In: Eisenberg MB, Al-Mefty O, eds. The Cavernous Sinus: a Comprehensive Text. Lippincott Williams & Wilkins;2000:21–33
13. Demonte F, Al-Mefty O. Cavernous sinus meningioma management with carotid preservation. In: Eisenberg MB, Al-Mefty O, eds. The Cavernous Sinus: a Comprehensive Text. Lippincott Williams & Wilkins; 2000:251–261
14. Al-Mefty O, Anand VK. Zygomatic approach to skull-base lesions. J Neurosurg 1990;73(5):668–673
15. Cushing H, Eisenhardt L. Meningiomas: Their Classification, Regional Behavior, Life History, and Surgical End Results. Charles C Thomas; 1938
16. Bonnal J, Thibaut A, Brotchi J, Born J. Invading meningiomas of the sphenoid ridge. J Neurosurg 1980;53(5):587–599
17. Ojemann R. Meningiomas: clinical features and surgical management. In: Wilkins R, Rengachary S, eds. Neurosurgery. McGraw-Hill; 1985:635–654
18. Al-Mefty O. Clinoidal meningiomas. J Neurosurg 1990;73(6):840–849
19. Al-Mefty O, Ayoubi S. Clinoidal meningiomas. Acta Neurochir Suppl (Wien) 1991;53:92–97

8 Surgical Treatment of Craniopharyngiomas

R. Michael Scott and Edward R. Smith

Craniopharyngiomas are tumors usually found in the region of the infundibulum, although they can develop anywhere along an axis from the nasophayrnx to the third ventricle. They comprise ~5 to 10% of pediatric brain tumors and present with signs and symptoms referable to their location, including visual loss, hormonal disturbances, hydrocephalus, and headache. The broad spectrum of management strategies employed in the treatment of these tumors—including surgical resection, radiation, and intratumoral delivery of chemotherapeutic agents or radioisotopes—underscores the difficulty of achieving successful cures with acceptable morbidity and has fostered considerable controversy among physicians involved in the care of children with these lesions. This chapter reviews the etiology, pathology, epidemiology, and presentation of these tumors, outlines relevant initial diagnostic evaluations, and summarizes the surgical management of craniopharyngioma.

◆ Etiology and Pathology

The term *craniopharyngioma* was coined by Harvey Cushing in 1932 to describe a class of tumors found in the sellar region that were first reported by Erdheim in 1904.[1,2] Microscopic examination has revealed that craniopharyngiomas comprise two distinct subtypes, adamantinomatous and papillary, which some consider to have separate—if related—embryologic origins (mixed subtypes of tumor, with both adamantinomatous and papillary regions, have also been described).[3–5] Evidence supports the premise that craniopharyngiomas originate from cells derived from the development of the adenohypophysis and tend to arise primarily from the region of the infundibulum.[6,7] At the end of the first month of gestation, part of the oral cavity (the stomodeum) projects up toward the brain (Rathke pouch). This tissue interfaces with the infundibulum: a downward projection of the brain. Over the next 2 weeks, the connection between the oral cavity and the brain (the pharyngohypophyseal stalk within the craniopharyngeal duct) involutes as the sphenoid bone grows and closes off the two spaces, while Rathke's pouch contributes to the development of the anterior pituitary gland.[1,6–8]

Craniopharyngiomas are thought to arise from remnants of Rathke's pouch and tissue from the craniopharyngeal duct.[9,10] In particular, there is some evidence suggesting that adamantinomatous lesions are derived from neoplastic transformation of epithelial remnants of the craniopharyngeal duct.[8,9] This is in contrast to the squamous papillary subtype of craniopharyngioma, which is considered to result from the metaplasia of adenohypophyseal cells.[8,11]

These tumor subtypes differ pathologically in several ways. Adamantinomatous craniopharyngiomas are most common in children and share characteristics with tooth enamel–forming and long-bone tumors of the skeletal system (the eponymous adamantinomas), including the tendency to produce calcified deposits intratumorally. The epithelial cells have a keratinized squamous layer that flakes off and degenerates into a characteristic cholesterol-rich "crank-case oil" fluid.[4,10,11] In contrast, the papillary subtype (also called squamous papillary), found nearly exclusively in adults (albeit still less frequently than adamantinomatous tumors), is characterized by stratified squamous epithelium that does not usually exhibit the calcification or cystic degeneration evident in the adamantinomatous tumors.[4,10–12]

Overall, most reports indicate that more than 90% of all pediatric craniopharyngiomas are adamantinomatous; fewer than 2% are purely papillary and the remainder exhibit mixed features.[10–13] In adults, approximately two-thirds (66%) of all cases are adamantinomatous, about one-fourth (27–28%) are papillary, and the remainder are mixed.[10–13]

Recent efforts in molecular biology have made inroads toward characterizing biological pathways involved in the genesis of these tumors. Disruptions in apoptotic pathways involving β-catenin and Wnt may contribute to the neoplastic transformation of craniopharyngiomas.[8] Of particular interest is the role that growth factors and angiogenic peptides such as cathepsins (proteinases that regulate tumor invasiveness and end-effector proteinases such as matrix metalloproteinases [MMPs]) and vascular endothelial growth factor (VEGF) play in craniopharyngioma growth and development.[8] These investigations are relevant not only because they shed light on the basic mechanisms of tumorigenesis but also because they facilitate the development of novel methods of tumor detection and follow-up; for example, recent data suggest that urine testing may be able to noninvasively detect brain tumors, including craniopharyngiomas.[14,15]

◆ Epidemiology

In the United States, ~340 craniopharyngiomas are diagnosed annually in the combined pediatric and adult population, of which 100 are in children between 0 and 14 years of age.[16] Craniopharyngioma has an incidence of 1.3 cases per million person-years, with no significant difference in presentation by sex or race.[16] As noted, about one-third of cases occur in children, and the remaining two-thirds present in adults.[1,16] This distribution manifests itself in a bimodal pattern, with the largest peak at 5 to 14 years of age and a smaller one at 50 to 74 years of age.[1,16] However, craniopharyngiomas have been diagnosed prenatally and in patients older than 70 years of age.[17–22]

Craniopharyngiomas represent 5 to 10% of all intracranial tumors in children in many series and more than half of all sellar region tumors in this population.[11,16,23] They are the most common nonglial intracranial tumors in children.[24] These tumors are comparatively less common in adults, comprising fewer than 5% of all brain tumors in this age group (with many reports indicating numbers closer to 1%).[16,23]

◆ Clinical Presentation

Although craniopharyngiomas can be discovered in the asymptomatic patient, the vast majority of cases are identified following the onset of characteristic signs and symptoms.[24] These are directly related to the location of the tumor, and variations in the site of origin help to explain variations in presentation. Generally, craniopharyngiomas exhibit one of three growth patterns: prechiasmatic (affecting the optic nerves and chiasm), retrochiasmatic (affecting the hypothalamus, optic tracts, and drainage of cerebrospinal fluid [CSF]), and sellar (affecting hormonal function). Overall, the most common clinical findings include sequelae of increased intracranial pressure due to mass effect and hydrocephalus (especially headache, nausea, and vomiting); visual loss; and/or endocrinologic dysfunction.[6,20,24] In the published series from Children's Hospital in Boston, findings resulting from increased intracranial pressure were the most common, leading to discovery of the tumor in 44% of patients.[24] Nearly one-fourth of patients with craniopharyngioma have hydrocephalus at presentation.[20] Visual deterioration can be quite severe before detection by the family or clinicians and may be asymmetric, depending on the growth pattern of the tumor.[24,25] Careful documentation of visual function is critical because it may substantially influence subsequent planning for operative approaches. Similarly insidious is the development of endocrine dysfunction, which may remain unnoticed for long periods of time owing to the often subtle onset of symptoms such as growth delay. Although a deficiency of growth hormone is the most common endocrinopathy found in the setting of craniopharyngioma (followed by hypothyroidism and diabetes insipidus), abnormalities of any and all of the pituitary hormones may be manifested, and careful retrospective analysis reveals some form of endocrine dysfunction in 60 to 90% of patients at diagnosis.[24,26] Hormonal symptoms can be compounded by effects of hypothalamic injury, including temperature intolerance and dysregulation, weight gain, and behavioral disturbances.

◆ Radiographic Evaluation and Differential Diagnosis

Recognition of the signs and symptoms described above prompts imaging studies of the brain to identify proximate causes. In the United States, computed tomography (CT) and magnetic resonance imaging (MRI) are commonly obtained. Tumors are usually large enough to be readily identified on standard studies, but in rare cases, smaller lesions may be missed if not specifically targeted. Multiplanar reconstructions and thin cuts through the region of the sella and infundibulum may help to reveal subcentimeter masses. MRI is particularly useful for the identification of tumors and delineation of the relationship of the tumor to surrounding neurovascular structures (including the carotids and their branches), optic apparatus, pituitary gland and stalk, and hypothalamus/ventricular system (**Fig. 8.1**). The tumor may appear heterogeneous, with cystic components bright on T1 and T2 and solid portions of the tumor exhibiting variable enhancement following administration of contrast (**Fig. 8.2**). MRI with axial, sagittal, and coronal planes with and without contrast is critical to preoperative planning and postoperative follow-up. Increasingly, MR angiography is helpful in delineating vascular anatomy for these same reasons.

We feel that CT is important in diagnosing and planning surgery for craniopharyngiomas. A distinguishing feature of these tumors is the presence of calcium, which may be difficult to detect on MRI (**Fig. 8.3**). Regions of calcification are present in the majority of pediatric tumors (up to 90%) and more than half of adult lesions.[10,23,27] Preoperative radiographic visualization of solid calcium deposits (when present) is invaluable to the surgeon in determining the feasibility of specific operative approaches. Moreover, CT is helpful in ascertaining the degree of pneumatization of the sphenoid, ethmoid, and frontal sinuses—relevant to transsphenoidal approaches for sellar tumors (sphenoid), drilling down the planum sphenoidale for frontal approaches (sphenoid/ethmoids), and bifrontal approaches for suprasellar tumors (frontal).

Preoperative angiography is generally not helpful in the evaluation of craniopharyngioma. The tumors are usually fed by small vessels that are difficult to visualize, even with a dedicated angiogram, and there is no role for preoperative embolization. Most of the relevant structural anatomy can be better delineated with MR angiography, which al-

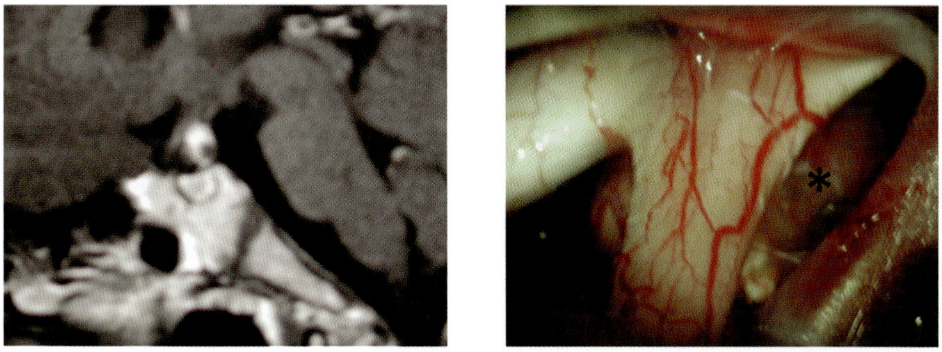

Fig. 8.1 Correlation between radiographic and operative visualization of craniopharyngioma (suprasellar/retrochiasmatic). The sagittal T1 enhanced MRI demonstrates a small tumor behind the optic apparatus (suprasellar/retrochiasmatic) with a small T1-hypointense cyst at the lower posterior margin. The intraoperative photograph reveals the tumor (*) as predicted, with the small cyst visible just below it (*) and a tiny calcified portion on the anterior portion of the tumor (between the optic nerve and carotid).

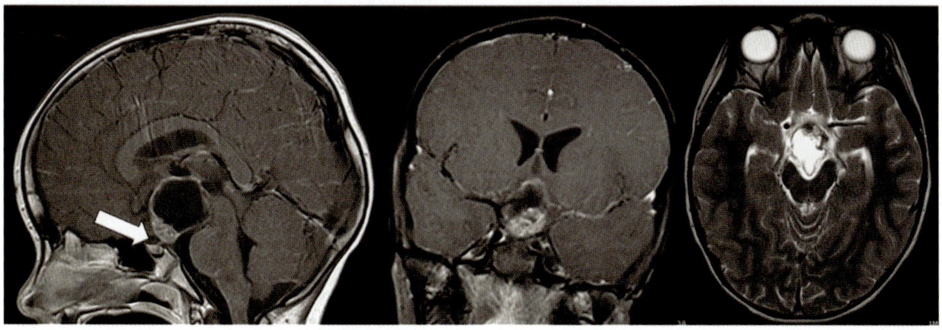

Fig. 8.2 MR appearance of craniopharyngioma. The sagittal and coronal T1 enhanced images reveal a large cystic lesion in the suprasellar region extending up toward the third ventricle with mixed imaging characteristics. Note the origin of the tumor from the region of the infundibulum above the pituitary gland (*arrow*). The axial T2 study demonstrates mixed signal, varying between the solid portions (darker) and the cyst (lighter).

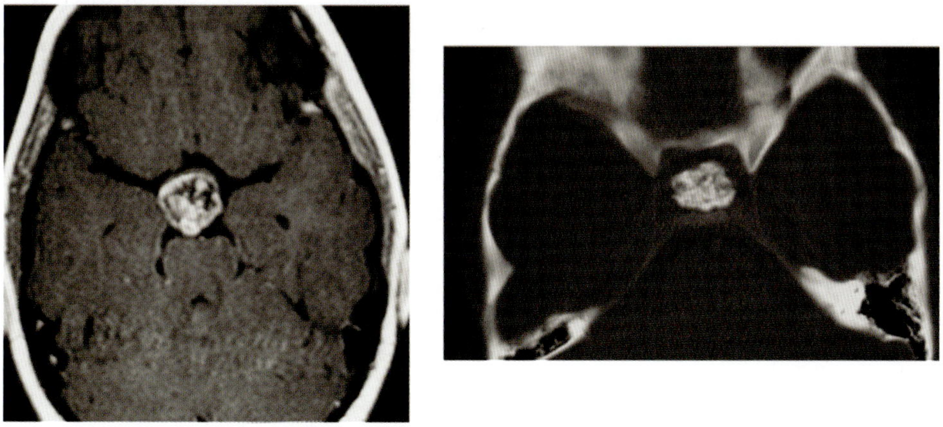

Fig. 8.3 Utility of CT for detecting calcification in craniopharyngioma. The axial T1 MRI on the left reveals the suprasellar craniopharyngioma, but it is difficult to ascertain what is calcified and what is mixed signal on T1. Using the axial CT (right), one can clearly identify a solid, calcified core to the tumor, a finding of substantial utility in formulating an appropriate treatment strategy.

lows visualization of the parenchyma and tumor side by side with associated vessels.

The differential diagnosis of tumors in the hypothalamic/sellar region is large and includes congenital lesions (Rathke cleft cyst, arachnoid cyst, dermoid/epidermoid cyst, hypothalamic hamartoma); tumors (pituitary adenomas, germinomas/nongerminomatous germ cell tumors, lymphoma, meningiomas, schwannomas of the cranial nerves, optic gliomas); vascular lesions (aneurysm, cavernous malformation); and inflammatory conditions (neurosarcoid, lymphocytic hypophysitis).[9,10,28] The characteristic calcification and cystic regions of craniopharyngiomas (especially in children) often help substantially with confirming the radiographic diagnosis. At our institution, we routinely obtain both CT and MRI in patients with suspected craniopharyngiomas.

◆ Initial Evaluation

In addition to the previously noted imaging, patients with craniopharyngioma should undergo preoperative endocrinologic assessment.[1,24,29] It is our practice to consult the endocrinology service before planned surgery and to obtain a panel of laboratory studies to evaluate pituitary function (**Table 8.1**). Deficient hormones are replaced as needed, with particular attention to cortisol deficiency: patients with craniopharyngioma should be considered in need of supplemental stress-dose steroids perioperatively.

When possible, a formal assessment of visual fields and an ophthalmologic examination should be performed before surgery.[24,25] This not only establishes a baseline, but also may help to guide the surgical approach if one optic

Table 8.1 Laboratory Tests for Endocrinology Evaluation

Prolactin
Thyroxine (T4), thyroid hormone binding ratio (THBR), thyroid-stimulating hormone (TSH), free T4
Insulin-like growth factor 1 (IGF-1), IGF-binding protein 3 (IGFBP-3)
Cortisol (if not receiving steroids)
DHEA (dehydroepiandrosterone) sulfate (if older than 6 years and not receiving steroids)
Follicle-stimulating hormone (FSH), luteinizing hormone (LH)
Estradiol (if female)
Testosterone (if male)
Electrolytes, blood urea nitrogen, creatinine, and serum osmolality
Bone age (at least by the time of hospital discharge)

nerve is substantially impaired and the other has retained function. Careful investigation and documentation of the patient's neurologic status is important for similar reasons. Lastly, although often not practical in the setting of an ill patient, those who present in a more elective fashion may be candidates for a detailed neuropsychological evaluation, allowing caregivers and families to more effectively follow changes over the course of treatment and develop more tailored coping strategies.[30,31]

For those patients who present when acutely ill, two conditions should be considered. First, hydrocephalus is a common cause for rapid deterioration in the setting of craniopharyngioma. If present, placement of an external ventricular drain can often immediately decrease intracranial pressure so that the patient can be stabilized until a definitive surgical treatment can be performed. On rare occasion, a large cyst within the tumor can be drained in this fashion to reduce mass effect. Second, as mentioned previously, many patients with craniopharyngioma are cortisol-deficient, and profound deterioration can occur from apparently minor physiologic stressors. Replacement of corticosteroids frequently averts disaster in these cases (we commonly administer dexamethasone 1–4 mg intravenously, although hydrocortisone 30 mg/m^2 is also effective).

◆ Treatment Strategies

Once identified, the primary objective of craniopharyngioma treatment is the restoration and preservation of neurologic function with minimal morbidity. There is substantial debate regarding the most effective method for achieving this goal. The difficulty in developing definitive guidelines for care stems in large part from the variability in presentation, the need for exceptionally long follow-up to assess efficacy, and the rarity of these tumors. The preferential use of specific treatments—radical surgery, subtotal resection, radiation, intracystic administration of chemotherapy—may be influenced by both published data and institutional bias. Here, we present an overview of surgical techniques used in the management of craniopharyngioma—approaches that are of use for both radical and subtotal resections.

Before an operation is undertaken, it is critical to define the goals of surgery. An important distinction is whether the objective is a complete resection or a planned subtotal debulking. This topic is controversial, and data exist supporting both strategies.[1,6,24,32–37] The policy at our institution is to attempt a total resection at initial presentation in most cases, but exceptions are made when preoperative imaging suggests that surgical morbidity would be unacceptable.[24] Radical resection can be attempted on repeat operations, but our experience has been that most successful reoperations occur when tumor was left behind initially because of poor visualization—a problem that can be remedied by altering the approach. In contrast, patients with tumors that were inextricably attached to vital neurovascular structures at the first operation are often poor candidates for gross total resection the second time around. Formulating goals for the surgery and planning an operative approach are difficult, and data support that surgeons with greater experience achieve better outcomes.[6,32,34] We routinely discuss cases among our group to draw upon the collective expertise of our practice. Unfortunately, even with careful planning, the nature of these tumors sometimes precludes achieving the expected preoperative objectives.

The primary goal of surgery is resection of the lesion with preservation of vital neural and vascular structures. Factors such as anatomic constraints imposed by these vital structures or characteristics of the tumor (eg, areas of calcification) may preclude a gross total resection, and secondary goals of surgery may include reducing mass effect, debulking the tumor so that it becomes more amenable to radiation therapy (either by reducing the size or creating margins around vital structures to minimize dose effect), restoring patterns of CSF flow, and establishing a tissue diagnosis with pathologic specimens. Review of the preoperative radiographic studies is invaluable in the selection of a surgical approach best suited to achieve these goals.

◆ Operative Approaches

Variation in the size and location of craniopharyngiomas, from small lesions located solely in the sella to huge tumors filling the third ventricle, has resulted in the development of numerous distinct surgical approaches. For many surgeons, familiarity with one method will often prompt its use in the majority of cases, and it can be difficult to balance the theoretic advantages of an alternative approach against the benefit afforded by experience. It is important to understand that there can be several equally valid approaches that may be efficacious for a given tumor. The growth pattern of an individual tumor can direct a surgeon to a particular approach. In general, craniopharyngiomas fall into three distinct groups: suprasellar/prechiasmatic, suprasellar/post-chiasmatic, and sellar. When viewed through this lens, it can be helpful to pair the common approaches (subfrontal, pterional, subtemporal, transcallosal/transventricular, and transsphenoidal) with specific growth patterns to maximize access to the tumor (**Table 8.2**).

Table 8.2 Potential Surgical Approaches Based on Craniopharyngioma Growth Patterns

1. Suprasellar
A. Primarily intraventricular: transcallosal/transventricular
B. Pre-chiasmatic: subfrontal
pterional
C. Post-chiasmatic: subfrontal
pterional
subtemporal
2. Sellar: transsphenoidal (microscopic/endoscopic)

Preoperative Avoidance of Complications: General Principles

Review of the case with nursing and anesthetic staff well beforehand allows anticipation of needed medications, hormone replacement, blood products, equipment, and potential emergencies. In addition to a discussion of the case with colleagues, a candid assessment of expected outcomes and risks of the surgery with the patient and family is vital. In the operating room, needs such as abdominal fat grafts, pericranial flaps to provide vascularized coverage of defects, and placement of ventricular or lumbar drains are best considered well in advance of the initial preparation. In planning operative approaches, it is useful to allow for additional exposure (through extension of the incision and bone flap) if possible. Although often not needed, the ability to improve access to the tumor intraoperatively can be invaluable.

Specific Approaches

Subfrontal

The subfrontal approach is commonly used in our institution. It allows excellent visualization of the optic nerves, carotids, and lamina terminalis. This approach is useful for most craniopharyngiomas, albeit less so for isolated sellar lesions. It affords wide access to the suprasellar region and can easily be combined with other approaches, such as the pterional, transcallosal/intraventricular, and even sellar (with drilling of the planum sphenoidale). The approach can be unilateral or bilateral, depending on the anatomy of the tumor. For retrochiasmatic and intraventricular tumors, removal of the superior orbital rim and roof improves visualization while minimizing retraction on the frontal lobes (**Fig. 8.4**).

Limitations of the approach include the risk for anosmia with injury to the olfactory nerves, the concern of venous congestion resulting from ligation of the superior sagittal sinus (which is usually minimal), and the extensive nature of the craniotomy; including violation of the frontal sinus with the attendant risk for CSF leak and mucocele.

In patients with hydrocephalus, placement of a preoperative drain may relax the brain and facilitate visualization with minimal retraction. A bicoronal incision is then marked out, with preparation of the surgical field to include the possibility of a pterional extension if needed. In patients with a large frontal air sinus, a site for an abdominal fat graft is readied. Anesthesia can be forewarned about the possibility of blood loss and air embolus if a bilateral exposure is planned and the sagittal sinus is to be exposed.

The patient is pinned in extension with the head midline to allow the frontal lobes to fall away from the floor of the anterior fossa. Following incision, the pericranium is preserved in elevating the scalp flap in anticipation of the need of a vascularized pedicle to cover the frontal sinus. In a unilateral case, the operating table can be rotated to vary lines of sight while the surgeon remains in a comfortable operating position, seated or standing. Dural opening should be low to the floor of the anterior fossa, and in the case of bilateral exposure, care should be taken to preserve at least one olfactory nerve.

If the orbital rim and roof are removed, the surgeon should attempt to avoid injury to the periorbita because the retraction of fat can be troublesome and can result in significant postoperative bruising. Gentle retraction on the orbit can greatly enhance visualization of the tumor, although some patients may experience bradycardia with compression of the eye. This will often resolve with slight repositioning of the retractor.

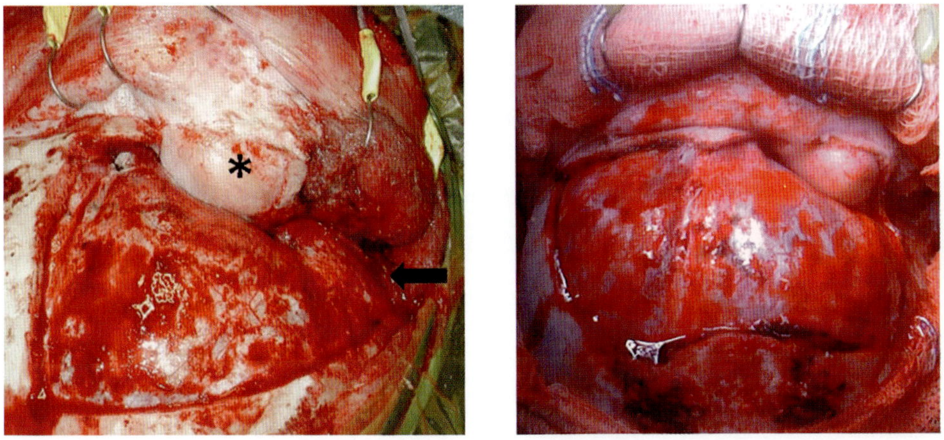

Fig. 8.4 Operative approaches (extradural). On the left, the unilateral subfrontal approach is demonstrated, with removal of the orbital roof (*). In addition, the craniotomy has been extended inferiorly to provide an element of a pterional approach (*arrow*), highlighting the versatility of these approaches and the importance of preserving flexibility in the operating room. The right image illustrates the bifrontal approach with removal of the right orbital roof.

Once intradural, the operating microscope is used and CSF cisterns are opened to further relax the brain. It is our practice to avoid the use of mannitol if possible, given the ability to achieve good relaxation with proper positioning and removal of CSF (and also given the potential issues with diabetes insipidus perioperatively). Drainage of cyst contents can aid in relaxation of the tight brain, although we prefer to maintain the tumor anatomy through the initial dissection, if possible, because the taut cyst provides good countertraction and a convenient dissection plane. Ultimately, however, cysts need to be drained, which can be accomplished with direct entry or aspiration with a fine needle. Placement of cottonoids around the cyst may help to prevent spread of the irritating cyst contents in the subarachnoid space, theoretically reducing the likelihood of chemical meningitis and tumor seeding.

In retrochiasmatic tumors, opening of the lamina terminalis can be useful. Care must be taken to avoid blind traction or injury to the walls of the third ventricle because hypothalamic injury can be devastating. Gentle downward pressure on the tumor from the lamina terminalis can deliver lesion into the more accessible subchiasmatic space. Use of a dental mirror or angled endoscope can substantially aid in visualization of difficult regions of the operative field. Drilling the planum sphenoidale can increase working room and afford greater access to the sella. When this is done, attention must be given to the possibility of entering the ethmoid or sphenoid sinus and appropriate steps taken to prevent CSF leak if a breach occurs (namely, packing the sinus with fat or muscle and covering the defect with tissue, preferably vascularized pericranium).

Pterional

The pterional approach is often used with suprasellar tumors that are both prechiasmatic and retrochiasmatic. It offers a more lateral view than the subfrontal route and can be combined with other approaches (subfrontal, subtemporal, transcallosal/transventricular) to expand access to larger masses. In addition to this versatility, it has the advantage of being familiar to many neurosurgeons. The primary limitation of the pterional approach is reduced visualization of the contralateral opticocarotid complex (**Fig. 8.5**).

At the Children's Hospital in Boston, we often employ this approach for small (usually incidentally discovered) tumors that are suprasellar. Our preference is to perform a right-sided craniotomy (assuming this to be the nondominant hemisphere), although we alter this based on tumor anatomy and function of the optic nerves. Should one optic nerve have markedly impaired function, we commonly approach from the side of the healthy nerve to better visualize and protect it.

The patient is positioned supine with the head extended and turned ~30 degrees away from midline. As with the subfrontal approach, the use of ventricular drainage may be helpful, although is it less likely to be needed with smaller tumors. Aspiration of CSF following the opening of CSF cisterns will nearly always enable excellent brain relaxation (again, without the need for the administration of hyperosmolar agents). Depending on the size of the tumor and the preference of the surgeon, the sylvian fissure can be opened to increase exposure at the bifurcation of the carotid.

Subtemporal

The subtemporal approach is employed primarily for access to suprasellar retrochiasmatic craniopharyngiomas that extend down toward the pons or laterally under the temporal lobe. The patient is placed in a supine or partially lateral position with the nose parallel to the floor. The vertex is tilted down toward the floor to allow the temporal lobe to fall away from the middle fossa. Upon opening the bone flap, it is helpful to use a drill or rongeur to remove bone flush with the floor of the middle fossa. Care must be taken to seal mastoid air cells with bone wax to prevent CSF leak postoperatively. Following gentle retraction on the temporal lobe, the tentorium can be divided to increase visualization of the interpeduncular and prepontine cisterns. It is important to preserve the trochlear nerve by cutting the tentorium behind the point at which they cross. Generally, the membrane of Liliequist will provide a barrier between the tumor and the basilar artery, although this is not an absolute constant, especially in reoperations.

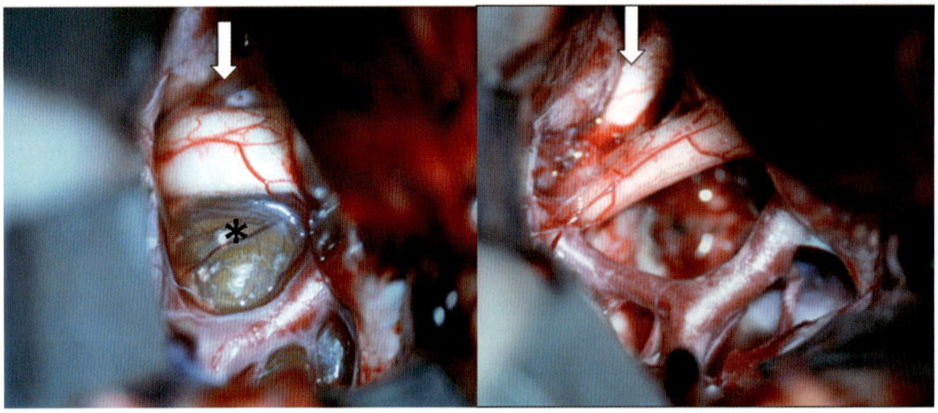

Fig. 8.5 Intraoperative view of craniopharyngioma (before and after resection). The left image demonstrates the view of a suprasellar/retrochiasmatic cystic craniopharyngioma as seen from a right pterional approach. Note the tumor (asterisk) in the opticocarotid triangle. The *arrow* points out the relatively limited access to the contralateral optic nerve—one shortcoming of this approach.

Transcallosal/Transventricular

Transcallosal/transventricular approaches are most helpful for tumors located high within the third or lateral ventricles. This route can be used independently or in combination with other approaches. The main limitation is the inability to visualize neurovascular structures near the sella. Generally, a craniotomy is made over the superior sagittal sinus with one-third posterior to the coronal suture, two-thirds anterior, and extension about 4 cm off midline toward the desired side. The white appearance of the corpus callosum must be identified, and frameless stereotaxy can be helpful in determining an entry point. A 2-cm opening in the callosum is made, and one can either carefully dissect between the fornices to enter the third ventricle directly or enter the frontal horn of the lateral ventricle, then open from the foramen of Monro posteriorly along the choroidal fissure. Care must be taken to avoid injury to the fornices and internal cerebral veins.

Transsphenoidal (Microscopic and Endoscopic)

The transsphenoidal approach has generally been employed in the removal of sellar craniopharyngiomas. Although it was traditionally limited to purely sellar lesions, surgeons have become increasingly capable of successfully resecting sellar lesions with suprasellar extension, with the improved visualization afforded by the operating endoscope. The main advantages of the transsphenoidal approach (either microscopic or endoscopic) include decreased surgical morbidity, shorter hospital stays, and improved access to sellar tumors. However, transsphenoidal surgery has markedly limited lateral exposure, minimal ability to control bleeding, and an increased risk for CSF leak/meningitis. Rare but catastrophic injury can occur following injuries to the carotid arteries and their major branches. Moreover, heavily calcified lesions are difficult to remove with the access provided from this route. Low tumors (particularly ones that are primarily midline, infradiaphragmatic, and cystic) are well suited to this approach.

Complication avoidance includes careful preselection of appropriate cases, as described above. In young children, the small working spaces and nonpneumatized sphenoid do not preclude this approach, but do require consideration. With children or in adults with small nares that might prevent the easy passage of surgical instruments, the translabial/transsphenoidal approach can be used to afford greater visualization and working access (**Fig. 8.6**). Image guidance, with either frameless stereotaxy and/or fluoroscopy, has proved useful in our institution (and others) to maintain a safe midline approach, especially in reoperated cases. On occasion, the decision to stage a procedure and perform a craniotomy at a subsequent date to remove suprasellar portions of a tumor may be prudent.

Following tumor removal, careful inspection of the cavity with an angled (30- or 70-degree) endoscope should be performed to assess the completeness of the resection and ensure the absence of injury. We routinely use a periumbilical incision to harvest abdominal fat grafts, which is less noticeable than lower quadrant sites. In patients with large tumors and evidence of a widened sella on preoperative imaging, the use of a lumbar drain may be helpful to prevent CSF leak and promote healing in the immediate postoperative period. Reconstruction of the sellar floor, often with a synthetic or bony graft, is important at the conclusion of the case.

Alternative Surgical Treatments

In addition to operative approaches targeted at removing the tumor, alternative surgical strategies exist to manage the issues caused by craniopharyngioma cysts and/or resultant hydrocephalus. In most cases, it is our practice to attempt to treat the underlying cause of the hydrocephalus before resorting to a ventriculoperitoneal shunt. In some craniopharyngiomas with large cystic components, placement of a catheter within the cyst can allow the delivery of sclerosing agents, such as bleomycin (an antibiotic that inhibits protein synthesis) or P^{32} (a radioactive isotope with limited penetration to surrounding tissues). Generally, these

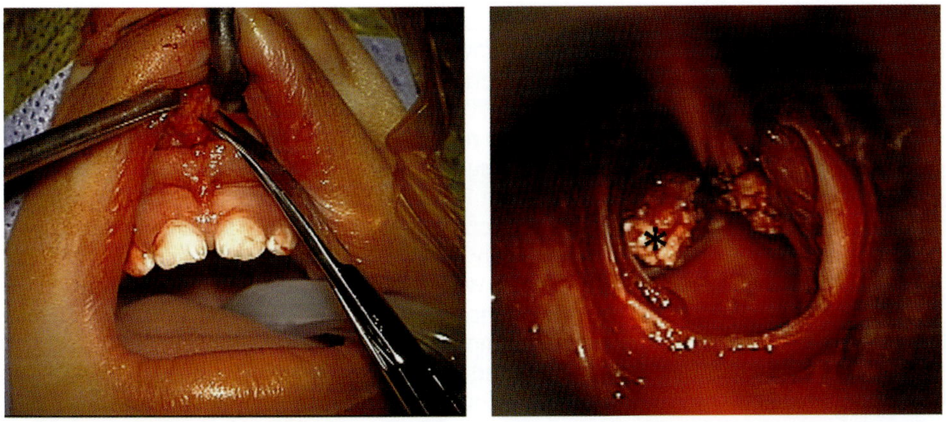

Fig. 8.6 Transsphenoidal approach (translabial/transsphenoidal). The transsphenoidal approach is most useful for sellar tumors confined to the midline. In young children or in adults with small nares, the translabial approach (left image) affords a wider viewing and working route. Care must be taken to leave a reasonable cuff of tissue above the gums to prevent injuring the nutrient vessels and nerves to the teeth. Once exposed, the tumor can be clearly identified (*) and removed. Maintaining the integrity of the diaphragma sellae reduces the risk for a postoperative CSF leak, and inspection of the operative field with an angled endoscope or dental mirror at the conclusion of the case can help to ensure a complete resection.

catheters are placed with stereotactic guidance because accuracy is of paramount importance. Leakage of toxic agents into the subarachnoid space or normal neural parenchyma is to be avoided. Often, contrast will be instilled through the catheter and an imaging study done to document the absence of a leak before delivery of the sclerosing agent.

Immediate Postoperative Care

Following surgical resection of a craniopharyngioma, patients are usually monitored in the intensive care unit. Primary concerns center on the management of hormonal replacement (especially with regard to diabetes insipidus and stress-dose corticosteroids), repeated assessment of visual function (monitoring for hemorrhage or blood pressure–dependent changes in eyesight), and documentation of the level of consciousness (watching for delayed hydrocephalus and effects of hypothalamic injury). As discussed below, postoperative imaging is useful. Continued discussion between intensive care unit staff, nursing, and the neurosurgical team is critical to maximize the likelihood of a successful outcome.

◆ Outcomes and Follow-up

Imaging

Postoperative imaging is critical to assess the extent of tumor resection and to establish a baseline for comparison in future studies. It is our practice to obtain an MRI with and without contrast either intraoperatively (with our operating room scanner) or within 72 hours following surgery. Increasingly, postoperative MR angiography is performed yearly to assess for the development of moyamoya, which is known to occur in this population and responds to surgical treatment if found.[38] The presentation of moyamoya can be delayed by years following surgery and should especially be considered in those patients who have also been treated with radiation. MR angiography can also help to identify fusiform dilatation of the carotid arteries, a phenomenon observed in ~10% of children after radical resection that appears to have a benign natural history.[39] CT is also performed postoperatively to ascertain whether any calcification remains in the operative bed, a finding considered by some to indicate residual tumor. It is our practice to consider reoperation only if the postoperative mass is unexpected and considered to be safe to resect. Calcified regions of tumor sometimes cannot be safely removed and so may deliberately be left in place. Small flecks of calcium—if found to be the only abnormality present on postoperative imaging—are often observed because their natural history as predictors of tumor recurrence is unclear.[40]

Endocrine, Metabolic, and Cognitive Issues

Endocrine dysfunction is common following the surgical treatment of craniopharyngiomas, with reports of diabetes insipidus occurring in more than 80% of patients and the need for hormone replacement in more than 90% of patients who underwent gross total resections.[20,26,27,29,34,35,41,42] Percentages are equally high for the replacement of thyroid hormone, sex hormones (following puberty), and corticosteroids.[29] Over half of all surgically treated children are candidates for growth hormone replacement.[29] Obesity resulting from hypothalamic injury is present in over half of children following resection.[29,36] For many of these patients, the deficits are permanent. As such, long-term endocrinologic follow-up is needed, with appropriate adjustments in hormone replacement (age-specific sex hormones, dosing of growth hormone, and careful monitoring of volume status for desmopressin replacement). Critically important is the recognition of the need for stress-dose corticosteroids in the setting of physiologic challenges such as illness and injury.

Increasingly appreciated are the consequences of the surgical treatment of craniopharyngioma on cognitive and emotional function. In the most severe state, akinetic mutism may render patients unable to function in society, but more subtle deficits in intelligence, emotion, and memory may add to the lifetime burden of this disease.[30,31] Awareness of these potential problems may facilitate appropriate referral for consultation with neuropsychology, psychiatry, and social work to provide additional support and coping mechanisms for affected patients.[20,31] The insidious nature of these deficits may cause them to be overlooked, particularly as the acute issues after surgery settle down with time, and thus mandate continued attention by the family and caregivers.

Long-term Issues and Recurrence

Craniopharyngiomas and the surgery to remove them can both produce long-term deleterious effects on the quality of life of affected patients.[30] The wide array of disorders associated with this tumor—endocrinologic, visual, metabolic, cognitive, and oncologic (among others)—has prompted our institution to adopt a model in which patients are treated and followed by a multidisciplinary team comprising specialists able to address each of these issues, a practice shared with other high-volume centers.[6,24]

We often obtain imaging every 3 to 6 months for the first 2 years, then space out to every 6 to 12 months up to the 5-year post-treatment time point. Several series report that average time to recurrence following operation with gross total resection is 2.5 to 3 years, with ~50% of patients remaining disease-free at 5 years, although these statistics remain controversial, with some reports indicating much better long-term disease-free intervals after gross total resection.[1,13,20,36,43] However, craniopharyngioma is notable for its capacity to recur decades after seemingly successful treatment and, as such, warrants prolonged monitoring.[24,33] Some reports note a 15 to 40% recurrence of tumor at 15 years, regardless of therapy administered.[1,24,44] If recurrence develops, it substantially reduces survival, even in delayed cases (10-year survival without recurrence is >99%, whereas patients with recurrence have a survival of <70% at 10 years).[20] We continue to monitor our patients with office visits and MRI studies beyond the 5-year postoperative time point, increasingly spacing out imaging to once every 5 years.

If recurrence is detected, the risks and benefits of treatment modalities must be weighed. In younger patients, there is often an impetus to attempt repeat surgical resection to avoid long-term risks of radiation (particularly in preschool-age children). Gross total resection at reoperation has been reported with rates ranging from 30 to 70%.[1,33,36,37] Prior radiation therapy and increasing size of tumor are noted as risk factors limiting the success of reoperation.[24,33,37] The practice at our institution is to attempt repeat resection if there is documented evidence of growth and the tumor appears to be accessible with minimal morbidity. The wide range of clinical and radiographic presentations of these tumors, coupled with the variety of treatments administered (surgery, radiation, radiosurgery, instillation of sclerosing agents), limits the ability to formulate general guidelines for the management of recurrent disease. As such, many patients are evaluated on a case-by-case basis, emphasizing the importance of providing treatment at an experienced center so that the treating surgeon can more accurately assess the likelihood of success.[33,34,37]

◆ Conclusion

The management of craniopharyngioma is challenging and best provided by surgeons who routinely treat these tumors at institutions with the resources to administer the required multidisciplinary care. Preoperative assessment should include both MRI and CT, coupled with a complete endocrinologic and visual evaluation. Operative approaches should be selected based on available anatomic routes of access, awareness of preexisting deficits to preserve remaining function, and the surgeon's experience. The goal of complete resection should be weighed against the risk for severe surgical morbidity and may sometimes prompt the abandonment of attempts at further tumor removal. Follow-up studies include immediate perioperative imaging and endocrinologic replacement as needed. Multidisciplinary care is helpful in the long-term management of these patients. Appreciation of the possibility of delayed recurrence, even decades later, should encourage continued monitoring well after the surgery has finished. The optimal management of patients affected by craniopharyngiomas remains controversial, and it is hoped that ongoing collaborative research will guide clinicians toward increasingly effective treatments.

References

1. Craniopharyngioma in children. 41st annual congress of the French Society of Neurosurgery. Lisbon, Portugal, 4-7 June 1991. Neurochirurgie 1991;37(Suppl 1):1–174
2. Lindholm J, Nielsen EH. Craniopharyngioma: historical notes. Pituitary 2009;12(4):352–359
3. Kleihues P, Burger PC, Scheithauer BW. The new WHO classification of brain tumours. Brain Pathol 1993;3(3):255–268
4. Louis DN, Ohgaki H, Wiestler OD, et al. The 2007 WHO classification of tumours of the central nervous system. Acta Neuropathol 2007;114(2):97–109
5. Kleihues P, Louis DN, Scheithauer BW, et al. The WHO classification of tumors of the nervous system. J Neuropathol Exp Neurol 2002;61(3):215–225, discussion 226–229
6. Jane JA Jr, Laws ER. Craniopharyngioma. Pituitary 2006;9(4):323–326
7. Kanter AS, Sansur CA, Jane JA Jr, Laws ER Jr. Rathke's cleft cysts. Front Horm Res 2006;34:127–157
8. Pettorini BL, Frassanito P, Caldarelli M, Tamburrini G, Massimi L, Di Rocco C. Molecular pathogenesis of craniopharyngioma: switching from a surgical approach to a biological one. Neurosurg Focus 2010;28(4):E1
9. Donovan JL, Nesbit GM. Distinction of masses involving the sella and suprasellar space: specificity of imaging features. AJR Am J Roentgenol 1996;167(3):597–603
10. Zada G, Lin N, Ojerholm E, Ramkissoon S, Laws ER. Craniopharyngioma and other cystic epithelial lesions of the sellar region: a review of clinical, imaging, and histopathological relationships. Neurosurg Focus 2010;28(4):E4
11. Miller DC. Pathology of craniopharyngiomas: clinical import of pathological findings. Pediatr Neurosurg 1994;21(Suppl 1):11–17
12. Crotty TB, Scheithauer BW, Young WF Jr, et al. Papillary craniopharyngioma: a clinicopathological study of 48 cases. J Neurosurg 1995;83(2):206–214
13. Weiner HL, Wisoff JH, Rosenberg ME, et al. Craniopharyngiomas: a clinicopathological analysis of factors predictive of recurrence and functional outcome. Neurosurgery 1994;35(6):1001–1010, discussion 1010–1011
14. Smith ER, Manfredi M, Scott RM, Black PM, Moses MA. A recurrent craniopharyngioma illustrates the potential usefulness of urinary matrix metalloproteinases as noninvasive biomarkers: case report. Neurosurgery 2007;60(6):E1148–E1149, discussion E1149
15. Smith ER, Zurakowski D, Saad A, Scott RM, Moses MA. Urinary biomarkers predict brain tumor presence and response to therapy. Clin Cancer Res 2008;14(8):2378–2386
16. Bunin GR, Surawicz TS, Witman PA, Preston-Martin S, Davis F, Bruner JM. The descriptive epidemiology of craniopharyngioma. J Neurosurg 1998;89(4):547–551
17. Freeman TB, Abati AD, Topsis J, Snyder JR, Beneck D, Lehman LB. Neonatal craniopharyngioma. N Y State J Med 1988;88(2):81–83
18. Joó JG, Rigó J Jr, Sápi Z, Timár B. Foetal craniopharyngioma diagnosed by prenatal ultrasonography and confirmed by histopathological examination. Prenat Diagn 2009;29(2):160–163
19. Lonjon M, Dran G, Casagrande F, Vandenbos F, Mas JC, Richelme C. Prenatal diagnosis of a craniopharyngioma: a new case with radical surgery and review. Childs Nerv Syst 2005;21(3):177–180
20. Karavitaki N, Brufani C, Warner JT, et al. Craniopharyngiomas in children and adults: systematic analysis of 121 cases with long-term follow-up. Clin Endocrinol (Oxf) 2005;62(4):397–409
21. Van Effenterre R, Van Effenterre G, Cabanis EA, Iba Zizen MT. Suprasellar tumors in patients over 70 years of age. Value of limited frontotemporal craniotomy. Visual results. Apropos of 5 cases. Neurochirurgie 1991;37(5):330–337
22. Sekiya T, Ito K, Akasaka K, Suzuki S. Two operated cases of craniopharyngioma in patients over 70 years old. No Shinkei Geka 1995;23(8):699–703
23. Samii M, Tatagiba M. Surgical management of craniopharyngiomas: a review. Neurol Med Chir (Tokyo) 1997;37(2):141–149
24. Scott RM. Craniopharyngioma: a personal (Boston) experience. Childs Nerv Syst 2005;21(8-9):773–777
25. Feletti A, Marton E, Mazzucco GM, Fang S, Longatti P. Amaurosis in infancy due to craniopharyngioma: a not-exceptional but often misdiagnosed symptom. Neurosurg Focus 2010;28(4):E7
26. Sanford RA, Muhlbauer MS. Craniopharyngioma in children. Neurol Clin 1991;9(2):453–465
27. Samii M, Bini W. Surgical treatment of craniopharyngiomas. Zentralbl Neurochir 1991;52(1):17–23
28. Smith MM, Strottmann JM. Imaging of the optic nerve and visual pathways. Semin Ultrasound CT MR 2001;22(6):473–487
29. Curtis J, Daneman D, Hoffman HJ, Ehrlich RM. The endocrine outcome after surgical removal of craniopharyngiomas. Pediatr Neurosurg 1994;21(Suppl 1):24–27

30. Waber DP, Pomeroy SL, Chiverton AM, et al. Everyday cognitive function after craniopharyngioma in childhood. Pediatr Neurol 2006;34(1):13–19
31. Müller HL, Bruhnken G, Emser A, et al. Longitudinal study on quality of life in 102 survivors of childhood craniopharyngioma. Childs Nerv Syst 2005;21(11):975–980
32. Wisoff JH. Craniopharyngioma. J Neurosurg Pediatr 2008;1(2): 124–125, discussion 125
33. Wisoff JH. Surgical management of recurrent craniopharyngiomas. Pediatr Neurosurg 1994;21(Suppl 1):108–113
34. Sanford RA. Craniopharyngioma: results of survey of the American Society of Pediatric Neurosurgery. Pediatr Neurosurg 1994;21 (Suppl 1):39–43
35. Merchant TE, Kiehna EN, Sanford RA, et al. Craniopharyngioma: the St. Jude Children's Research Hospital experience 1984–2001. Int J Radiat Oncol Biol Phys 2002;53(3):533–542
36. Hoffman HJ, De Silva M, Humphreys RP, Drake JM, Smith ML, Blaser SI. Aggressive surgical management of craniopharyngiomas in children. J Neurosurg 1992;76(1):47–52
37. Elliott RE, Hsieh K, Hochm T, Belitskaya-Levy I, Wisoff J, Wisoff JH. Efficacy and safety of radical resection of primary and recurrent craniopharyngiomas in 86 children. J Neurosurg Pediatr 2010;5(1):30–48
38. Scott RM, Smith ER. Moyamoya disease and moyamoya syndrome. N Engl J Med 2009;360(12):1226–1237
39. Elliott RE, Wisoff JH. Fusiform dilation of the carotid artery following radical resection of pediatric craniopharyngiomas: natural history and management. Neurosurg Focus 2010;28(4):E14
40. Elliott RE, Moshel YA, Wisoff JH. Minimal residual calcification and recurrence after gross-total resection of craniopharyngioma in children. J Neurosurg Pediatr 2009;3(4):276–283
41. Yang I, Sughrue ME, Rutkowski MJ, et al. Craniopharyngioma: a comparison of tumor control with various treatment strategies. Neurosurg Focus 2010;28(4):E5
42. Campbell PG, McGettigan B, Luginbuhl A, Yadla S, Rosen M, Evans JJ. Endocrinological and ophthalmological consequences of an initial endonasal endoscopic approach for resection of craniopharyngiomas. Neurosurg Focus 2010;28(4):E8
43. Kim SK, Wang KC, Shin SH, Choe G, Chi JG, Cho BK. Radical excision of pediatric craniopharyngioma: recurrence pattern and prognostic factors. Childs Nerv Syst 2001;17(9):531–536, discussion 537
44. Bülow B, Attewell R, Hagmar L, Malmström P, Nordström CH, Erfurth EM. Postoperative prognosis in craniopharyngioma with respect to cardiovascular mortality, survival, and tumor recurrence. J Clin Endocrinol Metab 1998;83(11):3897–3904

9 Surgical Treatment of Chordomas and Chondrosarcomas

Devyani Lal, Nancy J. Fischbein, and Griffith R. Harsh IV

Chordomas and chondrosarcomas are osteocartilaginous tumors that typically involve the skull base in a parasellar location. These tumors, often grouped together because of their similar osseous origins and location, are distinct in embryology, pathology, biological behavior, clinical features, and response to therapy. Chordomas arise from remnants of the embryonal notochord and are frequently located in the central skull base. Most grow slowly initially, but eventually their growth accelerates. They are locally invasive, and invasion, combined with rapid growth, often proves fatal. Chondrosarcomas originate from the chondral elements of bone. In the skull, they are often located in the paramedian sphenoid and the clival basiocciput. Most chondrosarcomas demonstrate slow, locally invasive growth. Many chondrosarcomas do not affect patient function or survival for decades.

◆ Incidence and Epidemiology

Chordomas and chondrosarcomas together account for ~0.2% of all intracranial tumors and 6% of all primary skull base tumors.[1,2]

Although chordoma is the most common extradural primary skull base tumor, its absolute incidence is low (<0.1 per 100,000 persons per year, or ~0.15% of all intracranial tumors).[3] Chordomas can occur at any age, but they peak in the fourth or fifth decade of life, with a median age at diagnosis of 46 years. Fewer than 5% arise in children.[4,5] There is no gender preponderance[2,6] or known association with exposure to radiation or environmental carcinogens. Chordomas occur in isolation and are not part of any known systemic syndrome. Although chordoma occurrence in one family has been linked to chromosome 7q33,[7] no gene mutation specific to chordoma has been identified.

Chondrosarcomas are even more rare, comprising only 0.02% of all intracranial neoplasms.[8] Although skull base chondrosarcomas can occur at any age, most patients present between 20 and 50 years of age[9]; the mean age at diagnosis is 40.7 years.[10] Chondrosarcomas are slightly more common in men.[11] Although they are usually isolated tumors, chondrosarcomas may occur in association with Paget disease, Ollier disease, or Maffucci syndrome.[12,13]

◆ Location

Chordomas occur at sites of embryonal remnants of the notochord: the sellar and parasellar region, clivus, spine, sacrum, and mediastinum. Thirty-five percent arise in the skull base, most commonly in the clival midline.[1,8] Classification of the tumor location as superior, middle, and/or inferior clival is helpful in planning surgical approaches.[14] With growth, chordomas expand and destroy bone and extend into extra-axial and intra-axial structures. Rostral notochord chordomas can often extend into the dorsum sellae and present in the sellar, suprasellar, or parasellar/cavernous sinus areas. These may compress the pituitary gland, optic nerves and chiasm, and midbrain.[15] Chordomas can extend ventrally through the clivus to present as a nasopharyngeal mass causing nasal obstruction or dysphagia.[16] Chordomas extending from the dorsal clivus can compress the midbrain, pons, and medulla. Tumors extending dorsolaterally can involve the petrous temporal bone. Although chordomas are usually extradural, they may infiltrate and penetrate the cranial dura; dural invasion usually occurs late in the course of aggressive tumors. Surgical durotomies may facilitate the intradural extension of chordomas. Chordomas very rarely arise as primary intradural intracranial neoplasms.[17,18] Metastasis usually occurs late in the course of the disease and is seen clinically in ~10 to 20% of cases.[19] Metastatic potential has not been correlated with any histologic or clinical features. The most common metastatic sites are skin, bone, lung, and lymph nodes. Intradural metastases of skull base chordomas are rare, and most occur following surgery.[20] Tumor recurrence may occur along routes of surgical access. Although metastases can be found in up to 40% of patients at autopsy,[19] local tumor growth is usually the predominant threat to patient function and survival.

Chondrosarcomas are mesenchymal, but their precise cell of origin is controversial; embryonal cartilaginous rests, mesenchymal pluripotent cells, and metaplastic fibroblasts have been proposed.[10,21] Although they can occur anywhere in the skull base, most cranial chondrosarcomas occur at skull base synchondroses,[22] notably those involving the clivus. Sixty-six percent are located at the petro-occipital junction (arising from the petroclival synchondrosis), 28% at the spheno-occipital synchondrosis, and 6% in the sphenoethmoid complex.[12] Isolated chondrosarcomas are usually paramedian, but when part of Ollier or Maffucci syndrome, they may be midline.[23] Chondrosarcomas originate as extradural tumors. Most grow slowly, destroy bone, and eventually extend into surrounding soft tissue. Most are low-grade malignancies[12] and have a much better prognosis than do chordomas.[24,25] The major concern after treatment is local recurrence.[26] Metastases occur late, if at all, and affect no more than 10% of patients.[11,22]

◆ Pathology

Small chordomas and chondrosarcomas appear to arise within cranial bone, and with growth, they erode normal bone structures, displace the overlying periosteum and dura, and develop a nodular surface. They are not encapsulated, but the thinned sheath of expanded periosteum and dura often forms a pseudocapsule. Ultimately, these tumors erode cranial foramina and compress cranial nerves, brain, and basal arteries.

Chordomas are grayish tan to bluish white, with a consistency that ranges from gelatinous to leathery and a texture that ranges from smooth to gritty. They may have soft foci of hemorrhagic necrosis or firm, calcium-dense areas. Histologically, chordomas are characterized by lobules and nests of large epithelium-like cells separated by fibrous strands. Tumor cells are arranged in sheets or cords in a background of myxoid stroma. They have abundant pink cytoplasm and moderately sized nuclei with mild to moderate atypia. Some cells have clear vacuoles, which impart a characteristic "bubbly" appearance to the cytoplasm. These "physaliferous" cells are large and vacuolated, and they contain mucus; they resemble the cells of the primitive notochord. Mitoses are limited and necrosis is common. Chordomas are immunohistochemically positive for cytokeratin, epithelial membrane antigen, carcinoembryonic antigen, and α-fetoprotein. Some chordomas stain positive for S-100 protein; this differentiates them from other sarcomatoid round cell or myxoid neoplasms.[1] Staining for brachyury, SOX-9, and podoplanin (markers for primitive notochord) helps distinguish chordoma from chondrosarcoma.[27]

Chondrosarcomas are osteocartilaginous tumors with varying grades of malignancy. Macroscopically, they are nodular and gray to tan-white. The tumor consistency can be mucinous, firm, or gritty. Large yellow-white or chalky areas of calcification may be present. Chondrosarcomas erode cancellous bone and extend peripherally into soft tissue. Microscopically, four classic types of chondrosarcoma have been described: conventional, clear cell, dedifferentiated, and mesenchymal.[12,28] Most skull base chondrosarcomas are of the conventional type. Conventional chondrosarcomas are composed of hyaline or myxoid cartilage or a combination of both. The neoplastic chondrocytes lie in clear lacunae within the hyaline matrix. Myxoid chondrosarcomas have bipolar or stellate neoplastic cells that float in a background of mucinous matrix. Tumor cells are arranged in a honeycomb of interconnecting strands and cords. They rarely have mitoses. As in chordomas, immunohistochemistry is positive for vimentin and S-100.[12] In contrast to chordomas, however, chondrosarcomas typically do not express epithelial markers such as keratin and epithelial membrane antigen[12] or markers for notochord differentiation.[27,29,30] Tumors are graded histologically (1–3) based on cellularity, mitotic activity, and nuclear atypia. Tumor grade is predictive of invasiveness, growth rate, metastatic potential, response to therapy, and outcome.[22,31–34] Grade 1 chondrosarcomas typically do not metastasize. Grade 2 chondrosarcomas have a higher metastatic tendency (10%), and grade 3 tumors have significant metastatic potential.

◆ Challenges

The sellar and parasellar location of chordomas and chondrosarcomas presents formidable challenges to effective treatment. The relative inaccessibility of these areas and the propensity for local invasion of tumor with involvement of critical neural and vascular structures pose technical challenges to surgical resection. Despite such challenges, the combination of surgery and radiation can offer cure for most low-grade chondrosarcomas and provide significant control of chordomas and high-grade chondrosarcomas.

◆ Clinical Presentation

Patients with a sellar or parasellar chordoma or chondrosarcoma typically present with headache and/or cranial neuropathies.[1,10,12,35,36] Unilateral abducens nerve palsy is the most common clinical sign. Hearing loss, dysphagia, dysarthria, and tongue weakness occur when the tumor extends to the basiocciput and affects the middle and lower cranial nerves.[9] Compression of the brainstem may manifest with sensory or motor signs. Endocrinopathies may result from involvement of the pituitary gland.

◆ Natural History

Patients with chordomas have a poor prognosis if untreated, with a mean duration of survival ranging from 6 to 28 months.[1,37] Patient age and gender, the histologic appearance of the tumor, the therapy received, and tumor recurrence have prognostic significance. Older patients generally do worse.[36] In one series, all patients with tumors diagnosed at age 40 years or younger were alive 5 years later, in contrast to only 22% of patients with tumors diagnosed at age older than 40 years.[38] Women have a poorer outcome than do men. A high mitotic rate also correlates with rapid growth and poor outcome. The natural history of chondrosarcomas is better, especially low-grade tumors. Nonetheless, most patients die without treatment.[10] Histologic grade is strongly correlated with survival; patients with grades 1, 2, and 3 tumors had 5-year survival rates of 90%, 81%, and 43% respectively.[33] The combination of surgery and radiation offers longer maintenance of neurologic function and survival. All patients warrant comprehensive evaluation, and most require aggressive treatment.

◆ Radiologic Investigations

Chordomas and chondrosarcomas are difficult to definitively distinguish radiologically.[39] Chordomas are typically centered in the midline, whereas chondrosarcomas are usually paramedian. Both tumors may compress, displace, invade, or envelop critical surrounding structures, such as cranial nerves, cavernous sinuses, vessels of the circle of Willis, and the brainstem.[40]

Radiologic evaluation narrows the differential diagnosis and facilitates treatment planning (**Table 9.1**). Computed tomography (CT), in both the axial and coronal planes, determines the extent of osseous erosion and depicts intratumoral calcification. On soft-tissue-window CT scans, involvement of adjacent structures can be identified to some extent, although magnetic resonance imaging (MRI) is far superior in this regard. Chordomas often appear to be of relatively low density on CT owing to their mucoid content, and they typically enhance only minimally or mildly after the administration of iodinated contrast material. Chondrosarcomas are typically not as low in density as chordomas, and they are more likely to enhance moderately after contrast administration, often in a "honeycomb" or "popcorn-like" pattern.

MRI is essential for accurate differential diagnosis and for defining the extent of the tumor (**Fig. 9.1**). Both chordomas and chondrosarcomas are usually hypointense or isointense to soft tissue on T1-weighted images and hyperintense on T2-weighted images.[41] Chondrosarcomas are more likely to have a speckled pattern of signal voids, indicative of tumor calcification, although occasionally re-

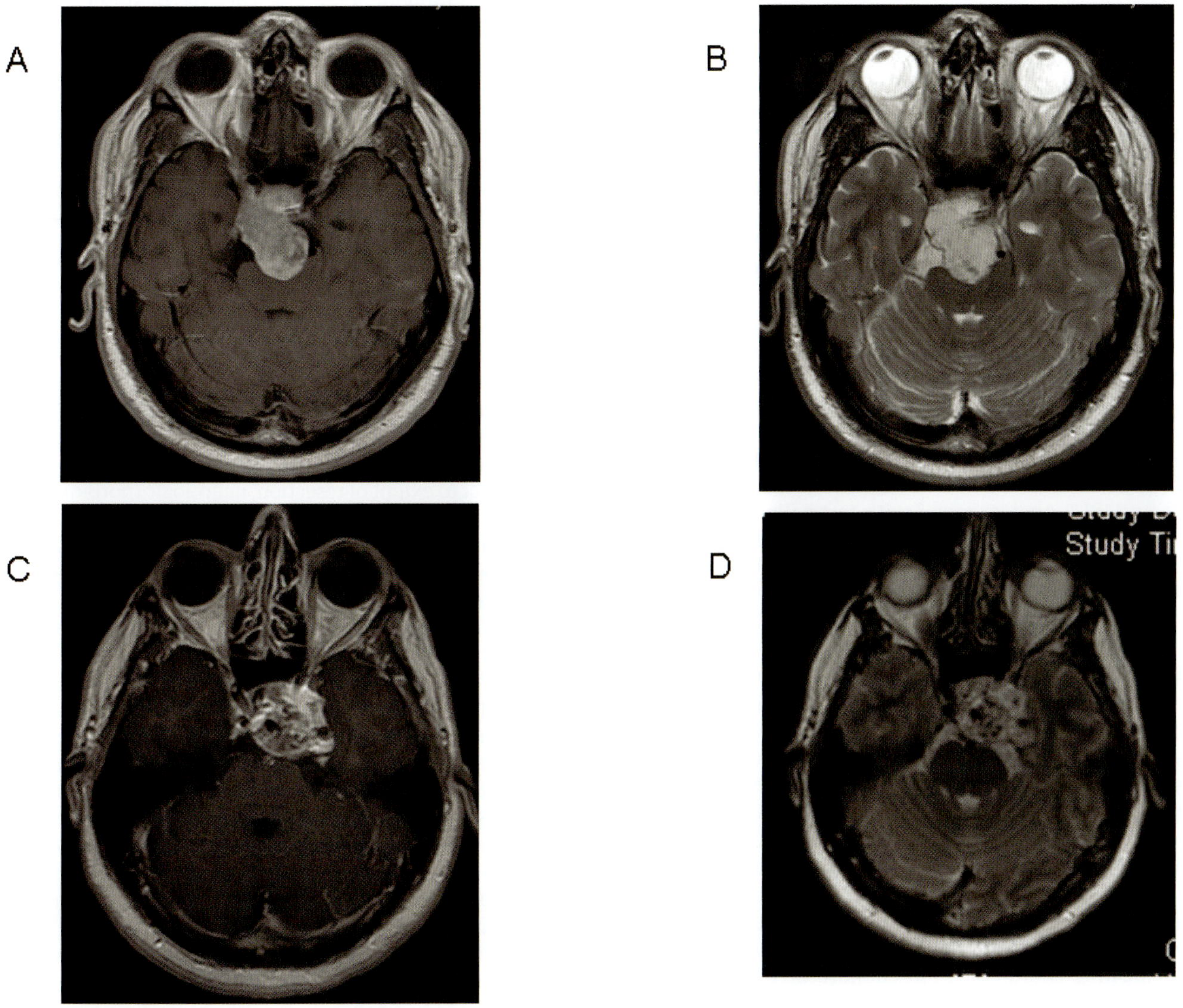

Fig. 9.1 **(A,B)** Chordoma and **(C,D)** chondrosarcoma. These can be difficult to distinguish radiologically. The chordoma is typically centered in the midline, is homogeneously bright on T2-weighted images, and enhances to a variable extent on post-gadolinium images; in this case, the enhancement is quite intense. The chondrosarcoma is more commonly centered off midline, although in this case its location is similar to that of most chordomas. The lesion shown here has areas of low signal on post-contrast and T2 images owing to intratumoral calcification. In the absence of calcification, chondrosarcomas are typically homogeneously bright on T2-weighted images and enhance intensely and homogeneously after gadolinium. **(A,C)** T1-weighted image with contrast. **(B,D)** T2-weighted image.

Table 9.1 Differential Diagnosis of Clival Masses

Chondroma
Chondrosarcoma
Chordoma
Craniopharyngioma
Eosinophilic granuloma
Fibrous dysplasia
Lymphoma
Meningioma
Metastases
Nasopharyngeal carcinoma
Neurofibroma
Osteoma
Osteoblastoma
Pituitary adenoma
Plasmacytoma/multiple myeloma

sidual fragments of bone may appear as signal voids on MRI in chordomas. Enhancement following the administration of a gadolinium-based contrast agent is almost always present.[42] Chordoma enhancement is variable and ranges from minimal to fairly intense; it often increases over time, such that the tumor will appear more intensely enhancing on delayed images. Chondrosarcoma enhancement is generally more intense than that of chordomas, and it can be heterogeneous owing to intermixed calcification. Tumor extension into the basal cisterns, cavernous sinuses, and adjacent regions such as the sella and nasopharynx is well delineated on MRI. The relationship of the tumor to the internal carotid and basilar arteries, especially any displacement or encasement, can be assessed by examining flow voids on MRI.[43] Angiography[10] with test balloon occlusion may be indicated if vessel sacrifice is contemplated.

◆ Treatment

Various options exist for the management of sellar and parasellar chordomas and chondrosarcomas. These include clinical and radiologic observation, biopsy followed by observation, biopsy followed by radiation, surgical removal, surgical removal followed by radiation, and chemotherapy. The appropriate choice of treatment requires confidence in the diagnosis, familiarity with the various treatment options, and predicted treatment outcome in the context of the individual patient.

The diagnosis of the tumor is usually based on characteristic radiographic features, as discussed above, although distinguishing chordoma from chondrosarcoma may not be possible without tissue sampling. Occasionally, a preliminary biopsy is indicated if the patient's age, medical condition, and neurologic deficits or the tumor's size and location contraindicate surgery and only radiation therapy will be offered. Additionally, a biopsy should be performed if other possibilities, such as metastasis, pituitary adenoma, and lymphoma, cannot be excluded on the basis of imaging alone. In this situation, the biopsy can often be performed at the start of an intended resection. Because chordomas and chondrosarcomas are predominantly extradural, standard stereotactic needle biopsy techniques may not be useful, and biopsy is more likely to be successfully performed through the nose.

Extensive resection and high-dose radiotherapy for both chordomas and chondrosarcomas are associated with better tumor control and longer patient survival[10,24,25,36,44] than is observation, surgery alone, or radiation alone. Patients should be evaluated by a multidisciplinary treatment team that includes a neurosurgeon, an otolaryngologist, and a radiation oncologist. A comprehensive treatment plan that maximizes tumor control and minimizes iatrogenic complications should be fashioned for each patient. Surgery is generally indicated as the first step toward the restoration or preservation of neurologic function, with radiation therapy to follow.

The surgical approach should be tailored to the goal chosen for each individual patient. The goal of surgical resection may vary from complete en bloc excision to piecemeal gross total resection of the tumor to radical subtotal removal that decompresses critical neurovascular structures and improves tumor geometry for postoperative radiotherapy. The choice of the surgical approach depends on the size, site of origin, and direction of expansion of the tumor; involvement of critical neurovascular structures; prior treatment; the patient's overall health; and the surgeon's technical expertise with the approach.

◆ Surgery

Surgery is usually the initial therapeutic modality for chordoma and chondrosarcoma. It is indicated to obtain diagnostic tissue, relieve neurologic symptoms, and resect tumor. Advances in skull base surgery have improved surgical outcome with respect to extent of resection, neurologic morbidity, and cosmesis (**Fig. 9.2**). For some tumors, staged operations via multiple approaches may be required to obtain satisfactory tumor exposure and removal. Microscopic and endoscopic techniques may both be helpful.[45] If reoperation is being planned, the sequelae of the earlier operation, such as scar tissue and distortion of the normal anatomy, must be taken into account. A fresh route of access is often preferred.

Many chordomas and chondrosarcomas of the sella and parasellar region pose significant challenges to complete resection by virtue of extensive bone involvement and their proximity to or envelopment of critical neural and vascular structures. The basic strategy is to maximize exposure of tumor and involved critical structures with minimal brain retraction. Coordination between neurosurgeons and otolaryngologists can achieve both improved exposure by traversing air sinuses or removing bone and more secure repair of the skull base defect with vascularized soft tissue flaps, which minimize the risks for cerebrospinal fluid (CSF) leakage and infection.

Surgical Approaches

The surgical approaches to chordomas and chondrosarcomas of the sella and parasellar region can be grouped according to whether they are exclusively midline or also

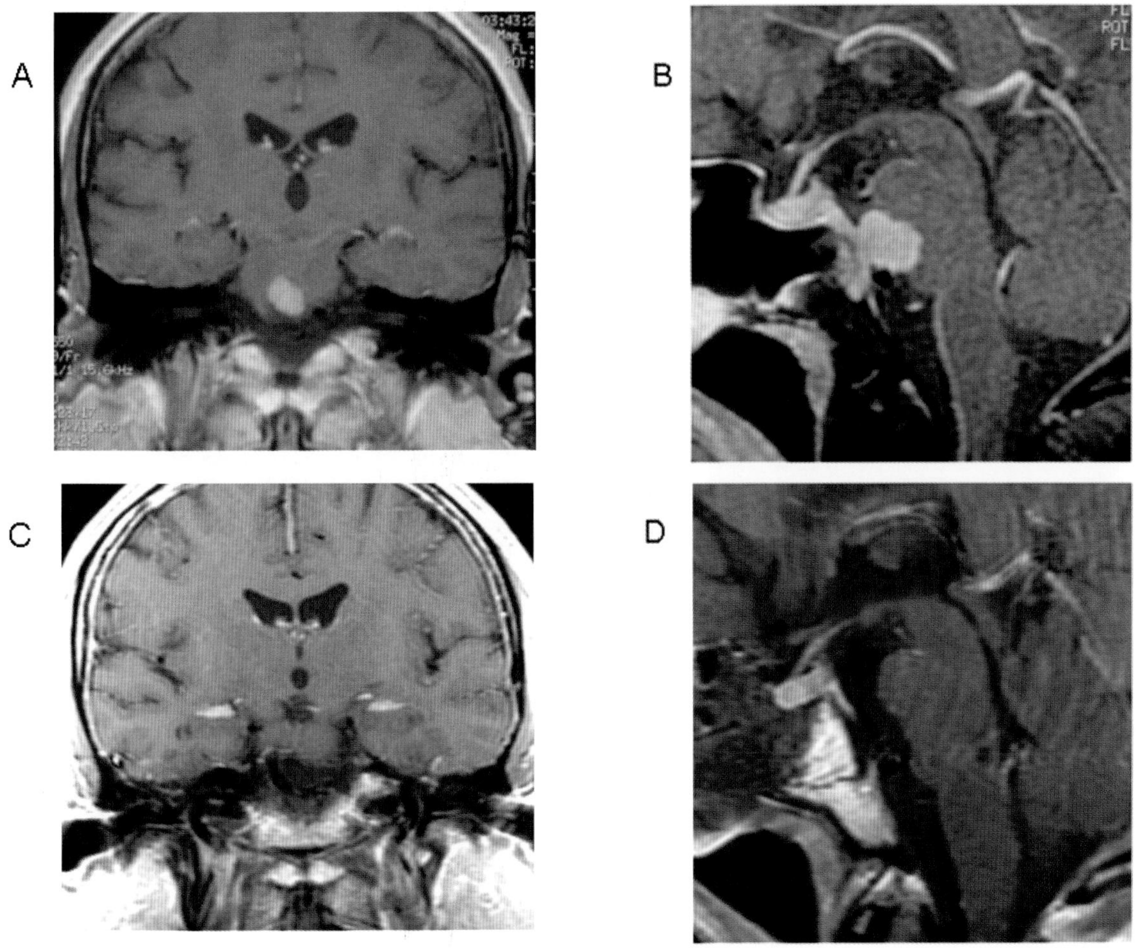

Fig. 9.2 Clival chordoma. (A,B) MRI before and (C,D) after resection. A 46-year-old man presented with diplopia and a right sixth nerve palsy. Preoperative MRI (coronal and sagittal T1-weighted images with contrast) shows a subsellar mass of clival origin with intradural extension compressing the pons above a horizontally oriented midbasilar segment. An endoscopic transsphenoidal approach was employed. Postoperative MRI (coronal and sagittal T1-weighted images with contrast) demonstrates gross total resection of tumor and expected postoperative changes in the sphenoid sinus and clivus.

have lateral extension[46] (**Table 9.2**). An extradural approach is generally used because most of these tumors are extradural.[47] This allows access to the bone of origin. When the overlying dura is infiltrated, the involved bone must be removed to approach the infiltrated dura. Tumor-infiltrated bone should always be drilled away, even if it is not restricting access to dural and intradural tumor.

Tumors limited to the sella and the immediately adjacent suprasellar, infrasellar, and cavernous sinus areas can be approached by a simple transsphenoidal approach.[48,49] A transnasal approach, or a combination of transnasal and transoral approaches, can be used to access the inferior midline extension of tumor down to the C1 vertebra. Suprasellar midline tumor extension that lies between the supraclinoidal internal carotid arteries can be accessed if the transsphenoidal approach is extended by removing the tuberculum sellae and adjacent planum (transtubercular, trans-planum). Even large, posteriorly directed intracranial extensions of the tumor that grow posteriorly through the dura to displace the brainstem can be removed by such extended transsphenoidal approaches.[50–56] Rigid endoscopes or the operating microscopes can be used. The endoscope's wide-angled view, illumination, and high magnification improve visualization of the surgical anatomy, and angled endoscopes can extend the surgical field laterally, superiorly, and inferiorly. Because this endoscopic view is two-dimensional, it requires supplementation with tactile and proprioceptive clues to depth (**Table 9.2**).

Suprasellar extension of firm tumor that extends lateral to the internal carotid arteries or incorporates cranial nerves or intracranial vessels usually warrants a craniofacial procedure. This combines the suprasellar exposure of a frontal craniotomy with the clival access of a transnasal, transsphenoethmoid approach. This approach can be endoscopically assisted. The transbasal and extended subfrontal approaches attempt to achieve a similar exposure from a single perspective.[14,57]

Parasellar tumors extending inferiorly in the midline and paramedian lower clivus are accessible through a transnasal, transsphenoidal, transclival approach. Even

Table 9.2 Surgical Approaches to Chordoma and Chondrosarcoma of the Sella and Parasellar Region

Location of tumor	Surgical approaches	Structures at risk	Complications
Sellar (midline)	• Transsphenoidal	Optic apparatus, ICA, CSF	Blindness, stroke, hypopituitarism, CSF fistula
Clival (midline)	• Transsphenoidal extended • Subfrontal	Optic, CNs VI and XII, pituitary, CSF, frontal lobe	Blindness, stroke, diplopia, hypopituitarism, CSF fistula, frontal hematoma
Sellar + suprasellar (midline)	• Transsphenoidal extended	Optic, ICA, pituitary, CSF	Blindness, stroke, hypopituitarism, CSF fistula
Sellar + infrasellar (midline)	• Transsphenoidal extended • Transethmoid (lateral rhinotomy) • Transoral	Optic, ICA, CNs VI and XII, pituitary, CSF	Blindness, stroke, diplopia, hypopituitarism, CSF fistula, epiphora
Sellar + inferior clival (midline)	• Transsphenoidal ± transoral	Optic, ICA, CNs VI and XII, pituitary, CSF	Blindness, stroke, diplopia, hypopituitarism, CSF fistula
Parasellar	• Frontotemporal • Transcavernous • Transnasal-maxillary	Optic; ICA; CNs III, IV, VI, and XII; pituitary; CSF	Blindness, stroke, diplopia, hypopituitarism, CSF fistula
Lateral sinus–pterygopalatine	• Transfacial • Transnasal-maxillary	Optic, ICA, CNs VI and XII, pituitary, CSF	Blindness, stroke, diplopia, hypopituitarism, CSF fistula
Petroclival (midline)	• Anterior transpetrosal (subtemporal)	Temporal lobe, ICA, CNs III–VI	Temporal hematoma, stroke, CN palsies
Petrous (posterior)	• Posterior transpetrosal (presigmoid)	CNs VI–XI, AICA, temporal lobe, brainstem	CN palsies, stroke, temporal hematoma, brainstem injury

Abbreviations: AICA, anterior inferior cerebellar artery; CNs, cranial nerves; CSF, cerebrospinal fluid; ICA, internal carotid artery.

further inferior extension to the craniovertebral junction, C1, and dens requires the addition of a transodontoid approach, which is usually transoral.[58] Tumors with significant lateral and inferior extension require the addition of a more oblique approach, such as the posterolateral or far lateral approach.[59]

The lateral extension of parasellar and midclival tumors anterior to the internal carotid arteries may be accessed by adding various degrees of maxillotomy to a more midline transnasal (endoscopic) or transfacial (microscopic or endoscopic) approach.[60] More posterior tumors with parasellar extension, especially when superior or lateral to the cavernous internal carotid artery, usually require a frontotemporal craniotomy; this may include dissection of the involved cavernous sinus.[61,62]

Parasellar tumor involving the petrous apex, tentorium, and subjacent posterior fossa can be exposed by a subtemporal, anterior transpetrosal route.[63,64] Larger tumors extending medially, inferiorly, and posteriorly usually require one of the posterior transpetrosal approaches. A presigmoid exposure is common to this group, but the extent of labyrinthectomy is dictated by the location, size, and consistency of the tumor and the status of the patient's hearing.[65] These lateral approaches have the advantage of avoiding the potentially contaminated nasal sinuses and oropharynx. In some cases, the risks for CSF leak and infection can be reduced by using a two-stage procedure: a lateral approach for removal of the intradural lateral tumor and dural repair followed by an anterior approach for the sellar midline tumor.

Surgical Technique

Chordomas often have two intermixed components: a soft, gelatinous portion within expanded bone or dura and a more sinewy part infiltrating and expanding the dura or extracranial soft tissue. The gelatinous part can be easily removed by suction or gentle dissection and curettage. The surrounding thickened arachnoid usually protects cranial nerves, brainstem, and vessels, except in reoperations, when this protection has been previously transgressed. In these reoperations, the tumor may surround cranial nerves and extend between brainstem arteries and the pia. Aggressive resection then risks cranial nerve injury and brainstem stroke from injury to perforating arteries. The sinewy portion requires more sharp dissection because the plane between tumor and the surrounding soft tissue is often obscured by tumor invasion. Whenever possible, thickened and thus potentially infiltrated dura and extradural soft tissue should be excised.

Chondrosarcomas are more discrete and thus often are more completely resectable than chordomas. Some chondrosarcomas may be heavily calcified and firmly fixed to the skull. These can be removed only by fragmenting them or by drilling. Before these calcified fragments are manipulated, it is essential to first identify and dissect tumor from adjacent cranial nerves and critical vessels. Incorporation of cranial nerves or vessels within the calcified tumor may warrant subtotal resection to preserve function.

Adherence to some basic principles helps reduce the incidence of surgical complications (**Figs. 9.3, 9.4,** and

9.5). First, removal of bone is almost always preferable to retracting brain as a means of gaining exposure, with the exposure only as large as is required to remove the tumor. The more extensive the dissection, the greater is the risk to cranial nerves, vessels, and dura (**Fig. 9.3**).

Second, for tumors with intradural extension, the dural defect must be closed securely, especially when the approach traverses the nose or oral cavity. Removal of involved bone and dura in transnasal, expanded, extended transsphenoidal approaches can often be complicated by CSF rhinorrhea and meningitis.[56] Historically, these occurred in 10 to 50% of patients who had tumors with a significant intradural component. These complications can be minimized by a meticulous, multilayered closure, preferably one in which at least one layer is vascularized. Dural openings should be sutured primarily if possible, or closed with autologous fascia or dural substitute if primary closure is not feasible. If a graft cannot be sewn in, an inlay graft of dural substitute or fascia should be placed such that its edges lie deep to the margins of the dural opening. This is then covered with a thin layer of tissue adhesive followed by an onlay graft of fascia or dural substitute. This onlay graft can be held snugly in gasket seal fashion by a firm plate (thin bone or cartilage, polyethylene glycol plate, or titanium wire mesh) wedged beneath the margins of the bone opening[66] (**Fig. 9.4**). The plate can then be covered with more tissue adhesive followed by vascularized soft tissue, such as the Hadad-Bassagasteguy flap (nasal septal pedicled mucosa fed by the posterior nasal artery)[67] in transnasal approaches, pericranium for subfrontal craniotomies, or temporalis fascia and muscle for lateral approaches (**Fig. 9.4**). Insecurely repaired large openings mandate temporary drainage of CSF through a ventriculostomy or lumbar drain.

Third, dissection should be meticulous. Approaches to these tumors frequently require maneuvering around the internal carotid and basilar arteries and cranial nerves. Adherence to microsurgical techniques, facilitated by endoscopic illumination, magnification, and angulation, permits safe tumor removal (**Fig. 9.5**). Inadvertent injury to the basilar and internal carotid arteries or their branches can be catastrophic. Similarly, the greatest care must be taken to avoid injury to the cranial nerves. Close attention to anatomic keys is essential.[60] Neuronavigation techniques are very helpful.[68] The pseudoencapsulated nature of both chordomas and chondrosarcomas and the soft consistency of the intradural extensions of chordomas facilitate separation of tumor from nerves and blood ves-

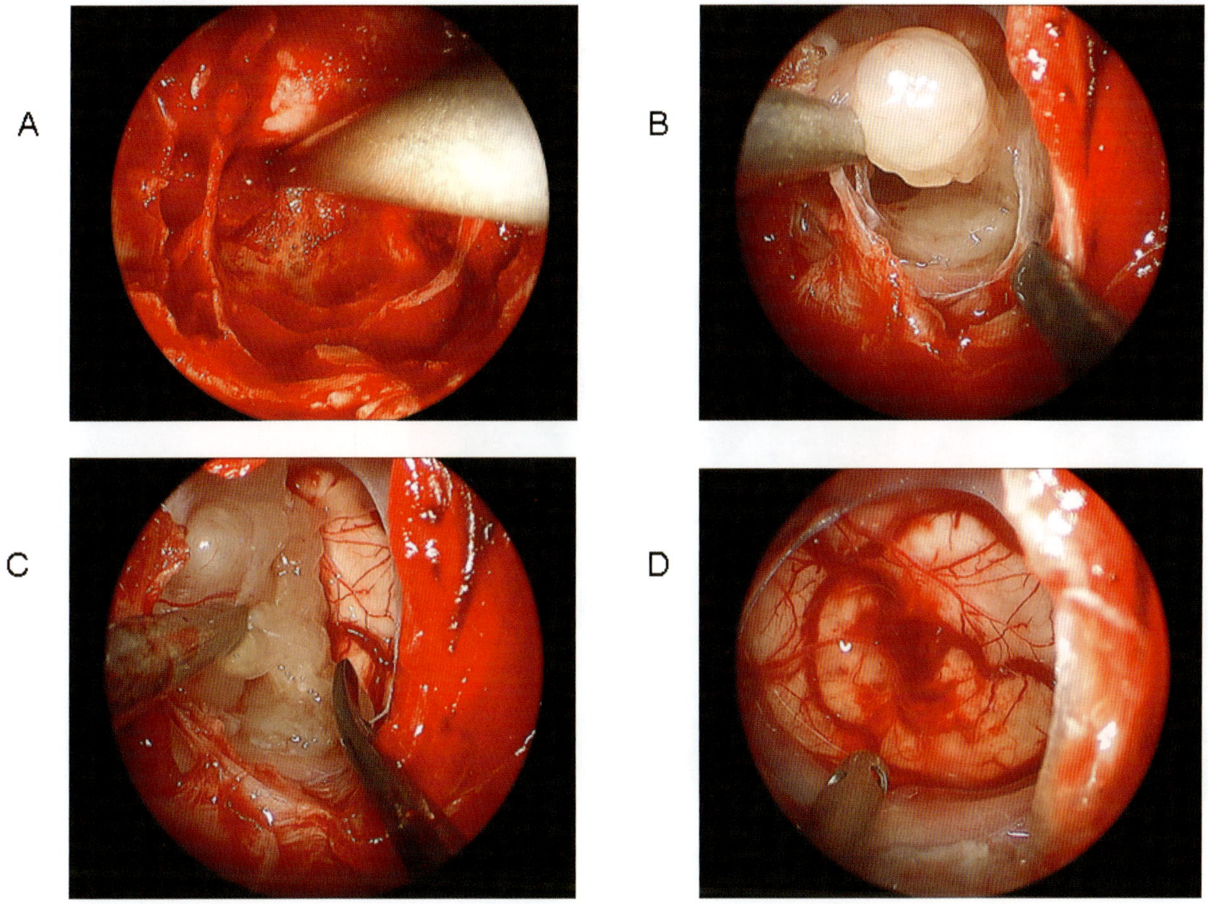

Fig. 9.3 Removal of a clival chordoma. **(A)** Extradural tumor (depicted radiographically in **Fig. 9.2**) is removed, and the mid clivus is drilled away. **(B)** The dura is opened, and intradural tumor is debulked. **(C)** Tumor is dissected from the brainstem. **(D)** Pons, after tumor removal, with basilar artery traversing inferiorly.

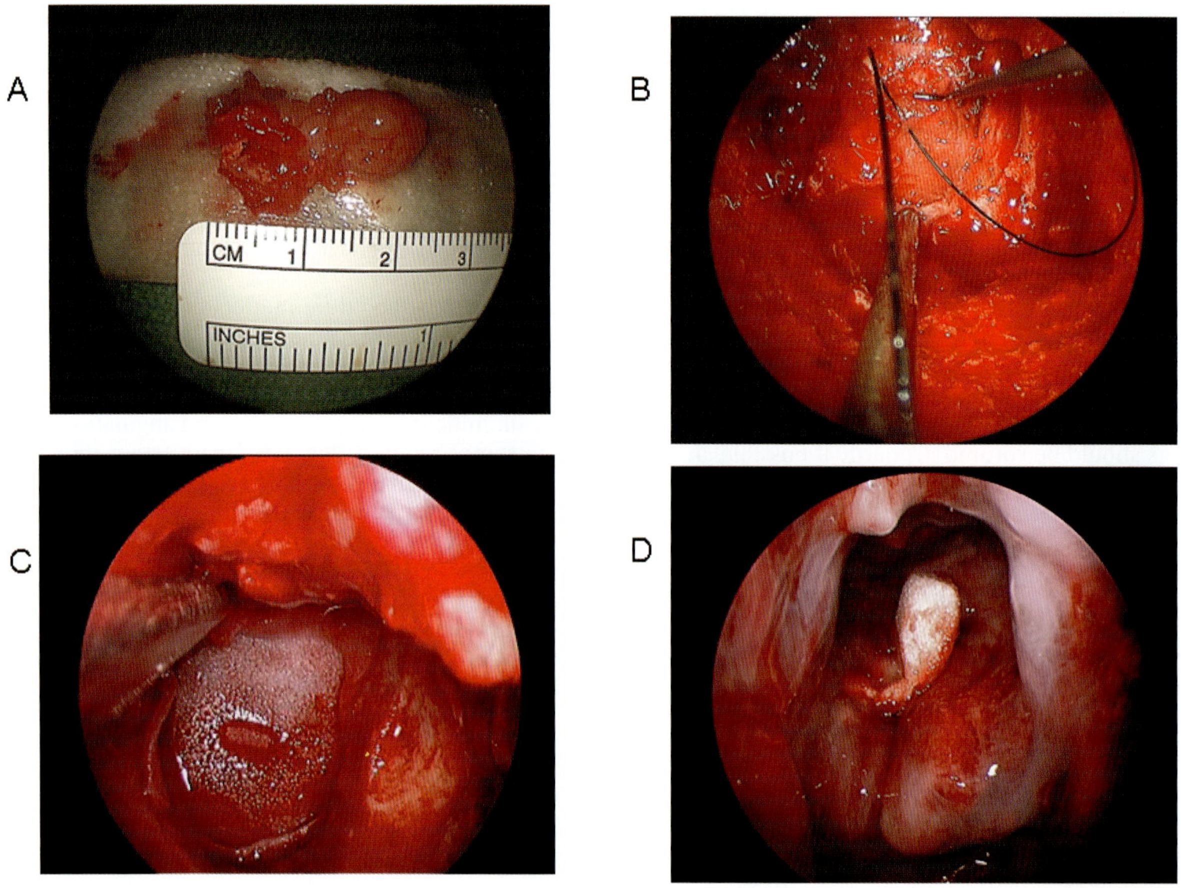

Fig. 9.4 Repair after resection of a clival chordoma. **(A)** Tumor specimen (removed as shown in **Fig. 9.3**). **(B)** Inlay graft of dural repair matrix. **(C)** A gasket seal closure with dural repair matrix and a polyethylene glycol plate. **(D)** A pedicled septal mucosal flap placed over the closure.

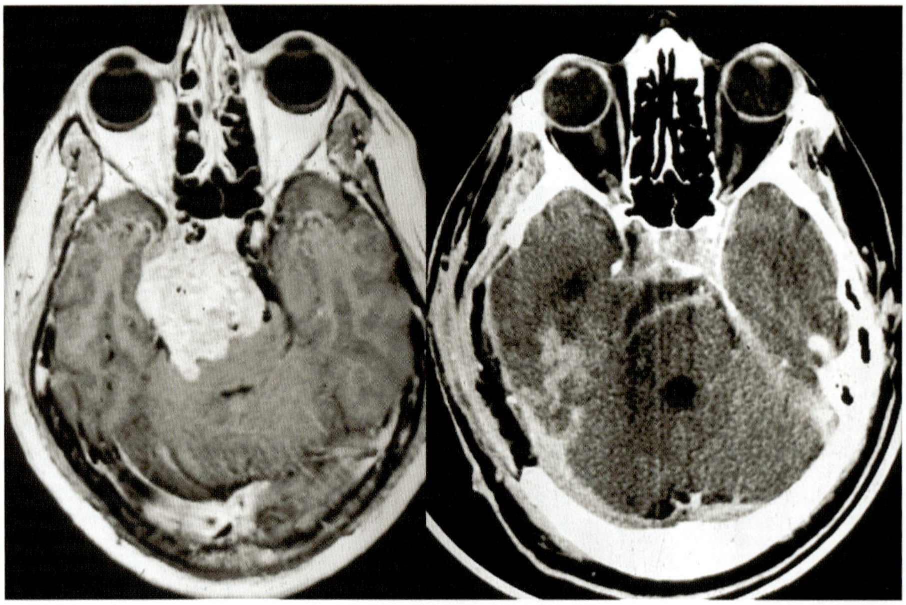

Fig. 9.5 Parasellar petroclival chondrosarcoma. **(A)** Contrast-enhanced axial preoperative MRI and **(B)** postoperative CT scans of a parasellar chondrosarcoma of the right posteroinferior cavernous sinus and petrous apex invaginating the pons and enveloping the basilar artery in a patient with intact hearing. The tumor was removed by a transpetrosal, retrolabyrinthine approach in which hearing was preserved.

sels. These structures are more likely to be displaced than invaded. The exception occurs at neural foramina, where nerves, surrounded by tumor-infiltrated bone, are most vulnerable to injury. Here and in the cavernous sinuses, it is sometimes preferable to leave small deposits of tumor rather than risk injury to a cranial nerve. Intentional sacrifice of a cranial nerve is almost never justified by a desire to obtain a complete resection of tumor because residual tumor can be treated by postoperative radiation therapy.

Fourth, the intent of surgery, as formulated preoperatively, must always be kept in mind. Not infrequently, the goal of surgery is to remove sufficient tumor to optimize the geometry of the tumor bed for subsequent radiation therapy. Because radiation exposure of the brainstem or optic pathways is the most common factor limiting the dose that can be given to these tumors, the primary indication of surgery is the removal of tumor invaginating the brainstem and in proximity to the optic nerves or chiasm (**Fig. 9.6**). Reduction of tumor mass is helpful in reducing radiation target volume, but the advantage conferred by reducing the tumor burden decreases at low tumor volumes[69] (**Table 9.3**). This diminishing return, coupled with the relatively indolent growth of low-grade chondrosarcomas and the microscopically invasive nature of chordomas and of higher-grade chondrosarcomas, makes aggressive efforts at total resection ill advised (**Fig. 9.7**).

Surgical Outcomes

Most studies of skull base chordomas and chondrosarcomas offer evidence that surgical resection helps extend survival.[22,36,57,70–76] Jawad and Scully[70] reviewed 962 treated chordomas. They found that size less than 8 cm, age younger than 59 years, Hispanic ethnicity, and surgical resection were all independent predictors of longer survival. Durations of survival were very similar for patients with "inoperable" disease and those for whom "surgery was recommended but not performed," suggesting that the benefits of surgery were not necessarily attributable to selection bias. In another series of 51 patients with intracranial chordomas, the 40 patients whose tumors were resected (partially or completely) were more likely to survive 5 years (55%) than were the 11 whose tumors were only biopsied (36%).[36] A more complete resection may also be associated with a better outcome than a less aggressive approach.[10,74] There are a few reports of long-term disease-free survival following radical resection alone.[10,77] These studies support attempting radical surgical resection in all patients in whom it is feasible.

Some surgical series in which radical resection was followed by radiation therapy report even better rates of tumor control. In one series of 60 patients (46 chordomas and 14 low-grade chondrosarcomas), no tumor recurrence was found in 80% at 3 years and 76% at 5 years after surgery.[10] Patients with chondrosarcomas did better than those with chordomas (5-year recurrence-free survival rates of 90% and 65%, respectively). However, 11 patients died during the postoperative follow-up period: 3 of systemic complications within 3 months of surgery, 5 of tumor recurrence, 1 of unrelated causes, and 2 of late complications of radiotherapy. The rates of nonlethal complications, such as CSF fistula, meningitis, and cranial nerve deficits, were also significant. This experience suggests that aggressive attempts to remove all tumor must be justified by both longer patient survival and avoidance of serious neurologic and functional compromise.[10,44]

Morbidity and mortality rates for surgical resection of chondrosarcomas are similar to those for chordomas. Some authors argue that complete excision of a low-grade chon-

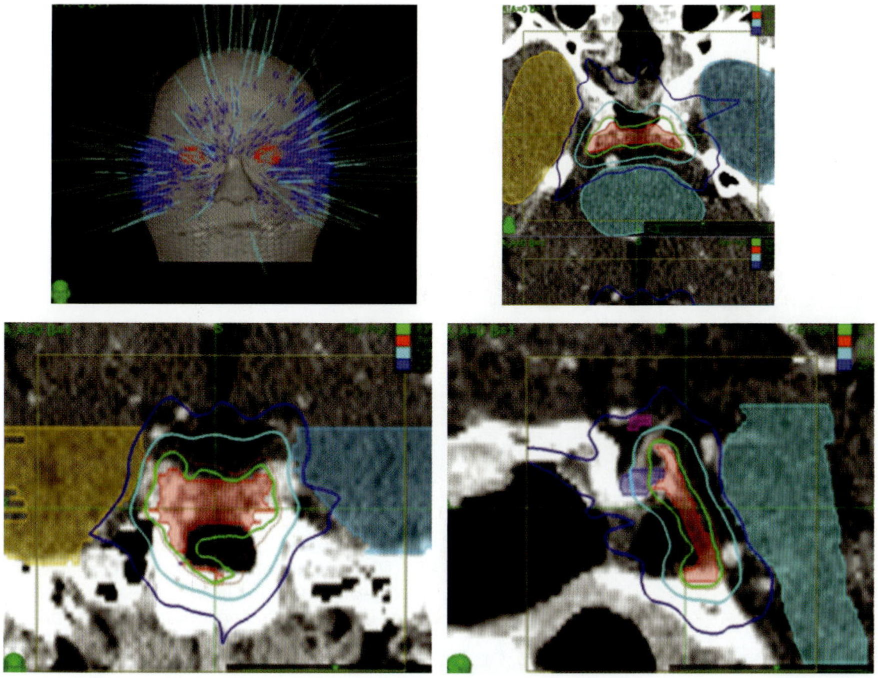

Fig. 9.6 Postoperative CyberKnife plan for chordoma. The resection field in the same patient shown in **Figs. 9.2** through **9.4** was treated with 35 Gy in five fractions, the equivalent of 80 Gy in 2-Gy fractions. Dose to the brainstem surface was less than 22 Gy in five fractions, the equivalent of 35 Gy in 2-Gy fractions.

Table 9.3 Surgical Series

No. patients	Tumor type(s)	Surgical resection	Radiation therapy	Complications	Outcome	Author (year)
38	Chordoma					Watkins et al (1993)
17	8 Chordoma 9 CS	GTR 53%	XRT 59%			Sen et al (1989)
60	46 Chordoma 14 CS	67% GTR or NTR	XRT 8%, P-P 10%, SRS 2%	30% CSF leak, 10% meningitis, 40% decreased Karnofsky score	84% recurrence-free for 5 years with TR, 64% with STR	Gay et al (1995)
51	Chordoma (19 chondroid)	11 BX 40 STR	XRT 76%		51% 5-year survival	Forsyth et al (1993)
25	Chordoma	GTR 43%, NTR 48%, STR 9%	P–P 74%, XRT 9%	Stroke, CN III palsy, hemianopia	4 died, 5 with recurrence, 16 recurrence-free	Al-Mefty & Borba (1998)
13	10 Chordoma 1 CS	Pedicled rhinotomy, subtotal	P-P	Palatal tear, CSF leak ± meningitis, lacrimal sac injury		Ojemann et al (1995)
36	Chordoma	GTR or NTR in 62%	22%	No CSF leak, meningitis, or new CN deficit	14% 5-year mortality, 19% recurrence	Menezes et al (1997)

Abbreviations: BX, biopsy; CN, cranial nerve; CS, chondrosarcoma; GTR, gross total resection; NTR, near-total resection; P-P, proton-photon radiotherapy; SRS, stereotactic radiosurgery; STR, subtotal resection; TR, total resection; XRT, conventional radiotherapy.

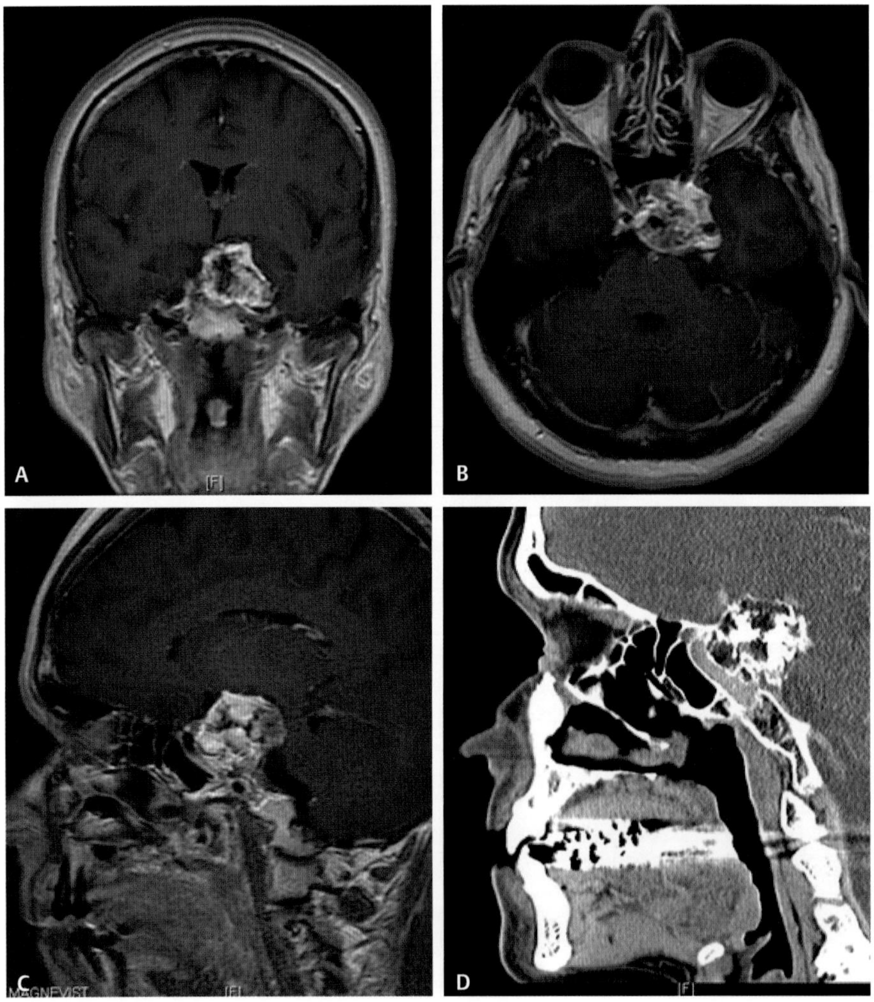

Fig. 9.7 Contraindications to surgery. Attachment of firm, calcified tumor to critical arteries can preclude safe total tumor removal. **(A–C)** MRI, T1 with contrast and **(D)** CT scan of sellar and parasellar chondrosarcoma. This lesion is heavily calcified, as evidenced by the low signal areas on MRI and the high density on CT. The left internal carotid artery is encased by tumor.

drosarcoma obviates the need for postoperative irradiation. Among patients who underwent complete resection of their tumor but not postoperative radiation therapy, 78.3% experienced 5 years of recurrence-free survival.[25,78] A superior outcome for even completely resected tumors following surgery and high-dose radiation therapy argues for the use of adjuvant radiotherapy.

◆ Radiation Therapy

The risk for microscopic residual tumor even after complete gross tumor resection is very high for almost all chordomas and for many chondrosarcomas. Local regrowth of these tumors in the skull base is not unusual, even after aggressive surgical treatment. Postoperative radiation therapy targeting the entire tumor volume is therefore indicated for all chordomas, incompletely resected low-grade chondrosarcomas, and higher-grade chondrosarcomas. Multiple clinical series document longer survival of patients with this approach.[1,5,6,10,36,79–87] One meta-analysis of 464 chordomas with a mean follow-up of 39 months found that younger age, chondroid histology, and treatment with surgery and radiation correlated with lower recurrence rates.[79]

The efficacy of radiation therapy of chordomas and chondrosarcomas is highly dependent on the dose delivered.[35,88,89] Lower doses of 45 to 60 Gy are associated with poor rates of progression-free and overall survival. Recurrence rates of 50 to 100% have been reported in chordomas treated with conventional irradiation.[85,86] Higher-dose radiation (66–84 Gy) can delay or prevent recurrence. The goal is to deliver these higher doses in a highly conformal way to maximally target tumor volume but spare adjacent radiosensitive structures from exposure beyond their tolerance. Exclusion of the optic nerve and chiasm at 55 to 60 CGE[90] (cobalt gray equivalent) may protect vision, and exclusion of the pituitary at 50 CGE may prevent endocrinopathies.[91]

Irradiation techniques include intensity modulation radiotherapy, conventionally fractionated radiotherapy, external beam photon radiation, particle beam radiotherapy, and stereotactic radiosurgery.

Intensity modulation radiotherapy modulates the dose intensity pattern of conventionally fractionated radiation to match the tumor shape. In one series of chondrosarcomas, postoperative fractionated radiotherapy provided a 5-year recurrence-free survival rate of 100%.[92]

Takahashi et al[81] reported the results of carbon ion radiation therapy in 9 of 32 patients following aggressive resection of a skull base chordoma. The 3-year recurrence-free survival rate following carbon ion therapy was 70%, compared with 57.1% after conventional radiotherapy and 7.1% in the untreated group.

Conformal proton radiation has been delivered to chordomas in high doses ranging from 66.6 to 79.2 CGE (median, 68.9 CGE).[87,92,93] A recent review of 416 chordomas treated with proton beam therapy in seven uncontrolled single-arm studies[87] found better outcomes and fewer complications for proton beam than had been reported for conventional radiation. In the largest single-institution proton beam series, the 5-year local tumor control rate was 54% for 125 chordomas and 98% for 130 low-grade chondrosarcomas.[93] Favorable prognostic factors for the long-term control of chordomas were male gender, small tumor volume, and high minimum dose. In another study, mixed photon-proton beam irradiation of chordomas to 75.6 to 82.9 CGE yielded 5- and 10-year local recurrence-free survival rates of 64% and 42%, respectively.[94] For chondrosarcomas treated with 66 to 83 CGE, the 5- and 10-year local recurrence-free survival rates were 97% and 92%, respectively.[94] In these proton series, relapse was overwhelmingly local. After local relapse, the actuarial rates of survival for patients with chordomas were 44% at 3 years and 5% at 5 years.[95]

Stereotactic radiosurgery targets high doses of X-rays from a linear accelerator (LINAC) or CyberKnife or gamma rays from cobalt sources (gamma knife) to a tumor in one to five treatment sessions. This precisely targets tumor very close (within 2–3 mm) to critical structures[96] (**Fig. 9.8**). Because the risk for injury rises with targeted volume, radiosurgery is usually limited to tumor volumes less than 10 cm^3. Radiosurgery may be particularly useful in treating small unresectable residual or recurrent chondrosarcomas or chordomas.[97]

Henderson et al[82] reported excellent outcomes following CyberKnife therapy of 24 tumors. They recommended a dose of 40 Gy in five sessions to the clinical treatment volume, defined as the gross tumor volume and a 1-cm margin. In another radiosurgical series including both types of tumor, 3 of 15 patients died of local tumor recurrence outside the target volume, and one died of intercurrent disease. Of the 11 surviving patients, 10 had tumors that were unchanged or smaller during the mean 4-year follow-up period. No neurologic or endocrine toxicity was observed.[96] This series highlights the challenges these tumors pose for radiosurgery. Unlike benign encapsulated tumors (eg, meningiomas and vestibular schwannomas) or metastases (which are usually spherical), chordomas and chondrosarcomas are irregularly invasive. These tumors are often quite large at diagnosis and even after aggressive resection may present a large volume at risk for recurrence. The microscopic and even gross tumor limits can be challenging to define radiographically. Once the target is determined, the irregular shape of the tumor and limits created by adjacent critical structures (optic pathways, brainstem) require complicated multiple isocenter treatment plans. Longer follow-up of larger number of patients is needed to confirm the role of radiosurgery in these tumors with a marked propensity to recur locally.

The risk for neurologic damage, such as brainstem injury and death, visual field loss, and hypopituitarism, is associated with all modalities of radiation therapy.[69,91,98] Although newer, more conformal radiation strategies improve efficacy and lower morbidity, local recurrence is common, and many patients, especially those with chordomas, will suffer from the side effects of treatment.

◆ Tumor Recurrence

Almost all chordomas and some chondrosarcomas recur despite radical resection and radiation therapy. In most cases, recurrence will eventually prove fatal. When tu-

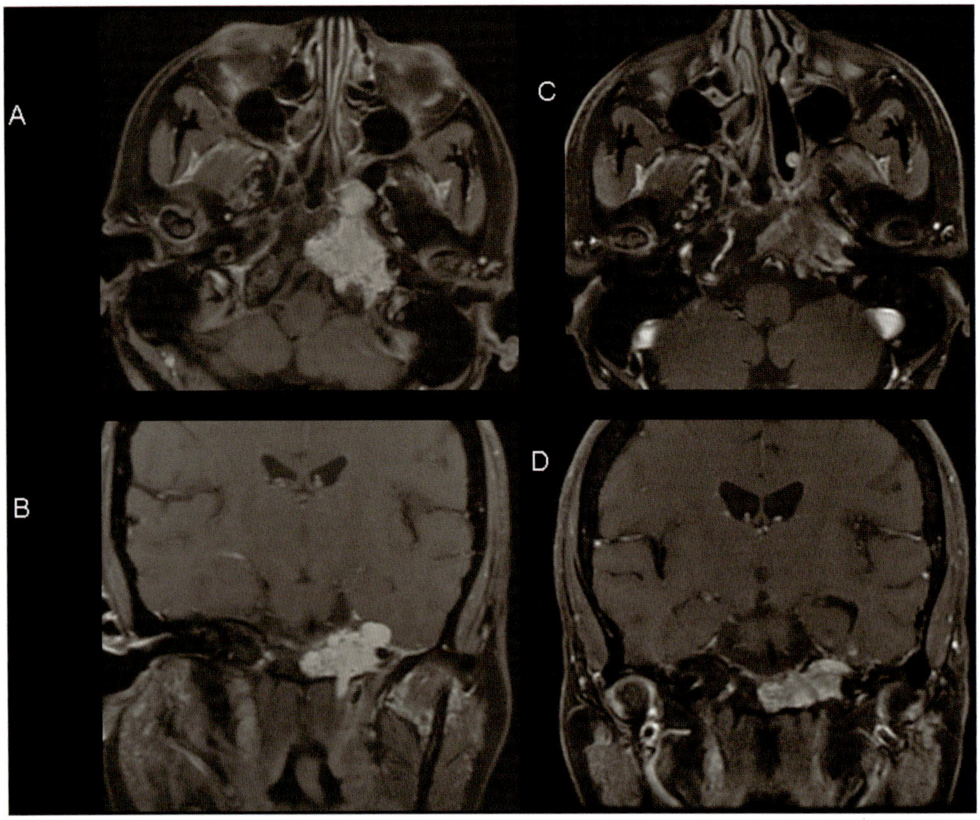

Fig. 9.8 Stereotactic radiosurgery for parasellar chondrosarcoma. Radiosurgery may be an alternative for tumors that cannot be removed safely. **(A,B)** MRI before and **(C,D)** 3 years after treatment with 30 Gy in five fractions shows a marked reduction in tumor bulk and intensity of enhancement, consistent with an excellent response to treatment.

mors recur, radiotherapy is offered for those that have not been previously irradiated. Repeat resection to reduce the tumor volume and alleviate brainstem compression may be needed. Surgery for previously resected tumors carries a higher incidence of complications,[10] but when previously irradiated tumors recur, repeat surgical resection is often the only choice. In one series, patients with relapse of any kind after proton radiation had actuarial survival rates of 43% at 3 years and 7% at 5 years. Local relapse carried actuarial survival rates of 44% at 3 years and 5% at 5 years and distant recurrence rates of 25% and 12%, respectively. Reoperation on 49 of 60 patients with locally recurrent tumor produced disease stabilization in 26 (53%) and yielded actuarial survival rates of 63% at 2 years and 6% at 5 years, compared with a 2-year survival rate of 21% for those receiving only supportive care.[95] Therefore, reoperation is of value in surgically accessible tumor recurrence, even though it is associated with greater risks and has less survival benefit than primary surgery. Stereotactic radiosurgery, too, may be useful for tumor recurrence. Ito et al[80] recently reported using gamma knife therapy in patients who had recurrent disease following aggressive resection of a clival chordoma. Among 19 patients who underwent surgery, 11 had recurrence. Patients with recurrent tumors, some of whom received reoperation, underwent gamma knife treatment. At a mean follow-up of 71 months, tumor control was achieved in all 11 patients with recurrence.

◆ Chemotherapy

Chemotherapy is usually reserved for surgically inaccessible, previously irradiated recurrent tumor or for metastatic disease. As advances in surgery and radiotherapy have improved rates of local control, the effective treatment of metastatic disease has become increasingly important. Up to one-third of patients with chordomas develop distant metastases,[19,99,100] most commonly to the lungs, liver, and bones.[2] Historically, chemotherapy has had poor efficacy.[101] Newer agents such as imatinib mesylate, a tyrosine kinase inhibitor that targets several enzymes and a growth factor expressed in chordomas, may offer improved outcomes.[102] A recent case report noted marked regression of a recurrent chordoma following intratumoral injection of carboplatinum.[103]

◆ Conclusion

Chordomas and chondrosarcomas of the sellar and parasellar region are rare (**Table 9.4**). The relative inaccessibility of these areas of the skull base, the proximity of the tumors to critical neurovascular structures, their relative insensitivity to radiation and chemotherapy, and their propensity to recur locally make them very challenging to treat. Treatment strategies are complex and require meticulous planning and execution of surgery and high-dose radiation therapy. Such an approach can offer cure for almost all low-grade chondrosarcomas and provide meaningful control of chordomas and high-grade chondrosarcomas.

Table 9.4 Key Points

• Chordomas and chondrosarcomas of the sella and parasellar areas are rare.
• Although they are often grouped together because of location and bony origin, chordomas and chondrosarcomas are distinct in embryology, pathology, clinical course, and response to therapy.
• The initial course of both tumors is insidious, reflecting slow, locally invasive growth; tumor enlargement threatens cranial nerve function and may compress the brainstem.
• A combination of surgery and high-dose postoperative radiation therapy is the preferred treatment; this cures almost all low-grade chondrosarcomas and controls many chordomas and higher-grade chondrosarcomas for a mean of ~5 years.
• Advances in skull base surgery, especially transnasal endoscopic approaches, provide improved access to tumors in these locations.
• Modern radiation techniques permit more conformal therapy, which results in greater efficacy with lower morbidity.
• Local recurrence is common for most chordomas and high-grade chondrosarcomas and is usually eventually lethal.
• Chemotherapy has historically been ineffective; newer agents targeting molecular mechanisms of tumor growth offer hope for improved efficacy.

References

1. Heffelfinger MJ, Dahlin DC, MacCarty CS, Beabout JW. Chordomas and cartilaginous tumors at the skull base. Cancer 1973; 32(2):410–420
2. O'Neill P, Bell BA, Miller JD, Jacobson I, Guthrie W. Fifty years of experience with chordomas in southeast Scotland. Neurosurgery 1985;16(2):166–170
3. McMaster ML, Goldstein AM, Bromley CM, Ishibe N, Parry DM. Chordoma: incidence and survival patterns in the United States, 1973–1995. Cancer Causes Control 2001;12(1):1–11
4. Wold LE, Laws ER Jr. Cranial chordomas in children and young adults. J Neurosurg 1983;59(6):1043–1047
5. Borba LA, Al-Mefty O, Mrak RE, Suen J. Cranial chordomas in children and adolescents. J Neurosurg 1996;84(4):584–591
6. Watkins L, Khudados ES, Kaleoglu M, Revesz T, Sacares P, Crockard HA. Skull base chordomas: a review of 38 patients, 1958-88. Br J Neurosurg 1993;7(3):241–248
7. Yang XR, Beerman M, Bergen AW, et al. Corroboration of a familial chordoma locus on chromosome 7q and evidence of genetic heterogeneity using single nucleotide polymorphisms (SNPs). Int J Cancer 2005;116(3):487–491
8. Borba LAB, Al-Mefty O. Skull base chordoma. Contemp Neurosurg 1998;20(13):1–6
9. Oguro K, Nakahara N, Yamaguchi Y, Shimabukuro H, Masuzawa T. Chondrosarcoma of the posterior fossa—case report. Neurol Med Chir (Tokyo) 1989;29(11):1030–1038
10. Gay E, Sekhar LN, Rubinstein E, et al. Chordomas and chondrosarcomas of the cranial base: results and follow-up of 60 patients. Neurosurgery 1995;36(5):887–896, discussion 896–897
11. Koch BB, Karnell LH, Hoffman HT, et al. National cancer database report on chondrosarcoma of the head and neck. Head Neck 2000;22(4):408–425
12. Rosenberg AE, Nielsen GP, Keel SB, et al. Chondrosarcoma of the base of the skull: a clinicopathologic study of 200 cases with emphasis on its distinction from chordoma. Am J Surg Pathol 1999;23(11):1370–1378
13. Korten AG, ter Berg HJ, Spincemaille GH, van der Laan RT, Van de Wel AM. Intracranial chondrosarcoma: review of the literature and report of 15 cases. J Neurol Neurosurg Psychiatry 1998; 65(1):88–92
14. Sekhar LN, Nanda A, Sen CN, Snyderman CN, Janecka IP. The extended frontal approach to tumors of the anterior, middle, and posterior skull base. J Neurosurg 1992;76(2):198–206
15. Thodou E, Kontogeorgos G, Scheithauer BW, et al. Intrasellar chordomas mimicking pituitary adenoma. J Neurosurg 2000;92(6): 976–982
16. Campbell WM, McDonald TJ, Unni KK, Laws ER Jr. Nasal and paranasal presentations of chordomas. Laryngoscope 1980;90(4):612–618
17. Steenberghs J, Kiekens C, Menten J, Monstrey J. Intradural chordoma without bone involvement. Case report and review of the literature. J Neurosurg 2002;97(1, Suppl):94–97
18. Inoue T, Takahashi N, Murakami K, Nishimura S, Kaimori M, Nishijima M. Osteochondroma of the sella turcica presenting with intratumoral hemorrhage. Neurol Med Chir (Tokyo) 2009;49(1):37–41
19. Laws ER. Parasellar lesions other than pituitary adenomas. In: The Management of Pituitary Tumors: a Handbook. Churchill-Livingstone; 1996:175–222
20. Krol G, Sze G, Arbit E, Marcove R, Sundaresan N. Intradural metastases of chordoma. AJNR Am J Neuroradiol 1989;10(1):193–195
21. Naumann S, Krallman PA, Unni KK, Fidler ME, Neff JR, Bridge JA. Translocation der(13;21)(q10;q10) in skeletal and extraskeletal mesenchymal chondrosarcoma. Mod Pathol 2002;15(5): 572–576
22. Hassounah M, Al-Mefty O, Akhtar M, Jinkins JR, Fox JL. Primary cranial and intracranial chondrosarcoma. A survey. Acta Neurochir (Wien) 1985;78(3-4):123–132
23. Tachibana E, Saito K, Takahashi M, Fukuta K, Yoshida J. Surgical treatment of a massive chondrosarcoma in the skull base associated with Maffucci's syndrome: a case report. Surg Neurol 2000;54(2):165–169, discussion 169–170
24. Crockard HA, Steel T, Plowman N, et al. A multidisciplinary team approach to skull base chordomas. J Neurosurg 2001;95(2):175–183
25. Crockard HA, Cheeseman A, Steel T, et al. A multidisciplinary team approach to skull base chondrosarcomas. J Neurosurg 2001;95(2):184–189
26. Stapleton SR, Wilkins PR, Archer DJ, Uttley D. Chondrosarcoma of the skull base: a series of eight cases. Neurosurgery 1993; 32(3):348–355, discussion 355–356
27. Oakley GJ, Fuhrer K, Seethala RR. Brachyury, SOX-9, and podoplanin, new markers in the skull base chordoma vs chondrosarcoma differential: a tissue microarray-based comparative analysis. Mod Pathol 2008;21(12):1461–1469
28. Richardson MS. Pathology of skull base tumors. Otolaryngol Clin North Am 2001;34(6):1025–1042, vii

29. Bouropoulou V, Bosse A, Roessner A, et al. Immunohistochemical investigation of chordomas: histogenetic and differential diagnostic aspects. Curr Top Pathol 1989;80:183–203
30. Brooks JJ, Trojanowski JQ, LiVolsi VA. Chondroid chordoma: a low-grade chondrosarcoma and its differential diagnosis. Curr Top Pathol 1989;80:165–181
31. Coltrera MD, Googe PB, Harrist TJ, Hyams VJ, Schiller AL, Goodman ML. Chondrosarcoma of the temporal bone. Diagnosis and treatment of 13 cases and review of the literature. Cancer 1986;58(12):2689–2696
32. Bourgouin PM, Tampieri D, Robitaille Y, et al. Low-grade myxoid chondrosarcoma of the base of the skull: CT, MR, and histopathology. J Comput Assist Tomogr 1992;16(2):268–273
33. Evans HL, Ayala AG, Romsdahl MM. Prognostic factors in chondrosarcoma of bone: a clinicopathologic analysis with emphasis on histologic grading. Cancer 1977;40(2):818–831
34. Finn DG, Goepfert H, Batsakis JG. Chondrosarcoma of the head and neck. Laryngoscope 1984;94(12 Pt 1):1539–1544
35. Raffel C, Wright DC, Gutin PH, Wilson CB. Cranial chordomas: clinical presentation and results of operative and radiation therapy in twenty-six patients. Neurosurgery 1985;17(5):703–710
36. Forsyth PA, Cascino TL, Shaw EG, et al. Intracranial chordomas: a clinicopathological and prognostic study of 51 cases. J Neurosurg 1993;78(5):741–747
37. Kamrin RP, Potanos JN, Pool JL. An evaluation of the diagnosis and treatment of chordoma. J Neurol Neurosurg Psychiatry 1964; 27:157–165
38. Mitchell A, Scheithauer BW, Unni KK, Forsyth PJ, Wold LE, McGivney DJ. Chordoma and chondroid neoplasms of the spheno-occiput. An immunohistochemical study of 41 cases with prognostic and nosologic implications. Cancer 1993;72(10): 2943–2949
39. Oot RF, Melville GE, New PF, et al. The role of MR and CT in evaluating clival chordomas and chondrosarcomas. AJR Am J Roentgenol 1988;151(3):567–575
40. Doucet V, Peretti-Viton P, Figarella-Branger D, Manera L, Salamon G. MRI of intracranial chordomas. Extent of tumour and contrast enhancement: criteria for differential diagnosis. Neuroradiology 1997;39(8):571–576
41. Larson TC III, Houser OW, Laws ER Jr. Imaging of cranial chordomas. Mayo Clin Proc 1987;62(10):886–893
42. Meyers SP, Hirsch WL Jr, Curtin HD, Barnes L, Sekhar LN, Sen C. Chordomas of the skull base: MR features. AJNR Am J Neuroradiol 1992;13(6):1627–1636
43. Goel A. Chordoma and chondrosarcoma: relationship to the internal carotid artery. Acta Neurochir (Wien) 1995;133(1-2):30–35
44. Almefty K, Pravdenkova S, Colli BO, Al-Mefty O, Gokden M. Chordoma and chondrosarcoma: similar, but quite different, skull base tumors. Cancer 2007;110(11):2457–2467
45. Frank G, Sciarretta V, Calbucci F, Farneti G, Mazzatenta D, Pasquini E. The endoscopic transnasal transsphenoidal approach for the treatment of cranial base chordomas and chondrosarcomas. Neurosurgery 2006;59(1, Suppl 1):ONS50–ONS57
46. Harsh GR IV, Joseph MP, Swearingen B, Ojemann RG. Anterior midline approaches to the central skull base. Clin Neurosurg 1996;43:15–43
47. Sen CN, Sekhar LN. An extreme lateral approach to intradural lesions of the cervical spine and foramen magnum. Neurosurgery 1990;27(2):197–204
48. Laws ER Jr. Transsphenoidal surgery for tumors of the clivus. Otolaryngol Head Neck Surg 1984;92(1):100–101
49. Fraioli B, Esposito V, Santoro A, Iannetti G, Giuffrè R, Cantore G. Transmaxillosphenoidal approach to tumors invading the medial compartment of the cavernous sinus. J Neurosurg 1995;82(1):63–69
50. Couldwell WT, Weiss MH, Rabb C, Liu JK, Apfelbaum RI, Fukushima T. Variations on the standard transsphenoidal approach to the sellar region, with emphasis on the extended approaches and parasellar approaches: surgical experience in 105 cases. Neurosurgery 2004;55(3):539–547, discussion 547–550
51. Laws ER, Kanter AS, Jane JA Jr, Dumont AS. Extended transsphenoidal approach. J Neurosurg 2005;102(5):825–827, discussion 827–828
52. Cavallo LM, Cappabianca P, Messina A, et al. The extended endoscopic endonasal approach to the clivus and cranio-vertebral junction: anatomical study. Childs Nerv Syst 2007;23(6): 665–671
53. Jho HD, Ha HG. Endoscopic endonasal skull base surgery: Part 3—The clivus and posterior fossa. Minim Invasive Neurosurg 2004; 47(1):16–23
54. Dehdashti AR, Karabatsou K, Ganna A, Witterick I, Gentili F. Expanded endoscopic endonasal approach for treatment of clival chordomas: early results in 12 patients. Neurosurgery 2008;63(2):299–307, discussion 307–309
55. Fatemi N, Dusick JR, Gorgulho AA, et al. Endonasal microscopic removal of clival chordomas. Surg Neurol 2008;69(4):331–338
56. Stippler M, Gardner PA, Snyderman CH, Carrau RL, Prevedello DM, Kassam AB. Endoscopic endonasal approach for clival chordomas. Neurosurgery 2009;64(2):268–277, discussion 277–278
57. Derome PJ. Surgical management of tumours invading the skull base. Can J Neurol Sci 1985;12(4):345–347
58. Crockard HA. The transoral approach to the base of the brain and upper cervical cord. Ann R Coll Surg Engl 1985;67(5):321–325
59. Babu RP, Sekhar LN, Wright DC. Extreme lateral transcondylar approach: technical improvements and lessons learned. J Neurosurg 1994;81(1):49–59
60. Kassam AB, Vescan AD, Carrau RL, et al. Expanded endonasal approach: vidian canal as a landmark to the petrous internal carotid artery. J Neurosurg 2008;108(1):177–183
61. Van Loveren HR, Mahmood A, Liu SS, Gruber D. Innovations in cranial approaches and exposures: anterolateral approaches. Clin Neurosurg 1996;43:44–52
62. Dolenc VV. Transcranial epidural approach to pituitary tumors extending beyond the sella. Neurosurgery 1997;41(3):542–550, discussion 551–552
63. Harsh GR IV, Sekhar LN. The subtemporal, transcavernous, anterior transpetrosal approach to the upper brain stem and clivus. J Neurosurg 1992;77(5):709–717
64. Kawase T, Shiobara R, Toya S. Middle fossa transpetrosal-transtentorial approaches for petroclival meningiomas. Selective pyramid resection and radicality. Acta Neurochir (Wien) 1994;129(3-4):113–120
65. Lawton MT, Daspit CP, Spetzler RF. Transpetrosal and combination approaches to skull base lesions. Clin Neurosurg 1996;43:91–112
66. Leng LZ, Brown S, Anand VK, Schwartz TH. "Gasket-seal" watertight closure in minimal-access endoscopic cranial base surgery. Neurosurgery 2008;62(5, Suppl 2):E342–E343, discussion E343
67. Hadad G, Bassagasteguy L, Carrau RL, et al. A novel reconstructive technique after endoscopic expanded endonasal approaches: vascular pedicle nasoseptal flap. Laryngoscope 2006;116(10): 1882–1886
68. Hwang PY, Ho CL. Neuronavigation using an image-guided endoscopic transnasal-sphenoethmoidal approach to clival chordomas. Neurosurgery 2007;61(5, Suppl 2):212–217, discussion 217–218
69. Hug EB, Loredo LN, Slater JD, et al. Proton radiation therapy for chordomas and chondrosarcomas of the skull base. J Neurosurg 1999;91(3):432–439
70. Jawad MU, Scully SP. Surgery significantly improves survival in patients with chordoma. Spine (Phila Pa 1976) 2010;35(1):117–123
71. Volpe R, Mazabraud A. A clinicopathologic review of 25 cases of chordoma (a pleomorphic and metastasizing neoplasm). Am J Surg Pathol 1983;7(2):161–170
72. Arnold H, Herrmann HD. Skull base chordoma with cavernous sinus involvement. Partial or radical tumour-removal? Acta Neurochir (Wien) 1986;83(1-2):31–37
73. Brooks JJ, LiVolsi VA, Trojanowski JQ. Does chondroid chordoma exist? Acta Neuropathol 1987;72(3):229–235
74. Sen CN, Sekhar LN, Schramm VL, Janecka IP. Chordoma and chondrosarcoma of the cranial base: an 8-year experience. Neurosurgery 1989;25(6):931–940, discussion 940–941
75. Rabadán A, Conesa H. Transmaxillary-transnasal approach to the anterior clivus: a microsurgical anatomical model. Neurosurgery 1992;30(4):473–481, discussion 482
76. Crockard A. Chordomas and chondrosarcomas of the cranial base: results and follow-up of 60 patients. Neurosurgery 1996;38(2):420
77. Kveton JF, Brackmann DE, Glasscock ME III, House WF, Hitselberger WE. Chondrosarcoma of the skull base. Otolaryngol Head Neck Surg 1986;94(1):23–32
78. Tzortzidis F, Elahi F, Wright DC, Temkin N, Natarajan SK, Sekhar LN. Patient outcome at long-term follow-up after aggressive mi-

crosurgical resection of cranial base chondrosarcomas. Neurosurgery 2006;58(6):1090–1098, discussion 1090–1098
79. Jian BJ, Bloch OG, Yang I, et al. Adjuvant radiation therapy and chondroid chordoma subtype are associated with a lower tumor recurrence rate of cranial chordoma. J Neurooncol 2010;98(1): 101–108
80. Ito E, Saito K, Okada T, Nagatani T, Nagasaka T. Long-term control of clival chordoma with initial aggressive surgical resection and gamma knife radiosurgery for recurrence. Acta Neurochir (Wien) 2010;152(1):57–67, discussion 67
81. Takahashi S, Kawase T, Yoshida K, Hasegawa A, Mizoe JE. Skull base chordomas: efficacy of surgery followed by carbon ion radiotherapy. Acta Neurochir (Wien) 2009;151(7):759–769
82. Henderson FC, McCool K, Seigle J, Jean W, Harter W, Gagnon GJ. Treatment of chordomas with CyberKnife: Georgetown University experience and treatment recommendations. Neurosurgery 2009;64(2, Suppl):A44–A53
83. Tai PT, Craighead P, Bagdon F. Optimization of radiotherapy for patients with cranial chordoma. A review of dose-response ratios for photon techniques. Cancer 1995;75(3):749–756
84. Thieblemont C, Biron P, Rocher F, et al. Prognostic factors in chordoma: role of postoperative radiotherapy. Eur J Cancer 1995; 31A(13–14):2255–2259
85. Catton C, O'Sullivan B, Bell R, et al. Chordoma: long-term follow-up after radical photon irradiation. Radiother Oncol 1996;41(1): 67–72
86. Cummings BJ, Hodson DI, Bush RS. Chordoma: the results of megavoltage radiation therapy. Int J Radiat Oncol Biol Phys 1983;9(5):633–642
87. Amichetti M, Cianchetti M, Amelio D, Enrici RM, Minniti G. Proton therapy in chordoma of the base of the skull: a systematic review. Neurosurg Rev 2009;32(4):403–416
88. Higinbotham NL, Phillips RF, Farr HW, Hustu HO. Chordoma. Thirty-five-year study at Memorial Hospital. Cancer 1967;20(11):1841–1850
89. Pearlman AW, Friedman M. Radical radiation therapy of chordoma. Am J Roentgenol Radium Ther Nucl Med 1970;108(2):332–341
90. Habrand IL, Austin-Seymour M, Birnbaum S, et al. Neurovisual outcome following proton radiation therapy. Int J Radiat Oncol Biol Phys 1989;16(6):1601–1606
91. Pai HH, Thornton A, Katznelson L, et al. Hypothalamic/pituitary function following high-dose conformal radiotherapy to the base of skull: demonstration of a dose-effect relationship using dose-volume histogram analysis. Int J Radiat Oncol Biol Phys 2001;49(4):1079–1092
92. Debus J, Hug EB, Liebsch NJ, et al. Brainstem tolerance to conformal radiotherapy of skull base tumors. Int J Radiat Oncol Biol Phys 1997;39(5):967–975
93. Terahara A, Niemierko A, Goitein M, et al. Analysis of the relationship between tumor dose inhomogeneity and local control in patients with skull base chordoma. Int J Radiat Oncol Biol Phys 1999;45(2):351–358
94. Munzenrider JE, Liebsch NJ. Proton therapy for tumors of the skull base. Strahlenther Onkol 1999;175(Suppl 2):57–63
95. Fagundes MA, Hug EB, Liebsch NJ, Daly W, Efird J, Munzenrider JE. Radiation therapy for chordomas of the base of skull and cervical spine: patterns of failure and outcome after relapse. Int J Radiat Oncol Biol Phys 1995;33(3):579–584
96. Muthukumar N, Kondziolka D, Lunsford LD, Flickinger JC. Stereotactic radiosurgery for chordoma and chondrosarcoma: further experiences. Int J Radiat Oncol Biol Phys 1998;41(2):387–392
97. Wanebo JE, Bristol RE, Porter RR, Coons SW, Spetzler RF. Management of cranial base chondrosarcomas. Neurosurgery 2006;58(2):249–255
98. Hug EB. Review of skull base chordomas: prognostic factors and long-term results of proton-beam radiotherapy. Neurosurg Focus 2001;10(3):E11
99. Chambers PW, Schwinn CP. Chordoma. A clinicopathologic study of metastasis. Am J Clin Pathol 1979;72(5):765–776
100. Sundaresan N, Galicich JH, Chu FC, Huvos AG. Spinal chordomas. J Neurosurg 1979;50(3):312–319
101. Castellano F, Ruggiero G. Meningiomas of the posterior fossa. Acta Radiol Suppl 1953;104:1–177
102. Casali PG, Messina A, Stacchiotti S, et al. Imatinib mesylate in chordoma. Cancer 2004;101(9):2086–2097
103. Guiu S, Guiu B, Feutray S, Chauffert B. Direct intratumoral chemotherapy with carboplatin and epinephrine in a recurrent cervical chordoma: case report. Neurosurgery 2009;65(3):E629–E630, discussion E630

10 Surgical Treatment of Rathke Cleft Cysts

Erin N. Kiehna, Spencer C. Payne, and John A. Jane Jr.

Luschka provided the earliest description of a Rathke cleft cyst (RCC) in 1860.[1] He described RCCs as "an epithelial area in the capsule of the human hypophysis resembling oral mucosa." Over the next century, they were alternately described as pituitary cysts, mucoid epithelial cysts, or colloid cysts until Frazier and Alpers finally identified them as a lesion of the Rathke cleft in 1934.[2] Just as the nomenclature varied, so did the theories of origin. RCCs were variously believed to have originated from neuroepithelium, endoderm, and metaplastic anterior pituitary cells[3–9] before they were finally identified as being derived from embryologic remnants of the Rathke pouch.[10–16]

It is now widely accepted that the Rathke pouch arises from a dorsal outpouching of the stomodeum that comes into contact with the downward outpouching of the neuroepithelium from the diencephalon. The pharyngohypophyseal trunk separates from the oral epithelium and is eventually completely severed by the sphenoid bone. The resulting pouch is lined by epithelial cells of ectodermal origin. The anterior and posterior walls become the pars distalis and pars intermedia, respectively, and the residual lumen involutes and normally regresses.[2,16] When it abnormally expands, it is known as an RCC.

On histopathologic specimen, the cyst wall is lined with a well-differentiated, ciliated columnar epithelium, which may contain goblet or ciliated cells. The cyst contents are primarily mucinoid, but appearances vary between lesions from nearly clear fluid to seemingly purulent material comprising necrotic debris.[17] Leakage of the cyst contents may result in inflammation that transforms the columnar epithelium into a stratified squamous epithelium more suggestive of a craniopharyngioma.[18,19]

◆ Prevalence

RCCs account for fewer than 1% of primary brain tumors.[20–22] The majority of RCCs are probably never symptomatic or diagnosed because there is a population incidence of 3 to 22% on autopsy studies.[1,9,15,21,23–27] Clinical series exhibit a nearly 2:1 female predominance, which is generally attributed to the fact that pituitary dysfunction is more readily apparent in females (ie, amenorrhea, galactorrhea).[15,23,24,28–31] This female predominance is not evident in autopsy series.[23] Symptomatic RCCs may be diagnosed at any age.[15,24,30,32,33]

◆ Diagnosis

Progressive enlargement of the cyst may result in symptoms of anterior lobe dysfunction, posterior lobe dysfunction, stalk compression/distortion, visual phenomena, and headaches (**Table 10.1**).[15] The duration of symptoms may range from a few days to years, with the more acute presentations likely secondary to intracystic hemorrhage or leakage of cyst contents resulting in acute inflammation.[18,29,34,35]

Headaches are generally the primary complaint in patients of any age, occurring in 70 to 85% of patients; they are most frequently frontal in location, with an average duration of 12 months before clinical diagnosis.[34–37] In their meta-analysis, Voelker et al found that children are more likely to present with hypopituitarism, including growth retardation and delay in sexual maturation, which take place over months to years.[15] Alternatively, adults usually present with symptoms of pituitary stalk, anterior pituitary, or posterior pituitary insufficiency. Men may develop decreased libido, decreased body hair, and fatigue. Premenopausal women may have amenorrhea (63%), galactorrhea (63%), or diabetes insipidus.[15,24,32,38,39] Conversely, postmenopausal women present with symptoms of panhypopituitarism, constitutional symptoms, and/or mental status changes.[15] Visual phenomena, including bitemporal hemianopsia, are also common in adults with symptoms of long-standing duration.[16] Hemianopsias or superior quadrantanopsias have been reported with RCCs as well.

◆ Endocrinologic Evaluation

Up to two-thirds of patients with RCC harbor endocrinopathies secondary to hypothalamic, adenohypophyseal, neurohypophyseal, and infundibular compression.[29,35] RCCs are associated with hyperprolactinemia secondary to pituitary stalk compression in as many as 18% of patients.[32,38,39] This is followed in frequency by hypocortisolism, hypo-

Table 10.1 Clinical Presentation and Symptomatology

Reference	Year	Headache*	Visual disturbance*	Anterior pituitary dysfunction*	Posterior pituitary dysfunction*	Hyperprolactinemia*
Voelker et al	1991	49	56	69	13	7
el-Mahdy and Powell	1998	46	46	50	14	29
Shin et al	1999	65	38	81	4	46
Benveniste et al	2004	71	20	55	5	42
Kim et al	2004	81	47	30	13	25
Weiss et al	2004	Unknown	49	53	0	18
Kanter et al	2004	86	37	60	10	22
Frank et al	2005	14	23	41	5	18
Aho et al	2005	Unknown	49	78	0	Unknown
Madhok et al	2009	81	Unknown	19	Unknown	Unknown
Kiehna et al	2010	68	21	58	0	31

*All numbers are percentages.

thyroidism, hypogonadism, and growth hormone deficiency. Hypopituitarism with more than one axis affected occurs in 10 to 15% of patients.[34] A thorough evaluation of the hypothalamic–pituitary–end-organ axis must be performed before surgery because hypocortisolemia and hypothyroidism can be associated with increased perioperative morbidity and mortality[16] (**Table 10.2**). Stress-dose hydrocortisone should be given to all patients with adrenal insufficiency at the time of surgery. Urine and serum electrolytes and osmolarity should be analyzed preoperatively and postoperatively to assess for diabetes insipidus. The hypothalamic–pituitary–end-organ axis should be checked serially in follow-up to ensure integrity.

Table 10.2 Preoperative Evaluation of Patients with Rathke Cleft Cyst

Imaging	Magnetic resonance imaging + gadolinium with pituitary sequences
	Computed tomography for bony architecture
Vision	Formal neuro-ophthalmologic examination
	Visual fields
Endocrine	Adrenocorticotropic hormone (ACTH)
	Cortisol (am)
	Follicle-stimulating hormone (FSH)
	Luteinizing hormone (LH)
	Growth hormone (GH), insulin-like growth factor 1 (IGF-1)
	Prolactin
	Thyroid-stimulating hormone (TSH), free thyroxine (T4)
	Basic metabolic panel
	Urine specific gravity and sodium

◆ Ophthalmologic Assessment

Up to one-third of patients with RCCs present with visual dysfunction.[29] Most commonly, this manifests as diminished acuity or a visual field deficit. All patients should undergo formal funduscopic, tangent screen, and perimetric testing to establish a visual baseline and assess for clinical signs of cyst growth and compression (**Table 10.2**).

◆ Diagnostic Imaging

The earliest reports of RCCs included skull radiographs demonstrating asymmetry of the sellar floor secondary to sellar erosion, with or without abnormal calcifications.[11,40,41] The advent of computed tomography (CT) more accurately depicted RCCs as well-circumscribed, hypodense to isodense cysts with rare calcification in the sella/suprasellar region.[42] Variances in densities within the cyst are likely due to variable concentrations of cholesterol crystals or mucinoid contents.[43–45] One-third to one-half of RCCs are found within the sella.[18,29,34,35] Only a small number are exclusively suprasellar.[46–49]

Magnetic resonance imaging (MRI) scan with fine cuts through the pituitary region should be performed to help differentiate an RCC from other similarly appearing lesions, such as epithelial cyst, dermoid cyst, epidermoid cyst, and craniopharyngioma.[50,51] An RCC appears as a characteristic hypointense to isointense homogeneous cyst on T1-weighted MRI that fails to enhance with contrast in the majority of patients[34,44] (**Figs. 10.1** and **10.2**). However, up to 25% of patients may show some contrast enhancement owing to cyst fluid extravasation and inflammatory changes in the capsule.[34] Hyperintense cyst fluid on T1-weighted (**Fig. 10.3**) and T2-weighted MRI often has a high protein content, and a fluid level may be present.[31,46,50,52] Patients with intracystic hemorrhage have cysts that are often hyperintense on T1 and hypointense on T2.[53] Recent studies

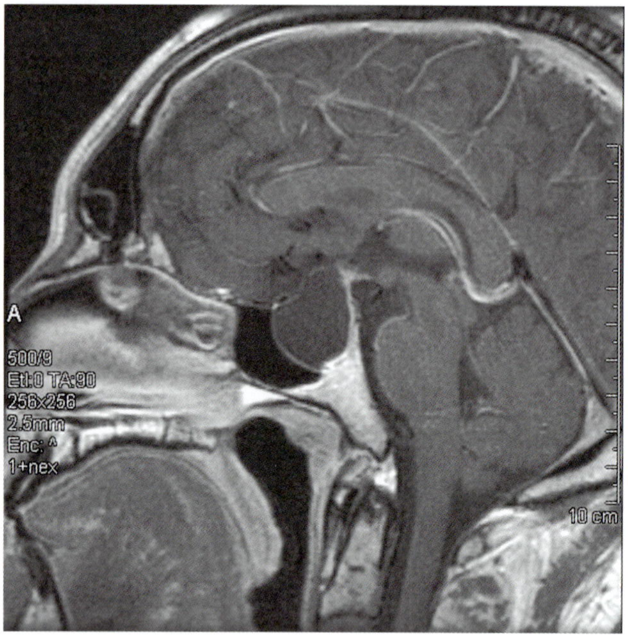

Fig. 10.1 Hypointense Rathke cleft cyst on T1-weighted MRI.

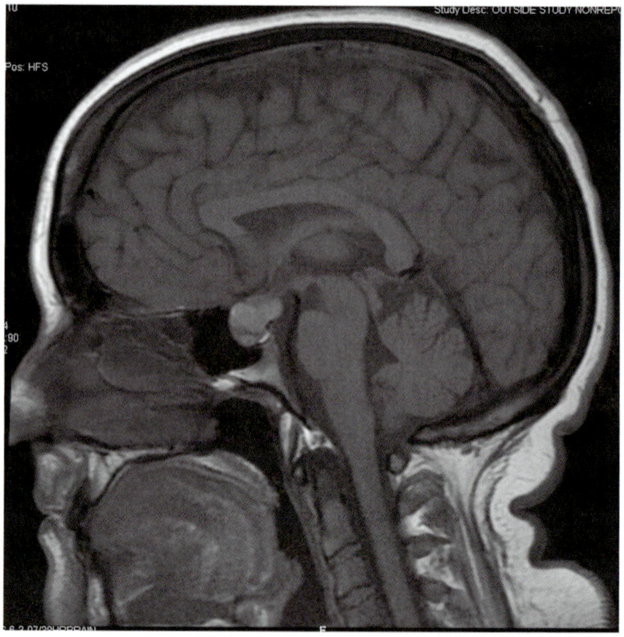

Fig. 10.2 Isointense Rathke cleft cyst on T1-weighted MRI.

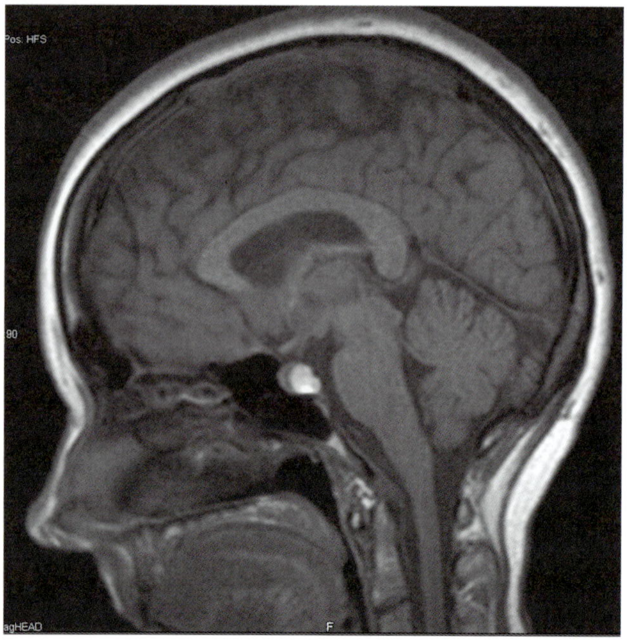

Fig. 10.3 Hyperintense Rathke cleft cyst on T1-weighted MRI.

have shown that RCCs are hypointense to brain parenchyma on diffusion-weighted imaging and have a higher apparent diffusion coefficient than do craniopharyngiomas and pituitary adenomas.[54] Most lesions are centrally located within the pituitary gland and are less than 1.5 cm in diameter.[31,55] Larger lesions may appear dumbbell-shaped as they extend into the suprasellar region.[15,42] If the cyst continues to expand and obstructs the foramina of Monro and the third ventricle, hydrocephalus may be present.[16]

In the modern treatment era, gadolinium-enhanced MRI should be performed with focused pituitary sequencing in three planes (**Table 10.2**). This aids in diagnosis and operative planning, allowing the surgeon to understand the relationship between the cyst and the optic nerves, chiasm, pituitary, infundibulum, hypothalamus, carotid arteries, and cavernous sinuses.[16,42,46] CT may also be of benefit for assessing the degree of calcification for diagnostic purposes, as well as planning transsphenoidal approaches.

◆ Indications for Surgery

Asymptomatic patients with an incidentally discovered cystic lesion in the sellar/suprasellar region should undergo the appropriate endocrine, ophthalmologic, and imaging evaluation, but treatment is rarely indicated. For patients who present with headaches as their sole complaint, a full headache evaluation and medical treatment should be employed initially. When a patient has a large but relatively asymptomatic cyst, serial imaging may be used to assess for further cyst expansion or compression of the optic chiasm. When a patient becomes symptomatic as a result of endocrinopathies or visual deficits, or if a patient has medically refractory headaches, surgical intervention is warranted.

◆ Operative Approaches

In 1934, Frazier and Alpers[2] performed the first successful craniotomy for resection of "tumor of the Rathke pouch." Their patient was "gainfully employed and asymptomatic" during the 3-year follow-up period. As such, RCCs were primarily resected via craniotomy until the 1970s, when

Hardy et al recommended the microsurgical transsphenoidal approach.[56,57] The incidence of aseptic meningitis secondary to rupture of cyst contents into the subarachnoid space during a craniotomy has declined with use of the transsphenoidal approach.[27,58]

With more modern neuroimaging techniques to assist in operative planning, newer techniques such as the direct endonasal and endoscopic transsphenoidal approaches have also proved to be safe and effective for fenestration and/or resection of RCCs.[59] Thus, the craniotomy is now reserved for lesions with suprasellar or parasellar components that would be difficult to access via the transsphenoidal route.[30,60] The surgical approaches are detailed in Chapters 11 ("Transsphenoidal Approaches to the Sellar and Parasellar Area") and 12 ("Transcranial Approaches to the Sellar and Parasellar Area").

◆ Surgical Techniques

There are two main surgical treatment strategies for symptomatic RCCs: simple fenestration and aggressive cyst wall resection.[16] The surgical decision making should take into account the patient's age, sex, desire for fertility, and comorbid medical conditions, in addition to the severity of symptoms.[61]

The most common strategy for the treatment of RCCs includes a fenestration of the cyst, evacuation of cyst contents, and biopsy of the cyst wall[11,15,23,24,29,30,43,62] (**Fig. 10.4**). Generally, there is little or no attempt to remove the cyst wall from the surrounding gland, and when possible, the sellar floor is not reconstructed, to allow the cyst to continue to drain into the sphenoid sinus.[29] This strategy allows relief of the symptomatology with little pituitary dysfunction but has previously been associated with a higher recurrence rate in the literature.[34–37,63]

A more aggressive strategy involves complete cyst wall resection. This technique has traditionally been associated with a lower recurrence rate;[16,61,64] however, it is associated with increased rates of postoperative cerebrospinal fluid (CSF) leaks and pituitary dysfunction, including diabetes insipidus.[35]

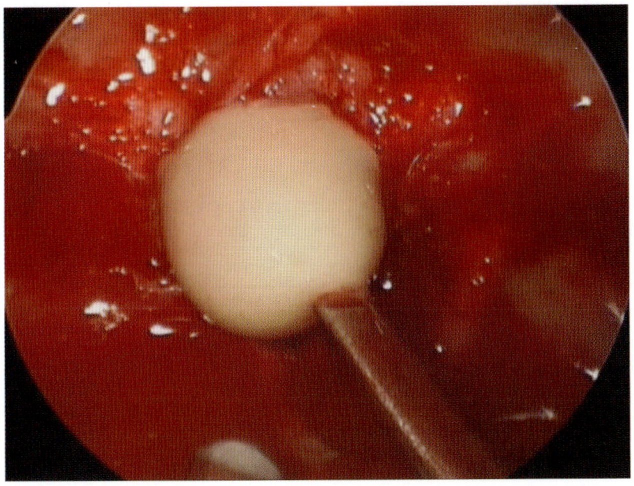

Fig. 10.4 Intraoperative endoscopic transsphenoidal view of a Rathke cleft cyst.

Microscopic Transsphenoidal

The transsphenoidal microsurgical approach has traditionally been the mainstay of the transsphenoidal surgical treatment of primarily intrasellar RCCs.[16] This may be performed via either a sublabial or an endonasal approach. Although the benefits include a three-dimensional view, the surgeon may be limited by a fixed view and smaller field. This approach continues to be favored for children, whose small nares may not allow passage of transsphenoidal instruments.

Endoscopic Transsphenoidal

The endoscopic transsphenoidal technique is used for the majority of RCC patients at our institution. In contrast to a microsurgical technique, the endoscope allows a wider field, angled viewpoints, and closer inspection.[22,63,65–67] The approach includes a two-nostril technique with wide exposure of the sphenoid sinus to maximize the surgeon's working space. The sella turcica is exposed widely with Kerrison rongeurs. For cysts with suprasellar extension and a prefixed chiasm, further removal of the tuberculum and a portion of the planum sphenoidale may be warranted and allows an extended transsphenoidal approach (although the increased risk for a postoperative CSF leak must be kept in mind).[68] When this more extended approach is to be performed and a CSF leak is anticipated preoperatively, a pedicled nasoseptal mucosal flap may be harvested at the beginning of the case to be used for the reconstruction.[69] Otherwise, attempts are made to preserve the nasoseptal artery on which this flap is based in the event an unexpected CSF leak is encountered and a "rescue" flap reconstruction may be necessary.[70]

The ability to switch between angled endoscopes allows the visual confirmation of complete removal of the cyst contents and provides a view of the internal cyst cavity. Following cyst collapse, in the absence of a CSF leak, we do not repair the sellar floor so as to allow continued drainage.[29]

◆ Outcomes

Clinical Outcomes

The surgical treatment of Rathke cleft cysts is associated with dramatic relief of headaches, visual dysfunction, and symptoms of hyperprolactinemia, including amenorrhea and galactorrhea[16] (**Table 10.3**). There is much less anticipated relief of the symptoms of hypopituitarism and diabetes insipidus after surgery.

Headaches are present in 44 to 81% of patients preoperatively, and modern studies show a 60 to 100% resolution rate.[15,34–36] Patients with persistent postoperative headaches tended to have chronic headaches preoperatively, whereas patients who presented with severe headache (possibly due to leakage of cystic contents and inflammation) were more likely to experience resolution.[35]

Visual loss is present in 11 to 67% of patients preoperatively on ophthalmologic examination, and as many as 92% of these patients have complete return of vision postop-

Table 10.3 Outcomes after Surgery for Rathke Cleft Cysts

		Percentage of patients with relief of				
Reference	Year	Headache*	Visual disturbance*	Anterior pituitary dysfunction*	Posterior pituitary dysfunction*	Hyperprolactinemia*
Voelker et al	1991	88	85	12	0	90
el-Mahdy and Powell	1998	70	67	15	25	63
Shin et al	1999	82	70	61	0	67
Benveniste et al	2004	91	96	28	0	Unknown
Kim et al	2004	93	64	63	29	77
Weiss et al	2004	Unknown	98	69	0	100
Kanter et al	2004	85	86	70	50	83
Frank et al	2005	100	100	Unknown	0	100
Aho et al	2005	Unknown	98	18	19	Unknown
Madhok et al	2009	96	Unknown	33	0	Unknown
Kiehna et al	2010	71	95	36	0	67

*All numbers are percentages.

eratively.[71] Modern series have not reported new cases of visual deficits postoperatively.

Endocrinopathies occur in 30 to 60% of patients preoperatively. A decrease in anterior pituitary dysfunction occurs in 15 to 70% of patients postoperatively, especially those with amenorrhea or galactorrhea.[18,23,34–38,72,73] Endocrine outcomes were best summarized by el-Mahady and Powell when they stated that patients with the poorest preoperative status have the poorest recovery rates.[29] As the RCC walls are intrinsically attached to the surrounding pituitary gland and stalk, dissection and resection of the cyst wall is associated with an increased incidence of postoperative diabetes insipidus and secondary hypopituitarism when compared with simple fenestration alone. Postoperative anterior pituitary dysfunction occurs in as many as 40 to 60% of patients,[35,63] and permanent postoperative diabetes insipidus occurs in as many as 40 to 50%.[35,37] It has been theorized that the high rate of diabetes insipidus in patients with RCCs is a result of inflammation and extension into the surrounding pituitary gland.[17] Only rarely does preoperative diabetes insipidus resolve after surgery.[16]

Relapse

Fenestration of the cyst is associated with a recurrence rate of ~10%[34–36,74] (**Table 10.4**). Other factors associated with relapse include cyst wall enhancement on MRI[34,50,51,56] and histopathology. Multiple authors have documented that squamous metaplasia on histopathology is associated with higher rates of relapse.[17,34] This suggests that even in cases in which the goal is fenestration alone, it is helpful to remove a small portion of the cyst wall for pathology review. Patients with squamous metaplasia should be followed more closely postoperatively because they may have a more aggressive lesion that can become re-encapsulated and reaccumulate cystic fluid.[16] Recurrence rates further vary based on the length of follow-up and the imaging schedule employed in follow-up. Over all, recurrence rates appear to be less than 20%, with Shin et al reporting the longest recurrence-free survival of 85% at 5 years and a few late recurrences resulting in a recurrence-free survival of 81% at 20 years.[31]

Table 10.4 Patient Outcomes by Surgical Approach

		Pediatric microscopic series	Adult endoscopic series		Adult microscopic transsphenoidal resection		
	Our series	Zada et al	Madhok et al	Frank et al	Aho et al	Benveniste et al	Sade et al
Patients, No.	8	9	35	22	118	62	10
Relief of headaches, %	75	88	96	100	—	91	75
New anterior pituitary dysfunction, %	0	30	0	41	2	10/67*	10
New posterior pituitary dysfunction, %	12.5	20	0	9	9/42*	6/50*	20
New visual disturbances, %	0	0	0	0	0	0	0
Recurrence, %	12.5	10	6	5	21/18*	0	0

*Indicates the percentage of patients with that outcome who underwent a simple decompression/attempted gross total resection.

◆ Complications

Postoperative complications of the surgical treatment of RCCs are related to the surgical approach and strategy. CSF rhinorrhea occurs in fewer than 3% of patients treated via a transsphenoidal approach and is almost exclusively a result of cyst wall dissection/resection.[30,35,37] It is treated surgically by repairing the sellar defect with abdominal fat, a bone, or a synthetic buttress to the floor of the sella and application of a glue or bonding agent. Conservative treatment measures include lumbar drainage.[16]

Meningitis is a rare consequence of RCC resections. Aseptic meningitis may be associated with leakage of the cyst contents into the subarachnoid[16] and can be managed with corticosteroids provided that meningitis related to infection is not present. CSF cultures should be obtained to rule out bacterial meningitis. Bacterial or fungal meningitis may result from a CSF leak related to a transsphenoidal approach. Treatment includes obtaining CSF cultures to isolate the offending organism, broad-spectrum intravenous antibiotics, and repair of any obvious CSF leak.[29,30,35–37]

◆ Follow-up

All patients should be followed closely by a multidisciplinary team consisting of a neurosurgeon, endocrinologist, and neuro-ophthalmologist at 8 to 12 weeks postoperatively and annually thereafter. Postoperative imaging should be obtained to establish a baseline after surgery and should be performed annually for the first several years before the time interval is increased. Ophthalmologic evaluations should be performed annually for patients who presented with visual deficits. Repeated recurrence of an RCC has been successfully treated with gamma knife radiosurgery.

◆ Conclusion

RCCs pose a challenging problem for the neurosurgeon whether they are managed surgically or conservatively. Transsphenoidal surgery has been established as the standard operative approach. The operative strategy, including the degree of surgical resection of the RCC, should be patient-specific, with a full discussion of the risks and benefits. Advancing technology, such as the three-dimensional endoscope, may continue to improve operative outcomes. Close follow-up with a multidisciplinary team is essential to recognize recurrences and the need for further treatment.

References

1. Shanklin WM. The incidence and distribution of cilia in the human pituitary with a description of microfollicular cysts derived from Rathke's cleft. Acta Anat (Basel) 1951;11(2–3):361–382
2. Frazier CH, Alpers BJ. Tumors of Rathke cleft (hitherto called tumors of Rathke's pouch). Arch Neurol Psychiatry 1934;32:973–984
3. Concha S, Hamilton BP, Millan JC, McQueen JD. Symptomatic Rathke's cleft cyst with amyloid stroma. J Neurol Neurosurg Psychiatry 1975;38(8):782–786
4. Leech RW, Olafson RA. Epithelial cysts of the neuraxis: presentation of three cases and a review of the origins and classification. Arch Pathol Lab Med 1977;101(4):196–202
5. Shuangshoti S, Netsky MG, Nashold BS Jr. Epithelial cysts related to sella turcica. Proposed origin from neuroepithelium. Arch Pathol 1970;90(5):444–450
6. Matsushima T, Fukui M, Fujii K, Kinoshita K, Yamakawa Y. Epithelial cells in symptomatic Rathke's cleft cysts. A light- and electron-microscopic study. Surg Neurol 1988;30(3):197–203
7. Palma L, Celli P. Suprasellar epithelial cyst. Case report. J Neurosurg 1983;58(5):763–765
8. Naiken VS, Tellem M, Meranze DR. Pituitary cyst of Rathke's cleft origin with hypopituitarism. J Neurosurg 1961;18:703–708
9. Rasmussen AT. Ciliated epithelium and mucus-secreting cells in the human hypophysis. Anat Rec 1929;41:273–283
10. Eisenberg HM, Weiner RL. Benign pituitary cysts. In: Wilkins RH, Rengachary SS, eds. Neuro-surgery. McGraw-Hill; 1985:932–934
11. Fager CA, Carter H. Intrasellar epithelial cysts. J Neurosurg 1966;24(1):77–81
12. Northfield DWC. Rathke-pouch tumours. Brain 1957;80(3):293–312
13. Smith RA, Bucy PC. Pituitary cyst lined with a single layer of columnar epithelium. J Neurosurg 1953;10(5):540–543
14. Yoshida J, Kobayashi T, Kageyama N, Kanzaki M. Symptomatic Rathke's cleft cyst. Morphological study with light and electron microscopy and tissue culture. J Neurosurg 1977;47(3):451–458
15. Voelker JL, Campbell RL, Muller J. Clinical, radiographic, and pathological features of symptomatic Rathke's cleft cysts. J Neurosurg 1991;74(4):535–544
16. Kanter A, Sansur C, Jane JA Jr, Laws ER Jr. Rathke's cleft cysts. In: Laws ER Jr, Sheehan JP, eds. Pituitary Surgery—a Modern Approach. Karger; 2006:127–157
17. Hama S, Arita K, Nishisaka T, et al. Changes in the epithelium of Rathke cleft cyst associated with inflammation. J Neurosurg 2002;96(2):209–216
18. Ikeda H, Yoshimoto T, Suzuki J. Immunohistochemical study of Rathke's cleft cyst. Acta Neuropathol 1988;77(1):33–38
19. Hunter IJ. Squamous metaplasia of cells of the anterior pituitary gland. J Pathol Bacteriol 1955;69(1-2):141–145
20. Mukherjee JJ, Islam N, Kaltsas G, et al. Clinical, radiological and pathological features of patients with Rathke's cleft cysts: tumors that may recur. J Clin Endocrinol Metab 1997;82(7):2357–2362
21. Teramoto A, Hirakawa K, Sanno N, Osamura Y. Incidental pituitary lesions in 1,000 unselected autopsy specimens. Radiology 1994;193(1):161–164
22. Zada G, Kelly DF, Cohan P, Wang C, Swerdloff R. Endonasal transsphenoidal approach for pituitary adenomas and other sellar lesions: an assessment of efficacy, safety, and patient impressions. J Neurosurg 2003;98(2):350–358
23. Isono M, Kamida T, Kobayashi H, Shimomura T, Matsuyama J. Clinical features of symptomatic Rathke's cleft cyst. Clin Neurol Neurosurg 2001;103(2):96–100
24. Baskin DS, Wilson CB. Transsphenoidal treatment of non-neoplastic intrasellar cysts. A report of 38 cases. J Neurosurg 1984;60(1):8–13
25. Bayoumi ML. Rathke's cleft and its cysts. Edinburgh Med J 1948;55(12):745–749
26. Gillman T. The incidence of ciliated epithelium and mucous cells in the normal Bantu pituitary. S Afr J Med Sci 1940;5:30–40
27. Steinberg GK, Koenig GH, Golden JB. Symptomatic Rathke's cleft cysts. Report of two cases. J Neurosurg 1982;56(2):290–295
28. Agnetti V, Carreras M, Rocca A, Turtas S, Viale GL. Epithelial cysts related to the Rathke's cleft. J Neurosurg Sci 1974;18(1):65–69
29. el-Mahdy W, Powell M. Transsphenoidal management of 28 symptomatic Rathke's cleft cysts, with special reference to visual and hormonal recovery. Neurosurgery 1998;42(1):7–16, discussion 16–17

30. Ross DA, Norman D, Wilson CB. Radiologic characteristics and results of surgical management of Rathke's cysts in 43 patients. Neurosurgery 1992;30(2):173–178, discussion 178–179
31. Shin JL, Asa SL, Woodhouse LJ, Smyth HS, Ezzat S. Cystic lesions of the pituitary: clinicopathological features distinguishing craniopharyngioma, Rathke's cleft cyst, and arachnoid cyst. J Clin Endocrinol Metab 1999;84(11):3972–3982
32. Tolis G, Somma M, Van Campenhout J, Friesen H. Prolactin secretion in sixty-five patients with galactorrhea. Am J Obstet Gynecol 1974;118(1):91–101
33. Berry RG, Schlezinger NS. Rathke-cleft cysts. Arch Neurol 1959;1:48–58
34. Kim JE, Kim JH, Kim OL, et al. Surgical treatment of symptomatic Rathke cleft cysts: clinical features and results with special attention to recurrence. J Neurosurg 2004;100(1):33–40
35. Benveniste RJ, King WA, Walsh J, Lee JS, Naidich TP, Post KD. Surgery for Rathke cleft cysts: technical considerations and outcomes. J Neurosurg 2004;101(4):577–584
36. Kanter AS, Diallo AO, Vance ML, Laws ER. Rathke's cleft cysts: a single center's experience. Presented at: American Association of Neurological Surgeons 2004 Conference; May 2004; Orlando, FL
37. Aho CJ, Liu C, Zelman V, Couldwell WT, Weiss MH. Surgical outcomes in 118 patients with Rathke cleft cysts. J Neurosurg 2005;102(2):189–193
38. Wenzel M, Salcman M, Kristt DA, Gellad FE, Kapcala LP. Pituitary hyposecretion and hypersecretion produced by a Rathke's cleft cyst presenting as a noncystic hypothalamic mass. Neurosurgery 1989;24(3):424–428
39. Woodruff WW Jr, Heinz ER, Djang WT, Voorhees D. Hyperprolactinemia: an unusual manifestation of suprasellar cystic lesions. AJNR Am J Neuroradiol 1987;8(1):113–116
40. Oka H, Kawano N, Suwa T, Yada K, Kan S, Kameya T. Radiological study of symptomatic Rathke's cleft cysts. Neurosurgery 1994;35(4):632–636, discussion 636–637
41. Verkijk A, Bots GTAM. An intrasellar cyst with both Rathke's cleft and epidermoid characteristics. Acta Neurochir (Wien) 1980;51(3-4):203–207
42. Nakasu Y, Nakasu S, Nakajima M, Itoh R, Matsuda M. Atypical Rathke's cleft cyst associated with ossification. AJNR Am J Neuroradiol 1999;20(7):1287–1289
43. Kucharczyk W, Peck WW, Kelly WM, Norman D, Newton TH. Rathke cleft cysts: CT, MR imaging, and pathologic features. Radiology 1987;165(2):491–495
44. Maggio WW, Cail WS, Brookeman JR, Persing JA, Jane JA. Rathke's cleft cyst: computed tomographic and magnetic resonance imaging appearances. Neurosurgery 1987;21(1):60–62
45. Nemoto Y, Inoue Y, Fukuda T, et al. MR appearance of Rathke's cleft cysts. Neuroradiology 1988;30(2):155–159
46. Barrow DL, Spector RH, Takei Y, Tindall GT. Symptomatic Rathke's cleft cysts located entirely in the suprasellar region: review of diagnosis, management, and pathogenesis. Neurosurgery 1985;16(6):766–772
47. Itoh J, Usui K. An entirely suprasellar symptomatic Rathke's cleft cyst: case report. Neurosurgery 1992;30(4):581–584, discussion 584–585
48. Rout D, Das L, Rao VR, Radhakrishnan VV. Symptomatic Rathke's cleft cysts. Surg Neurol 1983;19(1):42–45
49. Harrison MJ, Morgello S, Post KD. Epithelial cystic lesions of the sellar and parasellar region: a continuum of ectodermal derivatives? J Neurosurg 1994;80(6):1018–1025
50. Byun WM, Kim OL, Kim DS. MR imaging findings of Rathke's cleft cysts: significance of intracystic nodules. AJNR Am J Neuroradiol 2000;21(3):485–488
51. Hua F, Asato R, Miki Y, et al. Differentiation of suprasellar nonneoplastic cysts from cystic neoplasms by Gd-DTPA MRI. J Comput Assist Tomogr 1992;16(5):744–749
52. Hayashi Y, Tachibana O, Muramatsu N, et al. Rathke cleft cyst: MR and biomedical analysis of cyst content. J Comput Assist Tomogr 1999;23(1):34–38
53. Wagle VG, Nelson D, Rossi A, Uphoff D. Magnetic resonance imaging of symptomatic Rathke's cleft cyst: report of a case. Neurosurgery 1989;24(2):276–278
54. Kunii N, Abe T, Kawamo M, Tanioka D, Izumiyama H, Moritani T. Rathke's cleft cysts: differentiation from other cystic lesions in the pituitary fossa by use of single-shot fast spin-echo diffusion-weighted MR imaging. Acta Neurochir (Wien) 2007;149(8):759–769, discussion 769
55. Wen L, Hu LB, Feng XY, et al. Rathke's cleft cyst: clinicopathological and MRI findings in 22 patients. Clin Radiol 2010;65(1):47–55
56. Hardy J, Vezina JL. Transsphenoidal neurosurgery of intracranial neoplasm. Adv Neurol 1976;15:261–273
57. Cappabianca P, Cavallo LM, de Divitiis E. Endoscopic endonasal transsphenoidal surgery. Neurosurgery 2004;55(4):933–940, discussion 940–941
58. Shimoji T, Shinohara A, Shimizu A, Sato K, Ishii S. Rathke cleft cysts. Surg Neurol 1984;21(3):295–310
59. Madhok R, Prevedello DM, Gardner P, Carrau RL, Snyderman CH, Kassam AB. Endoscopic endonasal resection of Rathke cleft cysts: clinical outcomes and surgical nuances. J Neurosurg 2010;112(6):1333–1339
60. Day JD. Surgical approaches to suprasellar and parasellar tumors. Neurosurg Clin N Am 2003;14(1):109–122
61. Laws ER, Kanter AS. Rathke cleft cysts. J Neurosurg 2004;101(4):571–572, discussion 572
62. Kasperbauer JL, Orvidas LJ, Atkinson JLD, Abboud CF. Rathke cleft cyst: diagnostic and therapeutic considerations. Laryngoscope 2002;112(10):1836–1839
63. Frank G, Sciarretta V, Mazzatenta D, Farneti G, Modugno GC, Pasquini E. Transsphenoidal endoscopic approach in the treatment of Rathke's cleft cyst. Neurosurgery 2005;56(1):124–128, discussion 129
64. Eisenberg HM, Sarwar M, Schochet S Jr. Symptomatic Rathke's cleft cyst. Case report. J Neurosurg 1976;45(5):585–588
65. Cavallo LM, Prevedello D, Esposito F, et al. The role of the endoscope in the transsphenoidal management of cystic lesions of the sellar region. Neurosurg Rev 2008;31(1):55–64, discussion 64
66. Alfieri A, Schettino R, Tarfani A, Bonzi O, Rossi GA, Monolo L. Endoscopic endonasal removal of an intra-suprasellar Rathke's cleft cyst: case report and surgical considerations. Minim Invasive Neurosurg 2002;45(1):47–51
67. Kaptain GJ, Vincent DA, Sheehan JP, Laws ER Jr. Transsphenoidal approaches for the extracapsular resection of midline suprasellar and anterior cranial base lesions. Neurosurgery 2001;49(1):94–100, discussion 100–101
68. Laws ER. Endoscopic surgery for cystic lesions of the pituitary region. Nat Clin Pract Endocrinol Metab 2008;4(12):662–663
69. Pinheiro-Neto CD, Prevedello DM, Carrau RL, et al. Improving the design of the pedicled nasoseptal flap for skull base reconstruction: a radioanatomic study. Laryngoscope 2007;117(9):1560–1569
70. Rivera-Serrano CM, Carrau RL, Snuderman CH, Prevedello D, Kassam AB, Zanation A. Nasoseptal "rescue" flap: a novel modification of the nasoseptal flap technique for pituitary surgery. Presented at: Triological Society 2010 Annual Meeting; April 30, 2010; Las Vegas, NV
71. Rao GP, Blyth CPJ, Jeffreys RV. Ophthalmic manifestations of Rathke's cleft cysts. Am J Ophthalmol 1995;119(1):86–91
72. Landolt AM, Zachmann M. Results of transsphenoidal extirpation of craniopharyngiomas and Rathke's cysts. Neurosurgery 1991;28(3):410–415
73. Rottenberg GT, Chong WK, Powell MP, Kendall BE. Cyst formation of the craniopharyngeal duct. Clin Radiol 1994;49(2):126–129
74. Sade B, Albrecht S, Assimakopoulos P, Vézina JL, Mohr G. Management of Rathke's cleft cysts. Surg Neurol 2005;63(5):459–466, discussion 466

11 Transsphenoidal Approaches to the Sellar and Parasellar Area

Daniel M. Prevedello

The sinuses have been used as a corridor to access the pituitary fossa for over 100 years. From the beginning, surgeons appreciated the advantage of approaching the target from below and having direct access to the sella without manipulating the brain.[1] The technology at that time was very limited, however, and most surgeons did not feel it safe enough to perform major neurosurgical procedures through narrow nasal pathways. Harvey Cushing is probably the greatest example because he abandoned the transsphenoidal approach in 1927 owing in part to an inability to properly illuminate the surgical field.[2,3] Although Norman Dott, who had learned the technique from Cushing, employed a lighted speculum, it was only after the contributions of Gerard Guiot, who added fluoroscopy, and Jules Hardy, who added the operating microscope, that the transsphenoidal route became popular and was disseminated around the world.[1]

One of the limitations of the transsphenoidal approach performed with the microscope is the relative restriction of parasellar illumination and visualization. Although the sella can be well visualized, areas such as the cavernous sinus and anterior fossa region can be completely out of sight. With that in mind, some neurosurgeons started to add the endoscope to the scene in parallel with the microscope to augment visualization in these particular areas and so improve tumor resection and outcomes. Gerard Guiot was the first neurosurgeon to use the endoscope in the transsphenoidal route in the 1960s, but at that time the technology was still fairly primitive.[1] In the late 1970s, Apuzzo and colleagues,[4] as well as Bushe and Halves,[5,6] demonstrated the use of the endoscope as an adjunctive tool to remove pituitary lesions. Endoscopically "assisted" transsphenoidal microsurgery has since been reported by various authors, emphasizing its importance for tumors that extend beyond the sella.[7–12]

Surgeons progressively realized that the combination of speculum and endoscope is not ideal because one limits the other. Roger Jankowski and co-workers reported the first series of three cases in which an endoscopic transsphenoidal approach to the sella was used in 1992.[13] Ricardo Carrau and colleagues pursued a purely direct endoscopic endonasal approach to the pituitary fossa and described their experience in 1996,[14] followed by their first 50-patient series in 1997.[14–16] Paolo Cappabianca, Enrico de Divitiis, Luigi Cavallo, and colleagues developed appropriate surgical instrumentation and became a world reference for endoscopic pituitary surgery.[17–27]

At the same time that various surgeons were developing and demonstrating the feasibility of gaining access beyond the sella by using the transsphenoidal route, particularly to the midline anterior skull base with the microscope as the primary visualization tool,[7,8,28–32] Amin Kassam, Ricardo Carrau, Carl Snyderman, and colleagues defined and standardized modules of approaches to the skull base, expanded from the sella, while using the endoscope as the sole tool for illumination and visualization.[1,33,34]

Although it is still controversial whether the endoscope brings real advantages to dealing with sellar disease in relation to the microscope, the use of endoscopic endonasal techniques to reach the areas beyond the sella has become well accepted.[11,35–43]

◆ The Sella

The endonasal corridor is a median approach that is in the same axis as the sella and therefore represents an ideal route to reach the sella with no brain manipulation. Historically, craniotomies were the general approach used to deal with sellar disease. However, this concept was completely altered once Jules Hardy brought the operating microscope to the transsphenoidal operation.[44] Any transcranial approach requires some level of brain retraction and yields indirect visualization of the pituitary fossa, which is hidden by the planum sphenoidale.[45] Currently, fewer than 5% of patients with a pituitary adenoma have a craniotomy as an alternative approach for resection, and it is always related to an extrasellar tumor component.[45] There is a consensus that the sellar portion of tumor is better treated by a transsphenoidal route in an approach with the microscope, endoscope, or both.[45–50]

Microscopic Transsphenoidal Approach

The transsphenoidal approach has had some variations over the years. The initial description by Schloffer required a paranasal incision followed by a complete transethmoidal exposure to reach the sphenoid sinus and sella.[51] With the evolution of the technique, the approach has become progressively less invasive.

The procedure is performed with the patient under general anesthesia. The patient is positioned typically in a semirecumbent angle with the head tilted to the left.

There are three current variations of the transsphenoidal approach: sublabial, hemitransfixion, and direct endonasal, or "pushover."

Sublabial

From the time Cushing was using the technique until recently, the transsphenoidal approach was invariably performed as a sublabial procedure. Indeed, it is still performed that way in many centers around the world.[47,52]

An incision is made under the superior lip inside the mouth, and the mucoperiosteum is elevated from the bone at the piriform aperture. The plane between the mucoperichondrium and the mucoperiosteum posteriorly is encountered and the mucosa is separated from the septum on both sides. The septum is retracted, often to the left side, and a speculum is positioned and advanced until the rostrum of the sphenoid is well exposed in the center of the field. An anterior sphenoidectomy is performed with a rongeur. The sphenoid sinus is visualized, and the position of the sella is confirmed with lateral fluoroscopy or some other type of navigation.[53] The sella is opened either with a drill or with a chisel. Once the bone of the sellar face is removed and the dura is exposed, a knife, usually an 11-blade scalpel, is used to incise the dura. The sella is explored and the tumor can be removed, usually with ring curettes.

The sublabial approach has the advantage of creating a broad corridor, which can be as wide as the piriform aperture.[47] The disadvantage of the sublabial technique is related to potential complications of the approach. There is a higher incidence of anterior septal perforation with the sublabial approach. The superior anterior teeth can develop various grades of numbness, and saddle nose deformation due to anterior septum manipulation can also occur.

Endonasal

The other commonly used variations of the transsphenoidal route are endonasal procedures performed with the microscope. The transnasal hemitransfixion technique requires an incision in the septal mucosa ~1 cm behind the columella. The speculum is inserted directly in the nostril, and the plane between the mucoperiosteum and the septum is elevated posteriorly as in the sublabial approach. The rest of the procedure continues in a fashion similar to the sublabial approach.

The other variation is the direct endonasal ("pushover") technique. In this variant, the speculum is introduced earlier in the case, and the nasal pathway is followed directly until the posterior aspect of the septum. The mucosa is not elevated from the septum anteriorly. The middle turbinate is retracted laterally, and the posterior septum is dislocated to the opposite side. The mucosa is then disrupted very posteriorly at the bony septum area. The submucosal plane is elevated and the rostrum is exposed. The rest of the procedure follows the same technique as the sublabial one.

The advantage of the transnasal transsphenoidal approach is that it avoids manipulation of the anterior teeth and saddle nose deformities. On the other hand, it generates a narrower corridor, and the specula used need to be adapted for small nostrils. If the speculum is forced open during the procedure with the intent of creating better exposure, a nasal skin tear may occur. The other disadvantage is related to the fact that the speculum comes obliquely from one of the nostrils. This can generate a false impression of the midline, and the surgeon can inadvertently cross to the other side in the depths without appropriate awareness of the situation. This can be the scenario for a catastrophic complication because the surgeon can open the cavernous sinus directly in front of the internal carotid artery thinking that that is the midline.[54,55]

Endoscopic Endonasal Approach

Totally endoscopic transsphenoidal surgery started in the 1990s as a collaboration between otolaryngologists and neurosurgeons, with the goal of developing a less disruptive approach to the nasal structures.[1,13–16,23,56] It consists of a direct endonasal approach to the back of the nasal cavity, followed by identification of the sphenoid ostium. The anterior wall of the sphenoid sinus is opened, and the sinus can be visualized. Although there was an initial trend to perform this approach through only one nostril, currently most centers performing this procedure follow the binostril-bimanual technique, which allows much more freedom of movement.[33] A posterior septectomy is performed, communicating both nostrils posteriorly and creating a single working cavity.

The intrasphenoid septa are drilled, allowing broad visualization of all the sphenoid walls. At this point, the surgeon is able to determine with precision the skull base landmarks, particularly in well-pneumatized sinuses, which avoids the absolute need for fluoroscopy or image guidance (**Fig. 11.1**). Nonetheless, if the surgeons have easy access to image guidance, it is probably wise to use it for every endoscopic case because it is hard to predict in which cases it may be helpful to confirm a certain structure intraoperatively. Of course, cases of nonpneumatized sphenoid sinus clearly benefit from intraoperative image guidance. Such cases are simple to foresee based on preoperative computed tomography. However, cases with unexpected vascular complications or tumor-distorted anatomy can also benefit from intraoperative image guidance, even when there is a wide-open sphenoid sinus.

The face of the sella is then identified, and the bone is removed to expose the dura. The superior and inferior intercavernous sinuses and the face of the cavernous sinuses bilaterally are exposed. This relatively wide exposure coupled with an ample dural opening allows an unencumbered intrasellar dissection.

The dura of the sella is incised with a sharp blade that incises both layers of the dura but does not transgress the

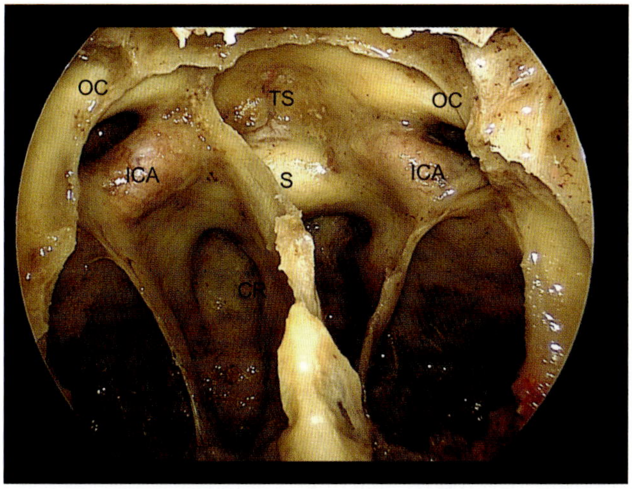

Fig. 11.1 Endoscopic visualization of the entire sphenoid sinus with a zero-degree endoscope in a cadaveric specimen demonstrating the wide exposure and the clear view of the main landmarks: the optic canals bilaterally (*OC*), the internal carotid arteries bilaterally (*ICA*), the tuberculum sellae recess (*TS*), the sella (*S*), and the clival recess (*CR*).

pituitary capsule. The dura is elevated from the sellar face, exposing the gland or tumor. An extracapsular resection of the tumor is always attempted, particularly in hyperfunctioning adenomas, to secure a complete resection. Even in cases in which the pituitary gland needs to be explored, in magnetic resonance imaging–negative cases of Cushing disease, for instance, an extracapsular resection of the hidden adenoma is attempted to permit a thorough resection of the functional adenoma and its margins because the pseudocapsule is indeed compact normal gland[46,57] (**Fig. 11.2**). Occasionally, the medial wall of the cavernous sinus needs to be resected to increase the chance of remission in more invasive adenomas. This affords an advantage of the endoscopic technique over the microscopic because the visualization offered by the endoscope laterally is far superior (**Fig. 11.3**).

Two surgeons perform the entire procedure. In our personal experience, because there are no data to support a significant difference in the literature, we believe that the visualization allowed by the endoscope is far superior to that from the operating microscope. Furthermore, the illumination and image captured by the endoscope are closer to the target, whereas with the microscope, the imaging is from a greater distance. This is particularly important because the surgeon's hands can block the view during microscopic surgery. The wide field of visualization provided by the endoscope allows dissection in the parasellar area, which is crucial to resect invasive pituitary adenomas from the cavernous sinus and to deal with extensive suprasellar projections of tumor, always under direct visualization and without the use of blind curettage (**Fig. 11.3**).

The most common indications for this approach are pituitary adenomas, intrasellar craniopharyngiomas, and Rathke cleft cysts.

◆ The Parasellar Areas

The use of microscope to reach areas around the sella is possible from a transsphenoidal approach. Because the light source is external, however, there are limitations for visualization of areas that are not in line with the approach. The surgeon often is obliged, in this scenario, to extend the size of the corridor by using a sublabial incision, which can be augmented laterally by a medial maxillectomy or a LeForte maxillary disarticulation.[58,59] The other aspect of limitation is related to the focal plane of the microscope, which becomes very constricted as the dissection is per-

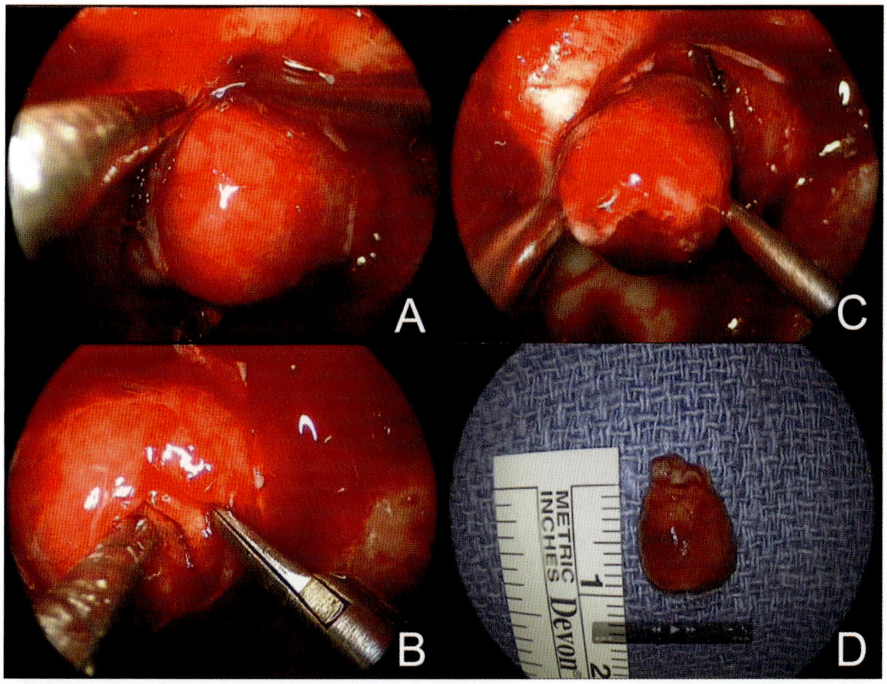

Fig. 11.2 Intraoperative photographs during an extracapsular resection of a pituitary adenoma in a patient with Cushing disease. **(A–C)** Intraoperative views with a zero-degree endoscope during an endoscopic endonasal transsellar approach. **(A)** Pituitary gland exposure. **(B)** Identification of the adenoma with visualization of the pseudocapsule. **(C)** Removal of the pituitary adenoma extracapsularly. **(D)** Specimen removed en bloc and sent to pathology (it proved to be an ACTH-staining adenoma).

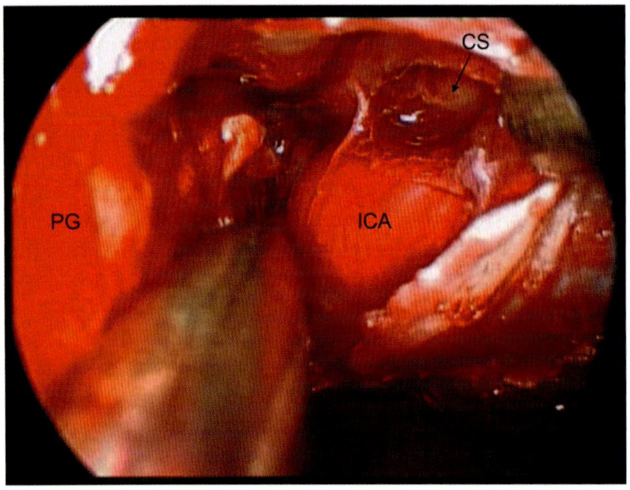

Fig. 11.3 Intraoperative photograph during a resection of a pituitary adenoma that was invading the left cavernous sinus. Note that the pituitary gland (*PG*) is protected on the right. The left medial wall of the cavernous sinus was opened by resection of the tumor that was invading the cavernous sinus (*CS*) and encasing the internal carotid artery (*ICA*). Once a tumor has been removed, the venous bleeding can be profuse, and one can see the roof of the cavernous sinus from below.

formed more deeply. To compensate for this limitation, the surgeon is required to move the microscope often to see areas of the skull base that are not located in the narrow microscopic field.

Based on the advantages of the endoscopic illumination and wide visualization, it becomes natural to use the endoscope to reach lesions located in the parasellar space. It is ideal when the sellar space is the primary source of the disease, as with pituitary adenomas. However, other lesions, like craniopharyngiomas, meningiomas, chordomas, chondrosarcomas, and schwannomas, may be present in these locations and may be treated by the endoscopic expanded endonasal approaches as well.[40,41,60–62] It is important to have dynamic endoscopic visualization to compensate for the lack of three-dimensional imaging obtained from a static endoscopic view.

Suprasellar and Anterior Fossa

Very often, a suprasellar tumor is the extension of a disease that started inside the sella, particularly in pituitary adenomas and some craniopharyngiomas. In these cases, most of the time, a sellar approach is sufficient to evacuate the tumor completely, starting with the sellar component and then following the tumor superiorly. Often, the superior tumor descends naturally as the sellar disease is removed. For these cases, a microscopic transsphenoidal approach is a feasible alternative; however, it becomes difficult to determine if there is any residual tumor superiorly at the end of the dissection. One alternative would be the use of interoperative MRI, or the insertion of an angled endoscope for investigation. Nevertheless, because the corridor is not prepared for an endoscopic approach, the surgeon often is able to see residua but ends up having difficulty reaching and removing such residua under direct visualization and frequently uses blind dissection at the corners with instruments like angled ring curettes, which carry some risk, even in experienced hands.

To reach tumors that originate or extend to the suprasellar space from the sella, we prefer an endoscopic endonasal transtuberculum and/or transplanum approach. This approach is defined by the removal of the tuberculum sellae and, depending on the anterior extension of the tumor, the planum sphenoidale. The optic canals mark the lateral limits for this approach. The suprasellar region is well reached through resection of the tuberculum sellae. For most of the macroadenomas that extend to the suprasellar space, a simple bony removal of the tuberculum sellae can be enough to allow the superior component to descend during surgery. Thus, the resection is inside out, and the diaphragma sellae and suprasellar arachnoid are often preserved, avoiding exposure of cerebrospinal fluid (CSF) spaces.

On the other hand, tumors like craniopharyngiomas (**Fig. 11.4**), tuberculum sellae meningiomas (**Fig. 11.5**), and some rare pituitary adenomas (**Fig. 11.6**) require a subarachnoid dissection to free them from critical suprasellar structures (**Fig. 11.7**).

The critical anatomic landmark for this approach is the medial optic carotid recess, which is the lateral aspect of the tuberculum sellae. It must be removed to allow adequate exposure of the suprasellar compartment. Once the bone is removed, the dura is opened above the superior intercavernous sinus, which is ligated only when there is disease that requires arachnoid dissection involving the sella and suprasellar space. The dural opening can occur from one internal carotid artery to the other with direct safe access to the medial aspect of the carotid cave and the optic canals. The opening is extended anteriorly in case the tumor is located above the planum sphenoidale.

Retrosellar Space and Clivus

Some pituitary macroadenomas can extend posteriorly over the dorsum sellae, reaching the retrosellar space. These lesions are virtually impossible to resect through a standard transsphenoidal microscopic approach. The alternatives are either a retromastoid posterior fossa approach or an endoscopic endonasal transclival approach.

An endonasal transclival approach can be performed in segmental portions (upper, middle, or lower thirds) or as complete removal of the clivus (panclivectomy). The upper third is related to the dorsum sellae in the midline and the posterior clinoids in the paramedian region. The posterior wall of the sella can be removed via a transsellar approach when the tumor has created intrasellar space, or after a pituitary transposition and ligation of the posterior intercavernous sinus.[63] The retrosellar bone can also be resected extradurally via a subsellar corridor after removal of the sellar bone and superior retraction of the sellar dura.[63] After transposition, the retrodorsal dura containing the basilar plexus is exposed. Dural opening with basilar plexus control provides access to the retrodorsal area and the interpeduncular cistern, surrounded laterally by the posterior communicating arteries and third cranial nerves and posteriorly by the basilar artery with its terminal branches.

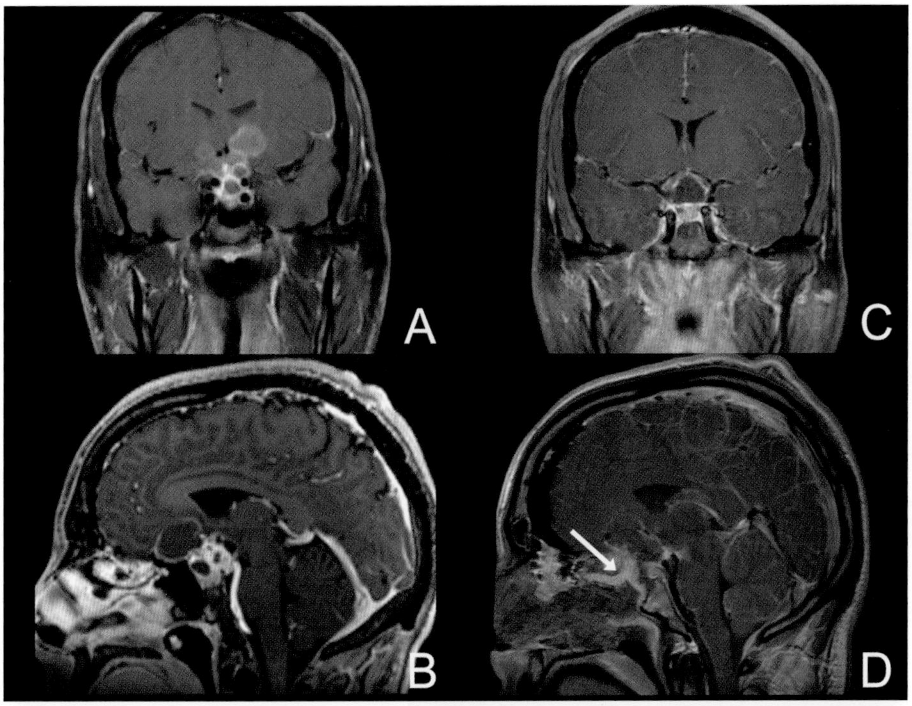

Fig. 11.4 **(A,B)** MRI with contrast of a 32-year-old man with a craniopharyngioma who presented with visual loss. The tumor has large components, both solid and cystic. **(A)** Coronal view. **(B)** Sagittal view. **(C,D)** Postoperative MRI with contrast 24 hours after an expanded endonasal transtuberculum and transplanum approach demonstrating complete resection of the craniopharyngioma. **(C)** Coronal view. **(D)** Sagittal view. Note the presence of an enhancing nasoseptal flap that was used for reconstruction (*black arrow*) and the preserved pituitary stalk.

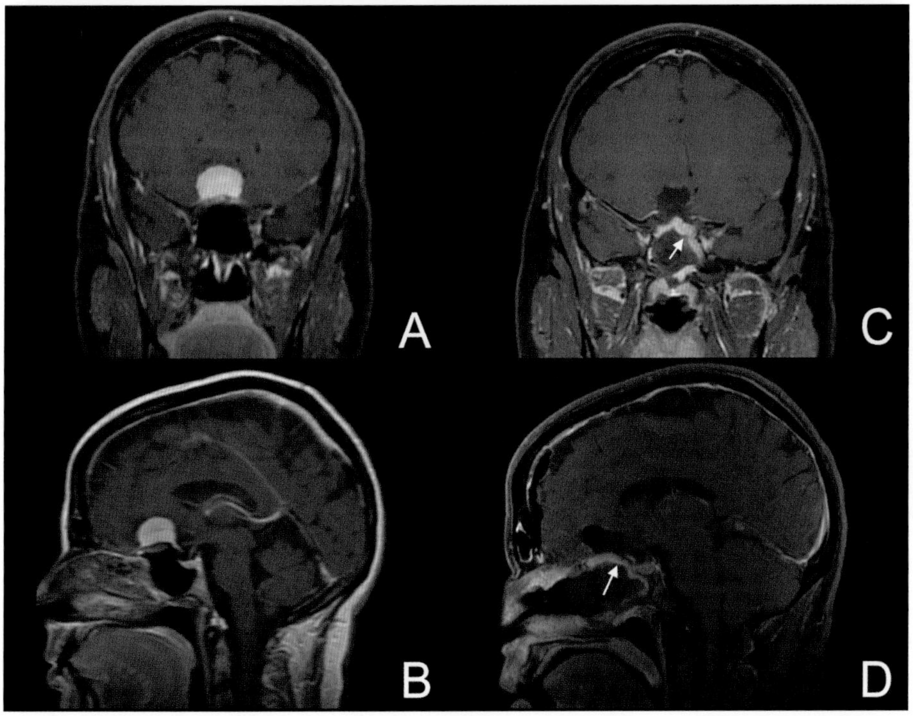

Fig. 11.5 MRI with contrast of a 39-year-old woman with a planum sphenoidale meningioma who presented with headaches and mild visual deterioration. **(A)** Coronal view. **(B)** Sagittal view. **(C,D)** Postoperative MRI with contrast 24 hours after an expanded endonasal transplanum approach demonstrating complete meningioma resection. **(C)** Coronal view. **(D)** Sagittal view. Note the presence of an enhancing nasoseptal flap that was used for reconstruction (*white arrows*) and the preserved pituitary gland and stalk.

Along with the indications for resection of macroadenomas invading the posterior fossa and the clivus, a transclival approach is frequently used for the resection of extradural and intradural diseases, such as chordomas and chondrosarcomas (**Fig. 11.8**). It is also used to access purely intradural disease anterior to the brainstem, such as meningiomas and craniopharyngiomas.

The middle clivus can be directly accessed at the posterior aspect of the sphenoid sinus, and its resection is limited laterally by both internal carotid arteries ascending in the paraclival areas. If the bone drilling continues inferiorly, the lower third of the clivus is restricted laterally by the fossa of Rosenmüller and the torus tubarius. Once intradural, a middle clivectomy gives access to the prepontine cistern and basilar artery, guarded laterally by the sixth cranial nerves. The inferior third gives access to the premedullary cistern, with the vertebral arteries posteriorly and the hypoglossal nerves limiting the approach laterally.

A panclivectomy can extend all the way from the dorsum sellae and posterior clinoids down to the basion at the foramen magnum.

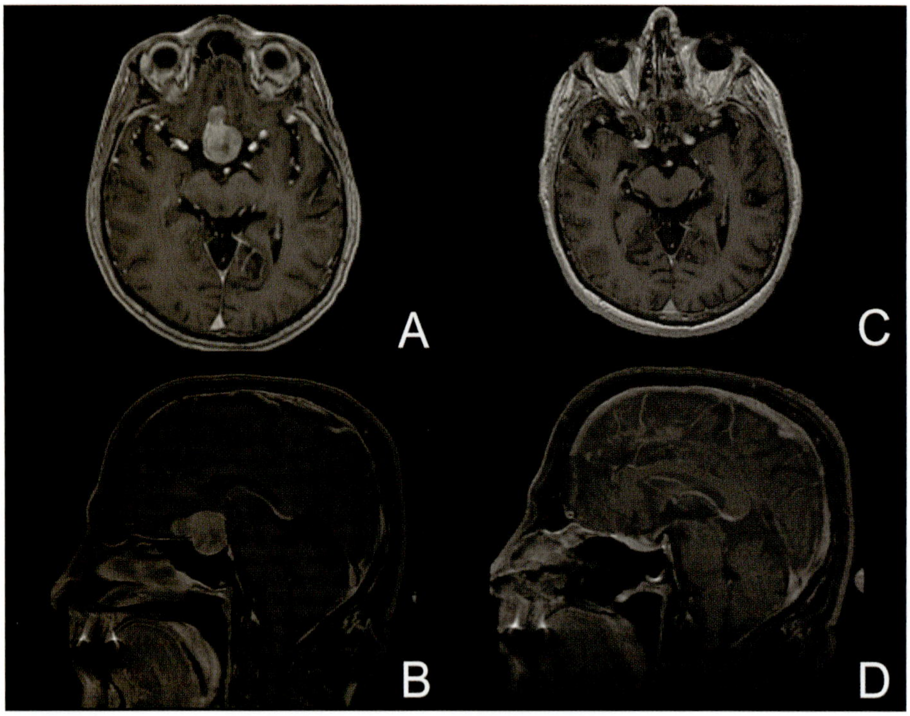

Fig. 11.6 MRI with contrast of a 56-year-old man with a pituitary macroadenoma with extension to the anterior fossa who presented with profound bitemporal hemianopsia. **(A)** Axial view. **(B)** Sagittal view. **(C,D)** Postoperative MRI with contrast at 3-month follow-up after an expanded endonasal transtuberculum and transplanum approach demonstrating complete adenoma resection. **(C)** Axial view. **(D)** Sagittal view.

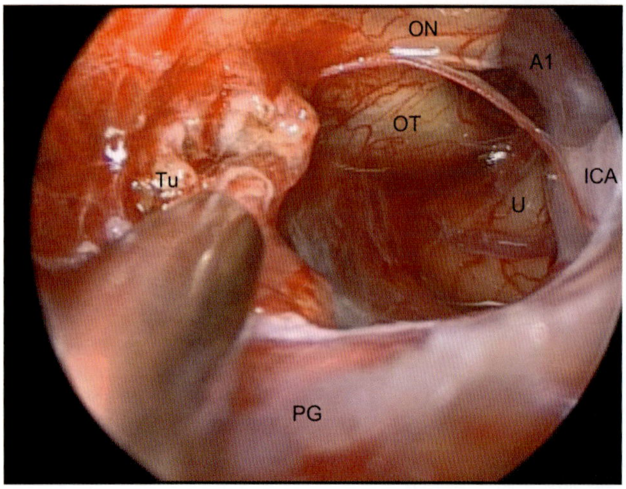

Fig. 11.7 Intraoperative view of the left suprasellar space with a zero-degree endoscope during dissection of a craniopharyngioma (*Tu*). Note that the tumor was dissected from the left internal carotid artery (*ICA*) and chiasmatic perforator, anterior cerebral artery (*A1*), left optic nerve (*ON*), and optic tract (*OT*). Note the anterior choroidal artery running on the surface of the uncus (*U*). PG, pituitary gland.

Cavernous Sinus and the Meckel Cave

Although pituitary macroadenomas often push the cavernous sinus wall laterally, respecting its limits, they may truly invade that space by crossing the plane of the medial cavernous sinus wall. There is debate in the literature regarding the pattern of this invasion. It is not clear if the invasiveness is a consequence of tumor cell characteristics or if it is related to the fact that some people may have a dehiscence of the medial wall of the cavernous sinus that facilitates adenoma penetration.[64] The reality is that any pituitary adenoma that disseminates into the cavernous sinus becomes a challenging entity to be cured, independently of the treatment strategy. Based on the potential morbidity, a surgical procedure, endonasal or craniotomy, will rarely be indicated for an invasive adenoma located inside the cavernous sinus. Radiosurgery and/or medical treatment, particularly in functional adenomas, are generally the most prudent options in these situations. However, there are circumstances in which a cavernous sinus approach is a reasonable option, such as when the patient develops cavernous sinus syndrome with florid cranial nerve neuropathy and decompression is indicated, which can be achieved with an endoscopic endonasal approach or a craniotomy with middle fossa peeling. Another reasonable indication is a patient with a functional pituitary adenoma that is limited to the medial compartment of the cavernous sinus. In this scenario, an endoscopic endonasal approach can be performed to resect the medial cavernous sinus wall and remove the disease located medial to the cavernous internal carotid artery (**Fig. 11.3**).

Other tumors can be present in these areas, such as meningiomas and schwannomas. When the disease is located lateral to the internal carotid artery in the middle fossa, filling the lateral compartment of the cavernous sinus and the Meckel cave, then a craniotomy with middle fossa skull base exposure becomes a reasonable surgical approach. However, when cavernous sinus meningiomas are resected, independently of the approach, the morbidity can be extremely high since they can invade cranial nerves.[65] Trigeminal schwannomas are usually not invasive and can be approached endonasally (**Fig. 11.9**) or by craniotomy.[62]

To reach the middle fossa through an endonasal corridor, a trans-pterygoid approach is performed. Initially, a maxillary antrostomy is developed, exposing the posterior wall

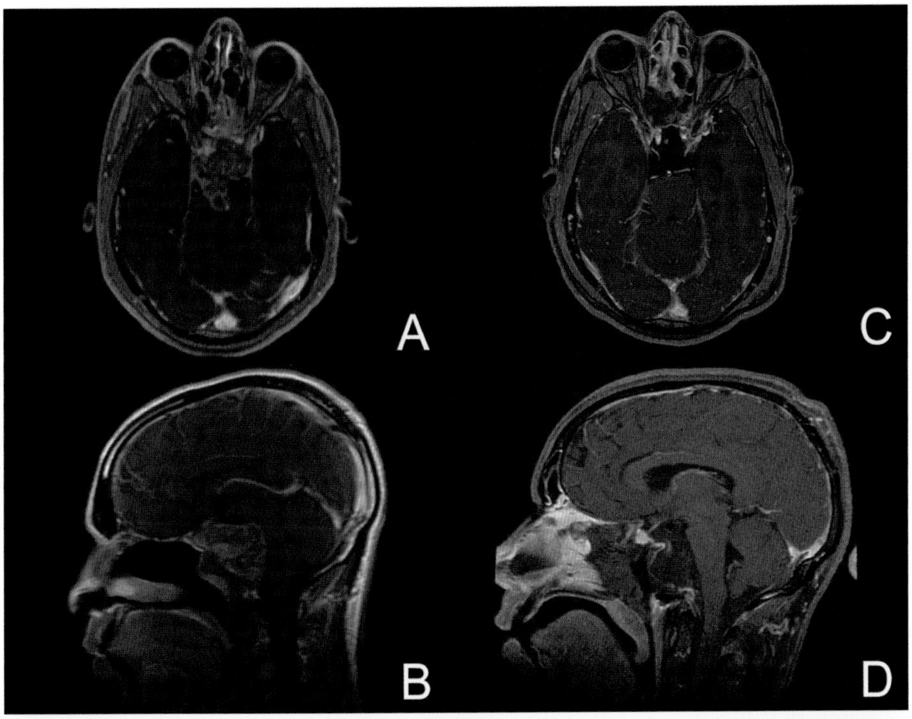

Fig. 11.8 MRI with contrast of a 28-year-old man with a recurrent clival chordoma who presented with right sixth cranial nerve palsy. **(A)** Axial view. **(B)** Sagittal view. **(C,D)** Postoperative MRI with contrast at 24 hours after an expanded endonasal transclival approach with intradural and extradural dissection demonstrating thorough chordoma resection. **(C)** Axial view. **(D)** Sagittal view. Note the preservation of the pituitary gland and stalk.

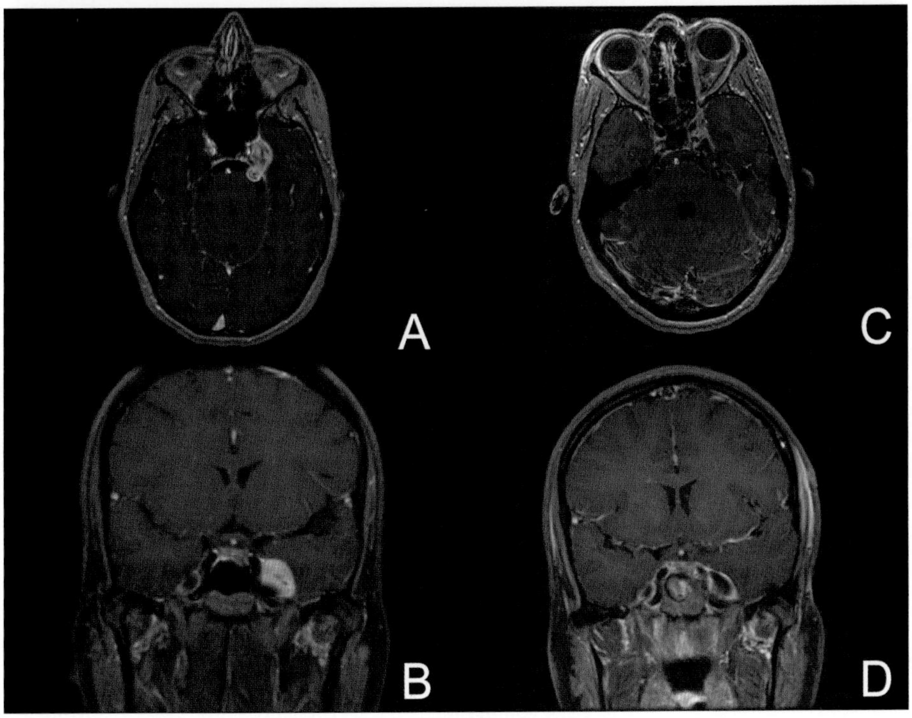

Fig. 11.9 MRI with contrast of a 20-year-old woman with a left trigeminal schwannoma who presented with left facial partial numbness. **(A)** Axial view. **(B)** Coronal view. **(C,D)** Postoperative MRIs with contrast at 24 hours demonstrating complete resection of the tumor via an endoscopic endonasal approach to Meckel's cave. **(C)** Axial view. Note that the left trigeminal nerve can now be visualized in normal position in the cistern. **(D)** Sagittal view.

of the maxillary sinus. The sphenopalatine artery is identified, and its branches are coagulated and ligated. The posterior wall of the maxillary sinus is removed, and the soft contents of the sphenopalatine fossa are retracted laterally. The vidian foramen and foramen rotundum are identified posteriorly in the sphenoid bone and preserved when possible. The lateral sphenoid recess can be completely exposed once the pterygoid base of the sphenoid plates is drilled. This exposure allows direct access to the middle fossa.

The quadrangular space is the front door to the Meckel cave.[22,62] This space is outlined by the horizontal petrous internal carotid artery inferiorly, the ascending vertical cavernous/paraclival internal carotid artery medially, the sixth cranial nerve superiorly in the cavernous sinus, and the maxillary division of the trigeminal nerve (V_2) laterally. The vidian nerve is followed posteriorly up to the level of the lacerum segment of internal carotid artery. Once the internal carotid artery is identified, it can be skeletonized if needed, depending on the pathology. The bone of the medial temporal fossa is drilled and the periosteum exposed and opened at the quadrangular space, as described above. Tumors commonly encountered in this region are invasive adenoid cystic carcinomas, juvenile nasal angiofibromas, meningiomas, schwannomas, and invasive pituitary adenomas.

The lateral compartment of the cavernous sinus is rarely approached because of the presence of cranial nerves coming and going to the superior orbital fissure. As we mentioned above, this area is explored surgically almost exclusively when the patient already has cranial nerve (III, IV, VI) deficits.

◆ The Reconstruction

Following the principles of reconstruction in open skull base surgery, we use vascularized tissue to rebuild the skull base defect. Hadad and Bassagasteguy, from Argentina, and colleagues developed a nasoseptal flap supplied by the posterior nasoseptal arteries, which are branches of the sphenopalatine artery.[66] This nasoseptal mucosal flap has been our preferred reconstruction technique.[67] The flap can be harvested initially in cases in which CSF exposure is likely, or as a rescue flap at the end of the procedure in cases in which there is an unsuccessful attempt to avoid an intraoperative CSF leak. In general, it is harvested on the side that requires less lateral exposure, contralateral to the lesion.[67]

During this reconstruction, the flap needs to be in contact with the denuded bone for proper defect closing, so all the sinus mucosa is removed.

Besides the nasoseptal flap, we use an inlay subdural graft of collagen matrix. Rarely, in cases in which the nasoseptal flap does not cover the entire defect, an additional onlay fascial graft and/or abdominal free fat is used. It is imperative to avoid any foreign body or nonvascularized tissue between the flap and the surrounding edges of the defect.

When a nasoseptal flap is not available, then other sources of vascularized tissue exist. Excellent alternatives can be encountered in the nasal cavity, such as an inferior turbinate flap, optimized for clival defects, or middle turbinate flaps for anterior fossa small defects.[1,68] In situations in which a vascularized flap is not available in the nasal cavity, such as after multiple surgical procedures or radiation, then healthy vascularized tissue can be elevated from outside and rotated into the nasal cavity to cover the defect. Examples of extranasal flaps that can be rotated into the nasal cavity are the trans-pterygoid temporoparietal fascia flap, based on the superficial temporal artery,[69] and a pericranial flap vascularized by the supraorbital artery, which can be elevated endoscopically and transferred to the nasal cavity through an opening in the nasal bone.[70]

Biological glue helps to fix the flap in place (but should not be overused), and nasal sponge packing or the balloon of a 12F Foley catheter is inserted to press the Hadad-Bassagasteguy flap against the defect. Inflation of the Foley balloon should be under microscopic or endoscopic observation to avoid overdistension and inadvertent compression of intracranial structures or flap vascular pedicle compromise.

◆ Conclusion

The microscopic transsphenoidal approach is the standard surgical technique for the resection of sellar lesions. However, its main limitation is related to the lack of appropriate visualization of areas distant to the sella. For those locations, the endoscopic endonasal approach is a great substitute based on the inherent characteristics of the endoscope, which allows broad-angle illumination and visualization. Although the endoscopic technique offers superior advantages over microscopic transsphenoidal surgery in dealing with parasellar lesions, it is not clear if the same is true for purely intrasellar lesions. However, the wide field given by the endoscope offers a comprehensive exposure of skull base landmarks, which allows a better surgical orientation and consequently a safer procedure.

References

1. Fortes FS, Carrau RL, Snyderman CH, et al. The posterior pedicle inferior turbinate flap: a new vascularized flap for skull base reconstruction. Laryngoscope 2007;117(8):1329–1332
2. Doglietto F, Prevedello DM, Jane JA Jr, Han J, Laws ER Jr. Brief history of endoscopic transsphenoidal surgery—from Philipp Bozzini to the First World Congress of Endoscopic Skull Base Surgery. Neurosurg Focus 2005;19(6):E3
3. Liu JK, Das K, Weiss MH, Laws ER Jr, Couldwell WT. The history and evolution of transsphenoidal surgery. J Neurosurg 2001; 95(6):1083–1096
4. Apuzzo ML, Heifetz MD, Weiss MH, Kurze T. Neurosurgical endoscopy using the side-viewing telescope. J Neurosurg 1977; 46(3):398–400
5. Bushe KA, Halves E. Modified technique in transsphenoidal operations of pituitary adenomas. Technical note (author's transl). Acta Neurochir (Wien) 1978;41(1–3):163–175
6. Halves E, Bushe KA. Transsphenoidal operation on craniopharyngiomas with extrasellar extensions. The advantage of the operating endoscope [proceedings]. Acta Neurochir Suppl (Wien) 1979;28(2):362
7. Dusick JR, Esposito F, Kelly DF, et al. The extended direct endonasal transsphenoidal approach for nonadenomatous suprasellar tumors. J Neurosurg 2005;102(5):832–841
8. Couldwell WT, Weiss MH, Rabb C, Liu JK, Apfelbaum RI, Fukushima T. Variations on the standard transsphenoidal approach to the sellar region, with emphasis on the extended approaches and parasellar approaches: surgical experience in 105 cases. Neurosurgery 2004;55(3):539–547, discussion 547–550
9. Frank G, Pasquini E, Mazzatenta D. Extended transsphenoidal approach. J Neurosurg 2001;95(5):917–918
10. Catapano D, Sloffer CA, Frank G, Pasquini E, D'Angelo VA, Lanzino G. Comparison between the microscope and endoscope in the direct endonasal extended transsphenoidal approach: anatomical study. J Neurosurg 2006;104(3):419–425
11. Frank G, Pasquini E, Doglietto F, et al. The endoscopic extended transsphenoidal approach for craniopharyngiomas. Neurosurgery 2006;59(1, Suppl 1):ONS75–ONS83
12. de Divitiis E, Cappabianca P. Microscopic and endoscopic transsphenoidal surgery. Neurosurgery 2002;51(6):1527–1529, author reply 1529–1530

13. Jankowski R, Auque J, Simon C, Marchal JC, Hepner H, Wayoff M. Endoscopic pituitary tumor surgery. Laryngoscope 1992;102(2):198–202
14. Carrau RL, Jho HD, Ko Y. Transnasal-transsphenoidal endoscopic surgery of the pituitary gland. Laryngoscope 1996;106(7):914–918
15. Jho HD, Carrau RL. Endoscopic endonasal transsphenoidal surgery: experience with 50 patients. J Neurosurg 1997;87(1):44–51
16. Litynski GS. Endoscopic surgery: the history, the pioneers. World J Surg 1999;23(8):745–753
17. Cappabianca P, Alfieri A, Colao A, et al. Endoscopic endonasal transsphenoidal surgery in recurrent and residual pituitary adenomas: technical note. Minim Invasive Neurosurg 2000;43(1):38–43
18. Cappabianca P, Frank G, Pasquini E, de Divitiis E, Calbucci F. Extended endoscopic endonasal transsphenoidal approaches to the suprasellar region, planum sphenoidale and clivus. In: de Divitiis E, Cappabianca P, eds. Endoscopic Endonasal Transsphenoidal Surgery. Springer-Verlag; 2003:176–187
19. Cavallo LM, Briganti F, Cappabianca P, et al. Hemorrhagic vascular complications of endoscopic transsphenoidal surgery. Minim Invasive Neurosurg 2004;47(3):145–150
20. Cavallo LM, Cappabianca P, Galzio R, Iaconetta G, de Divitiis E, Tschabitscher M. Endoscopic transnasal approach to the cavernous sinus versus transcranial route: anatomic study. Neurosurgery 2005;56(2, Suppl):379–389, discussion 379–389
21. Cavallo LM, Messina A, Cappabianca P, et al. Endoscopic endonasal surgery of the midline skull base: anatomical study and clinical considerations. Neurosurg Focus 2005;19(1):E2
22. Cavallo LM, Messina A, Gardner P, et al. Extended endoscopic endonasal approach to the pterygopalatine fossa: anatomical study and clinical considerations. Neurosurg Focus 2005;19(1):E5
23. Cappabianca P, Alfieri A, Thermes S, Buonamassa S, de Divitiis E. Instruments for endoscopic endonasal transsphenoidal surgery. Neurosurgery 1999;45(2):392–395, discussion 395–396
24. Cappabianca P, Cavallo LM, Mariniello G, de Divitiis O, Romero AD, de Divitiis E. Easy sellar reconstruction in endoscopic endonasal transsphenoidal surgery with polyester-silicone dural substitute and fibrin glue: technical note. Neurosurgery 2001;49(2):473–475, discussion 475–476
25. Cappabianca P, Cavallo LM, Valente V, et al. Sellar repair with fibrin sealant and collagen fleece after endoscopic endonasal transsphenoidal surgery. Surg Neurol 2004;62(3):227–233, discussion 233
26. Cappabianca P, de Divitiis E. Back to the Egyptians: neurosurgery via the nose. A five-thousand year history and the recent contribution of the endoscope. Neurosurg Rev 2007;30(1):1–7, discussion 7
27. de Divitiis E. Endoscopic transsphenoidal surgery: stone-in-the-pond effect. Neurosurgery 2006;59(3):512–520
28. Dumont AS, Kanter AS, Jane JA Jr, Laws ER Jr. Extended transsphenoidal approach. Front Horm Res 2006;34:29–45
29. Laws ER Jr. Transsphenoidal microsurgery in the management of craniopharyngioma. J Neurosurg 1980;52(5):661–666
30. Laws ER, Kanter AS, Jane JA Jr, Dumont AS. Extended transsphenoidal approach. J Neurosurg 2005;102(5):825–827, discussion 827–828
31. Kaptain GJ, Vincent DA, Sheehan JP, Laws ER Jr. Transsphenoidal approaches for the extracapsular resection of midline suprasellar and anterior cranial base lesions. Neurosurgery 2001;49(1):94–100, discussion 100–101
32. Kern EB, Laws ER Jr. The transseptal approach to the pituitary gland. Rhinology 1978;16(2):59–78
33. Kassam A, Snyderman CH, Mintz A, Gardner P, Carrau RL. Expanded endonasal approach: the rostrocaudal axis. Part II. Posterior clinoids to the foramen magnum. Neurosurg Focus 2005; 19(1):E4
34. Kassam A, Snyderman CH, Mintz A, Gardner P, Carrau RL. Expanded endonasal approach: the rostrocaudal axis. Part I. Crista galli to the sella turcica. Neurosurg Focus 2005;19(1):E3
35. de Divitiis E, Cappabianca P, Cavallo LM, Esposito F, de Divitiis O, Messina A. Extended endoscopic transsphenoidal approach for extrasellar craniopharyngiomas. Neurosurgery 2007;61(5, Suppl 2):219–227, discussion 228
36. de Divitiis E, Cavallo LM, Esposito F, Stella L, Messina A. Extended endoscopic transsphenoidal approach for tuberculum sellae meningiomas. Neurosurgery 2008;62(6, Suppl 3):1192–1201
37. Frank G, Sciarretta V, Calbucci F, Farneti G, Mazzatenta D, Pasquini E. The endoscopic transnasal transsphenoidal approach for the treatment of cranial base chordomas and chondrosarcomas. Neurosurgery 2006;59(1, Suppl 1):ONS50–ONS57
38. Kassam AB, Prevedello DM, Carrau RL, et al. The front door to Meckel's cave: an antero-medial corridor via expanded endoscopic endonasal approach- technical considerations and clinical series. Neurosurgery 2009;64(3, Suppl):71–82
39. Kassam AB, Vescan AD, Carrau RL, et al. Expanded endonasal approach: vidian canal as a landmark to the petrous internal carotid artery. J Neurosurg 2008;108(1):177–183
40. Prevedello DM, Thomas A, Gardner P, Snyderman CH, Carrau RL, Kassam AB. Endoscopic endonasal resection of a synchronous pituitary adenoma and a tuberculum sellae meningioma: technical case report. Neurosurgery 2007;60(4, Suppl 2):E401, discussion E401
41. Stippler M, Gardner PA, Snyderman CH, Carrau RL, Prevedello DM, Kassam AB. Endoscopic endonasal approach for clival chordomas. Neurosurgery 2009;64(2):268–277, discussion 277–278
42. Kassam AB, Mintz AH, Gardner PA, Horowitz MB, Carrau RL, Snyderman CH. The expanded endonasal approach for an endoscopic transnasal clipping and aneurysmorrhaphy of a large vertebral artery aneurysm: technical case report. Neurosurgery 2006;59(1, Suppl 1):E162–E165
43. Kassam AB, Snyderman C, Gardner P, Carrau R, Spiro R. The expanded endonasal approach: a fully endoscopic transnasal approach and resection of the odontoid process: technical case report. Neurosurgery 2005;57(1, Suppl):E213, discussion E213
44. Cappabianca P, de Divitiis E. Endoscopy and transsphenoidal surgery. Neurosurgery 2004;54(5):1043–1048
45. Youssef AS, Agazzi S, van Loveren HR. Transcranial surgery for pituitary adenomas. Neurosurgery 2005;57(1, Suppl):168–175
46. Prevedello DM, Pouratian N, Sherman J, et al. Management of Cushing's disease: outcome in patients with microadenoma detected on pituitary magnetic resonance imaging. J Neurosurg 2008;109(4):751–759
47. Kerr PB, Oldfield EH. Sublabial-endonasal approach to the sella turcica. J Neurosurg 2008;109(1):153–155
48. Cavallo LM, Prevedello D, Esposito F, et al. The role of the endoscope in the transsphenoidal management of cystic lesions of the sellar region. Neurosurg Rev 2008;31(1):55–64, discussion 64
49. Jane JA Jr, Han J, Prevedello DM, Jagannathan J, Dumont AS, Laws ER Jr. Perspectives on endoscopic transsphenoidal surgery. Neurosurg Focus 2005;19(6):E2
50. Nejadkazem M, Samii A, Fahlbusch R, Bidadi S. A simplified direct endonasal approach for transsphenoidal surgery. Minim Invasive Neurosurg 2008;51(5):272–274
51. Lindholm J. A century of pituitary surgery: Schloffer's legacy. Neurosurgery 2007;61(4):865–867, discussion 867–868
52. Er U, Gürses L, Saka C, et al. Sublabial transseptal approach to pituitary adenomas with special emphasis on rhinological complications. Turk Neurosurg 2008;18(4):425–430
53. Jagannathan J, Prevedello DM, Ayer VS, Dumont AS, Jane JA Jr, Laws ER. Computer-assisted frameless stereotaxy in transsphenoidal surgery at a single institution: review of 176 cases. Neurosurg Focus 2006;20(2):E9
54. Fatemi N, Dusick JR, de Paiva Neto MA, Kelly DF. The endonasal microscopic approach for pituitary adenomas and other parasellar tumors: a 10-year experience. Neurosurgery 2008;63(4, Suppl 2):244–256, discussion 256
55. Dusick JR, Esposito F, Malkasian D, Kelly DF. Avoidance of carotid artery injuries in transsphenoidal surgery with the Doppler probe and micro-hook blades. Neurosurgery 2007;60(4, Suppl 2):322–328, discussion 328–329
56. Cappabianca P, Alfieri A, de Divitiis E. Endoscopic endonasal transsphenoidal approach to the sella: towards functional endoscopic pituitary surgery (FEPS). Minim Invasive Neurosurg 1998;41(2):66–73
57. Oldfield EH, Vortmeyer AO. Development of a histological pseudocapsule and its use as a surgical capsule in the excision of pituitary tumors. J Neurosurg 2006;104(1):7–19
58. Carrabba G, Dehdashti AR, Gentili F. Surgery for clival lesions: open resection versus the expanded endoscopic endonasal approach. Neurosurg Focus 2008;25(6):E7
59. Al-Mefty O, Kadri PA, Hasan DM, Isolan GR, Pravdenkova S. Anterior clivectomy: surgical technique and clinical applications. J Neurosurg 2008;109(5):783–793
60. Zanation AM, Snyderman CH, Carrau RL, Gardner PA, Prevedello DM, Kassam AB. Endoscopic endonasal surgery for petrous apex lesions. Laryngoscope 2009;119(1):19–25

61. Gardner PA, Kassam AB, Thomas A, et al. Endoscopic endonasal resection of anterior cranial base meningiomas. Neurosurgery 2008;63(1):36–52, discussion 52–54
62. Kassam AB, Prevedello DM, Carrau RL, et al. The front door to Meckel's cave: an anteromedial corridor via expanded endoscopic endonasal approach- technical considerations and clinical series. Neurosurgery 2009;64(3, Suppl):71–82, discussion 82–83
63. Kassam AB, Prevedello DM, Thomas A, et al. Endoscopic endonasal pituitary transposition for a transdorsum sellae approach to the interpeduncular cistern. Neurosurgery 2008;62(3, Suppl 1):57–72, discussion 72–74
64. Prevedello DM, Jagannathan J, Jane JA Jr, Lopes MB, Laws ER Jr. Relevance of high Ki-67 in pituitary adenomas. Case report and review of the literature. Neurosurg Focus 2005;19(5):E11
65. Larson JJ, van Loveren HR, Balko MG, Tew JM Jr. Evidence of meningioma infiltration into cranial nerves: clinical implications for cavernous sinus meningiomas. J Neurosurg 1995;83(4): 596–599
66. Hadad G, Bassagasteguy L, Carrau RL, et al. A novel reconstructive technique after endoscopic expanded endonasal approaches: vascular pedicle nasoseptal flap. Laryngoscope 2006;116(10): 1882–1886
67. Kassam AB, Thomas A, Carrau RL, et al. Endoscopic reconstruction of the cranial base using a pedicled nasoseptal flap. Neurosurgery 2008;63(1, Suppl 1):ONS44–ONS52, discussion ONS52–ONS53
68. Prevedello DM, Barges-Coll J, Fernandez-Miranda JC, et al. Middle turbinate flap for skull base reconstruction: cadaveric feasibility study. Laryngoscope 2009;119(11):2094–2098
69. Fortes FS, Carrau RL, Snyderman CH, et al. Transpterygoid transposition of a temporoparietal fascia flap: a new method for skull base reconstruction after endoscopic expanded endonasal approaches. Laryngoscope 2007;117(6):970–976
70. Zanation AM, Snyderman CH, Carrau RL, Kassam AB, Gardner PA, Prevedello DM. Minimally invasive endoscopic pericranial flap: a new method for endonasal skull base reconstruction. Laryngoscope 2009;119(1):13–18

12 Transcranial Approaches to the Sellar and Parasellar Area

Bradley N. Bohnstedt, Todd Eads, R. Shane Tubbs, and Aaron A. Cohen-Gadol

The differential diagnosis of a mass within the parasellar space is vast. Common lesions include neoplastic extra-axial masses such as pituitary adenomas, craniopharyngiomas, and meningiomas, or rarely vascular lesions such as an aneurysm. An intra-axial tumor such as an astrocytoma may also be found in this region. Other lesions may be encountered, including Rathke cleft cyst, arachnoid cyst, germinoma, lymphoma, metastasis, abscess, sarcoidosis, histiocytosis, hypophysitis, infundibuloma, and neurocysticercosis, to name a few.[1] An in-depth understanding and familiarity with various transcranial approaches is necessary for neurosurgeons who are willing to tackle lesions within the parasellar region.

Although the transsphenoidal route is the preferred route for most patients with a pituitary adenoma, ~1 to 4% of pituitary tumors require surgical resection via a transcranial route.[2,3] Pituitary adenomas with a large suprasellar extension may be inaccessible through a purely transsphenoidal-transsellar route. Parasellar lesions extending into the cavernous sinus and dumbbell-shaped sellar lesions with a narrow neck across the diaphragma sellae may be approached through a transcranial route. Other contraindications to the transsphenoidal approach include active sinus infection, lesions that coexist with an adjacent aneurysm, and ectatic "kissing" carotid arteries or fibrous tumors with suprasellar extension. Some neurosurgeons have considered the uncertainty regarding the pathology of these lesions (ie, meningioma vs. adenoma) to be an indication for the transcranial route.[4] The most often cited reason for using the transcranial approach is a previously failed transsphenoidal exploration, which commonly results from a combination of the above-listed reasons. In addition, a lack of descent of the suprasellar component of a large pituitary macroadenoma after a transsphenoidal resection may lead the clinician to consider a transcranial approach from above. As a general rule, parasellar lesions that do not enlarge the sella, such as meningiomas and craniopharyngiomas, typically require a greater field of view than that provided through the transsphenoidal route and may be best approached through a transcranial corridor to ensure gross total resection with preservation of neighboring neurovascular structures.

Transcranial approaches provide a more panoramic view of critical neurovascular structures such as the carotid artery and optic nerves early in the dissection process, further protecting them from unsafe surgical manipulations. Conversely, transcranial approaches may pose increased surgical risks associated with a craniotomy, including frontal lobe injury due to retraction. When an approach to the sellar and parasellar regions is considered, the benefits of each approach should be carefully weighed against its inherent risks. When the neurosurgeon decides on a particular transcranial approach, he or she must take into account the specific features of the neuroanatomy of the lesion, including its size, location, relationship to the critical neurovascular structures, and predicted pathology.

◆ Preoperative Preparation

Before the incision is made for any of the approaches listed below, the patient is given an intravenous dose of an antibiotic (continued for 24 hours postoperatively) and an anticonvulsant (continued for 7 days postoperatively, unless a seizure disorder develops). The arterial P_{CO_2} is maintained at ~30 mm Hg throughout the case. The patient is also given 10 mg of dexamethasone and 1 g of mannitol per kilogram intravenously at the time of the incision. A lumbar drain or external ventricular drain is generally not required. However, an external ventricular drain may be placed when the patient has hydrocephalus or when peritumoral edema is significant enough to cause intracranial hypertension.

For all approaches, the head is held in position via a 3-pin Mayfield head holder or another fixation device. The head is positioned above the heart to encourage venous drainage, turned 20 to 30 degrees contralaterally, and slightly extended to keep the zygomatic arch as the highest point in the surgical field (**Fig. 12.1**). A minimal amount of hair is shaved, and the planned skin incision is infiltrated with lidocaine-epinephrine solution.

◆ Pterional Approach

The pterional craniotomy has been one of the workhorse approaches in neurosurgery for many years. Yasargil et al refined and described the intricacies of this approach.[5]

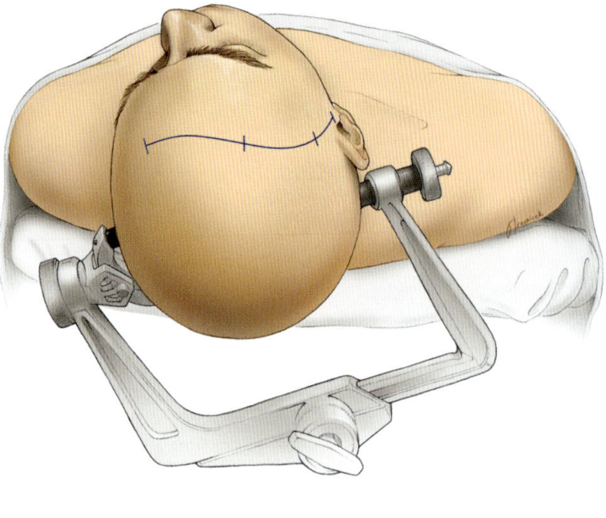

Fig. 12.1 For all approaches, the head is held in position via a three-pin Mayfield head holder. The head is positioned above the heart to encourage venous drainage, turned 20 to 30 degrees contralaterally, and slightly extended to keep the zygomatic arch as the highest point in the surgical field.

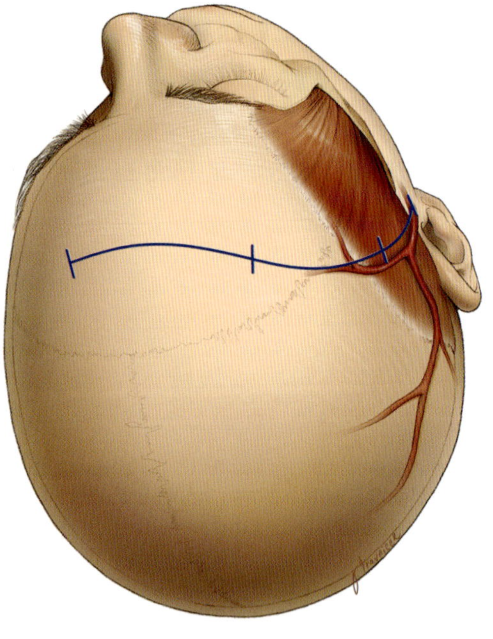

Fig. 12.2 A small area of hair is shaved along a standard pterional skin incision. The incision is begun at the zygomatic arch, 1 cm anterior to the tragus to avoid the superficial temporal artery, and is continued 1 to 2 cm behind the hairline to the contralateral midpupillary line.

Although commonly used for anterior circulation aneurysms, the pterional craniotomy also provides an excellent working corridor for resection of suprasellar and parasellar tumors. Of the transcranial approaches, it commonly affords one of the shortest operating distances to the lesion.[6] This approach displays familiar anatomy, provides efficient access to the sellar and parasellar regions, and is easily mastered. The senior author (ACG) most commonly uses this approach among the other transcranial routes for reaching parasellar lesions.

Once the decision has been made to use the pterional approach, laterality must be addressed. If the tumor extends significantly to one side, the tumor should be approached from that side. When lateral extension is not an issue, the approach is from the same side as the eye with the poorer vision. If the patient's vision is symmetrically affected, the approach is from the side of the nondominant hemisphere.

A small area of hair is shaved along a standard pterional skin incision. The incision is begun at the zygomatic arch, 1 cm anterior to the tragus to avoid the superficial temporal artery, and is continued 1 to 2 cm behind the hairline to the contralateral midpupillary line (**Fig. 12.2**). When reflecting the skin flap forward, the neurosurgeon should keep the plane of dissection below the plane of the superficial fat pad that rests above the temporal muscle and fascia. The frontal branch of the facial nerve travels through the superficial fascia of the fat pad and should be protected. The temporalis muscle is elevated from the bone with Bovie electrocautery and reflected with the scalp flap anteriorly in one musculocutaneous layer (**Fig. 12.3**).

A burr hole is placed just inferior to the posterior aspect of the superior temporal line, abutting the skin incision, and a standard pterional craniotomy flap is elevated and extended just lateral to the midpupillary line (**Fig. 12.4**). If the frontal sinus is violated, it is exenterated by thoroughly stripping its mucosa away to avoid formation of a mucocele, and the sinus ostium is plugged with pieces of temporalis muscle to avoid postoperative cerebrospinal fluid (CSF) rhinorrhea.

To maximize exposure and minimize frontal lobe retraction, the lateral aspect of the sphenoid ridge is drilled away as far as the superior orbital fissure. Furthermore, the edge of frontal bone over the lateral aspect of the roof of the orbit is drilled flush with the roof of the orbit by using a high-speed drill (**Figs. 12.5** and **12.6**). A Leksell rongeur is then used to remove additional temporal bone to expose the floor of the middle cranial fossa.

The dura is incised with a C-shaped durotomy (**Fig. 12.7**), reflected anteriorly, and tacked up with stitches to the galea of the retracted scalp flap. With an operating microscope, a retractor blade is gently placed subfrontally just anterior to the sphenoid ridge and lateral to the olfactory tract (**Fig. 12.8**). The olfactory tract is followed posteriorly until the arachnoid over the optic nerve and the internal carotid artery cisterns are identified. CSF can then be drained by opening these cisterns to further increase brain relaxation. When a large tumor completely fills these cisterns, preoperative placement of a lumbar drain or intraoperative placement of an external ventricular drain should be done through a frontal burr hole to increase brain relaxation and decrease the need for frontal lobe retraction for tumor exposure.

Retraction of the frontal and temporal lobes can be facilitated by opening the anterior limb of the sylvian fissure (**Fig. 12.9**). This maneuver will aid in reducing the retraction forces needed to obtain tumor exposure. The arachnoid of the sylvian fissure is dissected in a superfi-

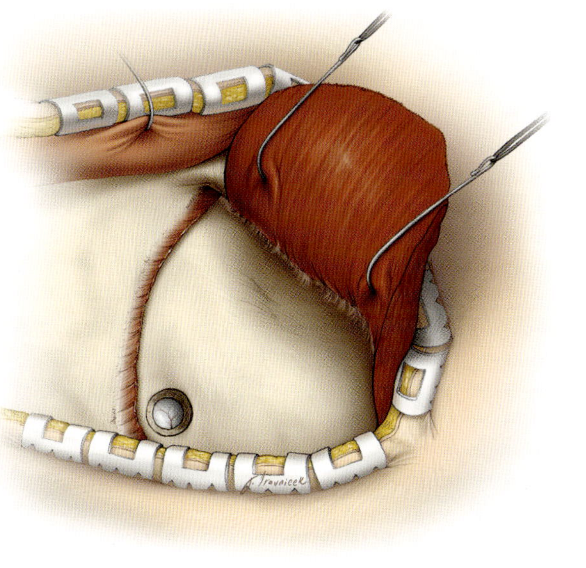

Fig. 12.3 The temporalis muscle is elevated from the bone with Bovie electrocautery and reflected with the scalp flap anteriorly in one musculocutaneous layer.

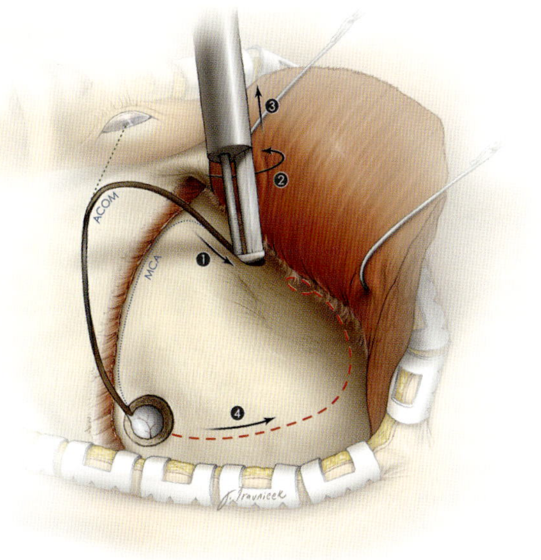

Fig. 12.4 A burr hole is placed just inferior to the posterior aspect of the superior temporal line, abutting the skin incision, and a standard pterional craniotomy flap is elevated and extended just lateral to the midpupillary line.

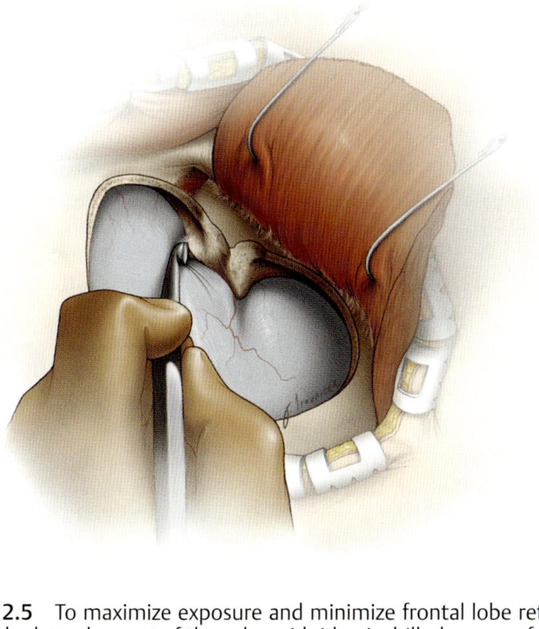

Fig. 12.5 To maximize exposure and minimize frontal lobe retraction, the lateral aspect of the sphenoid ridge is drilled away as far as the superior orbital fissure.

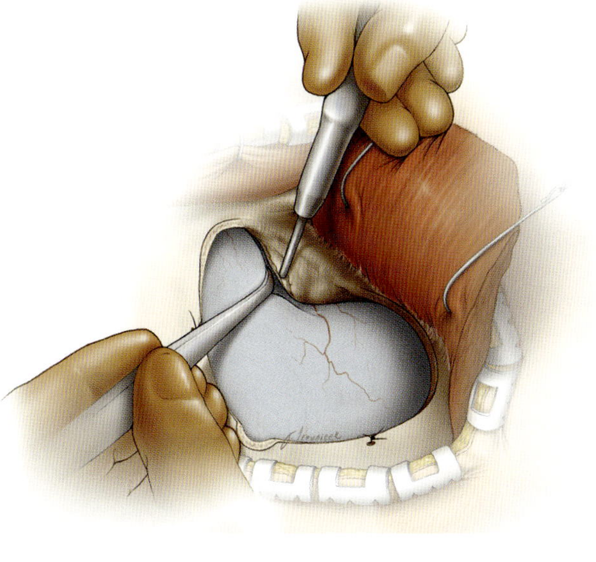

Fig. 12.6 The edge of frontal bone over the lateral aspect of the roof of the orbit is drilled flush with the roof of the orbit by using a high-speed drill.

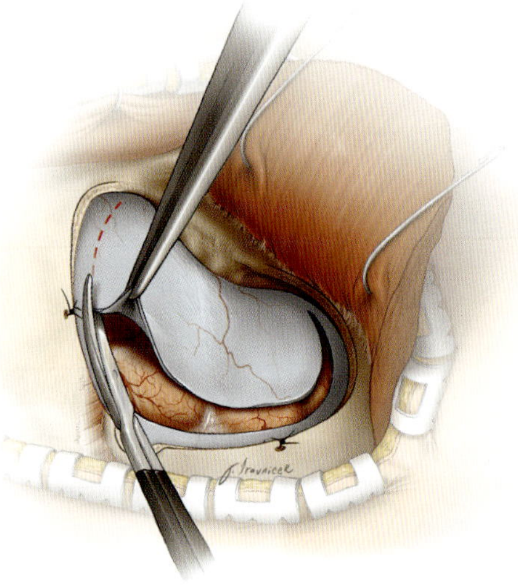

Fig. 12.7 The dura is incised by using a C-shaped durotomy.

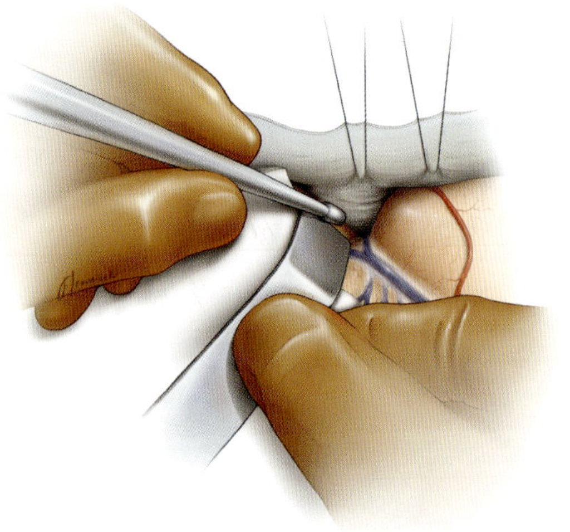

Fig. 12.8 With an operating microscope, a retractor blade is gently placed subfrontally just anterior to the sphenoid ridge and lateral to the olfactory tract.

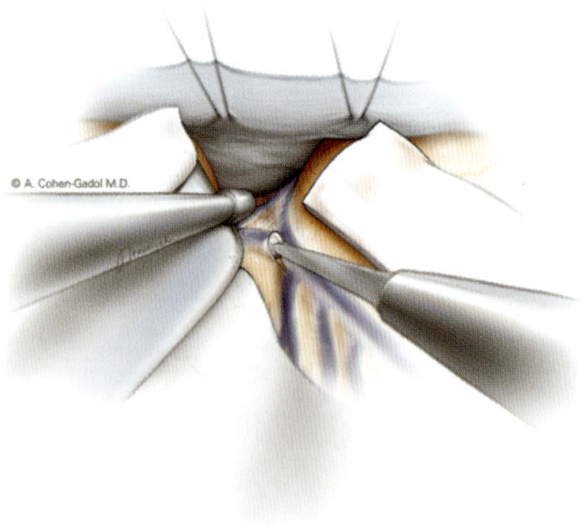

Fig. 12.9 Retraction of the frontal and temporal lobes can be facilitated by opening the anterior limb of the sylvian fissure.

cial to deep manner along its anterior limb (**Figs. 12.10** and **12.11**). The opening of the arachnoid nearest the lesion is of key importance for optimal exposure[7] (**Fig. 12.12**). The arachnoid is dissected by using a blunt fine-tip probe to separate the arachnoid from the entangled vessels and then sharply cut. Microscissors can be used to continue to open the arachnoid. Bleeding can generally be controlled with irrigation; however, the small bridging veins along the anterior limb of the sylvian fissure can be taken with little ill effect. The sylvian arteries should be preserved with their corresponding lobe as much as possible. The extent to which the fissure is split depends on and is tailored to the size of the lesion to be resected. The thicker arachnoid layers over the carotid artery and optic nerve are sharply cut (**Figs. 12.13** and **12.14**).

At this point, the neurosurgeon can work in several different corridors to access and resect the tumor, including the opticocarotid, prechiasmatic, and retrocarotid windows (**Fig. 12.15**). The lamina terminalis provides access to the third ventricular component of the lesion when necessary. Initially, only the ipsilateral optic nerve may be in view, but as tumor resection proceeds, identification of the contralateral carotid artery and optic nerve early in the dissection process is imperative to prevent their injury. Opening the falciform ligament will partly release the optic nerve and allow safer mobilization of the nerve to manipulate the tumor (**Fig. 12.16**). Tumor resection should begin with devascularization (especially for meningiomas) and as much intracapsular debulking as possible and then careful dissection of the tumor capsule away from the critical surrounding tissues (**Figs. 12.17, 12.18, 12.19,** and **12.20**). Further details concerning the treatment of individual pathologies can be found in Chapters 6 through 10.

The major disadvantage of the pterional approach becomes apparent in cases in which the optic chiasm is prefixed, allowing a very limited working channel. In addition, resection may become more difficult if the lesion extends far superiorly or posteriorly because of limited exposure through this basal frontal route. Complications associated with the pterional approach include infection, hematoma, CSF leakage, postoperative seizures, and frontal lobe edema from excessive retraction. Optic nerve damage may occur during surgery as a result of aggressive tumor resection or bipolar cauterization of the nearby perforating vessels. The perforating arteries supplying the optic apparatus arise from the anterior communicating artery and from underneath the chiasm and should be preserved. Hypothalamic and/or pituitary damage can also occur as the result of manipulation of these structures or their vascular supply. Pituitary dysfunction may manifest postoperatively as diabetes insipidus and should be treated accordingly.

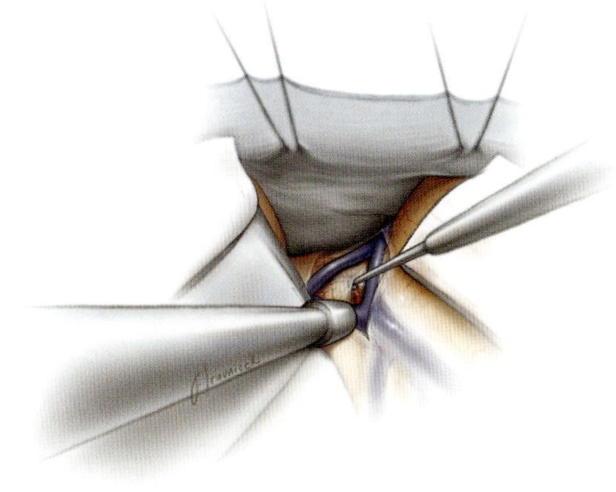

Fig. 12.10 The arachnoid of the sylvian fissure is dissected in a superficial to deep manner along its anterior limb.

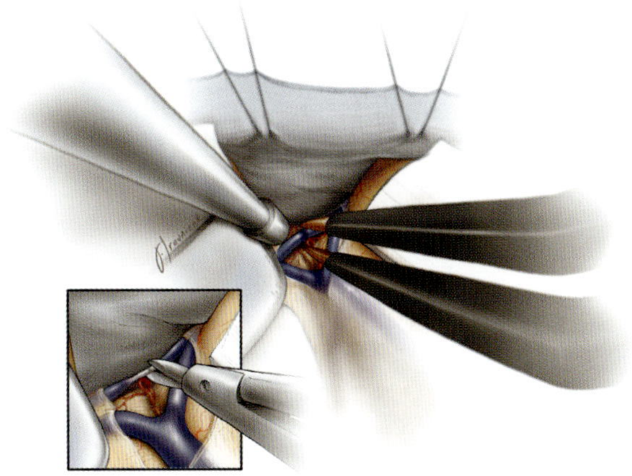

Fig. 12.11 Bridging veins are coagulated and cut.

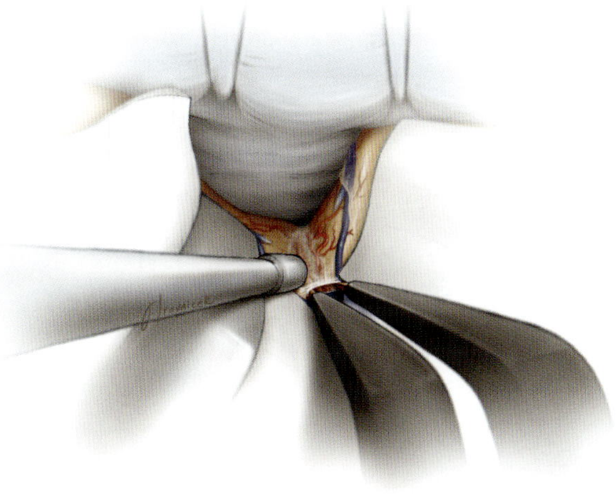

Fig. 12.12 The opening of the arachnoid nearest the lesion is of key importance for optimal exposure.

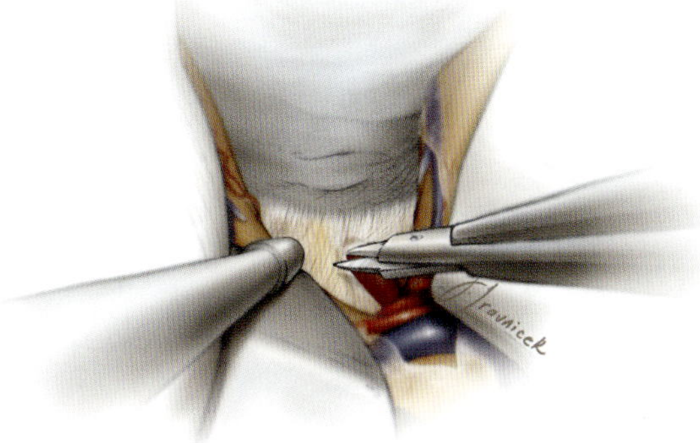

Fig. 12.13 The thicker arachnoid layers over the carotid artery and optic nerve are sharply cut.

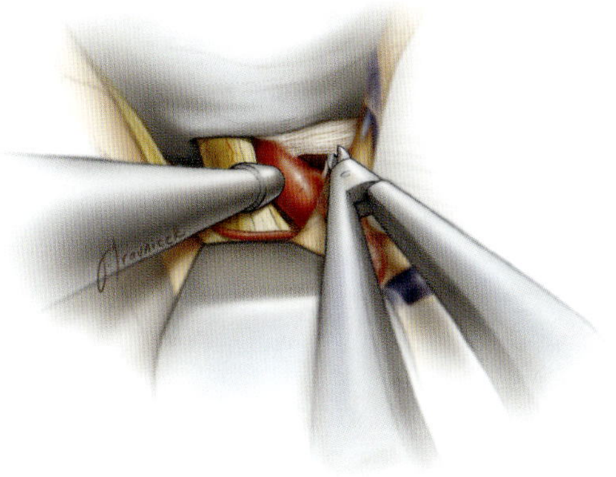

Fig. 12.14 Further arachnoid opening is completed.

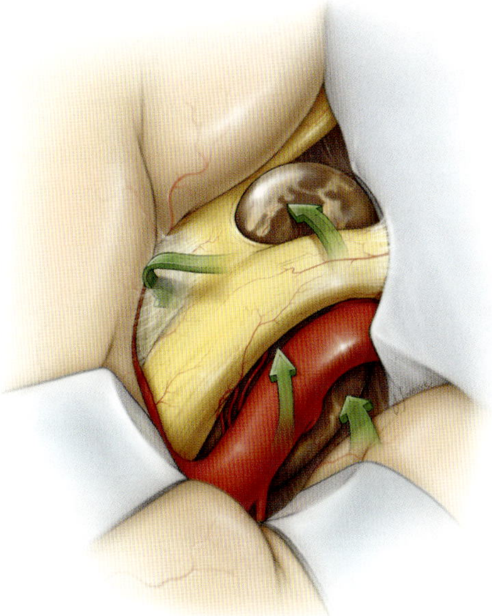

Fig. 12.15 The surgeon can work in several different corridors to access and resect the tumor, including the opticocarotid, prechiasmatic, and retrocarotid windows.

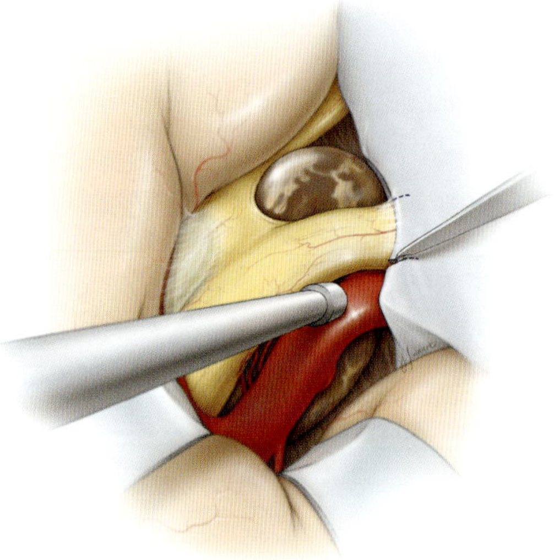

Fig. 12.16 Opening the falciform ligament will partly release the optic nerve and allow safer mobilization of the nerve to manipulate the tumor.

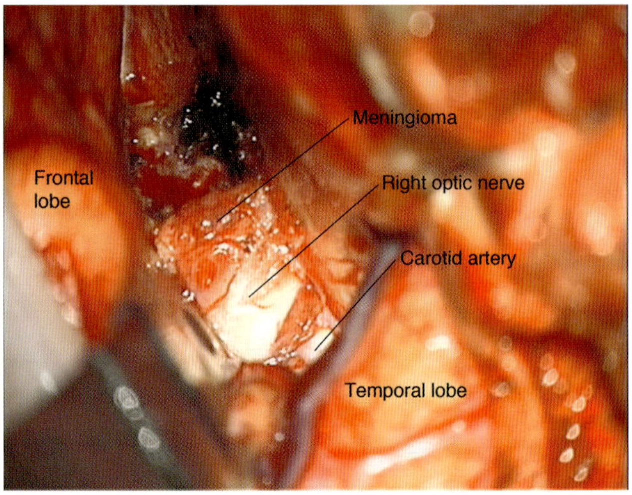

Fig. 12.17 Tumor resection should begin with devascularization (especially for meningiomas) and as much intracapsular debulking as possible and then careful dissection of the tumor capsule away from the critical surrounding tissues. These intraoperative images illustrate the steps involved in the removal of a suprasellar meningioma through a right pterional approach.

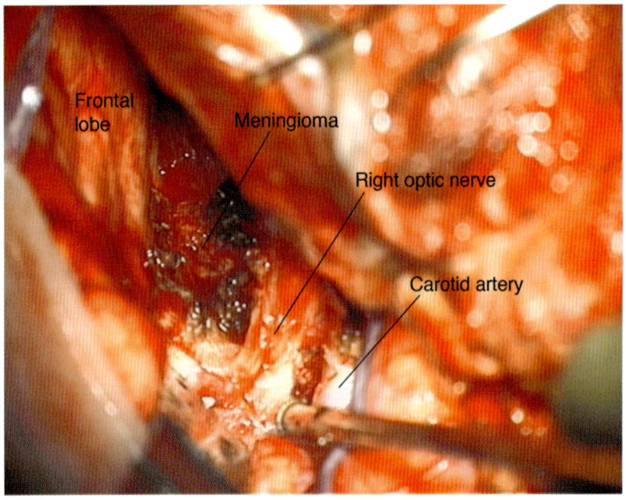

Fig. 12.18 The falciform ligament is incised, the optic nerve is released, and the tumor is debulked.

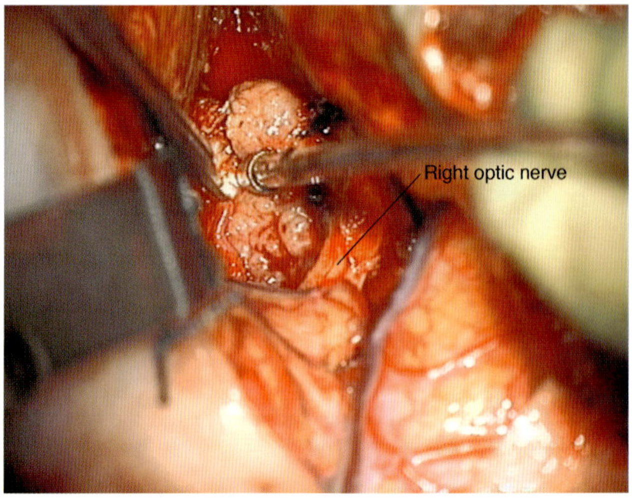

Fig. 12.19 Further tumor debulking is completed.

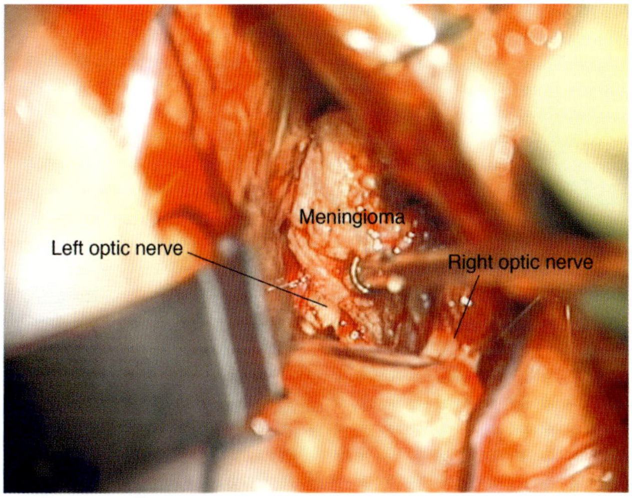

Fig. 12.20 Dissection around the posterior part of the tumor reveals the contralateral optic nerve at the level of the chiasm.

◆ Orbitozygomatic Approach

The orbitozygomatic (OZ) approach takes the pterional craniotomy one step further in terms of increasing visualization of the surgical corridor and decreasing the working distance of the operator by removing more of the skull base bone. The modified OZ craniotomy has been adequate for reaching parasellar lesions and is the preferred approach when additional bony removal is necessary for the resection of large lesions with superior and posterior extensions. This modified OZ approach is actually an extended frontotemporal craniotomy that includes a supraorbital osteotomy. The frontal and temporal bone flap, usually removed for a traditional pterional craniotomy, in this case also includes the orbital rim from just lateral to the supraorbital foramen/notch to as far as just inferior to the frontozygomatic suture. OZ craniotomy provides an expanded corridor in which to reach lesions involving the circle of Willis, including the orbit, paraclinoid and parasellar locations, cavernous sinus, and especially the more cranially located basilar apex region.

For the one-piece modified OZ osteotomy approach, the patient's head position is similar to the one used during the pterional approach, with the head rotated contralaterally ~15 degrees. An incision is begun at the inferior edge of the zygomatic bone 1 cm anterior to the tragus and carried to the contralateral midpupillary line just behind the hairline. The periosteum and superficial layer of the temporalis fascia (including the fat pad) are carried up in one layer with the skin flap by using an interfascial method. Care must be taken when working near the supraorbital notch to avoid cutting the supraorbital nerve and, instead, to release this nerve from its notch. Occasionally, a foramen (20–25%) may house this nerve, in which case the bone around the nerve should be drilled away. The nerve can then be reflected anteriorly along with the scalp flap. Dissection is continued along the orbital rim to the zygomatic process, allowing the scalp to be fully mobilized and reflected anteriorly along these bony edges. The superior and lateral periorbita is then carefully dissected away to a depth of ~1.5 to 2 cm. Care must be taken to keep the periorbita intact to lessen the chance of postoperative periorbital ecchymosis. The details of this modified OZ craniotomy have been previously described by Balasingam el al.[8]

Two burr holes are placed: one above the root of the zygoma and one at the keyhole. A craniotome is used to complete a frontotemporal craniotomy from the first burr hole above the zygoma toward the orbital rim just lateral to the supraorbital foramen/notch. However, further progress of the craniotome with the foot plate is stopped at the orbital roof (**Fig. 12.21**). The foot plate is then "turned around on itself" to expand the last few millimeters of bony cut to create enough space for removing the foot plate. Alternatively, the drill may be backed out along the calvarial bony cut back to the original burr hole and removed. A spatula may be used to protect the orbital contents during orbital osteotomy.

Next, the foot plate is removed and a straight side-cutting B1 drill bit (Midas Rex, Fort Worth, TX) is mounted on the drill to complete the *first orbital osteotomy* over the orbital rim (**Fig. 12.21**). Next, using a craniotome, the neurosurgeon will create a bony cut from the first burr hole at the root of the zygoma toward the keyhole (the cut is

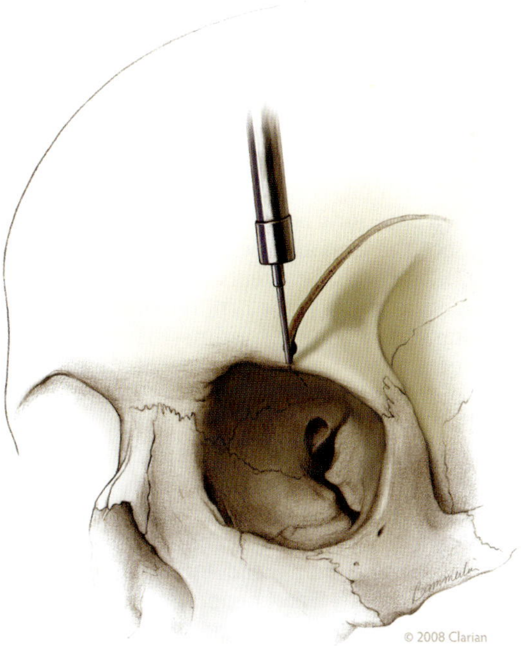

Fig. 12.21 A craniotome is used to complete a frontotemporal craniotomy from the first burr hole above the zygoma toward the orbital rim just lateral to the supraorbital foramen/notch; however, further progress of the craniotome with the foot plate is stopped at the orbital roof. (Used with permission from Clarian Health.)

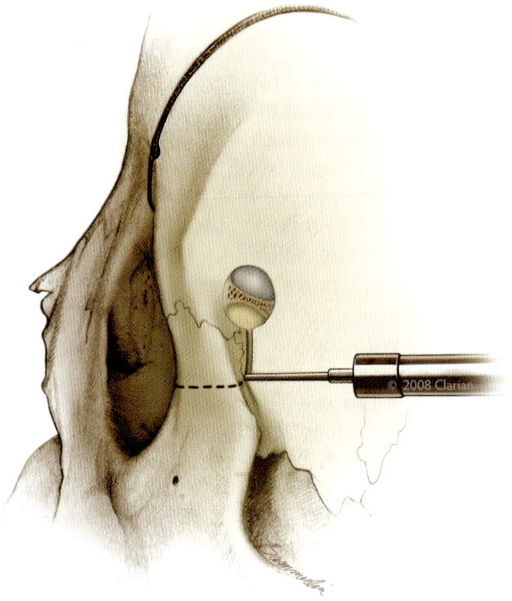

Fig. 12.22 The second orbital osteotomy involves making a cut (with the B1 drill bit) from the keyhole extending inferiorly and then anteriorly below the frontozygomatic suture to disconnect the frontal process of the zygomatic bone. (Used with permission from Clarian Health.)

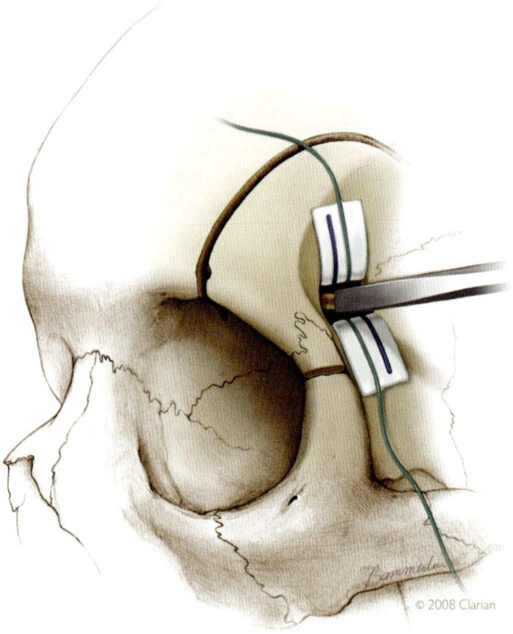

Fig. 12.23 Two cotton patties may be used to protect the frontal dura superiorly and periorbita inferiorly from the osteotome. (Used with permission from Clarian Health.)

bordered inferiorly by the temporalis muscle), and another cut from the keyhole backward toward the first burr hole (these latter two cuts are limited by the bone over the pterion, which may be thinned with the B1 bit).

The *second orbital osteotomy* involves making a cut (with the B1 drill bit) from the keyhole extending inferiorly and then anteriorly below the frontozygomatic suture to disconnect the frontal process of the zygomatic bone (**Fig. 12.22**). The orbital contents are again protected by a spatula, and the angle of the drill remains perpendicular to the plane of the bone at all times. The final and *third orbital osteotomy* will require the use of a thin, small osteotome to disconnect the orbital roof from the keyhole toward the first orbital osteotomy cut just lateral to the supraorbital foramen/notch. Two cotton patties may be used to protect the frontal dura superiorly and the periorbita inferiorly from the osteotome (**Fig. 12.23**). These three osteotomy cuts will disconnect the superior and lateral orbital attachments, allowing completion of a supraorbital osteotomy. The craniotomy bone flap is now reflected anteroinferiorly, and additional bony removal posteriorly along the roof of the orbit can be accomplished. The pterion is dilled away, and the dura is opened in a curvilinear fashion centered over the pterion. Inferior traction along the frontal dura over the orbit with tack-up sutures will gently depress the orbital contents inferiorly and allow an unobstructed view along the inferior frontal lobe toward the optic chiasm. Dissection, retraction, and tumor removal may proceed as in the pterional approach.

A transsylvian approach can be performed similarly to a pterional approach but can afford a shorter working distance with access to the parasellar region.[9]

Complications of the OZ approach are similar to those of the pterional route, although the risk for entry into the frontal sinus and cosmetic deformity is slightly higher. Removal of the lateral wall risks injury to the globe, and removal of the orbital roof risks injury to the optic nerve. Although providing superior visualization of the parasellar region and reducing frontal lobe retraction, this approach is also more time-intensive and is not performed as commonly as the pterional craniotomy.

◆ Bifrontal Approach

Most of the lesions in the parasellar space are approached through the pterional or OZ approaches. Large lesions with significant bilateral extension along the optic apparatus may be exposed by using the bifrontal approach. The potential advantage of this approach is the operative wide bilateral window it provides and the direct visualization of the anterior optic pathway and lamina terminalis.[6] The presence of a postfixed chiasm is another reasonable indication for this approach. However, we have rarely employed this route because the classic pterional approach is adequate to remove larger tumors. As tumor removal proceeds, the working corridor expands and additional exposure is not usually necessary.

After induction of general anesthesia and endotracheal intubation, the patient's head is fixed in a Mayfield head holder with the head extended 15 to 20 degrees to allow gravitational retraction of the frontal lobes. Lateral rotation of the head is not needed for this midline approach. A lumbar drain is generally placed before the surgery is begun.

The surgeon incises the scalp beginning 1 cm anterior to the tragus and continuing to 1 cm anterior to the opposite tragus, staying behind the hairline. The incision should be sinusoidal in shape and kept behind the hairline for cosmesis. An incision is made through the galea, which is then elevated from the pericranium with sharp dissection. It is necessary to maintain the periosteal layer intact because it will be used later to cover the frontal sinus. An attempt is also made to preserve the main trunk of the superficial temporal arteries bilaterally by dissecting through the superficial and subcutaneous layers of the skin within the first and last 3 cm of the incision. As separation of the galea and periosteum progresses anteriorly, the supraorbital nerves are carefully preserved and elevated as described above. An incision in the pericranium is made 5 cm superior to the supraorbital rim. A subperiosteal dissection is performed down over the frontal bone and laterally to the superior temporal lines, and a periosteal flap is reflected anteriorly while the supraorbital nerves are preserved. This creates a vascularized periosteal flap for covering the frontal sinus at the end of the procedure.

Two burr holes are placed in the region of the keyholes as well as one burr hole over the superior sagittal sinus ~3 cm anterior to the coronal suture (the superior extent of the craniotomy depends on the size of the lesion). Using a craniotome, the surgeon elevates a craniotomy as low and close to the orbital roof as possible. If the frontal sinus is large, a B1 bit without a foot plate may be used to complete the osteotomy over the anterior and posterior walls of the frontal sinus. The bone is removed in one piece, with the dura left intact. Attention is then turned to the frontal sinus. The sinus is exenterated from its mucosa, packed with muscle or fat, and covered with Tisseel (Baxter, Deerfield, IL).

The dura is incised in a U-shape with the base along the orbital floor. The anterior part of the sagittal sinus is ligated and coagulated along the superior edge of the craniotomy. The falx cerebri is cut, and the dura is retracted anteriorly with stay sutures.

A Greenberg retractor is affixed to the Mayfield head holder, and gentle retraction is placed on each frontal lobe as it is elevated. CSF may be drained in increments of 10 to 20 mL up to a total of 60 mL from the lumbar drain to afford more brain relaxation. The arachnoidal cistern surrounding the olfactory bulb and tracts can be opened to allow further drainage of CSF. Sharp dissection is then performed to release the olfactory nerves from the orbital surface of the frontal lobes to the level of the olfactory trigone. During this dissection, the olfactory artery arising lateral to the anterior cerebral artery or collateral branches distal to the anterior communicating artery should be preserved.[10] At the terminus of the olfactory nerve dissection, the basal interhemispheric fissure will demonstrate overhanging distal A2 segments of the anterior cerebral arteries. The chiasmatic and lamina terminalis cisterns can be exposed with sharp dissection. The anterior communicating artery and the optic chiasm will then come into view. Incision of the lamina terminalis will provide access to the tumor behind the optic chiasm and within the third ventricle. With the tumor now in view, careful dissection from the surrounding structures with incremental debulking may be conducted until adequate tumor resection is obtained. Further details concerning the treatment of individual lesions can be found in preceding chapters of this book.

Following resection of the tumor, meticulous hemostasis is obtained. Copious irrigation is performed to remove any residual blood. The dura is closed in a "watertight" fashion. A Gelfoam (Braun AG, Melsungen, Germany) sponge is placed extradurally. The frontal sinus is again inspected, packed with more muscle and bone, and covered with the pericranial flap. The bone is fixed with titanium Cranio-Fix plates (Aesculap AG, Tuttlingen, Germany). Finally, the galea is closed with interrupted sutures, and the skin is closed with staples. An optional subgaleal drain may be left in for 24 hours.

This approach may be modified to gain further visualization of more superiorly located tumors while minimizing frontal lobe retraction. The orbital roof just medial to the supraorbital notch may be osteotomized bilaterally with a craniotome. The orbital contents should be stripped from the bone to the depth of the posterior ethmoidal artery before this osteotomy. A vertical cut between the crista galli and the supraorbital bar defines the posterior edge of the extended bone flap. The inferior cut is through or just superior to the frontonasal suture. At the end of the procedure, the bone can be replaced with two 2-hole, low-profile titanium plates and titanium screws along the supraorbital bar.

The subfrontal approach also carries specific risks and challenges. The frontal sinus may be entered via this approach and should be exenterated as described above. The subfrontal approach also increases the risk for olfactory nerve injury, with the patient permanently anosmic postoperatively. The sacrifice of the superior sagittal sinus, although anterior to the coronal suture, may be associated with frontal lobe venous infarction. Retraction of both frontal lobes increases the risk for frontal lobe injury.

◆ Unilateral Subfrontal Approach

The unilateral subfrontal route has the advantages of requiring less surgical time to complete than the bilateral subfrontal approach and providing an anterior and nearly panoramic view of the sellar and parasellar lesions. This approach may be more appropriate for lesions that extend anteriorly or laterally on one side and is typically used for lesions located more anteriorly in the parasellar region, just above the pituitary gland and around the optic nerves. The unilateral subfrontal approach may provide adequate visualization of the anterior midline lesions, as does the bilateral subfrontal approach, without the need for ligation of the superior sagittal sinus or bilateral dissection of the olfactory bulb and tract.[7]

After induction of general anesthesia and intubation, the patient is positioned supine with the head in a Mayfield head holder and rotated between 10 and 30 degrees contralaterally. The head is extended ~30 degrees, with the zygoma elevated to the highest point. The skin incision starts 1 cm anterior to the tragus and 1 cm above the zygomatic arch and extends behind the hairline to the contralateral midpupillary line. The scalp flap is elevated with sharp dissection between the galea and periosteum. The superficial fat pad is elevated with the skin flap as in the pterional approach to preserve the temporal branch of the facial nerve. Dissection is continued to the supraorbital rim and the frontozygomatic suture. The temporalis muscle is separated from the anterior aspect of the superior temporal line and the frontozygomatic process. This muscle is then retracted posteriorly[11] and the pericranium is sharply removed from the bone, with its pedicle preserved anteriorly. This pericranium is preserved for potential use if the frontal sinus is violated.

A single burr hole is placed at the pterional keyhole. A craniotome is then used to cut along the supraorbital margin; the cut is stopped just lateral to the supraorbital notch and then extended as far superiorly as dictated by preoperative imaging. The inferior edge of the craniotomy is then completed close to the level of the orbital roof. If the frontal sinus is entered, exenteration as described above is performed. A U-shaped dural flap is cut so that the base is positioned inferiorly. The dura is then tacked up with stitches.

With the operating microscope, gentle elevation of the frontal lobe allows identification of the arachnoid attachments over the olfactory cistern, which is opened. The olfactory nerve is followed posteriorly until the anatomic windows of the subchiasmatic, opticocarotid, and retrocarotid cisterns are found. In the case of a prominent tuberculum sellae that limits visualization in the subchiasmatic space, a diamond burr drill can be used to drill down this bony structure to the level of the anterior intercavernous sinus. If necessary, the sphenoid sinus can be opened and the anterior wall of the sella turcica removed. With the tumor now in view, meticulous dissection from the surrounding structures with incremental debulking of the tumor will allow tumor removal.

Once the tumor resection is complete and hemostasis achieved, the dura is closed in a "watertight" fashion, and a Gelfoam sponge is placed extradurally. The frontal sinus is again inspected and, if violated, covered with the pericranial flap. Next, the bone flap is fixated with titanium CranioFix plates. The temporalis muscle is tacked back to the superior temporal line where a cuff of fascia was left intact. The scalp is closed with galeal sutures and the skin stapled. A subgaleal drain may also be placed before closure.

The complications associated with the unilateral subfrontal route are very similar to those described for the pterional craniotomy. As with the subfrontal approach, the chance of entering the frontal sinus and postoperative anosmia is greater than with the typical pterional approach

◆ Supraorbital Keyhole Approach

The supraorbital keyhole approach, developed most recently and similar to the unilateral subfrontal approach, is indicated for lesions superior to the pituitary gland and around the optic nerve. The advantages of this approach include minimal bone removal and a much smaller skin incision. However, the intracranial exposure afforded by this approach is more restrictive.

After induction of general anesthesia, intubation, and supine positioning of the patient, a Mayfield head holder is used to turn the head 15 to 60 degrees contralaterally, depending on the anatomy of the lesion according to preoperative imaging.[12] The head is extended slightly to place the zygoma at the highest point, thereby facilitating gravitational retraction of the frontal lobe.

The eye is lubricated and taped shut, and the skin is prepared. The eyebrow should not be shaved because of its slow regrowth. An incision is made within the eyebrow just lateral to the supraorbital notch and follows the orbital rim laterally and inferiorly to the end of the eyebrow. Medially, the incision is kept more superficial to avoid injury to the supraorbital nerve and artery. Careful dissection down through the layers of the galea to the periosteum is performed medially to identify and preserve the supraorbital nerve while maximizing the use and extent of the incision. Fish hooks are used to retract the superior skin flap and frontalis muscle, which has been sharply removed from the periosteum in a transverse direction. The orbicularis oculi muscle can be gently retracted inferiorly toward the orbit with retraction sutures. The pericranium is incised in a half moon shape with a base toward the orbit for later use if the frontal sinus is violated.[13] A short anterior segment of the temporalis fascia and muscle is released at the superior temporal line. Muscle and fascia are retracted inferolaterally to fully expose the frontozygomatic process and the keyhole.

A burr hole inferior to the superior temporal line and posterior to the keyhole is created with a high-speed drill. A half-moon–shaped craniotomy flap similar to that used in the unilateral subfrontal approach is then fashioned and may or may not include the lateral aspect of the orbital rim. An approximate size for this craniotomy is 10 to 15 mm by 15 to 25 mm. For further exposure, the orbital rim can be drilled down to better visualize the floor of the anterior cranial fossa.[13] The bony ridges over the anterior cranial fossa floor can also be drilled down to improve exposure.

The dura is opened in a U-shaped manner, with the base located inferiorly. With gentle elevation of the frontal lobe, the arachnoid cistern around the olfactory tract is visualized with the operating microscope and opened to allow adequate CSF drainage. The frontal lobe is gently elevated, and the olfactory tract is then traced back to the chiasmatic and carotid cisterns. After these arachnoid cisterns have been opened, the parasellar/suprasellar lesion should be within the field of view, and meticulous dissection from the surrounding structures with incremental debulking of the tumor can be conducted.

Following resection of the tumor, hemostasis is obtained, copious irrigation of the cisterns is performed, and the dura is closed with sutures. If the frontal sinus is violated, it can be addressed at this time, as described in previous sections of this chapter. A plate of Gelfoam is placed extradurally. The craniotomy is replaced and fixated with a burr hole cover plate and other combinations of low-profile titanium plates for cosmesis. The temporalis muscle and fascia are returned to their original positions and sewn to their corresponding fascial cuffs. If the pericranial flap was not used to close the frontal sinus, it is placed back over the bone. The scalp flap is closed with galeal and subcutaneous sutures, and a topical skin glue is placed on the skin.

The main disadvantage of the supraorbital keyhole approach is that it provides a much smaller working corridor and should not be used for large lesions. Injury to the supraorbital nerve may cause some numbness above the eyebrow. Frontalis palsy may be a more frequent complication of this exposure than of other approaches because of the location of the incision. A spacious frontal sinus appreciated on the preoperative computed tomographic scans and/or magnetic resonance (MR) images may be a contraindication to this form of craniotomy.

◆ Subtemporal Approach

The subtemporal approach is infrequently used for suprasellar and parasellar lesions but may be especially useful for those lesions that extend into the infratentorial space, are retrochiasmatic, or extend into the temporal fossa.[14] This route offers the most direct approach to remove the lesions in the often "difficult to reach" retrochiasmatic space. Preoperative MR venography may be useful to ensure that the vein of Labbé is not tethered anteriorly and therefore not vulnerable during elevation of the temporal lobe.

After induction of general anesthesia and intubation, a lumbar drain can be placed for CSF drainage and brain relaxation to minimize temporal lobe retraction. With the patient in a supine position and use of a Mayfield head holder, the patient's head is rotated 60 degrees away from the lesion and extended 30 degrees for optimal visualization of the sella and parasellar regions.[15]

A linear incision 1 cm anterior to the tragus is started 1 cm below the zygomatic arch and extended 1 cm above the superior temporal line. Preservation of the superficial temporal artery is attempted as dissection down to the zygomatic arch and the temporalis fascia is performed. The periosteum is incised over the zygomatic arch and exposed subperiosteally. Anterior and posterior osteotomies at the limits of the arch are then completed, and the arch is plated for later reattachment. Following this, the temporalis muscle is dissected parallel to the line of skin incision and retracted anteriorly and posteriorly with a cerebellar retractor.

A small temporal craniotomy is made with an anterior burr hole so that the inferior bony cut is flush with the floor of the middle cranial fossa. The middle meningeal artery can be coagulated and divided where it enters the middle cranial fossa through the foramen spinosum. A U-shaped dural flap is made with an inferior base and tacked out of the way with silk sutures. A wide, self-retaining retractor can then be inserted to gently retract the temporal lobe superiorly and provide exposure to the posterior parasellar area through the middle cranial fossa. Opening the basal cisterns along the third nerve will allow further CSF drainage and further brain relaxation. With the lesion now in view, dissection from the surrounding structures and incremental debulking of the tumor can proceed.

Following resection of the tumor, hemostasis is obtained, copious irrigation of the cisterns is performed, and the retractors are removed. The dura is closed with sutures, and a plate of Gelfoam is placed extradurally. The bone flap is fixated with titanium CranioFix plates, and the zygomatic arch is reattached with low-profile titanium plates. The muscle and scalp are closed in anatomic layers with interrupted sutures and staples.

Although the subtemporal approach offers a unique corridor to the retrochiasmatic tumor, it is limited by the restricted access it provides to the superior and anterior parasellar space. Postoperative difficulty in mandibular movement due to masseter and temporalis muscle dissection is frequent. In addition to the common risks of craniotomies mentioned in the section on the pterional approach, injury to the branches of the facial nerve just below the zygomatic arch is of unique concern with this approach. The significant temporal lobe retraction necessary during this surgery places the lobe at risk, and retraction injury can be especially symptomatic in the dominant hemisphere.

◆ Conclusion

The transcranial removal of parasellar lesions requires proficiency in microsurgical techniques. The neurosurgeon should not focus too much on the "exposure," but more on "what to do when we get there" in terms of handling the tumor and surrounding cerebrovascular structures. The classic pterional approach is a versatile route that allows safe exposure and removal of most parasellar lesions. One must at all times look out for the optic nerve and other adjacent cerebrovascular structures and remain patient while handling the tumor. "Pulling" the tumor indiscriminately and cutting without scrutinizing the tips of the microscissors can be regretted later. It is acceptable and preferable to say "here it is" and be wrong than to say "there it was" and be right.

References

1. Osborn A, Salzman KL, Barkovich AJ, et al. Diagnostic Imaging: Brain. 2nd ed. Amirsys; 2010
2. Wilson CB. A decade of pituitary microsurgery. The Herbert Olivecrona lecture. J Neurosurg 1984;61(5):814–833
3. Wilson CB. Endocrine-inactive pituitary adenomas. Clin Neurosurg 1992;38:10–31
4. Youssef AS, Agazzi S, van Loveren HR. Transcranial surgery for pituitary adenomas. Neurosurgery 2005;57(1, Suppl):168–175
5. Yasargil MG, Antic J, Laciga R, Jain KK, Hodosh RM, Smith RD. Microsurgical pterional approach to aneurysms of the basilar bifurcation. Surg Neurol 1976;6(2):83–91
6. Carmel P. Transcranial approaches. In: Apuzzo M, ed. Brain Surgery, vol. 1. Churchill Livingstone; 1993:339–357
7. Patterson R. Parasellar meningiomas. In: Apuzzo M, ed. Brain Surgery, vol. 1. Churchill Livingstone; 1993:219–230
8. Balasingam V, Noguchi A, McMenomey SO, Delashaw JB Jr. Modified osteoplastic orbitozygomatic craniotomy. Technical note. J Neurosurg 2005;102(5):940–944
9. Hakuba A, Liu S, Nishimura S. The orbitozygomatic infratemporal approach: a new surgical technique. Surg Neurol 1986;26(3):271–276
10. Dehdashti AR, de Tribolet N. Frontobasal interhemispheric translamina terminalis approach for suprasellar lesions. Neurosurgery 2005;56(2, Suppl):418–424

11. Fukushima T, Day JD. Surgical management of tumors involving the cavernous sinus. In: Schmidek H, Roberts D, eds. Schmidek and Sweet's Operative Neurosurgical Techniques, vol. 1. Saunders/ Elsevier; 2005:245–247
12. Reisch R, Perneczky A. Ten-year experience with the supraorbital subfrontal approach through an eyebrow skin incision. Neurosurgery 2005;57(4, Suppl):242–255
13. Fatemi N, Dusick JR, de Paiva Neto MA, Malkasian D, Kelly DF. Endonasal versus supraorbital keyhole removal of craniopharyngiomas and tuberculum sellae meningiomas. Neurosurgery 2009;64(5, Suppl 2):269–284, discussion 284–286
14. Al-Mefty O. Approach selection in juxtasellar surgery. In: Al-Mefty O, ed. Surgery of the Cranial Base. Kluwer; 1989:57–71
15. Deda H, Ugur HC. Zygomatic anterior subtemporal approach for lesions in the interpeduncular cistern. Skull Base 2001;11(4): 257–264

13 Radiation Therapy

Itai Pashtan, Kevin S. Oh, and Jay S. Loeffler

Radiation therapy has an important role in the local control of sellar and parasellar tumors that are not completely resected, recur after surgery, or are considered at high risk for recurrence despite surgical resection based on anatomic and/or biological factors. This chapter outlines the various delivery systems and fractionation schemes used in radiation therapy, as well as the data supporting its use in both benign and malignant conditions.

◆ Fractionation Schedules and Technology in Radiation Oncology

The term *fractionation* refers to the number of individual radiation treatments delivered. The total dose is the number of fractions multiplied by the dose per fraction. Clinical outcomes, such as local control, are heavily influenced by both the dose per fraction and total dose. For example, 50 Gy in 25 fractions may be equivalent in some tumors to 12 to 14 Gy in one fraction. Prolonging fractionation, by dividing the total dose into a larger number of fractions, has the potential to decrease late complications in normal tissue. This comes at the expense of a longer treatment time, which allows interfraction tumor repopulation and necessitates a higher total dose. The balance between these factors determines the relative benefits of conventional fractionated external beam radiation therapy (EBRT) versus those of stereotactic radiosurgery (SRS).

◆ Conventional Fractionated EBRT

The term *conventional fractionation* refers to the use of 1.8 to 2 Gy per day. As detailed in this chapter, the total doses for fractionated EBRT in the management of sellar/parasellar tumors range from 45 to 54 Gy, which implies 25 to 30 fractions, or 5 to 6 weeks of daily treatment. Treatment planning with three-dimensional conformal radiation therapy (CRT) is available in several commercially available software packages and typically requires at least three unopposed beams to reduce heterogeneity ("hot spots") and minimize dose in surrounding uninvolved tissue. A growing number of radiation oncology practices use inverse-planned intensity-modulated radiation therapy (IMRT) for cases with a difficult geometric relationship between target and normal tissue, such as tumor surrounding the optic nerve in a concave configuration. There are several methodologies for IMRT, but most commonly require the capacity to divide the primary beam into 5- to 10-mm beamlets and the use of software to iterate and evaluate fluence through these beamlets to achieve the plan objectives. In all cases of linear accelerator (LINAC)–based intracranial radiation therapy, beam energy should be 6 to 10 megavolts (MV).

◆ Stereotactic Radiosurgery

In SRS, a high dose can be delivered in a single fraction by using a highly accurate and reproducible three-dimensional coordinate system for localization. Typical SRS doses for intracranial tumors range from 12 to 35 Gy, delivered in one dose. Several stereotactic systems exist to achieve submillimeter precision, the most common of which are the gamma knife (Elekta, Stockholm, Sweden), CyberKnife (Accuray, Sunnyvale, CA), and linear accelerator–based systems. For example, the gamma knife uses a metal collimator helmet for patient immobilization and distancing from the treatment head, which consists of a hemispheric distribution of sources of cobalt 60 behind bores. Bores are systematically removed such that beam arrays converge at an isocenter. Several overlapping isocenters may be used for irregularly shaped targets. LINAC-based systems achieve immobilization with (1) a rigid frame secured to the calvarium by four pins above the level of the brow, (2) a mask that incorporates a bite piece that relies on the uniqueness of the patient's dental impression, or (3) a mask and image guidance system. The standard beam from a standard LINAC can be shaped by either cones or multileaf collimators (MLCs). A steep dose gradient between the target and adjacent normal tissues is created by (1) using multiple beam arrangements or arc therapy and (2) prescribing to the steepest portion of the beam profile, which is often the 50% isodose line (IDL) for gamma knife or the 80 to 90% IDL for LINAC-based SRS.

◆ Indications for SRS versus Conventional Fractionated EBRT

SRS has advantages over fractionated EBRT: convenience, the ability to spare normal tissue, and minimal toxicity.[1] For secretory pituitary adenomas, SRS may provide faster hormonal ablation.[2] However, many patients are not candidates for SRS because of unfavorable tumor size, irregular geometry, or tumor location. Although each case is considered individually, the dosimetric advantages of SRS generally decline when the tumor is larger than 3 cm. For tumors abutting critical organs at risk (OARs), it is often difficult to achieve sufficient dose falloff between the prescription dose and the tolerance of the OAR. For example, to keep the optic chiasm and nerves from receiving less than 8 to 10 Gy at typical SRS doses, the target should generally be located at least 3 to 5 mm away from the optic apparatus.

◆ Dose Limitations of the Optic Chiasm and Nerves

Historically, the 5-year risk for visual deficits from standard fractionated EBRT to the optic chiasm and nerves was believed to be 5% at 50 Gy and 50% at 65 Gy.[3] However, these guidelines were based on consensus agreement rather than actual clinical data. In 2010, the Quantitative Analysis of Normal Tissue Effects in the Clinic (QUANTEC) provided updated recommendations for safe irradiation of the optic nerve and chiasm, suggesting that radiation-induced optic neuropathy (RION) is extremely rare at less than 55 Gy with fraction sizes of 1.8 to 2 Gy per day. The risk increases to 3 to 7% at doses of 55 to 60 Gy, and to more than 7 to 20% at doses above 60 Gy.[4] Some series have suggested that tolerance may be lower and toxicity latency shorter in patients with pituitary tumors. Complications have been reported at doses as low as 46 Gy at 1.8 Gy per fraction, with average latencies of 10.5 and 31 months for pituitary and nonpituitary targets, respectively.[5–7] When radiation is delivered as a single fraction, several series have shown that that rate of RION is very low at doses of less than 8 to 10 Gy, increases with doses from 10 to 12 Gy, and reaches more than 10% at 12 to 15 Gy.[4,8] Therefore, the current recommendations for optic chiasm and nerve tolerance are below 55 Gy with standard fractionation and from below 8 to 10 Gy with SRS approaches. The brainstem tolerance is thought to be 12 Gy in a single fraction for 1 cm^3 or more of tissue.

◆ Proton Therapy

Protons and other positively charged heavy particles hold an inherent advantage over photon therapy in their ability to deliver an equivalent dose to the target while minimizing exit the dose. When protons interact with normal tissues, their velocity rapidly decreases near their end of range. As this occurs, the energy transferred increases exponentially until the particles come to rest. The region of maximum energy transfer is called the Bragg peak. Superimposing beams of successively lower energies and intensities creates a spread-out Bragg peak, which delivers the intended dose to a three-dimensional target. The primary dosimetric advantage of proton therapy is the minimization of low and medium doses to nearby normal brain tissue. The clinical implication in the treatment of brain tumors is the theoretic reduction in risk for neurocognitive deficits and second malignancy, which are believed to be associated with even low doses of radiation. Both of these late sequelae are particularly important in the pediatric population. Confirmatory prospective studies are sparse, but such studies are currently under way at Massachusetts General Hospital. Proton therapy can be used for both stereotactic radiosurgery (PSRS) and fractionated stereotactic radiation therapy (PSRT) with noninvasive immobilization devices in a manner analogous to photon-based therapy. In the current era, the widespread use of proton therapy is hampered by the expense associated with such facilities.

◆ Benign Tumors

Pituitary Adenomas

Radiation therapy plays a large role in the management of pituitary adenomas that have been incompletely addressed by surgical resection or have recurred biochemically or radiographically, and in the management of the rare medically inoperable patient. Extrasellar residual disease after resection and inadequate biochemical control with medications are common indications for radiation therapy. In the current era, SRS is preferable when the tumor geometry is favorable and the dose limitations to the optic apparatus and brainstem can be achieved. SRS is associated with faster biochemical normalization for secretory tumors.[1,2,9] The technique and outcomes of stereotactic approaches are discussed in Chapter 14. For tumors with considerable extrasellar extension or in close proximity to the optic apparatus or other OARs, fractionated EBRT should be considered the standard of care to minimize the risk for late complications.[9] The success of conventional fractionated EBRT in providing radiographic local control in nonfunctioning pituitary adenomas is ~95%. However, the actuarial rate of biochemical normalization of functioning tumors ranges from 50 to 100%, depending on histology.[10–12]

The first step in radiation planning is the definition of the target. The gross tumor volume (GTV) is the grossly visible pituitary adenoma by magnetic resonance imaging (MRI) and computed tomography (CT), which may extend outside the sella turcica into the cavernous sinus, sphenoid sinus, or intracranial parenchyma. The clinical target volume (CTV) encompasses the GTV as well as the extent of subclinical disease and typically includes the entire sella turcica and medial walls of the left and right cavernous sinuses. To create the planning target volume (PTV), the CTV is uniformly expanded by an additional margin to account for setup error and physiologic motion. The size of PTV expansion may range from 0 to 5 mm and depends on the reproducibility of the immobilization device used. Although there is 3 to 5 mm of setup uncertainty when a standard thermoplastic mask is used, when a stereotactic mask is used, the PTV expansion may be excluded altogether. OARs, such as the brainstem, optic apparatus, and temporal lobes, should also be defined. There are various dosimetric strategies available to achieve conformality to the target. Stereotactic radiosurgery (SRS) or stereotactic radiotherapy (SRT) techniques in which multiple non-coplanar arcs or pseudoarcs are used generally achieve the sharpest gradient between PTV and OARs. In centers without stereotactic capabilities, three-dimensional CRT with laterals, obliques, and/or a vertex field has been a standard approach for many years. Fractionated doses for pituitary adenomas range from 45 to 54 Gy, depending on tumor type.

Nonfunctioning Adenomas

Radiation therapy is indicated for patients who have nonfunctioning adenomas (NFAs) that are unresectable or subtotally resected and who are felt to be at high risk for impending symptoms. The goal of radiation in this setting is to halt radiographic progression and prevent the development of symptoms. Prophylactic radiation after gross total resection or near-total resection is not indicated because the risk for recurrence is very low.[13–16] If safe, repeat surgical debulking is often used as a strategy to delay radiotherapy (RT) and minimize the risk for hypopituitarism and other late sequelae.[15,16] Both fractionated and SRS approaches are associated with excellent rates of local control (95–100%) but should be used judiciously because of the risk for late effects.

Conventional fractionated EBRT at doses of 45 to 50.4 Gy in 1.8-Gy fractions has a long history of success in the treatment of NFAs. A retrospective experience of two hospitals in the United Kingdom, each with a different philosophy in management, included 126 patients with nonfunctioning pituitary adenomas.[17] One hospital routinely offered postoperative RT to 45 Gy in 30 to 33 fractions to its 63 patients, whereas the other did not. The 15-year progression-free survival (PFS) significantly favored the subgroup of patients who received RT (93 vs. 33%, $P < < 0.05$). Similarly, a group in the Netherlands compared 76 patients who received immediate postoperative RT ranging from 45 to 55.8 Gy at 1.8 to 2 Gy per fraction with 28 patients who were followed with a wait-and-see policy.[18] The 10-year local control rate was 95% for the RT group versus 22% for the wait-and-see group. Of note, there were no significant differences between the two groups with regard to need for hormonal supplementation or survival.

SRS can be used to successfully treat NFAs when they are geometrically favorable (eg, <3 cm in size and >5–10 mm from the optic chiasm). A review of 62 patients who received gamma knife radiosurgery with a median marginal dose of 16 Gy and follow-up of 64 months reported 3- and 7-year local control rates of 95%.[19] A prospective study that evaluated the efficacy of LINAC-based radiosurgery for non–surgically accessible adenomas included 37 patients with NFAs and reported 100% local control at a mean follow-up of 56.6 months and a dose of 13.4 Gy.[20]

If adequate sparing of normal tissue cannot be achieved with single-fraction SRS, fractionated SRT may be used because it combines the precise immobilization of SRS with the radiobiological benefits of standard fractionation on normal tissue. Colin et al reported a series of 63 patients with NFAs who were treated with fractionated SRT to 50.4 Gy at 1.8 Gy per fraction and followed for a median of 82 months; local control was 100%.[21] No late complications were reported, with the exception of pituitary deficiency in which the probability of requiring hormonal replacement was 28.5% at 4 years and 35% at 8 years.

In a limited number of centers, proton therapy is used to deliver treatment doses to gross disease while minimizing exit dose. In the Loma Linda experience, 24 patients with NFAs were treated to a median of 54 cobalt gray equivalents (CGE), with achievement of 100% local control at a median follow-up of 47 months.[22]

Functioning Adenomas

To achieve a relatively rapid biochemical remission, functioning adenomas typically require higher doses than NFAs. A dose response favoring the delivery of 45 Gy or more was reported in a retrospective review from Zierhut et al that included 139 patients with pituitary adenomas of various histologies;[12] however, this is not a universal finding.[23] The recommended fractionated EBRT dose is 45 to 54 Gy in 1.8- to 2-Gy fractions for acromegaly, Cushing disease, and prolactinoma. Because they are felt to be less radioresponsive, thyroid-stimulating hormone (TSH)–producing adenomas are often treated with a slightly higher dose (eg, 54 Gy). Preferences for SRS doses for functioning adenomas range widely, from 18 to 35 Gy in a single dose.

The latency period between treatment and biochemical normalization can be several years, during which medical suppression is required. When feasible, SRS is favored because of the shorter latency period required to achieve hormonal normalization. For example, a comparison of SRS versus standard fractionated EBRT in 29 hormonally active adenomas reported a mean time to normalization of 8.5 versus 18 months, respectively.[9]

Growth Hormone–Secreting Adenomas

RT is often used for patients with acromegaly who have suprasellar components that are unresectable or are incompletely controlled by surgery or medical therapy. Although radiographic local control may be quickly achieved with RT, biochemical and clinical normalization often requires many years. The most commonly accepted criteria for biochemical remission are normalization of insulin-like growth factor 1 (IGF-1; matched for age and gender) and a growth hormone (GH) level below 1 ng/mL after glucose challenge. There is wide variation in the reported biochemical remission rates for SRS and standard fractionated EBRT, but this likely reflects the long follow-up required to document maximized results, often 10 to 20 years.

Standard fractionated EBRT has been in routine use much longer than SRS, and this allows the literature to demonstrate the long-term follow-up required to maximize biochemical remission rates. The largest retrospective experience included 884 patients at 14 centers in the United Kingdom.[24] GH levels fell to below 2.5 ng/mL in 22%

at 2 years, 60% at 10 years, and 77% at 20 years. Sixty-three percent achieved normal IGF-1 levels at 10 years. Similarly, Barrande et al reported a long-term single-institution experience of 128 patients with acromegaly treated with fractionated radiation.[25] At a median follow-up of 11.5 years, basal levels of GH below 2.5 ng/mL were achieved in 7% at 2 years, 53% at 10 years, and 66% at 15 years. At last follow-up, 79% had achieved IGF-1 normalization. A smaller Dutch experience of 36 patients that used a median of 40 Gy reported IGF-1 normalization rates of 60%, 74%, and 84% at 5, 10, and 15 years, respectively, of follow-up.[26] Radiographic local control is immediate and almost universally achieved.[27,28]

Biochemical remission rates in large series of SRS range from 40 to 96%, but this wide variation likely reflects differences in defining biochemical remission and insufficient follow-up. A large systematic review of pituitary adenomas treated with SRS included 420 patients with acromegaly in 25 retrospective studies.[1] The mean marginal doses ranged from 15 to 34 Gy. Remission rates ranged from 0 to 100%, but the criteria were variable and often poorly defined. The use of somatostatin analogues during and after SRS often went unaccounted. The largest single series, published by Castinetti et al, included 82 patients treated with gamma knife to a marginal dose of 12 to 40 Gy.[29] At a mean follow-up of 50 months, 17% achieved a biochemical remission, defined as a GH level below 2 ng/mL and normalized IGF-1 after discontinuation of somatostatin agonists for at least 3 months. An additional 23% regained control of GH secretion with medical therapy. A study by Zhang et al included 68 patients with acromegaly treated with gamma knife to a mean marginal dose of 31 Gy.[30] Biochemical remission (generously defined as GH <12 ng/mL) was achieved in 40% at 12 months but reached 96% at 24 months. Kobayashi et al reviewed 67 patients treated with gamma knife to a mean marginal dose of 18.9 Gy.[31] At a mean follow-up of 63 months, GH levels significantly decreased (<5 ng/mL) in 41%. Serum IGF-1 levels also significantly decreased (<400 ng/mL) in 41% of cases.

Proton therapy is currently available in a selected few institutions for the treatment of acromegaly. The Massachusetts General Hospital experience included 22 patients treated with PSRS for refractory disease after transsphenoidal resection.[32] After delivery of a median dose of 20 CGE and 6.3 years of follow-up, 59% achieved biochemical complete response (CR), defined as sustained IGF-1 normalization without medical therapy. In these patients, the median time to CR was 3.5 years, suggesting a more rapid response with SRS compared with standard fractionated EBRT. The Loma Linda experience reported by Ronson et al included 11 patients with GH-secreting adenomas treated with fractionated proton therapy to a median dose of 54 CGE and documented biochemical normalization or improvement in 45% and 36%, respectively, at a median follow-up of 3.9 years.[22]

Predictors of biochemical response are poorly defined, but there is a suggestion that lower baseline IGF-1 and GH levels are associated with higher rates of normalization.[29,33,34] In SRS, there is some concern that the use of octreotide at the time of radiosurgery is associated with a longer latency period to biochemical response,[35] although this is not a universal finding.[29]

ACTH-Secreting Adenomas

In Cushing disease, RT is commonly used for patients with radiographic residual or recurrent disease after transsphenoidal surgery or in patients with no radiographic evidence of disease but with excessive hormone production. Biochemical remission is typically defined as normalization of urinary free cortisol (UFC) and serum adrenocorticotropic hormone (ACTH), but these criteria vary widely in the literature. Both standard fractionated EBRT and SRS appear to achieve biochemical remission rates of 50 to 80%.

Estrada et al included 30 patients with Cushing disease treated with 48 to 54 Gy and reported actuarial remission rates of 44% at 1 year and 83% at 3 years.[10] In 40 patients with Cushing disease treated with 45 to 100 Gy, Hughes et al reported an actuarial 10-year PFS rate of 59%.[36]

In the SRS literature, remission rates are 35 to 63% with shorter-term follow-up when compared with the standard fractionated EBRT literature. For example, Sheehan et al treated 43 patients who had refractory Cushing disease with gamma knife to a mean marginal dose of 20 Gy and achieved 63% biochemical normalization at a median follow-up of 44 months.[37] Although there have been no prospective comparisons, LINAC-based SRS and gamma knife SRS are believed to offer comparable results.[9,38]

Proton therapy seems to achieve remission rates similar to those of photon-based therapy while sparing normal tissue of exit dose. The Massachusetts General Hospital PSRS experience of 33 patients with ACTH-producing adenomas reported a 52% complete radiographic and biochemical response in patients off medical therapy after a median dose of 20 CGE at a median follow-up of 62 months.[39] In more than 50% of these patients, no tumor was present on MR at the time of the treatment. Older data from the Lawrence Berkeley Laboratory on the use of helium ions, another heavy charged particle, to treat 83 patients with Cushing disease with 30 to 150 Gy in three to four fractions demonstrated an 85% biochemical cure rate.[40]

Prolactinomas

RT for prolactin-secreting adenomas is very uncommon because the combination of medical therapy (eg, dopamine agonists) and surgery achieves biochemical remission and radiographic stability in the vast majority of cases.

In the event that either fractionated EBRT or SRS is required, their success without concurrent pharmacotherapy seems to be poorer than in other functional adenoma subtypes. Biochemical remission, often defined as normal serum prolactin of less than 20 to 25 ng/mL depending on sex, occurs in only 15 to 30% of cases with radiation alone and often requires a latency period of many years. For example, Littley et al reviewed the success of standard fractionated EBRT (20–42.5 Gy in eight to 15 fractions) in 58 patients and reported 71% prolactin normalization while they were on a dopamine agonist.[41] When medication was discontinued, only 21% remained normoprolactinemic.

In their comprehensive systematic review of SRS in pituitary adenomas, Sheehan et al included 393 prolactinomas across 22 series.[1] The single-fraction dose ranged from 13.3 to 33 Gy. Remission rates varied from 0 to 84%, but the majority of studies reported 15 to 30% endocrine cure rates in those that clearly defined their end points. All but one SRS series included 21 or fewer patients. The largest series included 128 patients treated with gamma knife to a marginal dose of 9 to 35 Gy and a median follow-up of 2.8 years.[42] Although radiographic control occurred in 98% of cases, only 13% of evaluable patients at 2 years had durable biochemical normalization off bromocriptine.

As in other functional adenomas, retrospective data in prolactinomas suggest a poorer response to radiation when patients are concurrently using pharmacotherapy. In a small gamma knife series of 20 patients, all five patients who achieved a complete biochemical remission were not on a concurrent dopamine agonist. Conversely, none of the nine patients using pharmacotherapy achieved a complete remission.[43]

These data should be interpreted with caution, given the low patient numbers in each of the retrospective studies. Nonetheless, the current literature suggests that although RT alone is sufficient to maintain radiographic stability, it rarely achieves biochemical normalization for prolactinomas. Radiation may be thought of as an adjunctive therapy to be used in combination with dopamine agonists and/or surgical resection.

Thyroid-Stimulating Hormone–Secreting Adenomas

TSH-secreting adenomas account for fewer than 1% of all functioning pituitary adenomas but are considered more resistant to all types of therapy. Transsphenoidal resection remains the most appropriate initial strategy but results in cure in only one-third of patients. Therefore, most patients will require pharmacotherapy, such as octreotide or bromocriptine, before and/or after surgery to maximize biochemical normalization. The data on RT for TSH-secreting adenomas are sparse. Because of their aggressive natural history, some would advocate radiation therapy to higher dose (54 Gy) in all cases of TSH-secreting adenomas.

Craniopharyngiomas

Craniopharyngiomas are benign cystic epithelial tumors that arise from the pars intermedia (remnant of the Rathke pouch) located between the anterior and posterior components of the pituitary gland. The bimodal distribution peaks at 5 to 14 and at 50 to 75 years of age. The majority are retrochiasmatic and may present with symptoms of increased intracranial pressure from compression of the third ventricle. Those that are prechiasmatic may lead to homonymous hemianopsia from compression of the optic chiasm.

Maximal safe resection is the first step in the management of craniopharyngiomas to confirm the diagnosis, rapidly relieve symptoms related to mass effect, and debulk tumor and cystic components to assist in radiation planning. Radiation alone should not be expected to reduce tumor/cyst size and symptoms. Historically, aggressive surgery was the preferred treatment strategy because when a gross total resection can be achieved, the 5-year PFS rate is 80 to 90%. However, aggressive surgery carries significant risk for cognitive decline, hypothalamic injury, optic nerve damage, diabetes insipidus, and other endocrinopathies. In the current era, most multidisciplinary teams favor maximal safe resection with postoperative RT (if residual disease remains), which offers similar PFS rates in comparison with gross total resection. Limited surgeries may include partial resections or cyst aspiration for relief of symptoms. Cognitive comparisons of patients undergoing either of the two approaches (extensive surgery vs. limited surgery + RT) performed at St. Jude Children's Research Hospital suggest that extensive surgery is associated with greater decline in full-scale IQ (9.8- vs. 1.25-point drop, $P < 0.063$) and quality of life.[44]

After subtotal resection alone, the 5-year PFS is less than 50%.[45,46] However, the addition of postoperative radiation improves 5-year PFS to 80 to 90%.[44,47,48] The Royal Marsden Hospital experience included 173 patients with craniopharyngioma treated between 1950 and 1986 with fractionated EBRT alone or with surgery. In this series, four underwent gross total resection. Median follow-up was 12 years. The 10- and 20-year PFS rates were 83% and 79%, respectively.[47] Overall survival (OS) rates were 77% and 66%, respectively.

The standard radiation dose for craniopharyngiomas is 50.4 to 54 Gy in 1.8-Gy fractions delivered to the tumor and cystic volumes after decompression. A margin of 1 to 2 cm may be added to include areas at high risk for microscopic extension. Three-dimensional CRT or IMRT should be used to minimize dose to adjacent normal tissues, including the optic chiasm, optic nerves, and brainstem.

SRS after limited surgery is another promising first-line or salvage option for those with favorable geometry. The University of Pittsburgh experience of 46 patients treated with gamma knife to a median marginal dose of 13 Gy (range, 9–20 Gy) demonstrated a 5-year PFS rate of 92% for the solid tumor component and 68% when the cystic components were included. Mean follow-up was 5.2 years.[49]

Acute clinical deterioration during or shortly after RT is uncommon, but it has been a well-documented phenomenon that is usually caused by rapid cyst reaccumulation. The Royal Marsden Hospital cohort included 26 patients (14%) whose condition acutely deteriorated 2 months before, during, or after RT. Cystic enlargement with or without hydrocephalus was the most common cause (62%); in an additional 23% of the cases, the cause was hydrocephalus without clear cystic enlargement.[50] All patients who received surgical intervention (eg, aspiration, resection, or shunt) survived the immediate period, whereas six of the seven without surgical intervention died. Therefore, early recognition and surgical intervention are paramount for the patient's success, leading some to advocate scheduled brain imaging at regular intervals during RT.

In summary, maximal safe resection is the initial step in the management of craniopharyngiomas for the establishment of a diagnosis, relief of compressive symptoms, and improvement of postoperative radiation dosimetry. When gross total resection can be safely achieved for small lesions, no postoperative RT is required. In larger tumors, limited surgery followed by standard fractionated EBRT is recommended to minimize late toxicities while preserving high rates of local control. SRS should be reserved for small or recurrent tumors at an adequate distance from the optic apparatus. Refractory cyst reaccumulation is often managed by intermittent aspiration or intralesional sclerosis with bleomycin or various β emitters. In very young children, attempts are often made to use limited surgeries and intralesional therapies as temporizing measures to delay RT and its neurocognitive late effects.

Meningiomas

Meningiomas arise from arachnoid cap cells between the dura and pia mater. When managed in a multidisciplinary setting, benign (World Health Organization [WHO] grade 1) meningiomas have a 90 to 95% local control rate and rarely limit life expectancy. As such, the management of benign meningiomas is a delicate balance between achieving long-term cure and minimizing treatment-associated toxicity. Special considerations are made for parasellar meningiomas, including those of the cavernous sinus, medial sphenoid wing, tuberculum sellae, and intracanalicular optic nerve sheath because of their intimate association with the optic apparatus. Because surgical biopsy carries high risk, RT is considered the primary therapy in these locations. Such lesions are typically diagnosed on radiographic appearance alone without tissue confirmation.

In general, RT is effective for benign meningiomas after subtotal resection. The University of California at San Francisco experience included 140 patients treated after subtotal resection with a median dose of 54 Gy.[51] This included 117 benign and 23 malignant tumors. With a median follow-up of 40 months, the 5-year PFS rate was 89% for all patients and 98% for those treated after the introduction of CT- or MRI-assisted treatment planning. Several other retrospective series of subtotally resected meningiomas have also reported 5-year PFS rates of 84 to 92%.[52–54] By comparison, SRT alone historically yields a 5-year PFS rate of 50 to 60%. SRS is another common treatment choice for small meningiomas that are located at a sufficient distance from the optic chiasm and nerves. Pollock et al retrospectively compared outcomes of benign meningiomas smaller than 3.5 cm treated with either surgical resection (n = 136) or SRS (n = 62) with a mean marginal dose of 17.7 Gy.[55] At mean follow-up of 5.3 years, there was no significant difference in 3- and 7-year PFS rates between SRS and Simpson grade 1 resections. When compared with less complete resections, SRS was associated with improved PFS. Proton therapy is used in a selected few institutions to deliver prescription doses to skull-based meningiomas while minimizing low- and medium-dose scatter to uninvolved brain tissue. Similar to the results in photon series, local control generally ranges from 90 to 100%, although most series have a short-term follow-up of 3 years or less.[56–58]

Higher-grade meningiomas have a much higher risk for recurrence after RT. Milosevic et al reported the Princess Margaret Hospital experience, which included 17 patients with atypical histology and 42 with malignant meningiomas based on brain invasion or histopathology.[59] A median dose of 50 Gy was administered to patients who previously had undergone gross total resection (29%), SRT (59%), or other (12%). Progression occurred in 66% after RT, of whom 92% died of meningioma. The 5-year cause-specific survival was only 34%.

The standard fractionated dose for benign meningiomas is 50.4 to 54 Gy in 1.8-Gy fractions. Retrospective data suggest better 5-year PFS rates with doses above 50 to 52 Gy.[51,59] Grades 2 and 3 meningiomas are often treated to 59.4 Gy. The radiation target conventionally includes (1) the dural tails and (2) a margin for microscopic extension along dural surfaces of 1 to 2 cm depending on aggressiveness of disease. For SRS, the recommended dose is 12 to 15 Gy for WHO grade 1 and more than 17 Gy when feasible for WHO grades 2 and 3 meningiomas. Radiation treatment planning is challenging for meningiomas of the parasellar region because the adjacent critical tissues (eg, optic chiasm and nerves) carry tolerances at or below the recommended radiation dose (see preceding section, "Dose Limitations of the Optic Chiasm and Nerves"). Therefore, optic nerve sheath meningiomas are not treated with SRS because a therapeutic dose (12 Gy × 1) would exceed optic chiasm and nerve tolerance (8–10 Gy). With fractionated EBRT, most radiation oncologists would advocate using 45 to 50.4 Gy for optic nerve sheath meningiomas to minimize the risk for radiation-induced optic neuropathy. Results with fractionated conformal radiation are quite impressive for tumor control and visual restoration.[60]

Meningiomas of the Cavernous Sinus and Medial Sphenoid Wing

Cavernous sinus meningiomas are rarely completely resectable and difficult to biopsy. Diagnosis relies heavily on radiographic findings. Because radiation alone offers excellent long-term local control of 93 to 100%,[61–65] attempts at resection should be avoided unless for palliative decompression in symptomatic patients.

A large experience from the University of Heidelberg included 57 patients treated with standard fractionated SRT as primary treatment (51%), following surgery (18%), or at the time of recurrence (32%); the median dose was 57.6 Gy.[63] With a median follow-up of 6.5 years, local control was 100% and 10-year survival was 95.5%. Selch et al reported a more modern series of 45 patients treated between 1997 and 2002 with CT- or MRI-assisted conformal RT to a median dose of 50.4 Gy.[64] RT was used as definitive, adjuvant, or salvage therapy. The overall 3-year PFS was 97.4%.

SRS is an option for cavernous sinus meningiomas that are considered geometrically favorable. Radiosurgery can also reverse cranial neuropathies more rapidly than fractionated schedules. SRS is associated with a 5-year PFS of 90 to 95%[66–71] and symptomatic improvement in 25 to 50%.[66,67,69,71] Lee et al reviewed 159 patients with cavernous sinus meningiomas treated with gamma knife SRS with or without prior subtotal resection.[67] The median marginal dose was 13 Gy. The 5- and 10-year local control rates were both 93%. Neurologic status improved in 29%. Another gamma knife series included 115 patients treated with a mean marginal dose of 13 Gy and reported 5- and 10-year local control rates of 94 and 92%, respectively.[66] Forty-three patients (46%) experienced neurologic improvement. A similar LINAC-based SRS series by Spiegelmann et al reviewed 42 patients treated to a mean marginal dose of 14 Gy. At a median follow-up of 3 years, the local control rate was 97.5%. Decreases in pretreatment neuropathies were noted in 29% of cranial nerve (CN) V, 22% of CN VI, and 13% of CN IV deficits. SRS for cavernous sinus meningiomas is associated with a low combined risk for complications ranging from 1 to 7%.[67–71] Of these, the most common risks include trigeminal neuropathy/neuralgia, diplopia, visual field deficits, and other manifestations of optic neuropathy.

Meningiomas of the Tuberculum Sellae or Optic Nerve Sheath

Other parasellar or suprasellar meningiomas, such as those arising from the tuberculum sellae or intracanalicular optic nerve sheath, are very rare. The tuberculum sellae is an osseous protuberance at the anterosuperior margin of the sella turcica that is covered by a layer of dura stretching as a roof over the sella toward the posterior clinoid. Anterior to this, optic nerve sheath meningiomas arise in the dural covering of the optic nerve and comprise only 1 to 2% of all intracranial meningiomas. Of these, the vast majority are intraorbital (92%), whereas 8% arise intracanalicularly.[72]

The published literature for these rare entities is scant. Available data suggest that maximal safe resection is possible in experienced hands and may be considered for symptomatic patients (ie, visual deficits) in need of immediate decompression. However, because of the likelihood of gross or microscopic residual disease, local recurrence is common. Chicani and Miller reported visual outcomes in 18 patients with suprasellar meningiomas treated at the Johns Hopkins Hospital.[73] Although there were mixed long-term results with respect to visual outcome, 39% developed radiographic recurrence at a mean time of 10.7 years. Over half of the recurrences occurred after gross total resection. Similarly, for optic nerve sheath meningiomas, a summary of the literature by Dutton reported an overall recurrence rate of 25% after surgery.[72] The operative complication rate was ~30%.

Fractionated radiation alone appears to provide excellent local control and preserve or improve vision in most cases. Turbin et al retrospectively reviewed 64 patients with primary optic nerve sheath meningiomas who were treated with surgery alone, surgery and RT, or RT alone to 40 to 55 Gy.[74] Mean follow-up was 12.5 years. There were no significant differences in visual acuity at baseline among the groups. After therapy, visual acuity significantly worsened in the surgery and surgery + RT groups but was unchanged in the RT-alone group. Complication rates were 62 to 68% in the surgical groups, but only 33% in the RT-alone group. Andrews et al reviewed 33 optic nerve sheath meningiomas treated with fractionated SRT to a median dose of 51 Gy with a median follow-up of 7.4 years.[75] Of 22 optic nerves with pretreatment function, vision was improved in 42% and at least preserved in 92%. Importantly, there were no local recurrences.

In contrast to SRS for cavernous sinus meningiomas, SRS for meningiomas of the tuberculum sellae or optic nerve sheath is not favored because the dose required for adequate local control (12–13 Gy) exceeds the optic chiasm and nerve tolerances (8–10 Gy). Therefore, high-precision fractionated SRT to 50.4 to 54 Gy should be considered the standard first-line therapy, given its favorable safety profile and success in local control.

Taken together, among patients with suprasellar lesions, very conservative resection may be considered for those who might gain visual benefit from immediate decompression. For those with optic nerve sheath meningiomas, any attempt at resection or even biopsy is associated with an enormous risk for immediate blindness of the affected eye. Postoperatively, there should be a low threshold for RT because of the likelihood of residual disease. For all others (including those who are asymptomatic or have preexisting severe/complete visual loss), high-precision fractionated SRT is emerging as the treatment of choice because of its favorable toxicity profile and excellent local control.

◆ Malignant Tumors

Optic Pathway Gliomas

Historically, optic pathway gliomas (OPGs) have been considered a unique entity from other gliomas because of their poor surgical accessibility, predilection for patients of a young age, and association with neurofibromatosis type 1 (NF1).[76] OPGs may occur in either the optic chiasm or nerves but often extend in an infiltrative pattern to the hypothalamus. Histology is typically a low-grade astrocytic tumor. They occur primarily in children, with 90% of cases occurring in patients younger than 20 years of age, and account for 5% of all pediatric central nervous system (CNS) tumors.[77] There is an association with the NF1 gene; between 25 and 40% of childhood optic pathway tumors occur in children with NF1.[78] The presenting symptom is most commonly visual loss, although children younger than 3 years of age are commonly brought to medical attention with proptosis, strabismus, nystagmus, or loss of developmental milestones.[78]

The overall management of OPGs draws from the principles used for other low-grade gliomas. Maximal safe resection should be considered initially to establish a diagnosis and provide immediate symptomatic relief if needed. Immediate postoperative radiation is often offered for those with symptomatic gross residual disease or at high risk for rapid progression. The timing of radiation should be determined on a patient-specific basis. A randomized trial of radiation given immediately after surgery versus at the time of progression found no difference in OS. However, immediate postoperative RT improved time to progression (4.8 years for adjuvant RT vs. 3.4 years for salvage RT).[79] Radiation doses typically range from 50.4 to 54 Gy in 1.8 Gy per fraction.[78] In adults with low-grade gliomas, randomized trials of 45 versus 59.4 Gy and of 50.4 versus 64.8 Gy have failed to demonstrate an improvement in 5-year OS with dose escalation.[80,81]

Age at diagnosis plays a crucial role in initial treatment decisions because RT in very young children is associated with neurocognitive late effects. Chemotherapy or close observation is often used to delay the need for RT to allow further brain maturation and obviate the side effects of treatment.[82] The standard first-line chemotherapy is the "Packer regimen" consisting of carboplatin and vincristine (CV).[83,84] Median delays in progression of 2.5 to 3 years can be achieved with chemotherapy, with 5-year PFS and OS rates of 56% and 90%, respectively.[85,86] A completed but unpublished phase III Children's Oncology Group trial (COG A9952) randomized patients between CV and TPCV (thioguanine, procarbazine, CCNU, and vincristine) in children younger than 10 years old with progressive or incompletely resected low-grade gliomas. Preliminary analysis suggests an overall response rate of ~60% with a 5-year event-free survival (EFS) of 35% for CV versus 48% for TPCV ($P = 0.11$).[83,87,88] Although the success of chemotherapy at delaying radiation is encouraging, it must be recognized that the majority of patients will have progression within 5 years and require radiation by that time. OPGs are historically associated with a higher risk for progression yet retain a very favorable OS rate.[89–91] This finding is likely related to the young patient demographics and the use of chemotherapy to delay RT, rather than intrinsic tumor behavior.

The association between NF1 and OPGs is well established.[92] OPG arising in the setting of NF1 is believed to have a more favorable natural history, and cases of spontaneous regression have been documented.[93–95] Study A9952 has preliminarily reported a 5-year OS of 98% in patients with NF, which compares favorably with 86% in the non-NF1 population ($P = 0.0017$).[87] However, radiation-related complications appear to be more common in the setting of NF1. In a series evaluating 58 patients with NF1 treated for optic gliomas, second primary tumors occurred in 9 of 18 (50%) following RT and in 8 of 40 (20%) without RT at a median of 12 years.[96] Moyamoya syndrome is characterized by the appearance of abnormal collateral vascular networks adjacent to spontaneously occluded vessels of the circle of Willis. Patients with NF1 are more likely to develop moyamoya syndrome, and at a lower radiation dose threshold.[97,98] These observations have led to a more conservative approach to the management of OPGs in NF1. Patients with asymptomatic OPGs are not treated—they are simply observed. Symptomatic patients receive chemotherapy as first-line therapy, with radiation reserved for truly refractory cases.

In the current era, advanced technologies have improved the ability to spare normal tissue, which is of particular importance in the pediatric population. These include three-dimensional treatment planning, stereotactic immobilization to reduce the margin required for setup uncertainty, and proton therapy to minimize exit dose. A prospective trial evaluating the use of SRT with only a 2-mm margin for low-grade gliomas achieved 8-year PFS of 65% and OS of 82%, with no marginal failures.[99]

Long-term outcomes after RT are very favorable in children with OPGs, with 10-year survival rates of 80 to 90% (**Table 13.1**). Because of the risks associated with RT, it may be reserved until the time of symptomatic or radiographic progression, and this timing is heavily based on the patient's age. Chemotherapy is often used as a strategy to delay RT and its potential neurocognitive effects. The primary role of surgery is for palliation of compressive symptoms and should be considered only on a patient-specific basis.

Germ Cell Tumors

Germ cell tumors are classified by the WHO system as pure germinomas (60% of intracranial germ cell neoplasms) and nongerminomatous germ cell tumors (NGGCTs, 40%). NGGCTs include teratomas, embryonal carcinomas, endodermal sinus tumors, choriocarcinomas, and mixed germ cell tumors.[100] The primary lesion is located between the suprasellar cistern and pineal gland in 95% of patients with intracranial germ cell tumors, with the majority of germinomas found in the suprasellar region and of nongerminomatous tumors in the pineal area.[100] Multiple midline germinomas are those that present with simultaneous involvement along the third ventricle, pineal, and suprasellar regions.[101,102] At presentation, a triad of diabetes insipidus, visual field abnormalities, and anterior hypopituitarism may be observed. Other common symptoms are related to increased intracranial pressure, including headache, nausea, vomiting, and lethargy.[103]

The differentiation between pure germinomas and NGGCTs is critical because this dramatically impacts prognosis and treatment decisions (**Table 13.2**). Complete staging

Table 13.1 Series of Optic Pathway Gliomas Treated with Radiotherapy

Reference	Authors	Year	N	Dose (median)	End point	Outcome	Follow-up (median)
151	Flickinger et al	1988	25	47 Gy (mean)	5-y OS, PFS	96%, 87%	10.2 y
					10-y OS, PFS	90%, 87%	
					15-y OS, PFS	90%, 87%	
152	Kovalic et al	1990	33	50.4 Gy	5-yOS	94%	12.3 y
					10-y OS	81%	
					15-y OS	74%	
153	Jenkin et al	1993	38	50 Gy	10-y OS, RFS	79%, 73%	11.5 y
154	Tao et al	1997	29	54 Gy	10-y OS, FFP	89%, 100%	9 y

Abbreviations: FFP, freedom from progression; OS, overall survival; PFS, progression-free survival; RFS, relapse-free survival.

Table 13.2 Series of Germinomas Treated with Radiotherapy with or without Chemotherapy

Reference	Authors	Year	N	Dose (median)	End point	Outcome	Median/mean follow-up
				Radiotherapy alone			
155	Haddock et al	1997	32	48.5 Gy (local), 30 Gy (CSI or WBRT)	5-y PFS	70%	5.5 y
					5-y OS	91%	
109	Hardenbergh et al	1997	40	52 Gy (local), 30 Gy (CSI)	5-y PFS	97%	5.2 y
					5-y OS	100%	
107	Bamberg et al	1999	11	50 Gy (local), 36 Gy (CSI)	5-y PFS	100%	5 y
					5-y OS	100%	
			49	45 Gy (local), 30 Gy (CSI)	5-y PFS	89%	
					5-y OS	92%	
156	Cho et al	2009	81	34.2→19.5 Gy (CSI)	10-y RFS	100%	10 y
				59→39.3 Gy (local)	10-y RFS	69%	
				Chemotherapy before radiotherapy			
114	Kretschmar et al	2007	12	GTV + 2 cm to 30.6 Gy if CR, 50.4 Gy if residual	5-y PFS	95%	5.5 y
					5-y OS	100%	

Abbreviations: CR, complete remission; CSI, craniospinal irradiation; GTV, gross tumor volume; OS, overall survival; PFS, progression-free survival; RFS, relapse-free survival; WBRT, whole-brain radiation therapy.

should include MRI of the brain and total spine with contrast, measurement of tumor markers including serum and cerebrospinal fluid (CSF) β-human chorionic gonadotropin (β-HCG) and α-fetoprotein (AFP), and CSF cytology. Pure germinomas often present with markers within normal limits; however, some may have β-HCG levels above 100 IU/L. Definitive diagnosis by surgical biopsy is recommended in most cases. However, if surgery is considered high-risk, then any patient with elevated AFP should be assumed to have NGGCT as opposed to pure germinoma.

RT has long been the standard treatment for pure germinomas and is an important component of multimodality therapy for NGGCTs.[78,104] Pure germinomas are extremely radioresponsive. When RT alone is used for localized disease, 10-year OS exceeds 90%. However, late effects of RT can impact the neuropsychological function and quality of life of these patients.[105] The historical treatment for pure germinomas has been craniospinal irradiation (CSI) to 36 Gy followed by a boost to the primary tumor to 50 to 54 Gy. However, the focus of treatment in recent years has shifted to decreasing the RT dose and volume while preserving curability. Debate continues over the most appropriate radiation volume. Choices include the local tumor only with a margin, tumor and third ventricle, whole ventricle, whole brain (WBRT), and full CSI. In a large meta-analysis of 754 patients, Rogers et al found that recurrence rates increased with smaller RT volumes: 4% following CSI, 8% following WBRT or whole-ventricle RT plus boost, and 23% following focal treatment alone.[106] Importantly, the frequency of spinal relapse did not significantly differ between the CSI group and the whole-brain/whole-ventricle group (1.2% vs. 2.9%, respectively) but was significantly higher in the focal radiation group (11.3%). MAKEI 83/86/89 was a prospective dose reduction study of intracranial germinoma. In this study, CSI to 30 Gy with a 15-Gy boost was compared with CSI to 36 Gy with a 14-Gy boost (all in 1.5-Gy fractions). There were no statistically significant differences in outcomes.[107] Complete remission was achieved in all 60 patients, with a 5-year relapse-free survival of 91% at a mean follow-up of 59.5 months. Currently, most advocate for treatment with whole-ventricle radiation doses of 21 to 24 Gy, with an additional boost to the primary tumor to 40 to 45 Gy. For patients with evidence of CSF dissemination at diagnosis, standard treatment remains CSI followed by a boost to the primary tumor and macroscopic metastases.[106,108,109]

Germinomas are highly responsive to chemotherapy, and this has led to combined-modality therapy trials attempting to further reduce the role of RT in low-risk subgroups. ACNS 0232 was a phase III trial that randomized children to RT alone versus chemotherapy followed by response-based RT. Patients with localized disease randomized to radiation alone received 21 Gy to the whole ventricle followed by a boost of 24 Gy to the primary site. Patients randomized to chemotherapy plus radiation received two to four cycles of chemotherapy (carboplatin, etoposide, cisplatin, and cyclophosphamide). If a complete response was achieved after two or four cycles, patients received 30

Gy to the involved field only. Unfortunately, the trial accrued poorly and closed early. Further studies are needed to determine whether the inclusion of chemotherapy will reduce the need for RT.

NGGCTs are much rarer than germinomas, and therefore their management is guided by far fewer available data. Outcomes of NGGCTs are worse than those for germinomas, and optimal radiation dose and volume remain controversial. The current standard of care requires multimodality therapy consisting of platinum-based chemotherapy, CSI, and consideration of second-look surgery for resection of gross residual disease. Series evaluating the use of RT alone (CSI plus boost) in children with NGGCTs reported poor rates of OS of 20 to 40%.[100,110,111] The use of neoadjuvant chemotherapy before RT has led to significant improvements, with survival rates of 60 to 70%.[112,113] In POG 9530, 14 patients who had NGGCTs or who had germinomas with elevated AFP or β-HCG received four cycles of cisplatin and etoposide alternating with vincristine and cyclophosphamide.[114] Five patients had a CR and received CSI to 30.6 Gy with boost to 50.4 Gy for local disease; nine patients had less than a CR and received CSI to 36 Gy with boost to 54 Gy. Probability of EFS was 79% at 58-month median follow-up. In the recently completed but unreported ACNS 0122, patients received carboplatin, VP-16, and ifosfamide followed by 36 Gy of CSI and an involved-field boost for a total dose of 54 Gy to the tumor bed. Second-look surgery was performed in those patients who did not achieve CR or partial response (PR) after neoadjuvant chemotherapy, and autologous peripheral blood stem cell transplantation was performed for persistently positive markers or evidence of residual malignant elements.

Mature teratomas are a distinct entity from other NGGCTs because they are theoretically benign and have a favorable prognosis. Most can be cured by complete resection.[103] When this cannot be achieved, treatment with adjuvant radiation to a dose of 50 Gy has shown survival of up to 93% at 10 years.[115]

RT plays an important role in the management of both pure germinomas and NGGCTs. Emerging technology in radiation oncology may be able to further spare normal brain tissue by using IMRT or proton radiotherapy while preserving oncologic outcomes.[116]

Chordomas and Chondrosarcomas

Chordomas and chondrosarcomas arising near the skull base are managed fairly similarly, although they originate from different cell types and have different prognoses. Chordomas are rare, slow-growing, locally aggressive tumors, thought to originate from notochord remnants within the axial skeleton. Approximately 35% arise within the skull base, 50% in the sacrococcygeal region, and 15% in the vertebral column.[117] Their metastatic potential is low, with reports ranging from ~5 to 20%. Failures are predominantly local in series with long-term follow-up.[118,119] Chondrosarcomas are malignant tumors of cartilage-forming cells and can arise in any bone preformed by cartilage. They most commonly arise in the humerus, femur, or bones of the pelvis but can originate in the skull base and represent ~5% of skull base tumors.[120] Skull-based chondrosarcomas are typically low-grade and progress slowly with relatively asymptomatic growth. This often leads to extensive locoregional infiltration by the time of diagnosis.

For both chordomas and chondrosarcomas, radical resection by an experienced surgeon is the single most important aspect of treatment because local progression rather than distant metastasis is the main contributor to morbidity and mortality. Gross total resection can be difficult to achieve because of the anatomic constraints to surgical access, as well as the proximity of adjacent critical normal tissues. The volume of residual disease is a strong predictor of local control. In a series by Berson et al, patients with low-volume disease (<20 cm^3) had a significantly higher local control rate after radiation than patients with larger-volume disease (80% vs. 33% at 5 years).[121] Similar findings were reported by Hug et al.[122] In patients with residual disease, postoperative radiation therapy is a vital component of care. In an early series of 155 patients with chordoma, there was a 1.5-year mean survival for patients who underwent surgery alone, compared with 5.2 years for those who underwent surgery followed by RT.[123] Even with the addition of adjuvant RT, the pattern of failure is predominantly local.[124]

Similar to surgery, RT should be consolidated at experienced centers because of the apparent benefit of high doses. Radiation targets are defined as (1) areas of gross disease on imaging, (2) areas occupied by tumor preoperatively, and (3) anatomic compartments at risk for harboring microscopic disease. The total dose appears to the most important determinant of local control after radiation therapy. Rates of local recurrence after doses below 60 Gy have been as high as 70 to 100%, with most patients dying of locally progressive disease.[119,125,126] In a more modern series, the use of advanced imaging and planning with doses of 50 to 64 Gy yielded 5-year PFS of only 23% and OS of 35%.[127] However, dose escalation is often limited by the proximity of critical normal tissues, such as the brainstem and cranial nerves. Hug et al reported decreased rates of 5-year local control for tumors with brainstem abutment compared with those located further away (53 vs. 94%, respectively).[122] When purposeful dose compromises are made at the tumor–critical structure interface, these "cold spots" within the tumor appear to be associated with the probability of recurrence.[128] Also, for unclear reasons, female patients have higher local failure rates than their male counterparts. At the present time, there are no reported prospective randomized trials evaluating the value of dose escalation in these tumors. A randomized trial (NCT00592748) stratifying patients into low- versus high-risk groups, with doses of 69.6 Gy (relative biological effectiveness [RBE]) or 75.6 Gy (RBE) in the low-risk group and with doses of 75.6 Gy (RBE) or 82.9 Gy (RBE) in the high risk group, is closed to accrual and not currently reported.

The use of charged particles, such as proton, helium, or carbon ion therapy, is strongly encouraged because of the ability to deliver high radiation doses to the tumor volume with minimal exit dose to critical structures. This strategy appears to improve local control compared with historical rates from photon therapy (**Table 13.3**). The treatment of macroscopic residual disease with conventional photon RT has yielded local control rates as poor as 27%.[125] In contrast, the Massachusetts General Hospital experience included 290 patients treated with proton with or without photon therapy to doses of up to 83 CGE.[129] At a median follow-up of 41 months, the 5- and 10-year local recurrence-free survival rates were 73% and 54%, respectively. The OS rates were 80% and 54%, respectively. Results from other experiences with charged particles have yielded similar results (**Table 13.3**). Series with modern photon techniques for dose escalation, such as SRT and three-dimensional CRT, suggest improved results for these in comparison with conventionally delivered photons. For example, Debus et al used stereotactic fractionated photons at a median dose of 66.6 Gy and reported 5-year local control rates of 50% for chordomas and 100% for chondrosarcomas.[130]

Late effects of RT are important to consider, given the long life expectancies that may be achievable with high-dose radiation therapy after safe maximal resection. Late

Table 13.3 Series of Chordomas and Chondrosarcomas Treated with Radiotherapy

Reference	Authors	Year	N	Histology	Dose (median)	End point	Outcome	Follow-up (median)
				Fractionated photons				
118	Forsyth et al	1993	39	Ch	50 Gy	5-y OS	51% (S, S+RT)	99 mo
						10-y OS	35%	
157	Tai et al	1995	159	Ch	55.8 Gy (mean)	5-y OS	20% S, 65% S+RT	4.1 y
						10-y OS	20% S, 50% S+RT	
125	Catton et al	1996	48	Ch	50 Gy	Median survival	62 months (4 S, 48 S+RT)	62 mo
				Stereotactic fractionated photons				
130	Debus et al	2000	45	Ch and Cs	66.6 Gy	5-y LC	Ch 50%, Cs 100%	27 mo (mean)
				Fractionated protons				
129	Munzenrider and Liebsch (MGH)	1999	519 (Ch 290, Cs 229)	Ch and low-grade Cs	66–83 CGE	5-y LRFS	Ch 73%, Cs 98%	41 mo
						10-y LRFS	Ch 54%, Cs 94%	
158	Hug et al (LLUMC)	2000	58	Ch and low-grade Cs	64.8–79.2 CGE	5-y LC	Ch 79%, Cs 100%	33 mo (mean)
159	Weber et al (PSI)	2005	29	Ch and low-grade Cs	Ch 74 CGE, Cs 68 CGE	3-y LC	Ch 87.5%, Cs 100%	29 mo
160	Noel et al (Orsay)	2005	100	Ch	67 CGE	4-y LC	54%	31 mo
161	Habrand et al	2008	30	Ch and low-grade Cs	68.4 CGE	5-y PFS	Ch 77%, Cs 81%	26.5 mo (mean)
162	Schulte et al (LLUMC)	2008	63	Cs	72 CGE	5-y LC	86%	84 mo
						10-y LC	83%	
				Gamma knife SRS				
163	Krishnan et al	2005	25	Ch	15 Gy	5-y LC	32%	58 mo
164	Martin et al	2007	28	Ch and Cs	16 Gy	5-y LC	Ch 63%, Cs 80%	88 mo
				LINAC-based SRS/SRT				
165	Chang et al	2001	10	Ch	19.4 Gy (mean)	LC	2/12	48 mo (mean)
				LINAC-based SRT				
166	Gwak et al	2005	9	Ch and Cs	21–43.6 Gy (3–5 fx)	2-y LC	89%	24 mo
				Other charged particles (carbon ion)				
167	Schulz-Ertner et al	2007	54	Cs, low- and intermediate-grade	60 GyE	4-y LC	90%	33 mo
168	Schulz-Ertner et al	2007	96	Ch	60 GyE	5-y LC	70%	31 mo (mean)

Abbreviations: CGE, cobalt gray equivalent; Ch, chordoma; Cs, chondrosarcoma; fx, fractions; Gy, gray; GyE, gray equivalent; LC, local control; LINAC, linear accelerator; LRFS, local relapse-free survival; LLUMC, Loma Linda University Medical Center; MGH, Massachusetts General Hospital; OS, overall survival; PFS, progression-free survival; PSI, Paul Scherrer Institut; RT, radiation therapy; S, surgery; SRS, stereotactic radiosurgery; SRT, stereotactic radiotherapy.

effects were reported in 8% of patients in a proton series at Massachusetts General Hospital, which included asymptomatic or symptomatic brain changes, unilateral or bilateral blindness, and unilateral deafness.[124] Temporal lobe damage has been reported in 7.6% of patients at 2 years and 13.2% at 5 years.[131]

In summary, the treatment of chordoma and chondrosarcoma should be consolidated within high-volume and experienced multidisciplinary teams that can safely offer radical surgery and high-dose RT. If available, strong consideration should be given to proton therapy to deliver conventionally fractionated doses of 72 Gy (RBE) for chondrosarcomas and 72 to 79 Gy (RBE) for chordomas.

Pituitary Carcinomas

Pituitary carcinomas are rare entities that comprise ~0.2% of pituitary tumors.[132] They are defined as pituitary tumors with metastasis outside the CNS or occurring as separate foci within the CNS. Histologic confirmation often reveals increased mitotic activity (6 per 10 hpf) and p53 overexpression.[133] Retrospective series suggest that ~75% are hormone-secreting and the remaining 25% nonfunctioning.[134] In a series of 15 patients, the mean latency period to metastasis was ~7 years, with greater tendency toward systemic metastasis than toward isolated craniospinal metastasis.[134]

Given their rarity, there is no consensus for treatment strategy. Outcomes are poor even after multimodality treatment, including surgery, radiation, and chemotherapy. Experience with fractionated involved-field radiation therapy (45–56 Gy) has been limited to case reports.[132,135] In a case report, a long-term survivor of pituitary carcinoma was initially treated with adjuvant RT to the sella to 56 Gy and at the time of recurrence 8 years later received WBRT to 24 Gy.[135]

Sellar Metastases

Large autopsy series report that 1 to 3% of patients with malignant tumors have pituitary metastases.[136–138] They are seen most commonly with breast cancer and lung cancer primaries but can originate from a wide variety of primary sites.[139,140] Neurohypophysial metastases are more common, although breast cancers appear to preferentially metastasize to the adenohypophysis.

Presenting symptoms most commonly include diabetes insipidus at rates between 29 and 71%.[138,139] Other symptoms may include anterior hypopituitarism, visual field defects, retro-orbital pain, and ophthalmoplegia.[141] In a series of 36 patients with pituitary metastases, such symptoms were the first sign of disease in 56%.[139] In this series from Morita et al, treatment was primarily surgical, and adjuvant RT to a median dose of 36 Gy was given to half of the patients. Median survival was ~6 months. Completeness of resection and radiation dose did not appear to be associated with OS. Kano et al reported an experience in which 18 patients were treated with gamma knife SRS to a median marginal dose of 13 Gy. The median survival was 5.2 months.[142] Following SRS, 50% of patients experienced relief of neurologic symptoms, and the condition of 43% of patients with preexisting diabetes insipidus was felt to have improved.

Decisions regarding choice of RT are largely driven by dosimetric considerations. Because of their close proximity to the optic chiasm, pituitary metastases are usually not amenable to SRS because therapeutic doses exceed chiasm tolerance. In the setting of multiple brain metastases, WBRT is recommended. If the sellar metastasis is solitary in nature or refractory to WBRT, then SRS, hypofractionated SRT, or involved-field RT may be considered as long as optic chiasm and nerve tolerances are respected.

◆ Late Effects of Radiation Therapy

The risk for late effects after radiation is always related to the adjacent normal tissue that receives a clinically relevant dose. In the sella and parasellar region, these "organs at risk" include the pituitary gland, optic chiasm, optic nerves, brain parenchyma, and contents of the cavernous sinus—namely, cranial nerves and carotid vessels. In the modern era, the sole purpose of advanced technology in radiation planning is to minimize dose to normal tissues and spare the patient both acute and late effects. These technologies include CT-based three-dimensional planning, IMRT, stereotactic approaches to minimize setup uncertainty, and proton therapy to minimize exit dose. Most of the available data below are drawn from the large experience in treating pituitary adenomas with standard fractionated EBRT and SRS.

Hypopituitarism

Hypopituitarism is a common late effect of RT when the prescribed dose to the sella is in the 45- to 54-Gy range used to treat most benign neoplasms. Because the sella is often the target, the risk for hypopituitarism is impossible to minimize. The risk for new hypopituitarism affecting at least one axis is 20 to 60% at 5 years for both standard fractionated EBRT and SRS.[10,11,37,143] For example, Estrada et al reported a 57% risk for new GH deficiency after treatment for Cushing disease.[10] With longer follow-up, Minniti et al reported new hypopituitarism in 85% at 15 years.[11] Hoybye et al reported 100% GH deficiency and 69% thyroid hormone deficiency with mean follow-up of 17 years after SRS for ACTH-secreting adenomas. More modern dosimetric analyses have attempted to identify predictors for hypopituitarism, such as dose parameters for the entire pituitary,[144] infundibulum,[145] and hypothalamus.[146]

Visual Deficits

At the recommended tolerance doses of less than 54 Gy in 1.8- to 2-Gy fractions and less than 8 to 10 Gy in a single SRS fraction, the risk for visual deficits is minimal. This is reviewed in the earlier section, "Dose Limitations of the Optic Chiasm and Nerves." Clinical data come from large series, including a compilation of 11 series involving 1388 patients treated with standard fractionated EBRT. The risk for visual injury was 1.7%.[147] Similarly, the Royal Marsden Hospital experience included 411 patients with pituitary adenomas treated with 45 to 50 Gy in 25 to 30 fractions and found a 1.5% incidence of visual deterioration at 20 years.[148] The largest SRS experience for adenomas included more than 1600 patients over 35 series and reported a 1% risk for visual changes.[1]

Second Malignancy

As in most disease sites, the risk for second malignancy after RT is difficult to measure because it is heavily dependent on dose, treatment volume, length of follow-up, and underlying host genetics. Radiation-induced tumors are most commonly meningiomas, gliomas, and sarcomas. Based on data from the literature for pituitary adenomas, the long-term risk for a second malignancy after standard fractionated EBRT is 1 to 3% at 20 years.[147–149] However, in a large review of SRS series including 1621 patients, there were no reported radiation-induced maligancies.[1] In addition to SRS, other modern technologies such as three-dimensional CRT and proton therapy provide a theoretic reduction in risk for second malignancy by reducing the volume of normal tissue exposed to radiation.

Radionecrosis

Radionecrosis within uninvolved brain parenchyma, such as the temporal lobes, is extremely uncommon when 45 to 54 Gy in 1.8- to 2-Gy fractions or standard SRS doses are delivered to the sella or parasellar region. The reported risk is less than 1%.[1,147]

Cerebrovascular Events

Radiation dose to the carotid vessels and circle of Willis has been associated with a small risk for subsequent vascular events. Brada et al reviewed 331 patients treated at the Royal Marsden Hospital between 1962 and 1986 for pituitary adenomas with RT.[150] The actuarial incidence rates for cerebrovascular accident were 4%, 11%, and 21% at 5, 10, and 20 years, respectively, from the date of RT. Compared with the general population in the United Kingdom, this was estimated to represent a relative risk increase of 4.1. However, this study did not include patient-related factors in the analysis, nor did it necessarily reflect modern radiation technologies and strategies.

◆ Conclusion

RT plays an important role in the management of benign and malignant tumors of the sellar and parasellar regions. In all of the neoplasms discussed in this chapter, there is a delicate balance between the benefits of local control and the risks for late complications of RT. Technology in radiation oncology is continuously evolving to improve the delivery of therapeutic doses to involved regions while minimizing dose to normal tissues. Most importantly, the optimal timing of RT is often difficult to ascertain and should be determined in a multidisciplinary setting.

References

1. Sheehan JP, Niranjan A, Sheehan JM, et al. Stereotactic radiosurgery for pituitary adenomas: an intermediate review of its safety, efficacy, and role in the neurosurgical treatment armamentarium. J Neurosurg 2005;102(4):678–691
2. Landolt AM, Haller D, Lomax N, et al. Stereotactic radiosurgery for recurrent surgically treated acromegaly: comparison with fractionated radiotherapy. J Neurosurg 1998;88(6):1002–1008
3. Emami B, Lyman J, Brown A, et al. Tolerance of normal tissue to therapeutic irradiation. Int J Radiat Oncol Biol Phys 1991;21(1):109–122
4. Mayo C, Martel MK, Marks LB, Flickinger J, Nam J, Kirkpatrick J. Radiation dose-volume effects of optic nerves and chiasm. Int J Radiat Oncol Biol Phys 2010;76(3, Suppl):S28–S35
5. van den Bergh AC, Dullaart RP, Hoving MA, et al. Radiation optic neuropathy after external beam radiation therapy for acromegaly. Radiother Oncol 2003;68(2):95–100
6. Aristizabal S, Caldwell WL, Avila J. The relationship of time-dose fractionation factors to complications in the treatment of pituitary tumors by irradiation. Int J Radiat Oncol Biol Phys 1977;2(7–8):667–673
7. Mackley HB, Reddy CA, Lee SY, et al. Intensity-modulated radiotherapy for pituitary adenomas: the preliminary report of the Cleveland Clinic experience. Int J Radiat Oncol Biol Phys 2007;67(1):232–239
8. Tishler RB, Loeffler JS, Lunsford LD, et al. Tolerance of cranial nerves of the cavernous sinus to radiosurgery. Int J Radiat Oncol Biol Phys 1993;27(2):215–221
9. Mitsumori M, Shrieve DC, Alexander E III, et al. Initial clinical results of LINAC-based stereotactic radiosurgery and stereotactic radiotherapy for pituitary adenomas. Int J Radiat Oncol Biol Phys 1998;42(3):573–580
10. Estrada J, Boronat M, Mielgo M, et al. The long-term outcome of pituitary irradiation after unsuccessful transsphenoidal surgery in Cushing's disease. N Engl J Med 1997;336(3):172–177
11. Minniti G, Osti M, Jaffrain-Rea ML, Esposito V, Cantore G, Maurizi Enrici R. Long-term follow-up results of postoperative radiation therapy for Cushing's disease. J Neurooncol 2007;84(1):79–84
12. Zierhut D, Flentje M, Adolph J, Erdmann J, Raue F, Wannenmacher M. External radiotherapy of pituitary adenomas. Int J Radiat Oncol Biol Phys 1995;33(2):307–314
13. Alameda C, Lucas T, Pineda E, et al. Experience in management of 51 non-functioning pituitary adenomas: indications for postoperative radiotherapy. J Endocrinol Invest 2005;28(1):18–22
14. Dekkers OM, Pereira AM, Roelfsema F, et al. Observation alone after transsphenoidal surgery for nonfunctioning pituitary macroadenoma. J Clin Endocrinol Metab 2006;91(5):1796–1801
15. Lillehei KO, Kirschman DL, Kleinschmidt-DeMasters BK, Ridgway EC. Reassessment of the role of radiation therapy in the treatment of endocrine-inactive pituitary macroadenomas. Neurosurgery 1998;43(3):432–438, discussion 438–439
16. Park P, Chandler WF, Barkan AL, et al. The role of radiation therapy after surgical resection of nonfunctional pituitary macroadenomas. Neurosurgery 2004;55(1):100–106, discussion 106–107
17. Gittoes NJ, Bates AS, Tse W, et al. Radiotherapy for non-function pituitary tumours. Clin Endocrinol (Oxf) 1998;48(3):331–337
18. van den Bergh AC, van den Berg G, Schoorl MA, et al. Immediate postoperative radiotherapy in residual nonfunctioning pituitary adenoma: beneficial effect on local control without additional negative impact on pituitary function and life expectancy. Int J Radiat Oncol Biol Phys 2007;67(3):863–869
19. Pollock BE, Cochran J, Natt N, et al. Gamma knife radiosurgery for patients with nonfunctioning pituitary adenomas:

results from a 15-year experience. Int J Radiat Oncol Biol Phys 2008;70(5):1325–1329
20. Voges J, Kocher M, Runge M, et al. Linear accelerator radiosurgery for pituitary macroadenomas: a 7-year follow-up study. Cancer 2006;107(6):1355–1364
21. Colin P, Jovenin N, Delemer B, et al. Treatment of pituitary adenomas by fractionated stereotactic radiotherapy: a prospective study of 110 patients. Int J Radiat Oncol Biol Phys 2005;62(2): 333–341
22. Ronson BB, Schulte RW, Han KP, Loredo LN, Slater JM, Slater JD. Fractionated proton beam irradiation of pituitary adenomas. Int J Radiat Oncol Biol Phys 2006;64(2):425–434
23. Murayama M, Yasuda K, Minamori Y, Mercado-Asis LB, Yamakita N, Miura K. Long term follow-up of Cushing's disease treated with reserpine and pituitary irradiation. J Clin Endocrinol Metab 1992;75(3):935–942
24. Jenkins PJ, Bates P, Carson MN, Stewart PM, Wass JA. Conventional pituitary irradiation is effective in lowering serum growth hormone and insulin-like growth factor-I in patients with acromegaly. J Clin Endocrinol Metab 2006;91(4):1239–1245
25. Barrande G, Pittino-Lungo M, Coste J, et al. Hormonal and metabolic effects of radiotherapy in acromegaly: long-term results in 128 patients followed in a single center. J Clin Endocrinol Metab 2000;85(10):3779–3785
26. Biermasz NR, van Dulken H, Roelfsema F. Long-term follow-up results of postoperative radiotherapy in 36 patients with acromegaly. J Clin Endocrinol Metab 2000;85(7):2476–2482
27. Milker-Zabel S, Debus J, Thilmann C, Schlegel W, Wannenmacher M. Fractionated stereotactically guided radiotherapy and radiosurgery in the treatment of functional and nonfunctional adenomas of the pituitary gland. Int J Radiat Oncol Biol Phys 2001;50(5):1279–1286
28. Minniti G, Jaffrain-Rea ML, Osti M, et al. The long-term efficacy of conventional radiotherapy in patients with GH-secreting pituitary adenomas. Clin Endocrinol (Oxf) 2005;62(2):210–216
29. Castinetti F, Taieb D, Kuhn JM, et al. Outcome of gamma knife radiosurgery in 82 patients with acromegaly: correlation with initial hypersecretion. J Clin Endocrinol Metab 2005;90(8):4483–4488
30. Zhang N, Pan L, Dai J, et al. Gamma knife radiosurgery as a primary surgical treatment for hypersecreting pituitary adenomas. Stereotact Funct Neurosurg 2000;75(2–3):123–128
31. Kobayashi T, Mori Y, Uchiyama Y, Kida Y, Fujitani S. Long-term results of gamma knife surgery for growth hormone-producing pituitary adenoma: is the disease difficult to cure? J Neurosurg 2005;102(Suppl):119–123
32. Petit JH, Biller BM, Coen JJ, et al. Proton stereotactic radiosurgery in management of persistent acromegaly. Endocr Pract 2007;13(7):726–734
33. Attanasio R, Epaminonda P, Motti E, et al. Gamma-knife radiosurgery in acromegaly: a 4-year follow-up study. J Clin Endocrinol Metab 2003;88(7):3105–3112
34. Littley MD, Shalet SM, Swindell R, Beardwell CG, Sutton ML. Low-dose pituitary irradiation for acromegaly. Clin Endocrinol (Oxf) 1990;32(2):261–270
35. Landolt AM, Haller D, Lomax N, et al. Octreotide may act as a radioprotective agent in acromegaly. J Clin Endocrinol Metab 2000;85(3):1287–1289
36. Hughes MN, Llamas KJ, Yelland ME, Tripcony LB. Pituitary adenomas: long-term results for radiotherapy alone and post-operative radiotherapy. Int J Radiat Oncol Biol Phys 1993;27(5):1035–1043
37. Sheehan JM, Vance ML, Sheehan JP, Ellegala DB, Laws ER Jr. Radiosurgery for Cushing's disease after failed transsphenoidal surgery. J Neurosurg 2000;93(5):738–742
38. Yoon SC, Suh TS, Jang HS, et al. Clinical results of 24 pituitary macroadenomas with linac-based stereotactic radiosurgery. Int J Radiat Oncol Biol Phys 1998;41(4):849–853
39. Petit JH, Biller BM, Yock TI, et al. Proton stereotactic radiotherapy for persistent adrenocorticotropin-producing adenomas. J Clin Endocrinol Metab 2008;93(2):393–399
40. Levy RP, Fabrikant JI, Frankel KA, et al. Heavy-charged-particle radiosurgery of the pituitary gland: clinical results of 840 patients. Stereotact Funct Neurosurg 1991;57(1–2):22–35
41. Littley MD, Shalet SM, Reid H, Beardwell CG, Sutton ML. The effect of external pituitary irradiation on elevated serum prolactin levels in patients with pituitary macroadenomas. Q J Med 1991;81(296):985–998
42. Pan L, Zhang N, Wang EM, Wang BJ, Dai JZ, Cai PW. Gamma knife radiosurgery as a primary treatment for prolactinomas. J Neurosurg 2000;93(Suppl 3):10–13
43. Landolt AM, Lomax N. Gamma knife radiosurgery for prolactinomas. J Neurosurg 2000;93(Suppl 3):14–18
44. Merchant TE, Kiehna EN, Sanford RA, et al. Craniopharyngioma: the St. Jude Children's Research Hospital experience 1984-2001. Int J Radiat Oncol Biol Phys 2002;53(3):533–542
45. Zhang YQ, Wang CC, Ma ZY. Pediatric craniopharyngiomas: clinicomorphological study of 189 cases. Pediatr Neurosurg 2002;36(2):80–84
46. Fahlbusch R, Honegger J, Paulus W, Huk W, Buchfelder M. Surgical treatment of craniopharyngiomas: experience with 168 patients. J Neurosurg 1999;90(2):237–250
47. Rajan B, Ashley S, Gorman C, et al. Craniopharyngioma—a long-term results following limited surgery and radiotherapy. Radiother Oncol 1993;26(1):1–10
48. Stripp DC, Maity A, Janss AJ, et al. Surgery with or without radiation therapy in the management of craniopharyngiomas in children and young adults. Int J Radiat Oncol Biol Phys 2004;58(3):714–720
49. Niranjan A, Kano H, Mathieu D, Kondziolka D, Flickinger JC, Lunsford LD. Radiosurgery for craniopharyngioma. Int J Radiat Oncol Biol Phys 2010;78(1):64–71
50. Rajan B, Ashley S, Thomas DG, Marsh H, Britton J, Brada M. Craniopharyngioma: improving outcome by early recognition and treatment of acute complications. Int J Radiat Oncol Biol Phys 1997;37(3):517–521
51. Goldsmith BJ, Wara WM, Wilson CB, Larson DA. Postoperative irradiation for subtotally resected meningiomas. A retrospective analysis of 140 patients treated from 1967 to 1990. J Neurosurg 1994;80(2):195–201
52. Glaholm J, Bloom HJ, Crow JH. The role of radiotherapy in the management of intracranial meningiomas: the Royal Marsden Hospital experience with 186 patients. Int J Radiat Oncol Biol Phys 1990;18(4):755–761
53. Miralbell R, Linggood RM, de la Monte S, Convery K, Munzenrider JE, Mirimanoff RO. The role of radiotherapy in the treatment of subtotally resected benign meningiomas. J Neurooncol 1992;13(2):157–164
54. Nutting C, Brada M, Brazil L, et al. Radiotherapy in the treatment of benign meningioma of the skull base. J Neurosurg 1999;90(5):823–827
55. Pollock BE, Stafford SL, Utter A, Giannini C, Schreiner SA. Stereotactic radiosurgery provides equivalent tumor control to Simpson Grade 1 resection for patients with small- to medium-size meningiomas. Int J Radiat Oncol Biol Phys 2003;55(4):1000–1005
56. Gudjonsson O, Blomquist E, Lilja A, Ericson H, Bergström M, Nyberg G. Evaluation of the effect of high-energy proton irradiation treatment on meningiomas by means of 11C-L-methionine PET. Eur J Nucl Med 2000;27(12):1793–1799
57. Noël G, Habrand JL, Mammar H, et al. Highly conformal therapy using proton component in the management of meningiomas. Preliminary experience of the Centre de Protonthérapie d'Orsay. Strahlenther Onkol 2002;178(9):480–485
58. Vernimmen FJ, Harris JK, Wilson JA, Melvill R, Smit BJ, Slabbert JP. Stereotactic proton beam therapy of skull base meningiomas. Int J Radiat Oncol Biol Phys 2001;49(1):99–105
59. Milosevic MF, Frost PJ, Laperriere NJ, Wong CS, Simpson WJ. Radiotherapy for atypical or malignant intracranial meningioma. Int J Radiat Oncol Biol Phys 1996;34(4):817–822
60. Arvold ND, Lessell S, Bussiere M, et al. Visual outcome and tumor control after conformal radiotherapy for patients with optic nerve sheath meningioma. Int J Radiat Oncol Biol Phys 2009;75(4):1166–1172
61. Brell M, Villà S, Teixidor P, et al. Fractionated stereotactic radiotherapy in the treatment of exclusive cavernous sinus meningioma: functional outcome, local control, and tolerance. Surg Neurol 2006;65(1):28–33, discussion 33–34
62. Dufour H, Muracciole X, Métellus P, Régis J, Chinot O, Grisoli F. Long-term tumor control and functional outcome in patients with cavernous sinus meningiomas treated by radiotherapy with or without previous surgery: is there an alternative to aggressive

tumor removal? Neurosurgery 2001;48(2):285–294, discussion 294–296
63. Milker-Zabel S, Zabel-du Bois A, Huber P, Schlegel W, Debus J. Fractionated stereotactic radiation therapy in the management of benign cavernous sinus meningiomas : long-term experience and review of the literature. Strahlenther Onkol 2006;182(11): 635–640
64. Selch MT, Ahn E, Laskari A, et al. Stereotactic radiotherapy for treatment of cavernous sinus meningiomas. Int J Radiat Oncol Biol Phys 2004;59(1):101–111
65. Maguire PD, Clough R, Friedman AH, Halperin EC. Fractionated external-beam radiation therapy for meningiomas of the cavernous sinus. Int J Radiat Oncol Biol Phys 1999;44(1):75–79
66. Hasegawa T, Kida Y, Yoshimoto M, Koike J, Iizuka H, Ishii D. Long-term outcomes of Gamma Knife surgery for cavernous sinus meningioma. J Neurosurg 2007;107(4):745–751
67. Lee JY, Niranjan A, McInerney J, Kondziolka D, Flickinger JC, Lunsford LD. Stereotactic radiosurgery providing long-term tumor control of cavernous sinus meningiomas. J Neurosurg 2002;97(1):65–72
68. Nicolato A, Foroni R, Alessandrini F, Bricolo A, Gerosa M. Radiosurgical treatment of cavernous sinus meningiomas: experience with 122 treated patients. Neurosurgery 2002;51(5):1153–1159, discussion 1159–1161
69. Roche PH, Régis J, Dufour H, et al. Gamma knife radiosurgery in the management of cavernous sinus meningiomas. J Neurosurg 2000;93(Suppl 3):68–73
70. Skeie BS, Enger PO, Skeie GO, Thorsen F, Pedersen PH. Gamma knife surgery of meningiomas involving the cavernous sinus: long-term follow-up of 100 patients. Neurosurgery 2010;66(4):661–668, discussion 668–669
71. Spiegelmann R, Nissim O, Menhel J, Alezra D, Pfeffer MR. Linear accelerator radiosurgery for meningiomas in and around the cavernous sinus. Neurosurgery 2002;51(6):1373–1379, discussion 1379–1380
72. Dutton JJ. Optic nerve sheath meningiomas. Surv Ophthalmol 1992;37(3):167–183
73. Chicani CF, Miller NR. Visual outcome in surgically treated suprasellar meningiomas. J Neuroophthalmol 2003;23(1):3–10
74. Turbin RE, Thompson CR, Kennerdell JS, Cockerham KP, Kupersmith MJ. A long-term visual outcome comparison in patients with optic nerve sheath meningioma managed with observation, surgery, radiotherapy, or surgery and radiotherapy. Ophthalmology 2002;109(5):890–899, discussion 899–900
75. Andrews DW, Faroozan R, Yang BP, et al. Fractionated stereotactic radiotherapy for the treatment of optic nerve sheath meningiomas: preliminary observations of 33 optic nerves in 30 patients with historical comparison to observation with or without prior surgery. Neurosurgery 2002;51(4):890–902, discussion 903–904
76. Parsons J. The Pathology of the Eye. Hodder and Stoughton; 1905:693–715
77. Dutton JJ. Gliomas of the anterior visual pathway. Surv Ophthalmol 1994;38(5):427–452
78. Halperin EC. Pediatric Radiation Oncology. 4th ed. Lippincott Williams & Wilkins; 2005
79. Karim AB, Afra D, Cornu P, et al. Randomized trial on the efficacy of radiotherapy for cerebral low-grade glioma in the adult: European Organization for Research and Treatment of Cancer Study 22845 with the Medical Research Council study BRO4: an interim analysis. Int J Radiat Oncol Biol Phys 2002;52(2):316–324
80. Karim AB, Maat B, Hatlevoll R, et al. A randomized trial on dose-response in radiation therapy of low-grade cerebral glioma: European Organization for Research and Treatment of Cancer (EORTC) Study 22844. Int J Radiat Oncol Biol Phys 1996;36(3):549–556
81. Shaw E, Arusell R, Scheithauer B, et al. Prospective randomized trial of low- versus high-dose radiation therapy in adults with supratentorial low-grade glioma: initial report of a North Central Cancer Treatment Group/Radiation Therapy Oncology Group/Eastern Cooperative Oncology Group study. J Clin Oncol 2002;20(9):2267–2276
82. Jahraus CD, Tarbell NJ. Optic pathway gliomas. Pediatr Blood Cancer 2006;46(5):586–596
83. Packer RJ, Ater J, Allen J, et al. Carboplatin and vincristine chemotherapy for children with newly diagnosed progressive low-grade gliomas. J Neurosurg 1997;86(5):747–754
84. Packer RJ, Lange B, Ater J, et al. Carboplatin and vincristine for recurrent and newly diagnosed low-grade gliomas of childhood. J Clin Oncol 1993;11(5):850–856
85. Packer RJ, Sutton LN, Bilaniuk LT, et al. Treatment of chiasmatic/hypothalamic gliomas of childhood with chemotherapy: an update. Ann Neurol 1988;23(1):79–85
86. Mahoney DH Jr, Cohen ME, Friedman HS, et al. Carboplatin is effective therapy for young children with progressive optic pathway tumors: a Pediatric Oncology Group phase II study. Neuro-oncol 2000;2(4):213–220
87. Ater J, Holmes E, Zhou T, et al. Results of COG Protocol A9952: a randomized phase 3 study of two chemotherapy regimens for incompletely resected low-grade glioma in young children. In: Abstracts from the Thirteenth International Symposium on Pediatric Neuro-Oncology; June 29-July 2, 2008; Chicago, IL (p 451)
88. Petronio J, Edwards MS, Prados M, et al. Management of chiasmal and hypothalamic gliomas of infancy and childhood with chemotherapy. J Neurosurg 1991;74(5):701–708
89. Gajjar A, Sanford RA, Heideman R, et al; Jude Children's Research Hospital. Low-grade astrocytoma: a decade of experience at St. J Clin Oncol 1997;15(8):2792–2799
90. Schomas D, Laack N, Schomberg P, Brown P. Pathologically diagnosed optic low-grade gliomas in children: long-term follow-up of the Mayo Clinic experience. In: Abstracts from the Thirteenth International Symposium on Pediatric Neuro-Oncology; June 29-July 2, 2008; Chicago, IL (p 449)
91. Janss AJ, Grundy R, Cnaan A, et al. Optic pathway and hypothalamic/chiasmatic gliomas in children younger than age 5 years with a 6-year follow-up. Cancer 1995;75(4):1051–1059
92. Davis F. Primary tumors of the optic nerve (a phenomenon of Recklinghausen's disease). Arch Ophthal 1940;23:735–821
93. Stern J, DiGiacinto GV, Housepian EM. Neurofibromatosis and optic glioma: clinical and morphological correlations. Neurosurgery 1979;4(6):524–528
94. Gottschalk S, Tavakolian R, Buske A, Tinschert S, Lehmann R. Spontaneous remission of chiasmatic/hypothalamic masses in neurofibromatosis type 1: report of two cases. Neuroradiology 1999;41(3):199–201
95. Parsa CF, Hoyt CS, Lesser RL, et al. Spontaneous regression of optic gliomas: thirteen cases documented by serial neuroimaging. Arch Ophthalmol 2001;119(4):516–529
96. Sharif S, Ferner R, Birch JM, et al. Second primary tumors in neurofibromatosis 1 patients treated for optic glioma: substantial risks after radiotherapy. J Clin Oncol 2006;24(16):2570–2575
97. Desai SS, Paulino AC, Mai WY, Teh BS. Radiation-induced moyamoya syndrome. Int J Radiat Oncol Biol Phys 2006;65(4):1222–1227
98. Kestle JR, Hoffman HJ, Mock AR. Moyamoya phenomenon after radiation for optic glioma. J Neurosurg 1993;79(1):32–35
99. Marcus KJ, Goumnerova L, Billett AL, et al. Stereotactic radiotherapy for localized low-grade gliomas in children: final results of a prospective trial. Int J Radiat Oncol Biol Phys 2005;61(2): 374–379
100. Jennings MT, Gelman R, Hochberg F. Intracranial germ-cell tumors: natural history and pathogenesis. J Neurosurg 1985;63(2): 155–167
101. Glenn OA, Barkovich AJ. Intracranial germ cell tumors: a comprehensive review of proposed embryologic derivation. Pediatr Neurosurg 1996;24(5):242–251
102. Rich TA, Cassady JR, Strand RD, Winston KR. Radiation therapy for pineal and suprasellar germ cell tumors. Cancer 1985;55(5):932–940
103. Melmed S. The Pituitary. 2nd ed. Blackwell; 2002
104. Wolden SL, Wara WM, Larson DA, Prados MD, Edwards MS, Sneed PK. Radiation therapy for primary intracranial germ-cell tumors. Int J Radiat Oncol Biol Phys 1995;32(4):943–949
105. Spiegler BJ, Bouffet E, Greenberg ML, Rutka JT, Mabbott DJ. Change in neurocognitive functioning after treatment with cranial radiation in childhood. J Clin Oncol 2004;22(4):706–713
106. Rogers SJ, Mosleh-Shirazi MA, Saran FH. Radiotherapy of localised intracranial germinoma: time to sever historical ties? Lancet Oncol 2005;6(7):509–519
107. Bamberg M, Kortmann RD, Calaminus G, et al. Radiation therapy for intracranial germinoma: results of the German cooperative prospective trials MAKEI 83/86/89. J Clin Oncol 1999; 17(8):2585–2592

108. Shirato H, Nishio M, Sawamura Y, et al. Analysis of long-term treatment of intracranial germinoma. Int J Radiat Oncol Biol Phys 1997;37(3):511–515
109. Hardenbergh PH, Golden J, Billet A, et al. Intracranial germinoma: the case for lower dose radiation therapy. Int J Radiat Oncol Biol Phys 1997;39(2):419–426
110. Matsutani M; Japanese Pediatric Brain Tumor Study Group. Combined chemotherapy and radiation therapy for CNS germ cell tumors—the Japanese experience. J Neurooncol 2001;54(3):311–316
111. Fuller BG, Kapp DS, Cox R. Radiation therapy of pineal region tumors: 25 new cases and a review of 208 previously reported cases. Int J Radiat Oncol Biol Phys 1994;28(1):229–245
112. Robertson PL, DaRosso RC, Allen JC. Improved prognosis of intracranial non-germinoma germ cell tumors with multimodality therapy. J Neurooncol 1997;32(1):71–80
113. Calaminus G, Bamberg M, Harms D, et al. AFP/beta-HCG secreting CNS germ cell tumors: long-term outcome with respect to initial symptoms and primary tumor resection. Results of the cooperative trial MAKEI 89. Neuropediatrics 2005;36(2):71–77
114. Kretschmar C, Kleinberg L, Greenberg M, Burger P, Holmes E, Wharam M. Pre-radiation chemotherapy with response-based radiation therapy in children with central nervous system germ cell tumors: a report from the Children's Oncology Group. Pediatr Blood Cancer 2007;48(3):285–291
115. Sano K. Pathogenesis of intracranial germ cell tumors reconsidered. J Neurosurg 1999;90(2):258–264
116. MacDonald SM, Trofimov A, Safai S, et al. Proton radiotherapy for pediatric central nervous system germ cell tumors: early clinical outcomes. Int J Radiat Oncol Biol Phys 2011;79(1):121–129
117. Dahlin DC, Unni KK. Bone Tumors: General Aspects and Data on 8,542 Cases. 4th ed. Charles C. Thomas Publisher; 1986
118. Forsyth PA, Cascino TL, Shaw EG, et al. Intracranial chordomas: a clinicopathological and prognostic study of 51 cases. J Neurosurg 1993;78(5):741–747
119. Rich TA, Schiller A, Suit HD, Mankin HJ. Clinical and pathologic review of 48 cases of chordoma. Cancer 1985;56(1):182–187
120. Kunanandam V, Gooding MR. Parasellar chondrosarcoma: total excision improves prognosis. Br J Neurosurg 1995;9(1):87–91
121. Berson AM, Castro JR, Petti P, et al. Charged particle irradiation of chordoma and chondrosarcoma of the base of skull and cervical spine: the Lawrence Berkeley Laboratory experience. Int J Radiat Oncol Biol Phys 1988;15(3):559–565
122. Hug EB, Loredo LN, Slater JD, et al. Proton radiation therapy for chordomas and chondrosarcomas of the skull base. J Neurosurg 1999;91(3):432–439
123. Heffelfinger MJ, Dahlin DC, MacCarty CS, Beabout JW. Chordomas and cartilaginous tumors at the skull base. Cancer 1973;32(2):410–420
124. Fagundes MA, Hug EB, Liebsch NJ, Daly W, Efird J, Munzenrider JE. Radiation therapy for chordomas of the base of skull and cervical spine: patterns of failure and outcome after relapse. Int J Radiat Oncol Biol Phys 1995;33(3):579–584
125. Catton C, O'Sullivan B, Bell R, et al. Chordoma: long-term follow-up after radical photon irradiation. Radiother Oncol 1996 ;41(1):67–72
126. Saxton JP. Chordoma. Int J Radiat Oncol Biol Phys 1981;7(7): 913–915
127. Zorlu F, Gürkaynak M, Yildiz F, Oge K, Atahan IL. Conventional external radiotherapy in the management of clivus chordomas with overt residual disease. Neurol Sci 2000;21(4):203–207
128. Terahara A, Niemierko A, Goitein M, et al. Analysis of the relationship between tumor dose inhomogeneity and local control in patients with skull base chordoma. Int J Radiat Oncol Biol Phys 1999;45(2):351–358
129. Munzenrider JE, Liebsch NJ. Proton therapy for tumors of the skull base. Strahlenther Onkol 1999;175(Suppl 2):57–63
130. Debus J, Schulz-Ertner D, Schad L, et al. Stereotactic fractionated radiotherapy for chordomas and chondrosarcomas of the skull base. Int J Radiat Oncol Biol Phys 2000;47(3):591–596
131. Santoni R, Liebsch N, Finkelstein DM, et al. Temporal lobe (TL) damage following surgery and high-dose photon and proton irradiation in 96 patients affected by chordomas and chondrosarcomas of the base of the skull. Int J Radiat Oncol Biol Phys 1998;41(1):59–68
132. Ragel BT, Couldwell WT. Pituitary carcinoma: a review of the literature. Neurosurg Focus 2004;16(4):E7
133. Kaltsas GA, Nomikos P, Kontogeorgos G, Buchfelder M, Grossman AB. Clinical review: Diagnosis and management of pituitary carcinomas. J Clin Endocrinol Metab 2005;90(5):3089–3099
134. Pernicone PJ, Scheithauer BW, Sebo TJ, et al. Pituitary carcinoma: a clinicopathologic study of 15 cases. Cancer 1997;79(4):804–812
135. Landman RE, Horwith M, Peterson RE, Khandji AG, Wardlaw SL. Long-term survival with ACTH-secreting carcinoma of the pituitary: a case report and review of the literature. J Clin Endocrinol Metab 2002;87(7):3084–3089
136. Abrams HL, Spiro R, Goldstein N. Metastases in carcinoma; analysis of 1000 autopsied cases. Cancer 1950;3(1):74–85
137. Kovacs K. Metastatic cancer of the pituitary gland. Oncology 1973;27(6):533–542
138. Max MB, Deck MD, Rottenberg DA. Pituitary metastasis: incidence in cancer patients and clinical differentiation from pituitary adenoma. Neurology 1981;31(8):998–1002
139. Morita A, Meyer FB, Laws ER Jr. Symptomatic pituitary metastases. J Neurosurg 1998;89(1):69–73
140. Teears RJ, Silverman EM. Clinicopathologic review of 88 cases of carcinoma metastatic to the putuitary gland. Cancer 1975;36(1): 216–220
141. Fassett DR, Couldwell WT. Metastases to the pituitary gland. Neurosurg Focus 2004;16(4):E8
142. Kano H, Niranjan A, Kondziolka D, Flickinger JC, Lunsford LD. Stereotactic radiosurgery for pituitary metastases. Surg Neurol 2009;72(3):248–255, discussion 255–256
143. Höybye C, Grenbäck E, Rähn T, Degerblad M, Thorén M, Hulting AL. Adrenocorticotropic hormone-producing pituitary tumors: 12- to 22-year follow-up after treatment with stereotactic radiosurgery. Neurosurgery 2001;49(2):284–291, discussion 291–292
144. Vladyka V, Liscák R, Novotný J Jr, Marek J, Jezková J. Radiation tolerance of functioning pituitary tissue in gamma knife surgery for pituitary adenomas. Neurosurgery 2003;52(2):309–316, discussion 316–317
145. Feigl GC, Bonelli CM, Berghold A, Mokry M. Effects of gamma knife radiosurgery of pituitary adenomas on pituitary function. J Neurosurg 2002;97(5, Suppl):415–421
146. Pai HH, Thornton A, Katznelson L, et al. Hypothalamic/pituitary function following high-dose conformal radiotherapy to the base of skull: demonstration of a dose-effect relationship using dose-volume histogram analysis. Int J Radiat Oncol Biol Phys 2001;49(4):1079–1092
147. Becker G, Kocher M, Kortmann RD, et al. Radiation therapy in the multimodal treatment approach of pituitary adenoma. Strahlenther Onkol 2002;178(4):173–186
148. Brada M, Rajan B, Traish D, et al. The long-term efficacy of conservative surgery and radiotherapy in the control of pituitary adenomas. Clin Endocrinol (Oxf) 1993;38(6):571–578
149. Tsang RW, Laperriere NJ, Simpson WJ, Brierley J, Panzarella T, Smyth HS. Glioma arising after radiation therapy for pituitary adenoma. A report of four patients and estimation of risk. Cancer 1993;72(7):2227–2233
150. Brada M, Burchell L, Ashley S, Traish D. The incidence of cerebrovascular accidents in patients with pituitary adenoma. Int J Radiat Oncol Biol Phys 1999;45(3):693–698
151. Flickinger JC, Torres C, Deutsch M. Management of low-grade gliomas of the optic nerve and chiasm. Cancer 1988;61(4):635–642
152. Kovalic JJ, Grigsby PW, Shepard MJ, Fineberg BB, Thomas PR. Radiation therapy for gliomas of the optic nerve and chiasm. Int J Radiat Oncol Biol Phys 1990;18(4):927–932
153. Jenkin D, Angyalfi S, Becker L, et al. Optic glioma in children: surveillance, resection, or irradiation? Int J Radiat Oncol Biol Phys 1993;25(2):215–225
154. Tao ML, Barnes PD, Billett AL, et al. Childhood optic chiasm gliomas: radiographic response following radiotherapy and long-term clinical outcome. Int J Radiat Oncol Biol Phys 1997;39(3): 579–587
155. Haddock MG, Schild SE, Scheithauer BW, Schomberg PJ. Radiation therapy for histologically confirmed primary central nervous system germinoma. Int J Radiat Oncol Biol Phys 1997;38(5):915–923

156. Cho J, Choi JU, Kim DS, Suh CO. Low-dose craniospinal irradiation as a definitive treatment for intracranial germinoma. Radiother Oncol 2009;91(1):75–79

157. Tai PT, Craighead P, Bagdon F. Optimization of radiotherapy for patients with cranial chordoma. A review of dose-response ratios for photon techniques. Cancer 1995;75(3):749–756

158. Hug EB, Slater JD. Proton radiation therapy for chordomas and chondrosarcomas of the skull base. Neurosurg Clin N Am 2000;11(4):627–638

159. Weber DC, Rutz HP, Pedroni ES, et al. Results of spot-scanning proton radiation therapy for chordoma and chondrosarcoma of the skull base: the Paul Scherrer Institut experience. Int J Radiat Oncol Biol Phys 2005;63(2):401–409

160. Noël G, Feuvret L, Calugaru V, et al. Chordomas of the base of the skull and upper cervical spine. One hundred patients irradiated by a 3D conformal technique combining photon and proton beams. Acta Oncol 2005;44(7):700–708

161. Habrand JL, Schneider R, Alapetite C, et al. Proton therapy in pediatric skull base and cervical canal low-grade bone malignancies. Int J Radiat Oncol Biol Phys 2008;71(3):672–675

162. Schulte RW, Kim D, Loredo LN, Slater JM, Slater JD. Proton Therapy for Chondrosarcomas of the Skull Base and Cervical Spine: Long-term Experience at Loma Linda University Medical Center. Int J Radiat Oncol Biol Phys 2008;72:S119

163. Krishnan S, Foote RL, Brown PD, Pollock BE, Link MJ, Garces YI. Radiosurgery for cranial base chordomas and chondrosarcomas. Neurosurgery 2005;56(4):777–784, discussion 777–784

164. Martin JJ, Niranjan A, Kondziolka D, Flickinger JC, Lozanne KA, Lunsford LD. Radiosurgery for chordomas and chondrosarcomas of the skull base. J Neurosurg 2007;107(4):758–764

165. Chang SD, Martin DP, Lee E, Adler JR Jr. Stereotactic radiosurgery and hypofractionated stereotactic radiotherapy for residual or recurrent cranial base and cervical chordomas. Neurosurg Focus 2001;10(3):E5

166. Gwak HS, Yoo HJ, Youn SM, et al. Hypofractionated stereotactic radiation therapy for skull base and upper cervical chordoma and chondrosarcoma: preliminary results. Stereotact Funct Neurosurg 2005;83(5-6):233–243

167. Schulz-Ertner D, Nikoghosyan A, Hof H, et al. Carbon ion radiotherapy of skull base chondrosarcomas. Int J Radiat Oncol Biol Phys 2007;67(1):171–177

168. Schulz-Ertner D, Karger CP, Feuerhake A, et al. Effectiveness of carbon ion radiotherapy in the treatment of skull-base chordomas. Int J Radiat Oncol Biol Phys 2007;68(2):449–457

14 Stereotactic Radiosurgery

Ricky Medel, Brian Williams, and Jason P. Sheehan

Tumors in and around the sella turcica represent some of the most challenging clinical entities that clinicians have dealt with over the past century. Nearly 100 years after Harvey Cushing's landmark work, *The Pituitary Body and Its Disorders: Clinical States Produced by Disorders of the Hypophysis Cerebri*,[1] pituitary adenomas, meningiomas, and other, rarer tumors of the parasellar and sellar region remain difficult to cure with microsurgical techniques alone. In fact, Harvey Cushing recognized the difficulties of conventional surgical approaches for treating intracranial tumors. Cushing and colleagues used a device called a radium bomb to deliver single-session, focused radiation to intracranial tumors.[2,3] At the time, the understanding of radiobiology and dosimetry was rather simplistic. Nevertheless, Cushing recognized the need for neurosurgeons to use radiation as an adjunct to the scalpel for treating intracranial tumors.

In 1951, stereotactic radiosurgery (SRS) was described by Lars Leksell as the "closed skull destruction of an intracranial target using ionizing radiation."[4] Leksell treated the first patient with a pituitary adenoma to undergo surgery with the gamma knife in 1968. Since that time, SRS has been used to treat thousands of patients with sellar and parasellar tumors. Radiosurgery can be used as an upfront treatment or to achieve control of recurrent or residual tumor.

Great attention and effort in the field of SRS have been placed on the preservation of surrounding neuronal, vascular, and hormonal structures. Refinement of the radiosurgical technique for parasellar and sellar tumors has been achieved through advances in radiobiology, neuroimaging, medical physics, and engineering. In this chapter, we review the role of SRS for the two most commonly treated tumors types in the parasellar and sellar region: pituitary adenomas and meningiomas.

◆ Radiosurgical Devices and Techniques

SRS involves focusing a high dose of radiation to the tumor while sparing surrounding structures significant doses of radiation. Radiosurgery is usually delivered in a single session but may be delivered in up to five sessions.[5] It uses a steep falloff of the radiation dose to the surrounding tissues. Patients are immobilized with rigid frames fixed to the skull or other immobilization devices (eg, aquaplast masks or bite blocks). Radiosurgery is image-guided and generally achieves submillimeter accuracy. Integrated imaging may be used to further track and compensate for potential sources of error.

There are several types of radiosurgical delivery devices, including the gamma knife, modified linear accelerators (LINACs), and proton beam units. Single-session radiosurgical doses for nonfunctioning adenomas are typically 12 to 18 Gy, and 15 to 30 Gy for functioning adenomas. Radiosurgical doses for World Health Organization (WHO) grade 1 meningiomas are typically 12 to 18 Gy. For multisession radiosurgery, these doses may be divided into two to five sessions or fractions.

Gamma knife radiosurgery involves the use of multiple isocenters of varying beam diameters to achieve a dose plan that conforms to irregular three-dimensional volumes. The number of isocenters varies based upon the size, shape, and location of the adenoma. In the current version of the gamma knife, each isocenter is comprised of eight independent sectors. Beam diameters for the current Gamma Knife Perfexion unit vary from zero (ie, blocked) to 16 mm in diameter.

Linear accelerator (LINAC)–based radiosurgery (eg, CyberKnife, Novalis Tx, Trilogy, Axesse) uses multiple radiation arcs to crossfire photon beams at a target.[6] Most systems use nondynamic techniques in which the arc is moved around its radius to deliver radiation that enters from many different vantage points. Technical improvements with LINAC-based radiosurgery include beam shaping, intensity modulation, minileaf collimation, and onboard computed tomography or fluoroscopic imaging.

Proton therapy is a method of external beam radiotherapy; it has been adapted as a radiosurgical tool for intracranial pathology. It takes advantage of the inherent superior dose distribution of protons compared with photons that is a consequence of the Bragg peak phenomenon.[7] Currently, there are a few centers where this treatment is available in the United States and abroad. The number of such centers is likely to increase in the coming years as compact proton units are developed and proton beam technology is applied to more types of intracranial and extracranial disease.

◆ Radiosurgery for Pituitary Adenomas

Pituitary adenomas are the most common intrasellar neoplasms and are found in 10 to 27% of the general population.[8,9] Microadenomas (<1 cm) may be discovered incidentally during magnetic resonance imaging (MRI) or may be diagnosed when a patient has symptoms of hormone hypersecretion. Macroadenomas may be diagnosed as a result of mass effect inducing hypopituitarism, elevation in prolactin, or a neurologic deficit (eg, cranial nerve dysfunction). The distribution of functioning and nonfunctioning microadenomas is equal. Among macroadenomas, nonfunctioning lesions occur with greater frequency (~80%).[8] Patients with pituitary adenomas often present with headache (40–60%), visual disturbance, hypopituitarism, or, less frequently, apoplexy.[8,9] Surgical intervention is currently the mainstay of treatment for nearly all lesions except prolactinomas. Patients with large or invasive lesions often require additional therapeutic modalities, and radiosurgery is an important part of their treatment.[9]

Nonfunctioning Pituitary Adenomas

Growth control following microsurgical resection will be achieved in 50 to 80% of patients with macroadenomas.[10] Radiosurgery provides an excellent therapeutic option for those with continued growth or evidence of recurrence. Worldwide, more than 11,000 patients have been treated, with the published literature supporting effective control of tumor growth and low rates of complications.[10]

Twenty-seven series were identified comprising 1009 patients with nonfunctioning adenomas[10–35] (**Table 14.1**). Follow-up (mean/median) ranged from 16.2 to 64 months, with an average rate of growth control of 96.8% (range, 92.2–100%; **Fig. 14.1**). The dose given to the tumor margin ranged from 12.3 to 26.9 gray (Gy). Neurologic deficits were uncommon (average, 4.0%; range, 0–17.6%), as was hypopitutarism (average, 6.4%; range, 0–40%). Pollock et al,[29] in their series of 62 patients, reported a rate of 27% experiencing new anterior pituitary deficiencies. There was no substantial difference in the dosimetry between those with and without hypopituitarism after radiosurgery; a median margin dose of 16 Gy was used in that series. However, they did demonstrate a significant relationship with the volume of the lesion treated; patients with a tumor volume of 4.0 cm^3 or less had a 5-year risk for developing a new hormonal deficit of 18%, whereas those with lesions larger than 4.0 cm^3 had a 5-year risk of 58% ($P = 0.02$). At our institution, we reported 90% tumor control in a series of 100 patients with nonfunctioning pituitary adenomas.[22] Tumor control was reduced when the margin dose to the tumor was less than 12 Gy. These data provide a basis upon which to provide patients with advice regarding the risks of intervention.

Secretory Pituitary Adenomas

Cushing Syndrome

In 80% of cases, endogenous Cushing syndrome results from hypersecretion of adrenocorticotropic hormone (ACTH), usually secondary to a pituitary corticotrope adenoma.[36] Although surgical resection remains the primary treatment for ACTH-secreting pituitary adenomas, invasion of the surrounding dura and/or cavernous sinus or the presence of a lesion undetectable on MRI makes surgical cure improbable. In these situations, radiosurgery serves as an invaluable adjunctive modality. What defines "cure" in Cushing syndrome remains the subject of some controversy. In 2003, the Endocrine Society published a consensus statement regarding the diagnosis and treatment of this disease, including the criteria for establishing biochemical remission or cure.[37] The guidelines were updated in 2008, and both versions suggest the use of morning postoperative serum cortisol levels.[36] Very low levels, less than 2 mcg/dL, predict a low rate of recurrence (~10% in 10 years). Most series use either mean serum free corti-

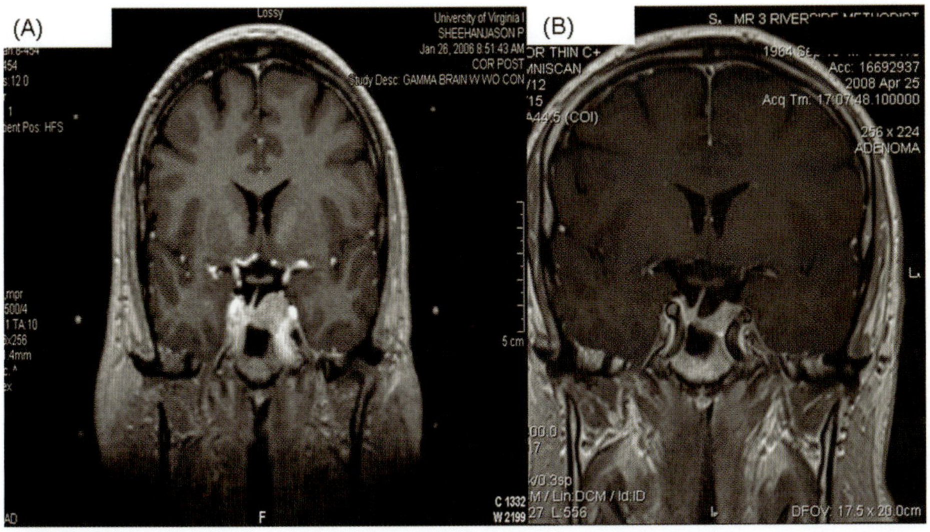

Fig. 14.1 A 41-year-old man who presented with a recurrent, nonfunctioning pituitary adenoma. **(A)** The patient underwent stereotactic radiosurgery in which 15 Gy was delivered to the tumor margin. **(B)** One and one-half years later, the pituitary adenoma has decreased substantially in size.

Table 14.1 Summary of the Literature Review for the Radiosurgical Management of Nonfunctioning Pituitary Adenomas

Year	Authors	Patients (N)	Mean/median follow-up (mo)	Mean/median margin dose (Gy)	Growth control (%) (1)	Neurologic deficit (%)†	Hypopituitarism (%)
1998	Lim et al	22	25.5*	25.4*	92.5*	1.7*	0
1998	Martinez et al	14	36*	15.8	100	3.4*	0
1998	Mitsumori et al	7	47*	NR	100	11.1	22.9
1998	Witt et al	24	32*	19.2*	94*	5.6*	0
1998	Yoon et al	8	49.2*	NR	96	0	29.2*
1998	Pan et al	17	29*	15.8	94.1	17.6	NR
1999	Hayashi et al	18	16.2*	22.5*	94.6	5.6	0
1999	Inoue et al	18	>24	20.2*	94.3*	0	NR
1999	Mokry et al	31	20.7	13.8	96.8	0	6.5
2000	Izawa et al	23	30.1	19.5	95.6	8.7	0
2000	Shin et al	3	18.7	16	100	6.3*	0
2002	Feigl et al	61	55.2*	15*	94*	NR	40*
2002	Sheehan et al	42	31.2	16	97.6	4.8	0
2002	Wowra and Stummer	30	57.7	16	93.3	0	10
2003	Muramatsu et al	8	30*	26.9	100	12.5	0
2003	Petrovich et al	52	34*	15*	100	3*	NR
2004	Losa et al	54	41.1	16.6	96.3	0	9.3
2004	Muacevic et al	51	21.7	16.5	95	0	3.9
2005	Kajiwara et al	14	32.1	12.6	92.9	7.1	7.1
2005	Picozzi et al	51	40.6	16.5	96.1	NR	NR
2005	Iwai et al	28	36.4	12.3	93	0	7
2006	Mingione et al	100	46.4	18.5	92.2	0	25
2006	Voges et al	37	56.6	13.4	100	4.2*	12.3*
2007	Liscák et al	140	60	20	100	0	1.4
2008	Pollock et al	62	64	16	96.8	1.6	27
2009	Hoybye and Rahn	23	78/97 (2)	20	100	4.3	0
2009	Kobayashi	71	50.2*		96.7	2.8	8.2
Total/Average		1009			96.8	4.0	6.4

(1) Classified as unchanged or reduced in size.
(2) Median duration of follow-up was 78 months for radiographic and 97 months for clinical follow-up.
* Data not available for separate group, only the cohort as a whole.
† Does not include asymptomatic diagnosis of radiation necrosis.

sol (5.4–10.8 mcg/dL), midnight salivary cortisol (normal, <4.2 nmol/L), or a urinary free cortisol (UFC) within the normal range. Nevertheless, there is significant variability in the exact testing and levels used to define biochemical remission.

A review of the radiosurgical literature revealed 36 studies comprising 671 patients with Cushing disease treated with radiosurgery, in most cases as an adjunct to operative resection[11–16,18,21,23,24,27,31–33,38–59] (**Table 14.2**). Most used 24-hour UFC or serum cortisol to assess remission. However, the criteria for defining remission were not reported for all series. The average rate of endocrine remission was 54.6%, with a range from 0 to 100% over a follow-up period (mean/median) from 16.2 to 94 months. In our experience, endocrine remission of Cushing disease was achieved on average ~12 months after SRS.[45] The rates of new neurologic deficit, including visual deterioration, were low (average, 2.5%), with some form of new anterior pituitary deficiency occurring in 23% of patients (range, 0–68.8%). Emphasizing the importance of long-term follow-up, late recurrence was also demonstrated in several series, with rates as high as 20%.[45,56]

Nelson Syndrome

In some patients, Cushing syndrome remains refractory to surgical resection and radiation therapy of pituitary lesion. In these patients, bilateral adrenalectomy remains a therapeutic option to induce remission of hypercorti-

Table 14.2 Summary of the Literature Review for the Radiosurgical Management of Cushing Syndrome

Year	Authors	Patients (N)	Mean/median margin dose (Gy)	Mean/median follow-up (mo)	Biochemical remission (%)‡	Neurologic deficit (%)†	Hypopituitarism (%)
1986	Degerbald et al	29	NR	> 36	76	0	41.4
1991	Levy et al	64	NR	NR	NR	4.8	33*
1993	Ganz et al	4	25	> 18*	50	NR	NR
1995	Seo et al	2	27.5	26.5	100	0	0
1998	Lim et al	4	25.4*	25.5*	25	1.7*	0
1998	Martinez et al	3	24	36*	66.7	3.4*	33.3
1998	Mitsumori et al	5	NR	47*	40	11.1*	22.9*
1998	Morange-Ramos et al	6	33.2	20*	66.6	16.7	16.7
1998	Pan et al	4	27.5	29*	100	0	NR
1998	Witt et al	25	19.2*	32*	52	5.6*	0
1999	Hayashi et al	10	22.5*	16.2*	10	0	0
1999	Inoue et al	3	20.2*	> 24	100	0	NR
1999	Mokry et al	5	17	56.3	33.3	0	40
1999	SH Kim et al	8	28.7*	26.9*	62.5	0	0
2000	Izawa et al	12	23.8*	26.4*	16.7	0	0
2000	Sheehan et al	43	20	39.1	63	2.3	16
2000	Shin et al	7	32.3	88.2	50	6.3*	16.7
2001	Hoybye et al	18	NR	16.8	44	0	68.8
2002	Feigl et al	4	15*	55.2*	60*	NR	40*
2002	Kobayashi et al	20	28.7	64	23.3	NR	NR
2002	Laws et al	40	20	NR	74	2.5	24
2002	Pollock et al	9	20	42.4*	78	22.2	16*
2003	Choi et al	7	28.5*	42.5*	55.6	0	0
2003	Petrovich et al	3	15*	34*	NR	3*	NR
2003	Wong et al	5	NR	38	100	0	20
2003	Witt	8	24*	24*	0	0	NR
2005	Devin et al	35	14.7	42	49	0	40
2006	Voges et al	17	16.4	58.7	52.9	4.2*	12.3*
2007	Castinetti et al	40	29.5	54.7	42.5	5	15
2007	Jagannathan et al	90	23	45	54	5	22
2007	Kajiwara et al	2	26	38.5	50	0	50
2007	Petit et al	33	20	62	52	0	52
2008	Pollock et al (1)	8	20	73	87	0	36*
2008	Tinnel et al	12	25	37	50	0	50
2009	Castinetti et al	18	28	94	50	5.3*	21*
2009	Wan et al	68	23	67.3	27.9	2.9	1.7*
Total/Average		671			54.6	2.5	23.0

(1) Contains patients included in the 2002 cohort by Pollock et al.
* Data not available for separate group, only the cohort as a whole.
† Does not include asymptomatic diagnosis of radiation necrosis.
‡ Percentage refers to all patients with remission, including those who subsequently experienced recurrence.

solemia. Although this procedure is effective, Nelson syndrome is a well-described complication, occurring in up to 23% of patients.[60] Characterized by elevated ACTH levels, hyperpigmentation, and progressive and often invasive tumors, this syndrome presents a therapeutic challenge of its own.

As opposed to the literature regarding the radiosurgical treatment of other pituitary adenomas, that for the use of radiosurgery in Nelson syndrome is fairly sparse. Ten series encompassing 94 patients have been published[32,43,47,49,61–66] (**Table 14.3**). Over an average follow-up period (mean/median) ranging from 18 to 84 months, normalization of ACTH occurred in only 24.3%; however, a significant reduction in hormone levels was more frequent. Control of tumor growth was achieved in the majority of cases (range, 82–100%). Overall, the paucity of literature prevents strong conclusions from being drawn, but it appears as if good tumor control with a reduction in ACTH levels is achievable with radiosurgery for patients with Nelson syndrome.

Acromegaly

Acromegaly occurs with a prevalence of ~60 per million and has significant associated morbidity and mortality (hypertension, diabetes, cardiomyopathy, and sleep apnea), with a standardized mortality ratio of 1.48.[67] Surgical resection is widely considered to be the first-line therapy; however, like patients with Cushing disease, those with invasion of surrounding structures (eg, the dura or the cavernous sinus) are unlikely to be cured. Although there exists some variation in the definition of biochemical cure, most consider a growth hormone (GH) level below 2.0 ng/mL to be appropriate because it has been associated with a reversal of the morbidity and mortality of the disease.[68] This GH level should occur with an insulin-like growth factor (IGF-1) level that is within the normal range for age and gender.

Forty-one series have been published comprising 1596 patients with acromegaly over a follow-up period (mean/median) ranging from 16.2 to 102 months[11–16,18,21,24,26,27,31–33,40,43,46,49,50,52,53,56–58,66,69–81] (**Table 14.4**). The rates of endocrine remission ranged from 0 to 100% (average, 43.8%). Several factors contributed to this considerable variation, including variation in the definition of remission, use of somatostatin analogues both during treatment and follow-up, and differences in treatment parameters. Radiosurgery was associated with a low incidence of adverse effects, with a reported 1.5% of patients developing new neurologic deficits, primarily changes in visual acuity or extraocular motility. Additionally, an average of 9.8% of patients developed some form of pituitary dysfunction following SRS. Of note, radiosurgically induced endocrine remission appears to occur later than in Cushing disease. Our center observed a mean time to endocrine remission of ~24 months after radiosurgery, compared with 12 months for a similarly treated cohort of patients with Cushing disease.[82] This and similar findings of a differential response of secretory pituitary adenomas to radiosurgery warrant further investigation in terms of the underlying radiobiology and ways to augment the effects of radiosurgery on more resistant types of secretory pituitary adenomas.[52]

Prolactinoma

Prolactinomas are the most common secretory pituitary adenomas and account for 44% of all pituitary microadenomas in autopsy series.[83] Unlike with other adenomas, observation is within the management paradigm, and when treatment is indicated, medical therapy remains the first-

Table 14.3 Summary of the Literature Review for the Radiosurgical Management of Nelson Syndrome

Year	Authors	Patients (N)	Mean/median follow-up (mo)	Mean/median margin dose (Gy)	Biochemical remission (%)‡	Growth control (%)
1991	Levy et al	17	NR	NR	NR	94
1993	Ganz et al	3	> 18*	NR	0	100
1998	Wolffenbuttel et al	1	33	12	0	100
1999	Laws et al	9	NR	NR	11	NR
2002	Pollock and Young	11	37	20	36.4	82
2002	Kobayashi et al	6	63	28.7	33	100
2006	Voges et al	9	63.1	15.3*	11.1	100
2007	Mauermann et al	23	20/50 (1)	25	17	91
2007	Petit et al	5	62	20	100	100
2009	Vik-Mo et al	10	84	26.2	10	100
Total/Average		94			24.3	96.3

(1) Median duration of follow-up was 20 months for radiographic and 50 months for endocrine follow-up.
* Data not available for separate group, only the cohort as a whole.
‡ Percentage refers to all patients with remission, including those who subsequently experienced recurrence.

Table 14.4 Summary of the Literature Review for the Radiosurgical Management of Acromegaly

Year	Authors	Patients (N)	Mean/median follow-up (mo)	Mean/median margin dose (Gy)	Biochemical remission (%)‡	Neurologic deficit (%)†	Hypopituitarism (%)
1991	Levy et al	318	NR	NR	NR	2.8	33*
1991	Thoren et al	21	64.4	NR	9.5	0	23.8
1993	Ganz et al	4	> 18*	20	25	NR	NR
1998	Landolt et al	16	16.8	25	68.8	0	0
1998	Lim et al	16	25.5*	25.4*	37.5	1.7*	6.3
1998	Martinez et al	7	36*	24.7	85.7	3.4*	0
1998	Morange-Ramos et al	15	20*	28.7	20	6.7	13.3
1998	Pan et al	15	29*	28.6	100	0	NR
1998	Witt et al	20	32*	19.2*	72	5.6*	0
1999	Hayashi et al	22	16.2*	22.5*	40.9	0	0
1999	Inoue et al	12	> 24	20.2*	58.3	0	NR
1999	Laws et al	56	NR	NR	25	NR	NR
1999	Mokry et al	16	45.9	16	31	0	18.8
1999	SHKim et al	11	26.9*	28.7	45.5	0	0
2000	Izawa et al	29	26.4*	23.8*	41.4	0	0
2000	Shin et al	6	42.7	34.4	66.7	6.3*	0
2000	Zhang et al	68	34	31.3	36.8 (3)	2.9	0
2001	Fukuoka et al	9	42	20	50	0	0
2001	Ikeda et al	17	55.8	25	82	0	0
2002	Feigl et al	9	55.2*	15*	60*	NR	40*
2002	Pollock et al	26	42.4*	20	42	0	16*
2003	Attanasio et al	30	46	20	23	0	6.6
2003	Choi et al	9	42.5*	28.5*	50	0	0
2003	Muramatsu et al	4	30*	27.5	50	0	0
2003	Petrovich et al	5	34*	15*	NR	3*	NR
2003	Witt	4	24*	24*	25	0	NR
2005	Castinetti et al	82	49.5	25	17	0	17.1
2005	Gutt et al	44	22.8	18	47.7	0	NR
2005	Kajiwara et al	2	53.5	13.5	0	0	0
2005	Kobayashi et al	67	63.3	18.9	4.8	11.1	14.6 (1)
2006	Jezkova et al	96	53.7	35	50	0	26
2006	Voges et al	64	54.3	16.5	37.5	4.2*	12.3*
2007	Pollock et al	46	63	20	50	2.2	33
2007	Roberts et al	9	25.4	21	44.4	0	33.3
2007	Vik-Mo et al	61	66	26.5	17	3.3	13.1
2008	Jagannathan et al	95	57	22	53	4.2	34
2008	Losa et al	83	69	21.5	60.2	0	8.5
2008	Pollock et al (2)	27	46.9	20	67	0	36*
2008	Tinnel et al	9	35	25	44.4	11	22
2009	Castinetti et al	43	102	24	42	5.3*	21*
2009	Wan et al	103	67.3*	21.4	36.9	1	1.7*
Total/Average		1596			43.8	1.5	9.8

(1) Includes one mortality secondary to hypopituitarism.
(2) Contains patients included in the 2002 cohort by Pollock et al.
(3) Of the 26 patients followed for longer than 36 months, 25 had normalization of their growth hormone levels.
* Data not available for separate group, only the cohort as a whole.
† Does not include asymptomatic diagnosis of radiation necrosis.
‡ Percentage refers to all patients with remission, including those who subsequently experienced recurrence.

line choice for most patients with prolactinomas. Concerning the definition of biochemical cure, most consider it to be a gender-appropriate normalization of serum prolactin levels. However, some studies have demonstrated that treatment may disrupt the pituitary stalk, leading to elevation in prolactin levels and falsely lowered rates of cure.[44]

A review of the literature revealed 32 radiosurgical series including 765 patients with a prolactin-secreting adenoma[11–18,21,23,24,27,32,33,35,40,43,46,49,50,52,53,56,57,66,70,84–89] (**Table 14.5**). Biochemical cure was realized in 30.8% of patients overall (0–83.3%) over a follow-up period (mean/median) of 19.5 to 75.5 months. Growth control rates were substantially better, with many achieving rates of 90% or greater. Here, as with other secretory adenomas, the use of medical therapy both during treatment and through follow-up had an effect on outcomes. The rates of adverse events remained low, with a mean of 2.1% (range, 0–9.1%) developing new neurologic deficits and 7.5% having some form of new pituitary dysfunction (range, 0–28%).

Biochemical Remission and Late Recurrence

Given the morbidity associated with hypersecretory lesions, radiosurgical intervention would ideally yield hormone normalization within a period of time similar to that seen after surgical extirpation.[90] Unfortunately, the period during which remission can occur is longer and demonstrates considerable variation, with reports of occurrence ranging from 3 months to 8 years.[31,55,79]

Concerning factors influencing remission, several groups have performed investigations designed to determine what if any variables may be used to predict or alter the efficacy of radiosurgery. Pollock et al[79] evaluated 46 patients with GH-secreting adenomas and identified two significant associations in both univariate and multivariate analysis. A preoperative IGF-1 level greater than 2.25 times the upper limit of normal was significantly associated with lower rates of biochemical cure (hazard ratio [HR], 2.9; 95% confidence interval [CI], 1.2–6.9), with this finding supporting the earlier reports by Castinetti and colleagues,[71] who identified a significant association between preoperative GH and IGF-1 levels and rates of remission.

The perioperative use of suppressive medications was also found to have an influence on remission (HR, 4.2; 95% CI, 1.4–13.2).[79] In patients with IGF-1 levels less than 2.25 times the upper limit of normal and those who were off somatostatin agonists at the time of radiosurgery, the rates of biochemical remission exceeded 80%. A similar finding was demonstrated by Landolt et al,[91] who showed that the remission rates fell from 60% to 11% for those using octreotide in the perioperative setting. Mechanisms underlying this result include a decreased radiosensitivity of tumor cells secondary to decreased cell division. Additionally, octreotide may act as a free radical scavenger, thereby decreasing the damage incurred by DNA following exposure to ionizing radiation. Importantly, this result is not exclusive to acromegaly. Landolt and colleagues[87] found a nonsignificant trend toward worse outcomes in patients treated with radiosurgery for prolactinomas while on dopamine agonists. Pouratian[89] et al, in their analysis of 23 patients with refractory prolactinomas, demonstrated a significant increase in the rates of remission for those patients off dopamine agonists at the time of treatment. We observed a similar improvement in endocrine remission in patients with acromegaly taken off pituitary-suppressive medications at the time of radiosurgery.[82]

There remains some controversy, however, as the literature has not been entirely consistent across series.[53,69,71,79,87,91] Two other groups analyzed remission rates after radiosurgery in the setting of somatostatin agonists, without an identifiable effect on outcome.[69,71] Several issues are postulated to account for this variability. First, the definition of cure is not entirely consistent across series, with some accepting GH values of less than 5 ng/mL.[50,72] Second, the rates of follow-up are inconsistent. Pollock et al[79] demonstrated that remission continued to occur for up to 5 years following radiosurgical treatment, whereas in the report by Castinetti and colleagues,[71] 44% of their patient population received the final endocrine evaluation less than 36 months following treatment. Despite inconsistent data, it is the practice at our center to discontinue the use of suppressive medications for 6 to 8 weeks around the period of radiosurgery, with the exact duration contingent on the specific pharmacokinetics of the specific substance used.

The rates of biochemical remission vary broadly across series, and one may note from the previously quoted results that a differential sensitivity to radiosurgery has been demonstrated for specific types of secretory pituitary adenomas.[17,32,52] In general, Cushing syndrome demonstrates the highest average rates of biochemical remission, followed by acromegaly, prolactinomas, and Nelson syndrome. This finding has been attributed to patient selection, tumor volume, radiation dose delivered, use of suppressive medications, and duration of follow-up.[17,52] In an attempt to control for such confounding variables, Pollock et al[52] reviewed a retrospective series of 46 patients similar in terms of the above-mentioned aspects. This analysis revealed an 87% remission rate for Cushing disease versus 67% for acromegaly and 18% for prolactinomas (HR, 4.4; 95% CI, 1.1–18.2; $P = 0.04$). Importantly, although only 18% of patients in this series with prolactinomas met the criteria for remission, the majority (82%) demonstrated symptomatic improvement. Concerning prolactinomas in particular, radiation-induced damage to the pituitary stalk may yield mild elevations of prolactin, resulting in falsely lowered rates of remission.[52] Although this supports the hypothesis that radiosensitivity varies with hormonal product, the etiology of this disparity remains obscure.

Over all, few cases of recurrence following documented biochemical remission are reported.[45,53] However, in these series, rates of up to 20% have been reported. This again serves to accentuate the necessity of long-term radiographic and endocrinologic follow-up after any therapeutic intervention for secretory pituitary adenomas.

Adverse Events

Adverse events following radiosurgery for a pituitary adenoma remain uncommon, with hypopituitarism occurring the most frequently. On average, 6 to 23% of patients

Table 14.5 Summary of the Literature Review for the Radiosurgical Management of Prolactinomas

Year	Authors	Patients (N)	Mean/median follow-up (mo)	Mean/median margin dose (Gy)	Biochemical remission (%)‡	Neurologic deficit (%)†	Hypopituitarism (%)
1991	Levy et al	20	NR	NR	60	NR	33*
1993	Ganz et al	3	> 18*	13.3	0	NR	NR
1998	Lim et al	18	25.5*	25.4*	55.6	1.7*	0
1998	Martinez et al	5	36*	33.2	0	3.4*	0
1998	Mitsumori et al	4	47*	NR	0	11.1*	22.9*
1998	Pan et al	27	29*	26	17.4	7.4	NR
1998	Witt et al	12	32*	19.2*	0	5.6*	0
1998	Yoon et al	11	49.2*	NR	81.8	0	29.2*
1999	Hayashi et al	13	16.2*	22.5*	15.4	7.7	0
1999	Inoue et al	2	> 24	20.2*	50	0	NR
1999	Laws et al	19	NR	NR	7	NR	NR
1999	Mokry et al	21	30.8	14.2	61.9	0	14.3
1999	Morange-Ramos et al	4	20*	28.8	0	0	25
1999	MS Kim et al	13	12*	22*	23.1	0	0
1999	SH Kim et al	18	26.9*	28.7*	16.7	0	0
2000	Izawa et al	15	26.4*	23.8*	20	6.7	0
2000	Landolt et al	20	28.5	25	25	5	NR
2000	Pan et al	128	33	31.2	52	0	NR
2002	Feigl et al	18	55.2*	15*	60*	NR	40*
2002	Pollock et al	7	42.4*	20	29	0	16*
2003	Choi et al	16	42.5*	28.5*	23.8	0	0
2003	Petrovich et al	12	34*	15*	83.3	3*	NR
2005	Kajiwara et al	3	35.7	14.3	33	0	9.5
2006	Pouratian et al	23	52	18.6	26	7	28
2006	Voges et al	13	56	13.5	15.4	4.2*	18.3
2007	Ma et al	51	37	26.1	40	NR	17.6
2008	Pollock et al (1)	11	48	25	18	9.1	36*
2008	Tinnel et al	2	19.5	19	50	0	0
2009	Castinetti et al	15	75	26	46.6	5.3*	21*
2009	Jezkova et al	35	75.5	34	37.1	0	14.3
2009	Kobayashi	30	37.4	18.4	43.5	0	0
2009	Wan et al	176	67.3	22.4	23.3	0	1.7*
Total/Average		765	19.5		30.8	2.1	7.5

(1) Contains patients included in the 2002 cohort by Pollock et al.
* Data not available for separate group, only the cohort as a whole.
† Does not include asymptomatic diagnosis of radiation necrosis.
‡ Percentage refers to all patients with remission, including those who subsequently experienced recurrence.

develop some form of anterior pituitary deficiency subsequent to treatment. This has been correlated with the tumor volume; those with a tumor volume of 4.0 cm^3 or less have a 5-year risk of 18%, versus 58% for those with larger lesions.[29] The incidence of postradiosurgical hypopituitarism is also likely to be related to the preradiosurgical status of the normal pituitary gland, type and timing of prior treatments, radiosurgical dose per volume delivered to the normal gland, and rigorousness and length of the follow-up assessment period. A safe radiosurgical dose or dose per volume below which hypopituitarism will not occur is unlikely to exist. However, a lower dose achieved in part through a steep gradient index is intuitively pleasing in terms of minimizing the risk for hypopituitarism.

The second most common side effect includes neuropathies of cranial nerves II, III, IV, V, and VI, which occur in 2% or fewer of all patients. Greater conformality and shielding strategies serve to minimize this risk.[92] Other rare side effects include radiation necrosis of the adjacent parenchyma,[32,52,53,57] internal carotid artery stenosis,[53,93] and secondary tumor formation.[94] Concerning radiosurgically induced neoplasia after the treatment of a pituitary tumor, no cases have been reported to date. Nevertheless, one must always be cognizant of this potential, especially when using radiosurgery in younger patients.

◆ Radiosurgery for Sellar and Parasellar Meningiomas

Meningiomas are common intracranial lesions, and although they are generally histologically benign, resection of skull base lesions can be associated with significant morbidity.[95–109] Given the intimate relationship of the sellar and parasellar region to critical neurovascular structures, tumor control and preservation of neurologic function have become the goals of therapy. Previously, external beam radiotherapy was the adjuvant treatment of choice following surgical resection. However, more recently, radiosurgery has replaced this modality and has even become an acceptable primary therapy in certain cases.

Tumor Control

For WHO grade 1 meningiomas, SRS results in control rates ranging from 86 to 100%,[110–138] with a recent series demonstrating 5- and 10-year progression-free survival rates of 95% and 69%, respectively[139] (**Fig. 14.2; Table 14.6**). Variability in tumor and treatment characteristics and the duration of follow-up are all partially responsible for the differential outcomes reported. Specific variables that have demonstrated statistical significance in predicting tumor control include tumor volume and patient age at the time of treatment, with a younger age portending a more favorable outcome. In our experience at the University of Virginia, those lesions larger than 5 cm^3 had an average peripheral dose of 12.7 Gy, compared with 15 Gy for smaller tumors ($P < 0.001$).[139] This finding serves as an impetus for cytoreductive surgery before radiosurgical therapy. When the sellar or parasellar meningioma is adjacent to critical, radiation-sensitive structures such as the optic apparatus despite maximal safe resection, multiple-session radiosurgery with LINAC-based systems or the Gamma Knife eXtend may achieve a high rate of tumor control and maintain neurologic function.[140]

As with pituitary adenomas, WHO grade 1 meningiomas are slowly progressive lesions, and long-term follow-up is necessary to adequately characterize treatment outcomes. There is evidence suggesting that meningiomas followed

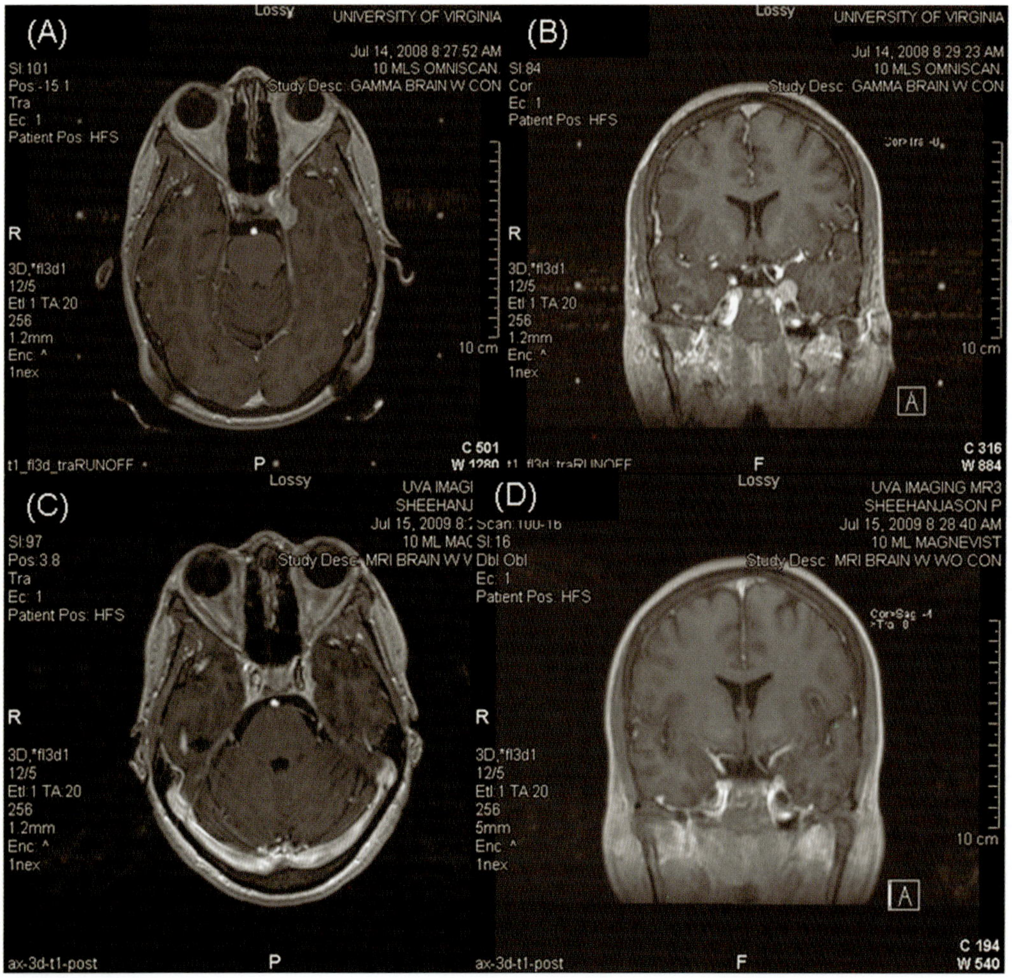

Fig. 14.2 A 36-year-old woman presented with worsening headaches and extraocular dysmotility. **(A)** Axial and **(B)** coronal postcontrast MR images of the brain revealed a left parasellar tumor consistent with a meningioma.The patient underwent stereotactic radiosurgery with a dose of 14 Gy to the tumor margin. **(C,D)** One year after radiosurgery, the patient's tumor was markedly smaller. In addition, her headaches and extraocular dysmotility resolved.

Table 14.6 Summary of the Literature Review for the Radiosurgical Management of Parasellar Meningiomas

Year	Author	Patients (N)	Mean follow-up (mo)	Actuarial tumor control (%)	Complications (%)
1997	Chang et al	55	48	98 (2 y)	4
2000	Roche et al	80	30.5	93 (5 y)	3.8
2002	Nicolato et al	138	48.5	97 (5 y)	1
2002	Lee et al	159	35	93 (5/10 y)	6.9
2002	Spiegelmann et al	42	38	97.5 (3/7 y)	7.1
2003	Iwai et al	43	49	92 (5 y)	0
2004	Selch	45	36	97.4 (3 y)	2.2
2005	Pollock et al	49	58	100 (1)	14
2007	Hasegawa et al	115	62	94 and 92 (5/10 y)	12
2008	Han (2)	63	77	90 (5 y)	15.9
2009	Kimball et al	49	50	100 and 98 (5/10 y)	2
2009	Takanashi	38	52	95.5	0
2010	U Virginia experience	138	84	95 and 71 (5/10 y)	10
Total/Average		1014		95.3	6.1

(1) Two patients underwent surgical resection for worsening symptoms 20 and 25 months after radiosurgery.
(2) Includes all skull base meningiomas and 12 cavernous sinus meningiomas.

for longer periods of time will either progress or decrease in size, whereas tumors with shorter follow-up remain constant in size.[22,139]

For patients with atypical and malignant meningiomas, SRS affords a much lower rate of tumor control.[141–144] In one study by Kano and colleagues, a margin dose exceeding 20 Gy to WHO grades 2 and 3 meningiomas was found to yield a higher chance of tumor control.[141] In general, SRS, like other treatment tools including resection, radiotherapy, and brachytherapy, offers a reasonable but far from perfect rate of local and distant tumor control for WHO grades 2 and 3 meningiomas. A higher margin dose should be delivered to the tumor during radiosurgery whenever possible.

Adverse Events

Cranial neuropathies were the most frequently observed adverse event (0–10%). These typically were secondary to tumor progression rather than to radiation-induced damage.[110–138] This compares favorably with the reported range of 18 to 41% following microsurgical resection.[95–109,145] Factors demonstrating an association with cranial neuropathy were those one would expect to be associated with tumor progression (larger volume, lower peripheral dose, and longer follow-up). In the series by Williams et al,[139] only tumor progression demonstrated significance on multivariate analysis, and 79% of patients who developed a new neurologic deficit did so in this setting. Contrary to what was demonstrated for pituitary adenomas, hypopituitarism was an infrequent finding.

◆ Conclusion

SRS has come to occupy an important role in the management of patients with parasellar and sellar tumors. Radiosurgery can be used after resection in patients with substantial residual tumor or tumor recurrence. It can also be used as an upfront treatment for some patients. Long-term tumor control is typically afforded by radiosurgery for those with pituitary adenomas and benign meningiomas. Neurologic function is generally preserved or improved, even when a tumor in the cavernous sinus is treated. Delayed tumor progression or radiation-induced complications are rare. However, lifelong follow-up of patients is generally recommended.

References

1. Cushing H. The Pituitary Body and Its Disorders: Clinical States Produced by Disorders of the Hypophysis Cerebri. J. B. Lippincott Company; 1912
2. Seymour ZA, Cohen-Gadol AA. Cushing's lost cases of "radium bomb" brachytherapy for gliomas. J Neurosurg 2010; 113(1):141–148
3. Schulder M, Loeffler JS, Howes AE, Alexander E III, Black PM. Historical vignette: The radium bomb: Harvey Cushing and the interstitial irradiation of gliomas. J Neurosurg 1996;84(3): 530–532
4. Leksell L. The stereotaxic method and radiosurgery of the brain. Acta Chir Scand 1951;102(4):316–319
5. Barnett GH, Linskey ME, Adler JR, et al; American Association of Neurological Surgeons; Congress of Neurolofical Surgeons Washington Committee Stereotactic Radiosurgery Task Force. Stereotactic radiosurgery—an organized neurosurgery-sanctioned definition. J Neurosurg 2007;106(1):1–5
6. Friedman WA, Foote KD. Linear accelerator radiosurgery in the management of brain tumours. Ann Med 2000;32(1):64–80
7. Chen CC, Chapman P, Petit J, Loeffler J. Proton radiosurgery in neurosurgery. Neurosurg Focus 2007;23(6):E5
8. Dekkers OM, Pereira AM, Romijn JA. Treatment and follow-up of clinically nonfunctioning pituitary macroadenomas. J Clin Endocrinol Metab 2008;93(10):3717–3726

9. Vance ML. Treatment of patients with a pituitary adenoma: one clinician's experience. Neurosurg Focus 2004;16(4):E1
10. Höybye C, Rähn T. Adjuvant gamma knife radiosurgery in nonfunctioning pituitary adenomas; low risk of long-term complications in selected patients. Pituitary 2009;12(3):211–216
11. Pan L, Zhang N, Wang E, Wang B, Xu W. Pituitary adenomas: the effect of gamma knife radiosurgery on tumor growth and endocrinopathies. Stereotact Funct Neurosurg 1998;70(Suppl 1):119–126
12. Feigl GC, Bonelli CM, Berghold A, Mokry M. Effects of gamma knife radiosurgery of pituitary adenomas on pituitary function. J Neurosurg 2002;97(5, Suppl):415–421
13. Hayashi M, Izawa M, Hiyama H, et al. Gamma knife radiosurgery for pituitary adenomas. Stereotact Funct Neurosurg 1999;72(Suppl 1):111–118
14. Inoue HK, Kohga H, Hirato M, et al. Pituitary adenomas treated by microsurgery with or without Gamma Knife surgery: experience in 122 cases. Stereotact Funct Neurosurg 1999;72(Suppl 1):125–131
15. Izawa M, Hayashi M, Nakaya K, et al. Gamma knife radiosurgery for pituitary adenomas. J Neurosurg 2000;93(Suppl 3):19–22
16. Kajiwara K, Saito K, Yoshikawa K, et al. Image-guided stereotactic radiosurgery with the CyberKnife for pituitary adenomas. Minim Invasive Neurosurg 2005;48(2):91–96
17. Kobayashi T. Long-term results of stereotactic gamma knife radiosurgery for pituitary adenomas. Specific strategies for different types of adenoma. Prog Neurol Surg 2009;22:77–95
18. Lim YL, Leem W, Kim TS, Rhee BA, Kim GK. Four years' experiences in the treatment of pituitary adenomas with gamma knife radiosurgery. Stereotact Funct Neurosurg 1998;70(Suppl 1):95–109
19. Liscák R, Vladyka V, Marek J, Simonová G, Vymazal J. Gamma knife radiosurgery for endocrine-inactive pituitary adenomas. Acta Neurochir (Wien) 2007;149(10):999–1006, discussion 1006
20. Losa M, Valle M, Mortini P, et al. Gamma knife surgery for treatment of residual nonfunctioning pituitary adenomas after surgical debulking. J Neurosurg 2004;100(3):438–444
21. Martinez R, Bravo G, Burzaco J, Rey G. Pituitary tumors and gamma knife surgery. Clinical experience with more than two years of follow-up. Stereotact Funct Neurosurg 1998;70(Suppl 1):110–118
22. Mingione V, Yen CP, Vance ML, et al. Gamma surgery in the treatment of nonsecretory pituitary macroadenoma. J Neurosurg 2006;104(6):876–883
23. Mitsumori M, Shrieve DC, Alexander E III, et al. Initial clinical results of LINAC-based stereotactic radiosurgery and stereotactic radiotherapy for pituitary adenomas. Int J Radiat Oncol Biol Phys 1998;42(3):573–580
24. Mokry M, Ramschak-Schwarzer S, Simbrunner J, Ganz JC, Pendl G. A six year experience with the postoperative radiosurgical management of pituitary adenomas. Stereotact Funct Neurosurg 1999;72(Suppl 1):88–100
25. Muacevic A, Uhl E, Wowra B. Gamma knife radiosurgery for nonfunctioning pituitary adenomas. Acta Neurochir Suppl (Wien) 2004;91:51–54
26. Muramatsu J, Yoshida M, Shioura H, et al. Clinical results of LINAC-based stereotactic radiosurgery for pituitary adenoma. Nippon Igaku Hoshasen Gakkai Zasshi 2003;63(5):225–230
27. Petrovich Z, Jozsef G, Yu C, Apuzzo ML. Radiotherapy and stereotactic radiosurgery for pituitary tumors. Neurosurg Clin N Am 2003;14(1):147–166
28. Picozzi P, Losa M, Mortini P, et al. Radiosurgery and the prevention of regrowth of incompletely removed nonfunctioning pituitary adenomas. J Neurosurg 2005;102(Suppl):71–74
29. Pollock BE, Cochran J, Natt N, et al. Gamma knife radiosurgery for patients with nonfunctioning pituitary adenomas: results from a 15-year experience. Int J Radiat Oncol Biol Phys 2008;70(5):1325–1329
30. Sheehan JP, Kondziolka D, Flickinger J, Lunsford LD. Radiosurgery for residual or recurrent nonfunctioning pituitary adenoma. J Neurosurg 2002;97(5, Suppl):408–414
31. Shin M, Kurita H, Sasaki T, et al. Stereotactic radiosurgery for pituitary adenoma invading the cavernous sinus. J Neurosurg 2000;93(Suppl 3):2–5
32. Voges J, Kocher M, Runge M, et al. Linear accelerator radiosurgery for pituitary macroadenomas: a 7-year follow-up study. Cancer 2006;107(6):1355–1364
33. Witt TC, Kondziolka D, Flickinger J, Lunsford LD. Gamma knife radiosurgery for pituitary tumors. In: Lunsford LD, Kondziolka D, Flickinger J, eds. Gamma Knife Brain Surgery. Karger; 1998:114–127
34. Wowra B, Stummer W. Efficacy of gamma knife radiosurgery for nonfunctioning pituitary adenomas: a quantitative follow up with magnetic resonance imaging-based volumetric analysis. J Neurosurg 2002;97(5, Suppl):429–432
35. Yoon SC, Suh TS, Jang HS, et al. Clinical results of 24 pituitary macroadenomas with linac-based stereotactic radiosurgery. Int J Radiat Oncol Biol Phys 1998;41(4):849–853
36. Biller BMK, Grossman AB, Stewart PM, et al. Treatment of adrenocorticotropin-dependent Cushing's syndrome: a consensus statement. J Clin Endocrinol Metab 2008;93(7):2454–2462
37. Arnaldi G, Angeli A, Atkinson AB, et al. Diagnosis and complications of Cushing's syndrome: a consensus statement. J Clin Endocrinol Metab 2003;88(12):5593–5602
38. Castinetti F, Nagai M, Dufour H, et al. Gamma knife radiosurgery is a successful adjunctive treatment in Cushing's disease. Eur J Endocrinol 2007;156(1):91–98
39. Castinetti F, Nagai M, Morange I, et al. Long-term results of stereotactic radiosurgery in secretory pituitary adenomas. J Clin Endocrinol Metab 2009;94(9):3400–3407
40. Choi JY, Chang JH, Chang JW, Ha Y, Park YG, Chung SS. Radiological and hormonal responses of functioning pituitary adenomas after gamma knife radiosurgery. Yonsei Med J 2003;44(4):602–607
41. Degerblad M, Rähn T, Bergstrand G, Thorén M. Long-term results of stereotactic radiosurgery to the pituitary gland in Cushing's disease. Acta Endocrinol (Copenh) 1986;112(3):310–314
42. Devin JK, Allen GS, Cmelak AJ, Duggan DM, Blevins LS. The efficacy of linear accelerator radiosurgery in the management of patients with Cushing's disease. Stereotact Funct Neurosurg 2004;82(5–6):254–262
43. Ganz JC, Backlund EO, Thorsen FA. The effects of gamma knife surgery of pituitary adenomas on tumor growth and endocrinopathies. Stereotact Funct Neurosurg 1993;61(Suppl 1): 30–37
44. Höybye C, Grenbäck E, Rähn T, Degerblad M, Thorén M, Hulting AL. Adrenocorticotropic hormone-producing pituitary tumors: 12- to 22-year follow-up after treatment with stereotactic radiosurgery. Neurosurgery 2001;49(2):284–291, discussion 291–292
45. Jagannathan J, Sheehan JP, Pouratian N, Laws ER, Steiner L, Vance ML. Gamma knife surgery for Cushing's disease. J Neurosurg 2007;106(6):980–987
46. Kim SH, Huh R, Chang JW, Park YG, Chung SS. Gamma knife radiosurgery for functioning pituitary adenomas. Stereotact Funct Neurosurg 1999;72(Suppl 1):101–110
47. Kobayashi T, Kida Y, Mori Y. Gamma knife radiosurgery in the treatment of Cushing disease: long-term results. J Neurosurg 2002;97(5, Suppl):422–428
48. Laws ER, Reitmeyer M, Thapar K, Vance ML. Cushing's disease resulting from pituitary corticotrophic microadenoma. Treatment results from transsphenoidal microsurgery and gamma knife radiosurgery. Neurochirurgie 2002;48(2–3 Pt 2):294–299
49. Levy RP, Fabrikant JI, Frankel KA, et al. Heavy-charged-particle radiosurgery of the pituitary gland: clinical results of 840 patients. Stereotact Funct Neurosurg 1991;57(1–2):22–35
50. Morange-Ramos I, Regis J, Dufour H, et al. Gamma-knife surgery for secreting pituitary adenomas. Acta Neurochir (Wien) 1998;140(5):437–443
51. Petit JH, Biller BMK, Coen JJ, et al. Proton stereotactic radiosurgery in management of persistent acromegaly. Endocr Pract 2007;13(7):726–734
52. Pollock BE, Brown PD, Nippoldt TB, Young WF Jr. Pituitary tumor type affects the chance of biochemical remission after radiosurgery of hormone-secreting pituitary adenomas. Neurosurgery 2008;62(6):1271–1276, discussion 1276–1278
53. Pollock BE, Nippoldt TB, Stafford SL, Foote RL, Abboud CF. Results of stereotactic radiosurgery in patients with hormone-producing pituitary adenomas: factors associated with endocrine normalization. J Neurosurg 2002;97(3):525–530

54. Seo Y, Fukuoka S, Takanashi M, Sasaki T, Suematsu K, Nakamura J. Gamma knife surgery for Cushing's disease. Surg Neurol 1995;43(2):170–175, discussion 175–176

55. Sheehan JM, Vance ML, Sheehan JP, Ellegala DB, Laws ER Jr. Radiosurgery for Cushing's disease after failed transsphenoidal surgery. J Neurosurg 2000;93(5):738–742

56. Tinnel BA, Henderson MA, Witt TC, et al. Endocrine response after gamma knife-based stereotactic radiosurgery for secretory pituitary adenoma. Stereotact Funct Neurosurg 2008;86(5):292–296

57. Wan H, Chihiro O, Yuan S. MASEP gamma knife radiosurgery for secretory pituitary adenomas: experience in 347 consecutive cases. J Exp Clin Cancer Res 2009;28:36

58. Witt TC. Stereotactic radiosurgery for pituitary tumors. Neurosurg Focus 2003;14(5):e10

59. Wong GK, Leung CH, Chiu KW, et al. LINAC radiosurgery in recurrent Cushing's disease after transsphenoidal surgery: a series of 5 cases. Minim Invasive Neurosurg 2003;46(6):327–330

60. Nagesser SK, van Seters AP, Kievit J, Hermans J, Krans HM, van de Velde CJ. Long-term results of total adrenalectomy for Cushing's disease. World J Surg 2000;24(1):108–113

61. Mauermann WJ, Sheehan JP, Chernavvsky DR, Laws ER, Steiner L, Vance ML. Gamma knife surgery for adrenocorticotropic hormone-producing pituitary adenomas after bilateral adrenalectomy. J Neurosurg 2007;106(6):988–993

62. Petit JH, Biller BMK, Yock TI, et al. Proton stereotactic radiotherapy for persistent adrenocorticotropin-producing adenomas. J Clin Endocrinol Metab 2008;93(2):393–399

63. Vik-Mo EO, Øksnes M, Pedersen P-H, et al. Gamma knife stereotactic radiosurgery of Nelson syndrome. Eur J Endocrinol 2009;160(2):143–148

64. Wolffenbuttel BH, Kitz K, Beuls EM. Beneficial gamma-knife radiosurgery in a patient with Nelson's syndrome. Clin Neurol Neurosurg 1998;100(1):60–63

65. Pollock BE, Young WF Jr. Stereotactic radiosurgery for patients with ACTH-producing pituitary adenomas after prior adrenalectomy. Int J Radiat Oncol Biol Phys 2002;54(3):839–841

66. Laws ER Jr, Vance ML. Radiosurgery for pituitary tumors and craniopharyngiomas. Neurosurg Clin N Am 1999;10(2):327–336

67. Melmed S. Medical progress: Acromegaly. N Engl J Med 2006;355(24):2558–2573

68. Growth Hormone Research Society; Pituitary Society. Biochemical assessment and long-term monitoring in patients with acromegaly: statement from a joint consensus conference of the Growth Hormone Research Society and the Pituitary Society. J Clin Endocrinol Metab 2004;89(7):3099–3102

69. Attanasio R, Epaminonda P, Motti E, et al. Gamma-knife radiosurgery in acromegaly: a 4-year follow-up study. J Clin Endocrinol Metab 2003;88(7):3105–3112

70. Castinetti F, Morange I, Dufour H, Regis J, Brue T. Radiotherapy and radiosurgery in acromegaly. Pituitary 2009;12(1):3–10

71. Castinetti F, Taieb D, Kuhn J-M, et al. Outcome of gamma knife radiosurgery in 82 patients with acromegaly: correlation with initial hypersecretion. J Clin Endocrinol Metab 2005;90(8):4483–4488

72. Fukuoka S, Ito T, Takanashi M, Hojo A, Nakamura H. Gamma knife radiosurgery for growth hormone-secreting pituitary adenomas invading the cavernous sinus. Stereotact Funct Neurosurg 2001;76(3-4):213–217

73. Ikeda H, Jokura H, Yoshimoto T. Transsphenoidal surgery and adjuvant gamma knife treatment for growth hormone-secreting pituitary adenoma. J Neurosurg 2001;95(2):285–291

74. Jagannathan J, Kanter AS, Olson C, Sherman JH, Laws ER Jr, Sheehan JP. Applications of radiotherapy and radiosurgery in the management of pediatric Cushing's disease: a review of the literature and our experience. J Neurooncol 2008;90(1):117–124

75. Jezkova J, Marek J, Hana V, et al. Gamma knife radiosurgery for acromegaly–long-term experience. Horumon To Rinsho 2006;64(5):588–595

76. Kobayashi T, Mori Y, Uchiyama Y, Kida Y, Fujitani S. Long-term results of gamma knife surgery for growth hormone-producing pituitary adenoma: is the disease difficult to cure? J Neurosurg 2005;102(Suppl):119–123

77. Landolt AM, Haller D, Lomax N, et al. Stereotactic radiosurgery for recurrent surgically treated acromegaly: comparison with fractionated radiotherapy. J Neurosurg 1998;88(6):1002–1008

78. Losa M, Gioia L, Picozzi P, et al. The role of stereotactic radiotherapy in patients with growth hormone-secreting pituitary adenoma [see comment]. J Clin Endocrinol Metab 2008;93(7):2546–2552

79. Pollock BE, Jacob JT, Brown PD, Nippoldt TB. Radiosurgery of growth hormone-producing pituitary adenomas: factors associated with biochemical remission. J Neurosurg 2007;106(5):833–838

80. Thorén M, Rähn T, Guo WY, Werner S. Stereotactic radiosurgery with the cobalt-60 gamma unit in the treatment of growth hormone-producing pituitary tumors. Neurosurgery 1991;29(5):663–668

81. Vik-Mo EO, Oksnes M, Pedersen P-H, et al. Gamma knife stereotactic radiosurgery for acromegaly. Eur J Endocrinol 2007;157(3):255–263

82. Jagannathan J, Sheehan JP, Pouratian N, Laws ER Jr, Steiner L, Vance ML. Gamma knife radiosurgery for acromegaly: outcomes after failed transsphenoidal surgery. Neurosurgery 2008;62(6):1262–1269, discussion 1269–1270

83. Klibanski A. Clinical practice. Prolactinomas. N Engl J Med 2010;362(13):1219–1226

84. Pan L, Zhang N, Wang EM, Wang BJ, Dai JZ, Cai PW. Gamma knife radiosurgery as a primary treatment for prolactinomas. J Neurosurg 2000;93(Suppl 3):10–13

85. Jezková J, Hána V, Krsek M, et al. Use of the Leksell gamma knife in the treatment of prolactinoma patients. Clin Endocrinol (Oxf) 2009;70(5):732–741

86. Kim MS, Lee SI, Sim JH. Gamma knife radiosurgery for functioning pituitary microadenoma. Stereotact Funct Neurosurg 1999;72(Suppl 1):119–124

87. Landolt AM, Lomax N. Gamma knife radiosurgery for prolactinomas. J Neurosurg 2000;93(Suppl 3):14–18

88. Ma ZM, Qiu B, Hou YH, Liu YS. Gamma knife treatment for pituitary prolactinomas. Zhong Nan Da Xue Xue Bao Yi Xue Ban 2006;31(5):714–716

89. Pouratian N, Sheehan J, Jagannathan J, Laws ER Jr, Steiner L, Vance ML. Gamma knife radiosurgery for medically and surgically refractory prolactinomas. Neurosurgery 2006;59(2):255–266

90. Jagannathan J, Smith R, DeVroom HL, et al. Outcome of using the histological pseudocapsule as a surgical capsule in Cushing disease. J Neurosurg 2009;111(3):531–539

91. Landolt AM, Haller D, Lomax N, et al. Octreotide may act as a radioprotective agent in acromegaly. J Clin Endocrinol Metab 2000;85(3):1287–1289

92. Jagannathan J, Yen C-P, Pouratian N, Laws ER, Sheehan JP. Stereotactic radiosurgery for pituitary adenomas: a comprehensive review of indications, techniques and long-term results using the Gamma Knife. J Neurooncol 2009;92(3):345–356

93. Lim YJ, Leem W, Park JT, Kim TS, Rhee BA, Kim GK. Cerebral infarction with ICA occlusion after Gamma Knife radiosurgery for pituitary adenoma: a case report. Stereotact Funct Neurosurg 1999;72(Suppl 1):132–139

94. Loeffler JS, Niemierko A, Chapman PH. Second tumors after radiosurgery: tip of the iceberg or a bump in the road? Neurosurgery 2003;52(6):1436–1440, discussion 1440–1442

95. Al-Mefty O, Smith RR. Surgery of tumors invading the cavernous sinus. Surg Neurol 1988;30(5):370–381

96. Cioffi FA, Bernini FP, Punzo A, Natale M, Muras I. Cavernous sinus meningiomas. Neurochirurgia (Stuttg) 1987;30(2):40–47

97. Cusimano MD, Sekhar LN, Sen CN, et al. The results of surgery for benign tumors of the cavernous sinus. Neurosurgery 1995;37(1):1–9, discussion 9–10

98. De Jesús O, Sekhar LN, Parikh HK, Wright DC, Wagner DP. Long-term follow-up of patients with meningiomas involving the cavernous sinus: recurrence, progression, and quality of life. Neurosurgery 1996;39(5):915–919, discussion 919–920

99. DeMonte F, Smith HK, al-Mefty O. Outcome of aggressive removal of cavernous sinus meningiomas. J Neurosurg 1994;81(2):245–251

100. Heth JA, Al-Mefty O. Cavernous sinus meningiomas. Neurosurg Focus 2003;14(6):e3

101. Kim DK, Grieve J, Archer DJ, Uttley D. Meningiomas in the region of the cavernous sinus: a review of 21 patients. Br J Neurosurg 1996;10(5):439–444

102. Klink DF, Sampath P, Miller NR, Brem H, Long DM. Long-term visual outcome after nonradical microsurgery patients with

parasellar and cavernous sinus meningiomas. Neurosurgery 2000;47(1):24–31, discussion 31–32
103. Knosp E, Perneczky A, Koos WT, Fries G, Matula C. Meningiomas of the space of the cavernous sinus. Neurosurgery 1996;38(3): 434–442, discussion 442–444
104. O'Sullivan MG, van Loveren HR, Tew JM Jr. The surgical resectability of meningiomas of the cavernous sinus. Neurosurgery 1997;40(2):238–244, discussion 245–247
105. Sekhar LN, Møller AR. Operative management of tumors involving the cavernous sinus. J Neurosurg 1986;64(6):879–889
106. Sekhar LN, Patel S, Cusimano M, Wright DC, Sen CN, Bank WO. Surgical treatment of meningiomas involving the cavernous sinus: evolving ideas based on a ten year experience. Acta Neurochir Suppl (Wien) 1996;65:58–62
107. Sekhar LN, Pomeranz S, Sen CN. Management of tumours involving the cavernous sinus. Acta Neurochir Suppl (Wien) 1991;53:101–112
108. Sekhar LN, Sen CN, Jho HD, Janecka IP. Surgical treatment of intracavernous neoplasms: a four-year experience. Neurosurgery 1989;24(1):18–30
109. Sindou M, Wydh E, Jouanneau E, Nebbal M, Lieutaud T. Long-term follow-up of meningiomas of the cavernous sinus after surgical treatment alone. J Neurosurg 2007;107(5):937–944
110. Chang SD, Adler JR Jr. Treatment of cranial base meningiomas with linear accelerator radiosurgery. Neurosurgery 1997;41(5):1019–1025, discussion 1025–1027
111. Chang SD, Adler JR Jr, Martin DP. LINAC radiosurgery for cavernous sinus meningiomas. Stereotact Funct Neurosurg 1998;71(1):43–50
112. Chang SD, Doty JR, Martin DP, Hancock SL, Adler JR. Treatment of cavernous sinus tumors with linear accelerator radiosurgery. Skull Base Surg 1999;9(3):195–200
113. Chen JC, Giannotta SL, Yu C, Petrovich Z, Levy ML, Apuzzo ML. Radiosurgical management of benign cavernous sinus tumors: dose profiles and acute complications. Neurosurgery 2001;48(5):1022–1030, discussion 1030–1032
114. Duma CM, Lunsford LD, Kondziolka D, Harsh GR IV, Flickinger JC. Stereotactic radiosurgery of cavernous sinus meningiomas as an addition or alternative to microsurgery. Neurosurgery 1993;32(5):699–704, discussion 704–705
115. Friedman WA, Murad GJ, Bradshaw P, et al. Linear accelerator surgery for meningiomas. J Neurosurg 2005;103(2):206–209
116. Hasegawa T, Kida Y, Yoshimoto M, Koike J, Iizuka H, Ishii D. Long-term outcomes of gamma knife surgery for cavernous sinus meningioma. J Neurosurg 2007;107(4):745–751
117. Iwai Y, Yamanaka K, Ishiguro T. Gamma knife radiosurgery for the treatment of cavernous sinus meningiomas. Neurosurgery 2003;52(3):517–524, discussion 523–524
118. Johnson MD, Sade B, Milano MT, Lee JH, Toms SA. New prospects for management and treatment of inoperable and recurrent skull base meningiomas. J Neurooncol 2008;86(1):109–122
119. Kida Y, Kobayashi T, Tanaka T, Oyama H, Niwa M, Maesawa S. Radiosurgery of cavernous sinus meningiomas with gamma-knife. No Shinkei Geka 1996;24(6):529–533
120. Kimball MM, Friedman WA, Foote KD, Bova FJ, Chi YY. Linear accelerator radiosurgery for cavernous sinus meningiomas. Stereotact Funct Neurosurg 2009;87(2):120–127
121. Kuo JS, Chen JC, Yu C, et al. Gamma knife radiosurgery for benign cavernous sinus tumors: quantitative analysis of treatment outcomes. Neurosurgery 2004;54(6):1385–1393, discussion 1393–1394
122. Kurita H, Sasaki T, Kawamoto S, et al. Role of radiosurgery in the management of cavernous sinus meningiomas. Acta Neurol Scand 1997;96(5):297–304
123. Lee JY, Niranjan A, McInerney J, Kondziolka D, Flickinger JC, Lunsford LD. Stereotactic radiosurgery providing long-term tumor control of cavernous sinus meningiomas. J Neurosurg 2002;97(1):65–72
124. Liscák R, Simonová G, Vymazal J, Janousková L, Vladyka V. Gamma knife radiosurgery of meningiomas in the cavernous sinus region. Acta Neurochir (Wien) 1999;141(5):473–480
125. Malik I, Rowe JG, Walton L, Radatz MW, Kemeny AA. The use of stereotactic radiosurgery in the management of meningiomas. Br J Neurosurg 2005;19(1):13–20
126. Maruyama K, Shin M, Kurita H, Kawahara N, Morita A, Kirino T. Proposed treatment strategy for cavernous sinus meningiomas: a prospective study. Neurosurgery 2004;55(5):1068–1075
127. Nicolato A, Foroni R, Alessandrini F, Bricolo A, Gerosa M. Radiosurgical treatment of cavernous sinus meningiomas: experience with 122 treated patients. Neurosurgery 2002;51(5):1153–1159, discussion 1159–1161
128. Nicolato A, Foroni R, Alessandrini F, Maluta S, Bricolo A, Gerosa M. The role of gamma knife radiosurgery in the management of cavernous sinus meningiomas. Int J Radiat Oncol Biol Phys 2002;53(4):992–1000
129. Pamir MN, Kiliç T, Belirgen M, Abacioğlu U, Karabekiroğlu N. Pituitary adenomas treated with gamma knife radiosurgery: volumetric analysis of 100 cases with minimum 3 year follow-up. Neurosurgery 2007;61(2):270–280, discussion 280
130. Pendl G, Schröttner O, Eustacchio S, Ganz JC, Feichtinger K. Cavernous sinus meningiomas—what is the strategy: upfront or adjuvant gamma knife surgery? Stereotact Funct Neurosurg 1998;70(Suppl 1):33–40
131. Pollock BE, Stafford SL. Results of stereotactic radiosurgery for patients with imaging defined cavernous sinus meningiomas. Int J Radiat Oncol Biol Phys 2005;62(5):1427–1431
132. Pollock BE, Stafford SL, Utter A, Giannini C, Schreiner SA. Stereotactic radiosurgery provides equivalent tumor control to Simpson Grade 1 resection for patients with small- to medium-size meningiomas. Int J Radiat Oncol Biol Phys 2003;55(4): 1000–1005
133. Roche PH, Régis J, Dufour H, et al. Gamma knife radiosurgery in the management of cavernous sinus meningiomas. J Neurosurg 2000;93(Suppl 3):68–73
134. Shin M, Kurita H, Sasaki T, et al. Analysis of treatment outcome after stereotactic radiosurgery for cavernous sinus meningiomas. J Neurosurg 2001;95(3):435–439
135. Spiegelmann R, Nissim O, Menhel J, Alezra D, Pfeffer MR. Linear accelerator radiosurgery for meningiomas in and around the cavernous sinus. Neurosurgery 2002;51(6):1373–1379, discussion 1379–1380
136. Tishler RB, Loeffler JS, Lunsford LD, et al. Tolerance of cranial nerves of the cavernous sinus to radiosurgery. Int J Radiat Oncol Biol Phys 1993;27(2):215–221
137. Villavicencio AT, Black PM, Shrieve DC, Fallon MP, Alexander E, Loeffler JS. Linac radiosurgery for skull base meningiomas. Acta Neurochir (Wien) 2001;143(11):1141–1152
138. Ziyal IM, Sekhar LN, Salas E. Radiosurgery: an effective treatment for cavernous sinus meningiomas? Crit Rev Neurosurg 1999;9(2):107–115
139. Williams B, Yen CP, Starke R, et al. Gamma knife radiosurgery for parasellar meningiomas: long-term results including complications, predictive factors, and progression free survival. J Neurosurg 2010; in press
140. Adler JR Jr, Gibbs IC, Puataweepong P, Chang SD. Visual field preservation after multisession cyberknife radiosurgery for perioptic lesions [reprint in Neurosurgery 2008;62(Suppl 2):733–743; PMID: 18596432]. Neurosurgery 2006;59(2):244–254
141. Kano H, Takahashi JA, Katsuki T, et al. Stereotactic radiosurgery for atypical and anaplastic meningiomas. J Neurooncol 2007;84(1):41–47
142. Rosenberg LA, Prayson RA, Lee J, et al. Long-term experience with World Health Organization grade III (malignant) meningiomas at a single institution. Int J Radiat Oncol Biol Phys 2009;74(2):427–432
143. Huffmann BC, Reinacher PC, Gilsbach JM. Gamma knife surgery for atypical meningiomas. J Neurosurg 2005;102(Suppl):283–286
144. Harris AE, Lee JY, Omalu B, Flickinger JC, Kondziolka D, Lunsford LD. The effect of radiosurgery during management of aggressive meningiomas. Surg Neurol 2003;60(4):298–305, discussion 305
145. Landeiro JA, Ribeiro CH, Lapenta MA, Flores MS, Lopes CA, Marins J. Meningiomas of the cavernous sinus: the surgical resectability and complications. Arq Neuropsiquiatr 2001;59(3-B):746–753

15 Intracavitary Radiation for Cystic Craniopharyngiomas

L. Dade Lunsford, Ajay Niranjan, Hideyuki Kano, Peter Kang, and Douglas Kondziolka

Despite the major advances of skull base microsurgical techniques, as well as expanded endoscopic techniques, craniopharyngiomas continue to be difficult to remove totally with acceptable morbidity. Ideally, surgical techniques result in total removal, maintenance of visual function, sparing of endocrinologic loss, and absence of delayed recurrence. Even when feasible, radical resection continues to be associated with unsatisfactory long-term outcomes, often because of residual neurobehavioral disorders, cognitive impairment, the long-term need for replacement hormone therapy, and hypothalamic obesity.

Realizing the morbidity of surgical techniques for craniopharyngioma in the early 1950s, both Leksell et al and Wycis et al proposed the implantation of a β-emitting isotope into cystic craniopharyngiomas.[1,2] Isotope implantation was designed to lead to slow involution of the cyst wall by delivery of a tumoricidal dose to the thin epithelial layer of the cyst. Since that time, selected pioneers in Europe have continued to apply the instillation of radioactive isotopes into craniopharyngioma cysts. Efforts in Europe, especially in Stockholm under the direction of Erik-Olof Backlund, demonstrated that intracavitary irradiation provides an effective and safe technique in the management of cystic craniopharyngiomas.[3–5] Leksell and Backlund used both radioactive phosphorus 32 (in colloidal chromic solution) and yttrium 90.[1,3] In the United States, the unavailability of ^{90}Y has led to the primary use of ^{32}P. Stereotactic insertion of the isotope with fine-needle technique is critical.

◆ Rationale for Intracavitary Irradiation

The treatment of cystic brain tumors using radioactive isotopes is based on the concept that continued cyst enlargement is the result of secretion from the thin epithelial cyst layer. Most craniopharyngiomas in fact have solid components, and subsequently develop cystic changes over the course of time. The cyst gradually enlarges like a bubble blown off a piece of bubblegum. By the time of clinical presentation, the cyst may range in volumes as small as 1 mL to as large as 126 mL. Depending upon its location and volume, the enlarging cyst results in endocrine loss, progressive visual dysfunction, and neurocognitive and intellectual deficits.

Intracavitary irradiation uses stereotactic precision to puncture the cyst and instill the isotope volume designed to deliver 180 to 250 Gy of radiation over five half-lives of the isotope.[6–8] Because the half-life of ^{32}P is 14 days, it takes ~70 days to deliver the full isotope effect. As a pure β emitter, the falloff of radiation from the decay of the isotope is very steep. The radiation dose falls off in accordance with the inverse square law, which refers to the fact that reduction in activity is proportional to 1 divided by the square of the distance from the source. The half-value tissue penetrance of ^{32}P is 0.9 mm, indicating that most of the radiation effect by far is delivered within several millimeters of the cyst wall. Implantation of the isotope leads to a "coating out" of the internal cyst wall and slow delivery of the radiobiological effect of the ^{32}P decay. This dose range appears to be sufficient to lead to cyst involution in the vast majority of cases. Long-term outcome studies from multiple centers are now available to demonstrate the benefit of intracavitary management of cystic craniopharyngiomas. Because current magnetic resonance imaging (MRI) confirms that most patients have solid and cystic tumors, many will require multimodality management. Successful strategies require cyst control, solid tumor management by microsurgery or endoscopic surgery, and stereotactic radiosurgery.[9,10] A combination of such techniques may be best to achieve the best outcomes for patients with these strategically located tumors capable of producing visual, endocrinologic, and cognitive dysfunction.

◆ Initial Experience

After the primary author returned from his Van Wagenen–sponsored fellowship at the Karolinska Institute in 1981, an initial, cautious trial of the role of intracavitary radiosurgery was pursued at the University of Pittsburgh Center for Image-Guided Neurosurgery. In the 28-year interval from 1980 to 2003, 61 patients with craniopharyngioma (33 males and 28 females) underwent intracavitary radiation after the initial diagnosis or recognition of a recurrent craniopharyngioma.[6] All patients had their tumor confirmed initially (before

1991) with computed tomography (CT) and with magnetic resonance imaging (MRI) afterward. The ages of the patients in this initial experience ranged from 4 to 74 years (mean, 28 years), and the calculated cyst volumes ranged from 1.8 to 126 mL. All patients underwent preoperative endocrinologic assessment, visual acuity and formal visual field examinations, and overall neurologic assessment. The majority of the patients had undergone multiple prior surgical procedures, including one or more craniotomies and transsphenoidal resection, and seven patients had had ventriculoperitoneal shunts placed for hydrocephalus management. Fractionated external beam radiation therapy, the role of which has declined over the last 10 years, had been previously administered to 11 patients.

◆ Stereotactic Technique for Intracavitary Irradiation

We select patients with monocystic or multicystic craniopharyngiomas. After review of the preoperative CT scan or MRI, we can estimate the cyst volume for the nuclear pharmacist. Using a simple calculation, $\pi/6 \times (X \times Y \times Z)$, we determine the volume of an oblate spheroid. X, Y, and Z are the diameters of the lesion in the three cardinal planes; × denotes multiplication. The nuclear pharmacist orders colloidal chromic phosphate ^{32}P in a stock solution dose. This is assayed on the day of delivery and reassayed on the day of the operation. If the cyst volume is less than 20 cm^3, the suspension is usually diluted with a 30% glucose solution to facilitate delivery of the isotope.

All patients are brought to the operating room for the surgical procedure, which is done under mild conscious sedation. The Leksell Model G stereotactic head frame (Elekta Instruments, Stockholm, Sweden) is attached to the patient's head with the use of local anesthesia. High-resolution axial CT (2.5-mm configured axial slices, 512 × 512 matrix) is performed with a dedicated intraoperative CT scanner in our image-guided operating room suite. The cyst area in square centimeters is calculated on each slice by tracing the cyst volume after intravenous iodinated contrast is administered. The sum of each slice is then multiplied by the slice thickness (2.5 mm) to calculate the cystic tumor volume in cubic centimeters. The calculated cyst volume is called to the nuclear pharmacist, who prepares the isotope and calculates the volume of P^{32} necessary to provide a dose of 180 to 250 Gy over five half-lives (~70 days).

The patient is advanced through the opening of the CT scanner, and the head is prepared with alcohol and draped. A frontal coronal suture twist drill craniostomy is performed with the arc attached at the chosen X, Y, and Z coordinates for a central puncture of the cyst. The trajectory is plotted in advance to reduce the number of pial transgressions and, when feasible, the ventricular entry. The target point is usually 7 to 10 mm inferior to the dorsal margin of the cyst, as it is sometimes necessary to puncture the cyst sharply and depress the cyst briefly before the 0.9-mm-outer-diameter sharp-tipped needle is inserted into the center of the cyst (**Fig. 15.1**). The 0.9-mm sharp-tipped needle is passed through a 15-cm stabilizing cannula after closed-skull percutaneous twist drill craniostomy and puncture of the dura. Once the target is reached, the stylet is removed and a three-way stopcock is attached (**Fig. 15.2**). Using a tuberculin syringe, we generally withdraw 1 mL of cyst fluid. A neuropathologist examines the fluid with polarized light microscopy to detect cholesterol crystals. Two tuberculin syringes are attached to the three-way stopcock (**Fig. 15.3**). The nuclear pharmacist and the radiation safety officer deliver the calculated volume of ^{32}P, usu-

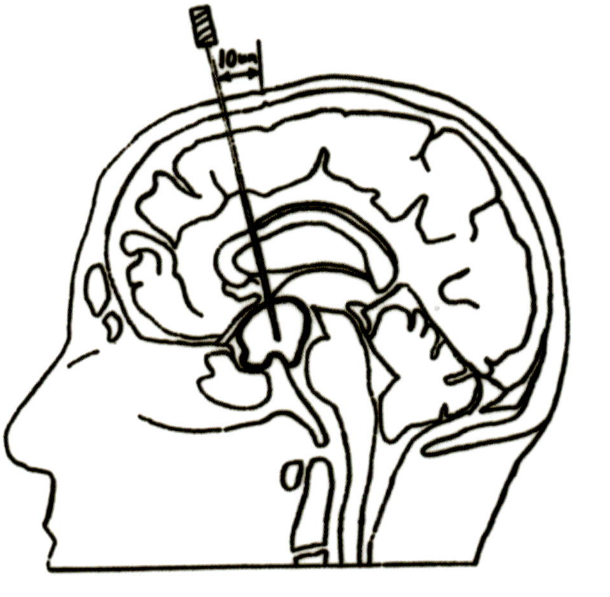

Fig. 15.1 In the transfrontal stereotactic approach to a suprasellar cystic craniopharyngioma, the twist drill craniostomy is placed near the coronal suture, and fine-needle technique (0.9-mm outer-diamenter needle) is used to puncture the cyst (as depicted in a drawing by Erik-Olof Backlund, a pioneer in stereotactic techniques and disciple of Lars Leksell).

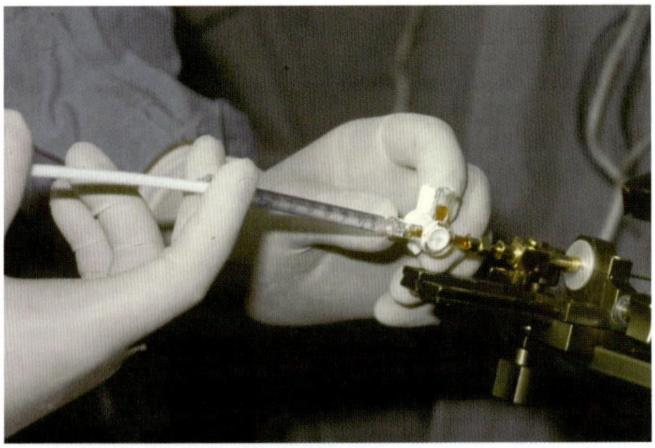

Fig. 15.2 Once the target is reached, the fine-needle stylet is removed and a three-way stopcock is attached to the needle hub. A tuberculin syringe is used to withdraw generally 1 mL of cyst fluid, which is sent to neuropathology to assess for the presence of cholesterol crystals under polarized light microscopy.

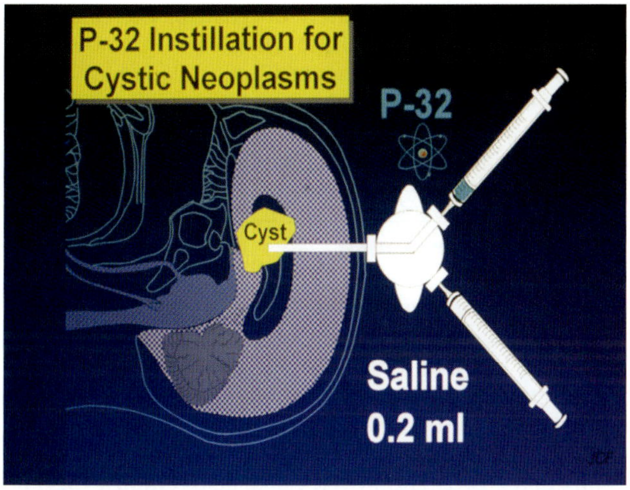

Fig. 15.3 Phosphorus 32 is injected into the cyst after attachment of a tuberculin syringe containing the predetermined amount of isotope, designed to deliver 250 Gy to the internal cyst wall over five half-lives of isotope decay (70 days). The isotope and cyst fluid are mixed by a barbotage method of withdrawal and the injection repeated five or more times. After this, 0.2 mL of sterile saline is injected via the other stopcock port to clear the needle of remaining isotope. The needle and stopcock are cleared of the isotope by the radiation safety officer, and that activity is subtracted from the calculated amount delivered to provide a final isotope volume.

ally in the range of 0.6 to 0.8 mL. The isotope contained in the syringe is injected through the stopcock into the cyst, and a barbotage method is used to ensure mixture. After this, the residual isotope is flushed out of the needle with 0.2 mL of sterile saline.

The goal is to restore the cyst volume to that of the original calculation. Collapse of the cyst induces a potential for internal wrinkling, which may suboptimally cause areas of the wrinkled cyst wall to receive an insufficient therapeutic dose of the β-emitting isotope. After the final isotope injection, the residual activity of ^{32}P (as well as all instruments and supplies used) is assayed by the nuclear pharmacist. Any activity is subtracted from the dose administered to the patient. Using our intraoperative CT, we do an immediate postoperative head scan and usually observe a small air bubble at the anterior margin of the cyst (the patients are supine on the CT scanner table). All patients are kept in the hospital for a one-night stay. In our experience, the mean radiation dose delivered is 224 Gy (range, 189–250 Gy to the cyst wall). The median cyst volume is 7.0 cm^3 (range, 2.0–20 cm^3).

◆ Follow-up

Clinical follow-up and imaging are obtained from each patient and the referring physicians. When possible, patients are contacted by telephone to determine their long-term outcomes. CT or MRI studies are normally performed at 3 months after the procedure and at quarterly intervals during the first year. In the next 5 years, they are requested annually. Formal neuro-ophthalmologic evaluations, as well as periodic endocrinologic assessments, are also performed.

◆ Results

In this review of 61 patients treated before 2008, 12 of the 61 patients eventually died as a result of tumor progression and eight were lost to follow-up (**Table 15.1**). The mean follow-up interval after diagnosis was 82 ± 14 months (47 ± 8 months after intracavitary irradiation). Actuarial survival rates after diagnosis were 90% at 5 years and 80% at 10 years. We noted a trend toward increased survival in children younger than 16 years of age. Among 53 patients who had long-term follow-up, treatment with ^{32}P intracavitary irradiation was considered to have failed in eight. The results of cyst response after intracavitary irradiation are shown in **Table 15.2**. In 15 patients with predominantly mono- or multicystic tumors, 80% of the tumors became smaller after treatment. In 37 patients with mixed solid and cystic tumors, 65% of the tumors became smaller after treatment. Cystic control was not associated with the patient's sex or age, tumor type (ie, mono- or multicystic tumor, mixed tumor with solid components), primary versus

Table 15.1 Patient Characteristics

Characteristics		No. patients (N = 61)	Percentage (%)
Sex	Male	33	54
	Female	28	46
Age	Mean	28	
	Range	3–74	
	Adults	38	62
	Children	23	38
Prior treatment	No treatment	29	48
	Craniotomy	26	43
	RT	13	21
	Aspiration	4	7
	CHT	1	2
Initial symptom	Headache	38	62
	Visual disturbance	28	46
	Lethargy	12	20
	Nausea	13	21
	Memory disturbance	4	7
	Amenorrhea	4	7
	Obesity	3	5
	Growth reduction	2	3
	Galactorrhea	1	2
	Mental disorder	1	2
	Seizure	1	2
	NA	3	5

Abbreviations: CHT, intracavitary chemotherapy with bleomycin; NA, not available; RT, fractionated radiation therapy.

Table 15.2 Tumor Cyst Response after Phosphorus 32 Intracavitary Irradiation

	No. (%)	
	Mono- or multicystic	Mixed cystic/solid
Response	(n = 15)	(n = 37)
Disappeared	3 (20%)	5 (14%)
Decreased	9 (60%)	19 (51%)
Unchanged	1 (7%)	4 (11%)
Increased	2 (13%)	9 (24%)

adjuvant treatment, cyst volume, radiation dose, preoperative visual acuity or field, or preoperative pituitary function. During follow-up, six patients developed new cystic tumors. Illustrative cases of tumor reduction are shown (**Figs. 15.4** and **15.5**).

◆ Additional Treatment

Among the 53 patients with long-term follow-up, treatment with intracavitary radiation failed in eight. Seventeen patients (32%) required additional cyst aspiration after intracavitary irradiation because of persistent symptoms related to larger cyst volume (**Fig. 15.6**). The median interval between intracavitary irradiation and additional cyst aspiration was 0.5 months (range, 0.2–18 months). Early cyst decompression is especially important in patients with progressive optic neuropathy. Although spontaneous cyst regression is the rule, it may take several months. Early cyst aspiration at 2 to 6 weeks after implantation may be necessary to achieve the best early response. In such patients, the procedure is repeated with stereotactic technique. After cyst puncture with fine-needle technique, we gently aspirate approximately one-half of the calculated volume. We assay the fluid to make sure that no significant isotope has been removed. Even if planned reaspiration is performed within 2 weeks of the ^{32}P instillation, a relatively small percentage of isotope can be recovered as it presumably adheres to the internal cyst wall.

◆ Clinical Response

Among our patients who underwent primary management with intracavitary irradiation for a monocystic craniopharyngioma, 48% had improved visual acuity and 52% had improved visual fields. Among patients who were treated as part of a multimodality strategy (intracavitary irradiation was an adjuvant strategy), 28% had improved visual acuity and 25% had improved visual fields (**Tables 15.3** and **15.4**). Three patients developed the new onset of visual abnormalities despite documented tumor regression. One of these patients underwent stereotactic radiosurgery to the solid component of the residual tumor. In these patients, visual dysfunction was thought to be related to a potentially adverse effect of ^{32}P irradiation.

◆ Endocrinologic Response

Among patients treated with primary monocystic intracavitary irradiation, 52% continue to have normal pituitary function, but 48% have had one or more axes of pituitary function loss. In the adjuvant treatment group, only 19% of patients had preserved endocrine function before the procedure, and 81% had documented loss of pituitary function in one or more axes. Three patients developed pituitary dysfunction as a consequence of cystic recurrence. Four patients developed diabetes insipidus after treatment with ^{32}P intracavitary radiation.

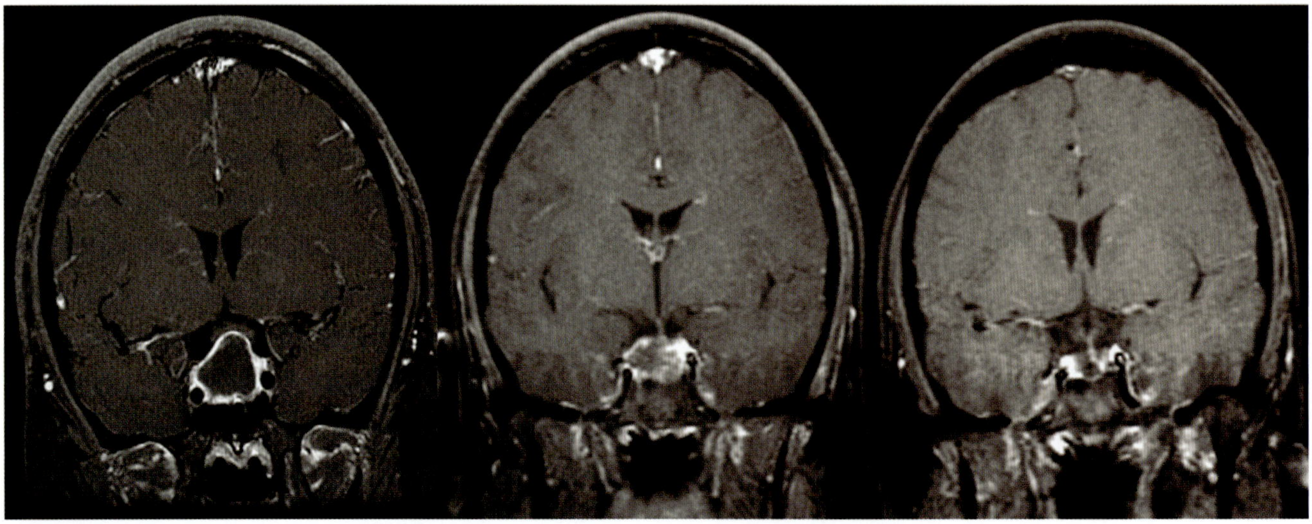

Fig. 15.4 Coronal gadolinium-enhanced MRI obtained in a 14-year-old boy with a cystic craniopharyngioma, intrasellar and suprasellar in location, compressing the overlying optic apparatus at the time of stereotactic P^{32} intracavitary irradiation as initial treatment (*left*). Coronal gadolinium-enhanced MRI obtained three months after stereotactic P^{32} irradiation, revealing reduction in the cystic tumor (*center*). Coronal gadolinium-enhanced MRI obtained three years after P^{32} irradiation, revealing complete cyst regression (*right*).

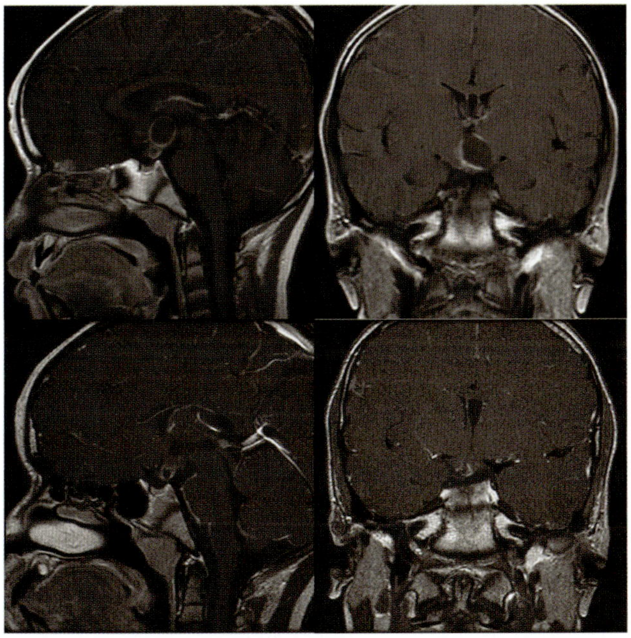

Fig. 15.5 Sagittal and coronal gadolinium-enhanced MRI obtained in a 5-year-old boy with a mixed solid and cystic craniopharyngioma, intrasellar and suprasellar in location, compressing the overlying optic apparatus at the time of stereotactic intracavitary irradiation as an initial treatment (*top*). Sagittal and coronal gadolinium-enhanced MRI obtained 2 years after stereotactic irradiation, revealing marked reduction in the cystic portion of the tumor (*bottom*).

◆ Other Complications

In our total 28-year experience, only one patient developed an early postoperative complication. A patient with a mixed multicystic and solid craniopharyngioma underwent multiple endoscopic skull base procedures but developed a tumor cyst of the third ventricle. Before the planned procedure, the cyst spontaneously ruptured into the ventricle and decompressed. However, within a matter of months, the cyst re-formed, and intracavitary stereotactic irradiation was performed. Several days after this procedure, the patient was readmitted with headache, low-grade fever, stiff neck, and cerebrospinal fluid (CSF) pleocytosis. No radioactivity was confirmed in the CSF. The patient had an aseptic meningitic reaction that resolved with corticosteroids. This patient has undergone additional surgical procedures followed by gamma knife stereotactic radiosurgery.[9,10]

◆ Discussion

Patients who are eligible for radical gross total resection of a craniopharyngioma may have the best long-term response in terms of tumor control.[11–19] However, such patients often pay a significant price that may include endocrinologic, cognitive, behavioral, and visual difficulties.[20,21] Craniopharyngiomas remain one of the most difficult tumors for neurosurgeons to manage. For patients, the side effects of surgery are often significant. Because of the attachment of these tumors to critical neurovascular, endocrine, and visual structures, patients are often unable to undergo radical resection with an acceptable morbidity. For most of these patients, multimodality management, administered over the course of years, is frequently necessary.[10,22] The options for craniopharyngioma management include fractionated radiation therapy,[22] cyst management with intracavitary irradiation, intracystic chemotherapy with bleomycin,[23–28] endoscopic resection, and, more recently, phase I trials with interferon.

Because craniopharyngiomas frequently are detected in childhood, we generally try to withhold conventional fractionated radiation therapy, even when it can be administered with modern techniques of image-guided radiation therapy.[22] Intracavitary irradiation with ^{32}P is an additional tool for treating patients with cystic craniopharyngiomas. Using modern imaging techniques, we find that most patients have a solid, small tumor component with one or more cysts arising from it. Intracavitary irradiation provides symptomatic cyst control in a high percentage of patients, but it does not solve the ultimate progression of the solid component of the tumor. It also does not prevent the formation of new tumor cysts. In

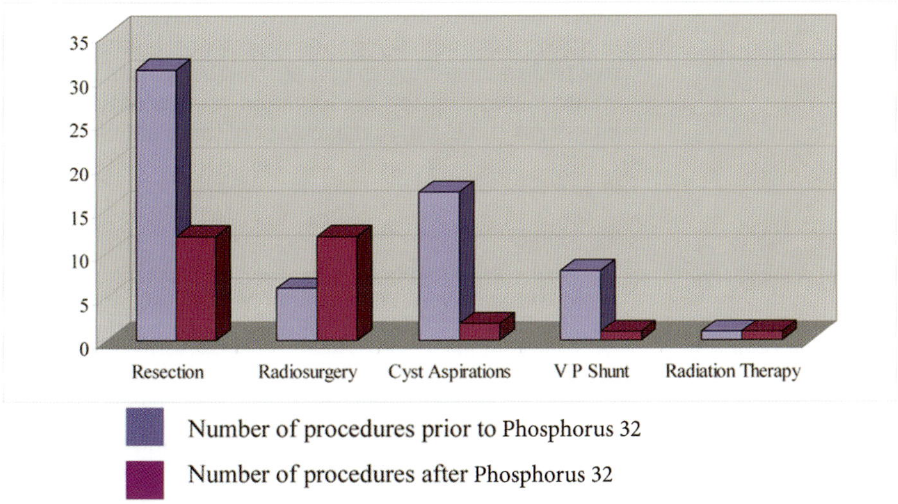

Fig. 15.6 Surgical procedures before and after P^{32} intracavitary irradiation in patients with cystic craniopharyngioma. In a comparison of the numbers of procedures performed before and after intracavitary radiation, the number of additional procedures tended to decrease after intracavitary radiation.

Table 15.3 Preoperative Visual and Endocrine Function

	No. patients (%)	
	Primary treatment	**Adjuvant treatment**
Characteristics	(n = 29)	(n = 32)
Visual acuity		
Normal	17 (59%)	12 (38%)
Decreased	10 (34%)	8 (25%)
Blind	0 (0%)	10 (31%)
NA	2	2
Visual field		
Normal	8 (28%)	10 (31%)
Field cut	18 (62%)	21 (66%)
NA	3	1
Endocrine function		
Normal	15 (52%)	6 (19%)
Stalk effect[a]	4 (14%)	0 (0%)
Partial[b]	5 (17%)	9 (28%)
Panhypopituitarism	4 (14%)	15 (47%)
Diabetes insipidus	4 (14%)	18 (56%)
NA	2	2

Abbreviation: NA, not available.
[a]Patients with increased prolactin.
[b]Patients with deficiency of one to three anterior pituitary hormones.

Table 15.4 Postoperative Visual and Endocrine Function

	No. patients (%)	
	Primary treatment	**Adjuvant treatment**
Characteristics	(n = 29)	(n = 32)
Visual acuity		
Normal	15 (52%)	9 (28%)
Decreased	7 (24%)	11 (34%)
Delayed worsening	5 (17%)	5 (16%)
NA	2	7
Visual field		
Normal	16 (55%)	8 (25%)
Unchanged	5 (17%)	10 (31%)
Delayed worsening	6 (21%)	7 (22%)
NA	2	7
Endocrine function		
Normal	11 (38%)	4 (13%)
Stalk effect[a]	0 (0%)	0 (0%)
Partial[b]	6 (21%)	5 (16%)
Panhypopituitarism	10 (34%)	17 (53%)
Diabetes insipidus	8 (28%)	15 (47%)
NA	2	6

Abbreviation: NA, not available.
[a]Patients with increased prolactin.
[b]Patients with deficiency of one to three anterior pituitary hormones.

such patients, repeat surgery or stereotactic radiosurgery may be necessary.[9,10]

The continuing goals for the management of craniopharyngioma include preservation of visual and endocrine function and reduction in the risk for delayed cognitive dysfunction. Intracavitary irradiation with ^{32}P has more than a 60-year history and remains a valuable tool. The use of this tool requires training and expertise, as emphasized by Leksell et al[1] and Backlund.[3] Access to pure β emitters is critical to the successful continued management of tumor cysts when they develop. The need for delayed stereotactic aspiration with precise frame-based imaging guidance, especially when tumors are wrapped around critical vascular and optic nerve structures, is critical.

◆ Conclusion

Stereotactic ^{32}P intracavitary irradiation has a relatively low risk. It is an effective strategy for the primary treatment of monocystic craniopharyngiomas and for the adjuvant management of the cystic component of multicystic or mixed solid craniopharyngiomas. Craniopharyngiomas are one of the most difficult tumors that neurosurgeons encounter. Efforts to minimize morbidity from the tumor or from its treatment can reduce the significant dysfunction that patients with cranopharyngioma experience. Minimally invasive treatment strategies that pursue the goals of cognitive, endocrine, and vision preservation remain critical to the long-term successful management of these patients.

References

1. Leksell L, Backlund EO, Johansson L. Treatment of craniopharyngiomas. Acta Chir Scand 1967;133(5):345–350
2. Wycis HT, Robbins R, Spiegeladolf M, Meszaros J, Spiegel EA. Studies in stereoencephalotomy III; treatment of a cystic craniopharyngioma by injection of radioactive P32. Confin Neurol 1954;14(4):193–202
3. Backlund EO. Studies on craniopharyngiomas. 3. Stereotaxic treatment with intracystic yttrium-90. Acta Chir Scand 1973;139(3):237–247
4. Van den Berge JH, Blaauw G, Breeman WA, Rahmy A, Wijngaarde R. Intracavitary brachytherapy of cystic craniopharyngiomas. J Neurosurg 1992;77(4):545–550
5. Voges J, Sturm V, Lehrke R, Treuer H, Gauss C, Berthold F. Cystic craniopharyngioma: long-term results after intracavitary irradiation with stereotactically applied colloidal beta-emitting radioactive sources. Neurosurgery 1997;40(2):263–269, discussion 269–270
6. Hasegawa T, Kondziolka D, Hadjipanayis CG, Lunsford LD. Management of cystic craniopharyngiomas with phosphorus-32 intracav-

itary irradiation. Neurosurgery 2004;54(4):813–820, discussion 820–822

7. Lunsford LD, Pollock BE, Kondziolka DS, Levine G, Flickinger JC. Stereotactic options in the management of craniopharyngioma. Pediatr Neurosurg 1994;21(Suppl 1):90–97
8. Pollock BE, Lunsford LD, Kondziolka D, Levine G, Flickinger JC. Phosphorus-32 intracavitary irradiation of cystic craniopharyngiomas: current technique and long-term results. Int J Radiat Oncol Biol Phys 1995;33(2):437–446
9. Chiou SM, Lunsford LD, Niranjan A, Kondziolka D, Flickinger JC. Stereotactic radiosurgery of residual or recurrent craniopharyngioma, after surgery, with or without radiation therapy. Neuro-oncol 2001;3(3):159–166
10. Niranjan A, Kano H, Mathieu D, Kondziolka D, Flickinger JC, Lunsford LD. Radiosurgery for craniopharyngioma. Int J Radiat Oncol Biol Phys 2010;78(1):64–71
11. Abe T, Lüdecke DK. Transnasal surgery for infradiaphragmatic craniopharyngiomas in pediatric patients. Neurosurgery 1999;44(5):957–964, discussion 964–966
12. Duff JM, Meyer FB, Ilstrup DM, Laws ERJ, Schleck CD, Scheithauer BW. Long-term outcomes for surgically resected craniopharyngiomas. Neurosurgery 2000;46(2):291–302, discussion 302–305
13. Fahlbusch R, Honegger J, Paulus W, Huk W, Buchfelder M. Surgical treatment of craniopharyngiomas: experience with 168 patients. J Neurosurg 1999;90(2):237–250
14. Honegger J, Buchfelder M, Fahlbusch R. Surgical treatment of craniopharyngiomas: endocrinological results. J Neurosurg 1999;90(2):251–257
15. Isaac MA, Hahn SS, Kim JA, Bogart JA, Chung CT. Management of craniopharyngioma. Cancer J 2001;7(6):516–520
16. Kalapurakal JA, Goldman S, Hsieh YC, Tomita T, Marymont MH. Clinical outcome in children with recurrent craniopharyngioma after primary surgery. Cancer J 2000;6(6):388–393
17. Khafaga Y, Jenkin D, Kanaan I, Hassounah M, Al Shabanah M, Gray A. Craniopharyngioma in children. Int J Radiat Oncol Biol Phys 1998;42(3):601–606
18. Kim SK, Wang KC, Shin SH, Choe G, Chi JG, Cho BK. Radical excision of pediatric craniopharyngioma: recurrence pattern and prognostic factors. Childs Nerv Syst 2001;17(9):531–536, discussion 537
19. Wang KC, Kim SK, Choe G, Chi JG, Cho BK. Growth patterns of craniopharyngioma in children: role of the diaphragm sellae and its surgical implication. Surg Neurol 2002;57(1):25–33
20. Caldarelli M, di Rocco C, Papacci F, Colosimo C Jr. Management of recurrent craniopharyngioma. Acta Neurochir (Wien) 1998;140(5):447–454
21. Fisher PG, Jenab J, Goldthwaite PT, et al. Outcomes and failure patterns in childhood craniopharyngiomas. Childs Nerv Syst 1998;14(10):558–563
22. Habrand JL, Ganry O, Couanet D, et al. The role of radiation therapy in the management of craniopharyngioma: a 25-year experience and review of the literature. Int J Radiat Oncol Biol Phys 1999;44(2):255–263
23. Cavalheiro S, Sparapani FV, Franco JO, da Silva MC, Braga FM. Use of bleomycin in intratumoral chemotherapy for cystic craniopharyngioma. Case report. J Neurosurg 1996;84(1):124–126
24. Hader WJ, Steinbok P, Hukin J, Fryer C. Intratumoral therapy with bleomycin for cystic craniopharyngiomas in children. Pediatr Neurosurg 2000;33(4):211–218
25. Haisa T, Ueki K, Yoshida S. Toxic effects of bleomycin on the hypothalamus following its administration into a cystic craniopharyngioma. Br J Neurosurg 1994;8(6):747–750
26. Hetelekidis S, Barnes PD, Tao ML, et al. 20-year experience in childhood craniopharyngioma. Int J Radiat Oncol Biol Phys 1993;27(2):189–195
27. Jiang R, Liu Z, Zhu C. Preliminary exploration of the clinical effect of bleomycin on craniopharyngiomas. Stereotact Funct Neurosurg 2002;78(2):84–94
28. Savas A, Arasil E, Batay F, Selcuki M, Kanpolat Y. Intracavitary chemotherapy of polycystic craniopharyngioma with bleomycin. Acta Neurochir (Wien) 1999;141(5):547–548, discussion 549

16 Chemotherapy Options for Sellar and Parasellar Tumors

Arnaldo Neves Da Silva and David Schiff

Among the sellar and parasellar tumors that may be amenable to treatment with chemotherapy are pituitary carcinomas, craniopharyngiomas, germ cell tumors, chordomas, plasmacytomas, meningiomas, and primary central nervous system (CNS) lymphomas of the pituitary. Even though these tumors all together account for a very small fraction of intracranial neoplasms, they deserve special attention because of their location, which may result in endocrine and visual disturbances.

◆ Pituitary Carcinomas

Pituitary carcinomas are extremely rare and aggressive tumors, accounting for only 0.1 to 0.2% of all pituitary tumors.[1–3] The hallmark of these tumors is concomitant metastasis, either outside the CNS or in noncontiguous foci within the CNS.

The mainstay of the treatment of pituitary carcinoma remains surgery, with either conventional or focused adjuvant radiation therapy modalities that have been well discussed in other chapters of this book. However, when the tumor is a carcinoma, disease generally progresses despite these interventions. Cytotoxic chemotherapy is usually employed as a last resort, and several single case reports and small series of pituitary carcinomas treated with chemotherapy have been published[2,4–18] (**Table 16.1**).

◆ Temozolomide

Temozolomide (TMZ) is an imidazotetrazine derivative that acts as a DNA-methylating agent. It is absorbed rapidly after oral administration and crosses the blood-brain barrier.[20] TMZ in addition to radiation therapy is the standard treatment for glioblastoma (GBM).[21,22] The effect of TMZ depends on methylation of a specific guanine in DNA. MGMT (O-6-methylguanine-DNA methyltransferase) is a DNA repair enzyme removing the alkyl group from the guanine.[23,24] A high level of expression of MGMT in gliomas implicates a poor response to TMZ.[23] McCormack et al, analyzing MGMT expression in 88 pituitary tumor samples, found low MGMT expression in only 13% of the cases and did not find a significant difference between MGMT expression in invasive and noninvasive tumors, or in recurrent and nonrecurrent tumors.[25]

TMZ is usually administered at a dose of 200 mg/m^2 per day for 5 days in cycles of 28 days, as for high-grade gliomas. Recently, a multicenter Phase II study by the Spanish Neuro-Oncology Group using extended-schedule dose-dense TMZ in refractory gliomas (85 mg/m^2 per day for 21 consecutive days in 28-day cycles until disease progression or unacceptable toxicity) showed activity deserving further evaluation in larger cohorts.[26] The rationale for the protracted schedule is the continuous depletion of MGMT, enhancing the cytotoxicity of TMZ.[27,28]

Fadul et al in 2004 reported in abstract form two cases of pituitary carcinoma that responded partially to TMZ. The first patient, who had a prolactin-secreting tumor, received 10 cycles of TMZ with reduction of prolactin levels and control of pain caused by metastasis to the cervical and thoracic spine; treatment was stopped secondary to persistent fatigue. The second patient, who had a nonsecreting pituitary carcinoma and local invasion plus multiple drop metastases to the cervical and thoracic spinal cord, received 12 cycles of TMZ with improvement of visual fields and magnetic resonance imaging (MRI) showing reduction of the metastasis volume until treatment was discontinued secondary to lymphopenia.[29] Also in 2004, Zhu et al reported the successful use of TMZ in a patient with refractory malignant prolactinoma.[30]

Another reported case summarized the course of a 72-year-old man who had a prolactin-secreting pituitary carcinoma treated with TMZ during 24 months, with stabilization of his prolactin levels, marked reduction of the size of the cerebellopontine angle and cervical metastatic deposits, and a remarkable functional recovery.[31] Kovacs et al reported a case of a prolactin-secreting pituitary carcinoma treated with TMZ with decrease of serum prolactin levels and clinical improvement.[32] Kovacs et al also demonstrated hemorrhage, necrosis, fibrosis, and shrinkage in the tumor after TMZ treatment. Neuronal transformation was also seen, a process described in various tumor types including pituitary adenomas, mainly growth hormone (GH)–producing tumors.[33,34] The cause of the neuronal transformation is unknown, and the authors believe that TMZ may act similarly to nerve growth factor, causing neuronal metaplasia, which is the transformation of pituitary tumor cells to nerve cells.

Table 16.1 Single Case Reports and Small Series of Pituitary Carcinomas Treated with Chemotherapy before Temozolomide

Reference	Tumor/ hormone	Site of metastases	Chemotherapy	Outcome
Kaiser et al, 1983	ACTH	Liver, lung, mediastinum, ilium, hip, sacral and lumbar spine	Cyclophosphamide + Adriamycin + 5-FU (5 cycles)	Disease control
Vaughan et al, 1985	ACTH	Invasive ACTH	Procarbazine + VP + CCNU (12 weeks)	Disease control
Hashimoto et al, 1986	GH	Left occipital lobe, pons, both cerebellopontine angles, spinal cord	Cisplatin + vinblastine + bleomycin (3/52)	No response
Kasperlik-Zaluska et al, 1987	GH	Invasive, not malignant	Doxorubicin + CCNU (4 cycles)	Disease control
Asai et al, 1988	GH	Right frontal lobe	Methotrexate + 5-FU	Follow-up of 2 years, no recurrence
Nawata et al, 1990	ACTH	Liver, lung, olfactory bulb	Mitotane + carmofur (derivative of 5- FU)	Disease progression, death within 4 months of chemotherapy
Petterson et al, 1992	PRL	Frontal lobe, lateral ventricle, cerebellopontine angle, left vertebral artery	CCNU + procarbazine + VP	Initial response but then disease progression
Walker et al, 1993	PRL	Liver, lungs, hilar nodes	CCNU + 5-FU + folinic acid	Disease progression, death within a month
Walker et al, 1993	PRL	Thoracic and lumbar vertebrae, femur	CCNU + 5-FU + folinic acid	Disease progression, death within weeks
Mixson et al, 1993	TSH	Base of brain, lung, liver, abdominal cavity, bone	5-FU + Adriamycin + cyclophosphamide	Initial response but death within 5 months of treatment
Beauchesne et al, 1995	FSH	Thoracic and lumbar spine, lymph nodes, frontal lobe	VP-16 + cisplatin	Disease progression
Gollard et al, 1995	PRL	Recurrence in transsphenoidal surgery tracts, lymph nodes, ovary, uterus	Cisplatin + VP (2 cycles) Procarbazine + CCNU + vincristine (2 cycles) + tamoxifen	Alive 20 months after initial presentation
Pernicone et al, 1997	PRL	Oral submucosa, ovaries, myometrium, lymph nodes	Cisplatin + procarbazine + CCNU + vincristine	No response
Pernicone et al, 1997	PRL	Spinal subarachnoid	Cisplatin + procarbazine + CCNU + vincristine	No response, died within 15 months
Pernicone et al, 1997	Null cell	Femur, liver	Cisplatin + procarbazine + CCNU + vincristine	No response, death within 4 years
Kaltsas et al, 1998	GH	Extension to right cavernous sinus	CCNU + 5-FU (2 cycles)	Alive 5 years after initiation of chemotherapy
Kaltsas et al, 1998	PRL	Pituitary fossa, liver, lungs	CCNU + 5-FU (2 cycles)	Death 4 weeks after liver metastases noted (3 months after initiation of chemotherapy)
Kaltsas et al, 1998	PRL	Pituitary fossa, thoracic and lumbar spine	CCNU + 5-FU (1 cycle)	Death 5 months after spinal metastases noted (6 months after initiation of chemotherapy)
Kaltsas et al, 1998	PRL	Frontal lobe, parietal lobe, left orbit	CCNU + 5-FU (6 cycles) Carboplatin (5 cycles) Carboplatin (3 cycles) 5-FU/INF-a (8 cycles) Carboplatin/INF-a (4 cycles)	Death 11 months after CNS metastases noted (11 years after chemotherapy)
Kaltsas et al, 1998	ACTH	Thoracic spine, liver	CCNU + 5-FU (6 cycles) Carboplatin (6 cycles) DTIC (2 cycles)	Death 18 months after spinal metastases noted (3 years after chemotherapy)
Kaltsas et al, 1998	PRL	Retrosellar and brainstem extensions	CCNU + 5-FU (2 cycles)	Death from other cause (6 months after initiation of chemotherapy)
Kaltsas et al, 1998	ACTH	Pituitary fossa, both cavernous sinuses	CCNU + 5-FU (4 cycles) Carboplatin + 5-FU (6 cycles)	Alive 4 years after initiation of chemotherapy
McCutcheon et al, 2000	FSH/ LH	Left cavernous sinus, left frontal lobe, Meckel's cave, petrous apex	Cyclophosphamide + Adriamycin + diethyltriazinoimidazole + carboxamide (7 cycles)	Died of fungal septicemia 9 months after last resective surgery (17 months after discovery of dural metastasis)

Abbreviations: ACTH, adrenocorticotropic hormone; CCNU, lomustine; DTIC, dacarbazine; FSH, follicle-stimulating hormone; 5-FU, 5-fluorouracil; GH, growth hormone; INF, interferon; LH, luteinizing hormone; PRL, prolactin; TSH, thyroid-stimulating hormone; VP, etoposide.

Source: Adapted from Kaltsas et al.[19]

Hagen et al reported two patients with invasive pituitary macroadenoma and one patient with pituitary carcinoma treated with TMZ who experienced a significant decrease in tumor volume, hormone hypersecretion, and symptoms. All three patients were tested for MGMT expression; this was negative in two patients, and only a few nuclei stained positive in the third patient, potentially explaining the favorable treatment response.[24]

Neff et al reported a patient who had an invasive prolactinoma treated with TMZ, with marked decrease and stabilization of the prolactin levels and continuous tumor bulk reduction on follow-up imaging over 26 cycles of TMZ.[35]

Moyes et al reported a case of a patient with Nelson syndrome, an aggressive ACTH-secreting macroadenoma, in addition to high levels of ACTH and skin hyperpigmentation, treated successfully with TMZ. The ACTH levels fell from 2472 to 389 pmol/L, and follow-up imaging confirmed marked shrinkage of the tumor after 4 cycles of TMZ.[36] Immunostaining was negative for MGMT, again perhaps explaining the favorable tumor response.

Mohammed et al published three cases of aggressive pituitary macroadenomas treated with TMZ. The first two patients had ACTH-secreting macroadenomas of the Crooke's cell variant, and the third patient harbored GBM with an incidental pituitary tumor. The first two patients had radiologic evidence of tumor shrinkage and clinical improvement during treatment. One of these patients had a diagnosis of Nelson syndrome. The third patient underwent radiation therapy and TMZ for GBM, and pituitary tumor reduction was also noticed on follow-up scans, with collapse of the suprasellar component into the sella despite the sellar area not having been included in the radiation treatment field.[37]

Recently, Thearle et al reported a patient with an invasive ACTH-secreting macroadenoma who failed conventional treatment and developed rapid tumor growth leading to the compromise of multiple cranial nerves. This patient was treated with a combination of TMZ and capecitabine (Xeloda), with a marked tumor burden reduction and a decrease in ACTH levels of more than 90%. The tumor recurred after 5 months with a hypermetabolic positron emission tomography (PET) scan, suggesting transformation into a more aggressive histology.[38] Capecitabine is an oral chemotherapeutic agent that is converted to 5-fluorouracil (5-FU) in vivo by the enzyme thymidine phosphorylase.[39] 5-FU is metabolized to 5-dUMP, which produces a deficiency of thymidylate by inhibiting thymidylate synthase (TS). This leads to a decrease in DNA synthesis and inhibition of cell division by reducing the conversion of UMP to dTMP by TS, leading to thymidylate deficiency. TMZ causes DNA damage at any point in the cell cycle through base pair mismatch of O-6-methylguanine with thymidine in the sister chromatid instead of cytosine, which arises because the mismatch repair enzymes misread the methylated guanine as an adenosine and place thymidine in the sister chromatid. The basis of the use of capecitabine for 10 days before the addition of TMZ is that decreased thymidine levels intracellularly accentuate the mismatch repair process leading to a break in DNA, which is a potent stimulus for apoptosis.[38,39]

Bush et al reported a retrospective series of seven patients with aggressive pituitary tumors treated with TMZ.[40] MGMT promoter methylation and MGMT expression in 14 surgical specimens from these seven patients were compared and correlated with the clinical response to TMZ. Clinically significant tumor reduction was observed in two patients, a 20% tumor reduction in one, stable disease in three, and progressive metastatic disease in one patient. The DNA promoter site for MGMT was unmethylated, and variable amounts of MGMT expression were seen in all 14 specimens. The authors could not find any correlation between MGMT expression and clinical outcomes but concluded that TMZ is a valuable alternative in the management of aggressive pituitary tumors.

Laws et al in 2003 published the results of a Phase I study of transsphenoidal post-resection implantation of Gliadel wafers in nine patients with aggressive pituitary adenomas.[41] Gliadel is a polymer wafer impregnated with BCNU (bis-chloroethyl-nitrosurea), an alkylating agent, designed to capitalize on the concept of delivering local treatment to brain tumors, avoiding the toxic effects of systemic treatment and bypassing the blood-brain barrier.[42,43] Three patients were disease-free after a mean follow-up of 19 months, two had stable residual disease, one had disease progression, two patients died secondary to disease progression, and one died because of a stroke. The study concluded that Gliadel implantation into the sella turcica for aggressive pituitary tumors is safe.[41] No further studies of this agent in pituitary adenomas have been reported.

With respect to ongoing studies, presently there is one Phase II study evaluating the safety and efficacy of TMZ in the treatment of invasive pituitary tumors (NCT00601289). In addition, there is one study investigating the use of lapatinib in slowing the growth rate of pituitary tumors. Lapatinib is an FDA-approved drug used to treat breast cancer and has been shown to inhibit both epidermal growth factor receptor (EGFR) and erbB2 tyrosine kinases, which are overexpressed in pituitary adenomas.

◆ Craniopharyngiomas

Craniopharyngiomas are benign tumors of the sellar and parasellar region that may be solid, cystic, or a combination of the two. Their treatment poses a challenge because the tumors are difficult to completely resect, and recurrence, even in instances of presumed gross total resection, is common. Craniopharyngiomas are the most common suprasellar tumor in the pediatric age group and the most common nonglial primary intracranial tumor in children.[44,45]

The treatment of craniopharyngiomas is multidisciplinary, involving surgical resection by craniotomy or the transsphenoidal route, fractionated radiation therapy, and radiosurgery for residual tumor.[44] In patients with primarily cystic tumors, recurrent tumors, and/or tumors with a difficult surgical approach, and in young patients, for whom postponing more aggressive treatment such as radiation therapy or surgery is desirable, the use of intracavitary bleomycin has a role.[46] Bleomycin, an antibiotic produced from the fungus *Streptomyces verticillus*, induces single-strand and double-strand DNA breaks.[46–48] The double-strand breaks and resulting loss of chromosome fragments probably account for bleomycin cytotoxicity.[46,49]

Takahashi et al in 1985 reported the first seven cases of craniopharyngiomas treated with intracavitary bleomycin administered through an Ommaya reservoir inserted into the cyst.[50] Among these patients, those with cystic tumors had a better outcome than the ones with solid or combination lesions.[50] This initial publication was supported by several others.[51–60]

Hargrave in 2006, analyzing the data of those publications, found that stable disease (stable cyst volume reduction) was achieved in 57% of the patients, with an obviously better response seen in cystic craniopharyngiomas. The median dose of bleomycin was 5 mg (2–15 mg). Seventy-one percent of the patients received 3 doses per week (1–7 doses); the median number of doses was 8 (1–30). The median cumulative dose was 53 mg (5–150 mg).[61] The major side effects directly attributed to bleomycin were headaches (42%), fever (36%), nausea and vomiting (21%), endocrine manifestations (16%), somnolence (15%), infarct/hemorrhage (10%), personality changes, vision changes (7%), and hearing problems, seizures, and death related to bleomycin therapy (1%).[61]

Hukin et al recently reported the Canadian experience with intracystic bleomycin.[62] Seventeen patients were reported, of whom 12 were treated at the time of diagnosis and five at recurrence. Five patients achieved a complete response and six a partial response, and five had a minor response to intracystic bleomycin. The treatment protocol varied between centers, with most following a thrice-weekly regimen. The course of treatment averaged 4 weeks (range, 2–15 weeks), and the median dose per course was 36 mg (range, 15–75 mg). The median dose per instillation was 3 mg (range, 2–5 mg), and the median dose per week was 9 mg (range, 4–20 mg). In a single injection, the median drug concentration within the cyst was 0.09 mg/mL per dose (range, 0.01–2 mg/mL per dose). The median follow-up was 4 years (range, 0.5–10.2 years), and the median progression-free survival (PFS) was 1.8 years (range, 0.3–6.1 years). Observed complications included transient symptomatic peritumoral edema in two patients, precocious puberty in one patient, and panhypopituitarism in two patients.

Bleomycin is a neurotoxic drug; if leakage occurs, severe complications may develop, such as hypothalamic toxicity causing hypersomnia, personality changes, memory impairment, and thermal dysfunction,[60] and even death.[57]

Lactate dehydrogenase (LDH) activity in craniopharyngioma fluid is elevated typically to ~3000 units, and the LDH isoenzyme pattern shows elevation of L4 and L5 fractions. Repeated injection of bleomycin causes a gradual clearing of the motor oil–colored cystic fluid, with a decrease in LDH activity (<1000 units), and the L4 and L5 fractions show a flat pattern.[50,63]

Laws et al treated one patient who had craniopharyngioma with Gliadel placement after transsphenoidal tumor resection. This patient had previously undergone three transsphenoidal resections, one craniotomy, and one gamma knife radiosurgery; at recurrence, the patient was treated with a new transsphenoidal tumor resection and placement of three Gliadel wafers. After 6 months of follow-up, no tumor recurrence was seen.[41]

Jakacki et al reported a Phase II evaluation of systemic interferon alfa-2a (IFN-α-2a) in patients with progressive and/or recurrent craniopharyngiomas.[64] The rationale for using IFN-α-2a is that the drug shows activity against squamous cell skin carcinoma, which is believed to have the same embryologic origin as craniopharyngioma.[65,66] IFNs exert antitumor activity through direct antiproliferative, cytotoxic, and maturational effects, and they also modulate the immune response.[64,67,68] IFN-α-2a was administered in a dose of 8 million units (MU) per square meter daily for 16 weeks (induction phase), followed by the same dose three times per week for 32 weeks (maintenance phase). Fifteen patients received the drug, but only 12 could be followed with imaging. Radiologic response was seen in three patients with predominantly cystic tumors.

Intratumoral IFN-α was used in nine patients, with complete disappearance of the tumor in seven and partial reduction in two. Mean follow-up was 1 year and 8 months (range, 1–3.5 years), and the doses ranged from 18 to 36 MU. The most frequent side effects of IFN-α are fatigue, fever, weight loss, loss of appetite, and behavioral changes.[59]

IFN-α also seems to reduce the size of cystic craniopharyngiomas by activating the Fas apoptotic pathway. Twenty-one patients with cystic craniopharyngiomas received intracystic IFN-α; the tumor size of all patients and the apoptotic factor soluble FasL (sFasL) concentration in eight patients were monitored. A complete response (tumor reduction) was observed in 11 patients (52.4%), a partial response in seven (33.3%), and a minor response in three (14.3%). The concentration of sFasL was increased in all eight patients, and it was examined concomitantly with tumor reduction. The mean follow-up was 27 months (range, 6 months to 4 years). Two patients underwent surgical resection, and tumor removal was easier than in the ones who had received chemotherapy preoperatively.[69]

◆ Pituitary Lymphomas

Although particularly rare, primary central nervous system lymphomas (PCNSLs) arising from the sellar and parasellar region are one of the causes of hypothalamic-pituitary dysfunction.[70] In a series of 1120 patients with pituitary tumors resected via the transsphenoidal route, only one case (0.1%) was diagnosed as a pituitary lymphoma.[71] In another series of 353 patients with pituitary masses, pituitary lymphoma was found in one case (0.3%).[72] The majority of PCNSLs are B-cell lymphomas, and besides acquired immunodeficiency syndrome (AIDS) and other immunodeficiency conditions, lymphocytic hypophysitis and pituitary adenomas have been implicated as risk factors for pituitary lymphomas.[73]

The treatment of PCNSL traditionally combines whole-brain radiation therapy (WBRT) and chemotherapy with methotrexate (MTX) alone or in combination with other agents. MTX is a folate antagonist and has limited penetration in the CNS because of its high degree of ionization at a physiologic pH; high doses (≥ 3.5 g/m^2) are used to achieve cytotoxic intratumoral concentrations.[74] We extrapolate the treatment of PCNSL anywhere in the CNS to lesions arising in the sellar and parasellar areas.

Several combination regimens of WBRT and MTX are associated with reasonable response rates.[75–80] The combination of MTX, procarbazine, and vincristine (MPV) followed by WBRT and cytarabine after radiation is associated with an overall response rate of 91%, a PFS of 24 months, and an overall survival of 36.9 months.[81] In another important study, rituximab, a chimeric monoclonal antibody against the protein CD20, which is primarily found on the surface of B cells, was tested with MPV followed by a lower dose of WBRT (23.4 Gy for patients who had complete response to chemotherapy or 45 Gy for patients who did not have a complete response).[77] The overall response rate was 93%, and the 2-year median PFS rate was 57%. No treatment-related neurotoxicity was observed. The authors concluded that the addition of rituximab to MPV (R-MPV) increased the risk for significant neutropenia requiring routine growth factor support, that additional cycles of R-MPV nearly doubled the complete response rate, and that reduced-dose WBRT was not associated with neurocognitive decline.

Chemotherapy protocols without WBRT were designed to avoid the delayed cognitive effects associated with radiation therapy, particularly in patients older than 60 years of age and in those with underlying vascular risk factors, with radiation therapy reserved for an eventual relapse.[74] Intravenous MTX alone, 8 g/m^2, was used in 25 patients, with a complete response achieved in 52% of the patients, a median PFS of 12.8 months, and a median overall survival of 55.4 months.[82,83] Interestingly, 5 of 25 patients in this trial treated with MTX alone achieved a complete response and, after a median follow-up of 6.8 years, had not had a relapse. Several other drugs, including rituximab, have been added to MTX therapy in regimens that do not include WBRT,[84,85] with the intent to achieve a more durable response.

The blood-brain barrier can limit the diffusion of MTX into brain and tumor. The blood-brain barrier can be disrupted with the use of osmotic agents (ie, mannitol), enhancing drug delivery to the tumor. A multicenter analysis of 149 patients treated with blood-brain barrier disruption and intra-arterial MTX over 23 years showed an overall response rate of 81.9% (57.8% complete response), a median overall survival of 3.1 years (25% estimated survival at 8.5 years), a median PFS of 1.8 years, a 5-year PFS rate of 31%, and a 7-year PFS rate of 25%.[86] Focal seizures (9.2%) were the most frequent side effect, and no long-term sequelae were reported. The study concluded that tumor control and outcomes were comparable or superior to those achieved with other PCNSL treatment regimens.

Intrathecal chemotherapy is reserved for patients with concomitant leptomeningeal lymphoma, although prospective[87–89] and retrospective[90,91] studies indicate that intrathecal chemotherapy does not improve outcomes in patients who received MTX-based therapy.[75] Additionally, some studies indicate that systemic MTX eradicates neoplastic cells from the cerebrospinal fluid (CSF).[92,93] Other aspects should be taken into consideration before intrathecal chemotherapy is started, including the risks for complications of Ommaya reservoir placement, chemical meningitis, drug leakage outside the CNS, and infection. Several clinical trials have included intrathecal chemotherapy.[78,79,84,85]

Patients with relapse of PCNSL after an initial response to therapy have a median survival of ~4.5 months, posing a challenge to the clinician. WBRT alone is associated with a radiographic response in 74 to 79% of patients, with a median survival after radiation of 10.9 to 16 months; patients younger than 60 years of age tend to perform better.[74] Several chemotherapeutic agents have been used for relapsed PCNSL. Intraventricular rituximab is an alternative for patients who did not receive it as an initial therapy.[94] A trial comparing intraventricular rituximab and intraventricular MTX in patients with relapsed PCNSL is ongoing.

◆ Germ Cell Tumors

Primary intracranial germ cell tumors account for 1% of all primary brain tumors in adults and are divided into five types: germinomas (65%), teratomas (18%), embryonic carcinomas (5%), choriocarcinomas (5%), and endodermal sinus tumors (7%).[95,96] Germinomas are more often located in the suprasellar region than in the pineal region.[97]

Germinomas are extremely radiosensitive tumors; patients have 5-year survival rates of more than 90% with radiation therapy alone.[98–101] In contrast, tumors containing nongerminomatous malignant elements are less radiosensitive; studies including radiation therapy with or without chemotherapy show a 5-year survival rate of 20 to 76%.[102–104]

Results of the Third International CNS Germ Cell Tumor Study, designed to demonstrate the efficacy of a chemotherapy-only protocol in avoiding the additional morbidity caused by radiation therapy of germ cell tumors, were recently published.[105] Twenty-five patients with newly diagnosed germ cell tumors were treated with one of two risk-tailored chemotherapy regimens. Regimen A consisted of 4 to 6 cycles of carboplatin/etoposide alternating with cyclophosphamide/etoposide for patients who had low-risk localized germinoma with normal CSF and serum tumor markers. Regimen B consisted of 4 to 6 cycles of carboplatin/cyclophosphamide/etoposide for patients who had intermediate-risk germinoma, positivity for human chorionic gonadotropin β (HCG-β) and/or CSF HCG-β below 50 mIU/mL, and high-risk biopsy-proven nongerminomatous malignant elements or elevated serum/CSF α-fetoprotein and/or serum/CSF HCG-β above 50 mIU/mL. The 6-year event-free and overall survival rates were 45.6% and 75.3%, respectively. The study concluded that chemotherapy-alone regimens are less effective than regimens including radiation therapy. The authors recommended radiation therapy, either alone or with chemotherapy, as the standard treatment for pure germinomas and radiation plus chemotherapy for tumors with nongerminomatous malignant elements.

◆ Chordomas

Chordomas are very rare tumors that arise from the remnants of the embryonic notochord; they are characterized by slow growth, a long natural history, frequent local recurrences, and an axial skeleton location (sacrum, skull base, and spine). They are considered low-grade malignancies, but they have the capacity to metastasize to distant organs. Chordomas were diagnosed in 10 patients in a series of 1120 sellar masses treated with transsphenoidal surgery.[71]

Classically, the treatment of skull base chordomas consists of surgery to reduce tumor volume and, if possible, establish a safety margin for irradiation between the tumor and neurovascular structures. This is followed by some form of radiation therapy or stereotactic radiosurgery.[106,107]

Historically, chemotherapy has not played a role in the treatment of chordomas, and reports of tumor responses to anthracyclines, cisplatin, and alkylating agents have been anecdotal. In rare instances, chordomas can transform into high-grade sarcomas, becoming a potential target for chemotherapy.[76]

Recently, a strong expression of EGFR and C-met (mesenchymal-epithelial transition factor) was reported in a series of 12 chordomas.[108] In addition, platelet-derived growth factor receptor β (PDGFR-β) was overexpressed in a series of 31 chordomas.[109] Because chordomas seem to express EGFR and PDGFR, these tumors may be amenable to treatment with currently available targeted therapy. Several cases of the successful use of imatinib and erlotinib, tyrosine kinase inhibitors, have reported.[110–112]

◆ Meningiomas

Meningiomas are one of the more common brain tumors in adults. About 90% of them are World Health Organization (WHO) grade 1 (benign), 5 to 7% are WHO grade 2 (atypical), and only 3% are WHO grade 3 (malignant or anaplastic).[113]

Historically, the gold standard treatment for meningiomas has been complete surgical resection. Chemotherapy is reserved for more aggressive tumors, recurrent tumors, or those localized in areas of difficult surgical approach; it is also used after radiation therapy when other options have been exhausted. Although chemotherapy is sometimes useful, reliable, effective agents are lacking and remain an area of investigation.

Chamberlain reported a series of 14 patients who had malignant meningiomas treated with adjuvant chemotherapy that included cyclophosphamide, Adriamycin, and vincristine (CAV); the patients showed a modest improvement in survival when compared with patients treated with surgery alone.[114] In a prospective Phase II study of TMZ in 16 patients with refractory meningiomas, no patient demonstrated PFS at 6 months; therefore, the study was terminated, and the conclusion was that TMZ is ineffective in meningiomas.[115] In a study investigating the MGMT promoter methylation status in 36 meningiomas, none of the specimens showed MGMT gene promoter methylation, providing a rationale for TMZ ineffectiveness.[116]

Twelve patients with recurrent postoperative residual masses or inoperable meningiomas were treated with INF-α and followed with PET. In five patients treated from 9 months to 8 years, INF-α seemed to be an effective oncostatic drug, deserving of further studies.[117]

Irinotecan (CPT-11), a topoisomerase I inhibitor, demonstrated growth-inhibiting effects in primary meningioma cultures and in malignant cell lines in vitro and in vivo, but the drug proved ineffective in a Phase II study.[118,119]

Several successful reports of hydroxyurea, an oral ribonucleotide reductase inhibitor against meningiomas, have been published.[120–125] Schrell at al, after demonstrating that hydroxyurea inhibits growth of cultured human meningioma cells and meningioma transplants in nude mice by inducing apoptosis,[124] reported a successful outcome in four patients who had recurrent and/or unresectable meningiomas treated with hydroxyurea.[125] In another study, of 21 patients with recurrent and progressive meningiomas treated with fractionated three-dimensional conformal radiation therapy and concurrent hydroxyurea, disease stabilization was achieved in 14 patients (66%). Progression-free survival rates at 1 and 2 years were 84% and 77% respectively.[121] A Phase II study to further evaluate the role of hydroxyurea in meningiomas (SWOG-S9811) has been completed, but the results have not yet been reported.

PDGF and its receptor PDGFR are frequently co-expressed in meningiomas. A Phase II study of imatinib mesylate (a PDGFR inhibitor) for recurrent meningiomas accrued 23 patients (13 with benign, five with atypical, and five with malignant meningiomas), of whom 22 were eligible. Overall median PFS was 2 months (0.7–34 months), and the 6-month PFS rate was 29.4%. For benign meningiomas, median PFS was 3 months (1.1–34 months), and the 6-month PFS rate was 45%. For atypical and malignant meningiomas, median PFS was 2 months (0.7–3.7 months), and the 6-month PFS rate was zero. Imatinib was well tolerated but did not show any significant activity against recurrent meningiomas.[126]

Meningiomas also overexpress EGFR. Based on this observation, a Phase II study with the EGFR inhibitors gefitinib and erlotinib for recurrent meningiomas was conducted. The study accrued 25 patients. Sixteen patients (64%) received gefitinib, and nine patients (36%) received erlotinib. Eight patients (32%) had benign tumors, nine (36%) atypical meningiomas, and eight (32%) malignant meningiomas. No objective imaging responses were seen, but eight patients (32%) maintained stable disease. The study concluded that although well tolerated, neither gefitinib nor erlotinib appears to be effective against recurrent meningiomas.[127]

Clinical trials of treatments for recurrent meningiomas, including target therapies with bevacizumab (a monoclonal antibody against vascular endothelial growth factor [VEGF]), sorafenib, sunitinib, and vatalanib (targets VEGFR and PDGFR), are under way.

◆ Plasmacytomas

Intrasellar plasmacytomas are rare and can mimic nonfunctional pituitary adenomas clinically and radiologically. Plasmacytomas can progress to multiple myeloma, or multiple myeloma can be diagnosed simultaneously.[128]

Traditionally, plasmacytomas have been treated with surgery and radiation therapy for local or residual disease. Chemotherapy is added for systemic myeloma treatment.

Sinnott et al, in a review of 22 cases of intrasellar plasmacytomas reported in the literature, found that radiation therapy was administered to the sellar lesion in 71% of the patients after surgery and systemic chemotherapy was administered to 29% of the patients following the diagnosis of multiple myeloma.[128]

Patients undergoing chemotherapy for multiple myeloma comprise two groups: those who are candidates for autologous hematopoietic cell transplantation (HCT) and those who are not candidates for HCT.

In patients who were not candidates for HCT, three randomized trials demonstrated superior PFS in those treated with melphalan, prednisone, and thalidomide (MPT) versus patients treated with melphalan and prednisone.[129–132] Bortezomib, melphalan, and prednisone (VMP) are an alternative to MPT.[133,134]

In patients who are candidates for HCT, induction chemotherapy with thalidomide and dexamethasone is the standard treatment.[135,136] Lenalidomide (a thalidomide analogue) combined with dexamethasone seems to be an alternative and is highly effective and well tolerated.[137] Bortezomib with dexamethasone is also a well-tolerated and effective alternative.[138]

The term *hematopoietic cell transplantation* indicates transplantation of progenitor (stem) cells from any source (eg, bone marrow, peripheral blood, cord blood), and HCT may be the only treatment with a chance of producing cure.

◆ Conclusion

Although not a first-line treatment for most sellar and parasellar tumors, chemotherapy remains a valuable option for selected patients. The histology, grade, and behavior of the tumor will shape the decision to employ chemotherapy and the type of agents used.

References

1. Ragel BT, Couldwell WT. Pituitary carcinoma: a review of the literature. Neurosurg Focus 2004;16(4):E7
2. Pernicone PJ, Scheithauer BW, Sebo TJ, et al. Pituitary carcinoma: a clinicopathologic study of 15 cases. Cancer 1997;79(4):804–812
3. Kaltsas GA, Nomikos P, Kontogeorgos G, Buchfelder M, Grossman AB. Clinical review: Diagnosis and management of pituitary carcinomas. J Clin Endocrinol Metab 2005;90(5):3089–3099
4. Asai A, Matsutani M, Funada N, Takakura K. Malignant growth hormone-secreting pituitary adenoma with hematogenous dural metastasis: case report. Neurosurgery 1988;22(6 Pt 1): 1091–1094
5. Harris PE, Bouloux PM, Wass JA, Besser GM. Successful treatment by chemotherapy for acromegaly associated with ectopic growth hormone releasing hormone secretion from a carcinoid tumour. Clin Endocrinol (Oxf) 1990;32(3):315–321
6. Walker JD, Grossman A, Anderson JV, et al. Malignant prolactinoma with extracranial metastases: a report of three cases. Clin Endocrinol (Oxf) 1993;38(4):411–419
7. Kaiser FE, Orth DN, Mukai K, Oppenheimer JH. A pituitary parasellar tumor with extracranial metastases and high, partially suppressible levels of adrenocorticotropin and related peptides. J Clin Endocrinol Metab 1983;57(3):649–653
8. Vaughan NJ, Laroche CM, Goodman I, Davies MJ, Jenkins JS. Pituitary Cushing's disease arising from a previously non-functional corticotrophic chromophobe adenoma. Clin Endocrinol (Oxf) 1985;22(2):147–153
9. Hashimoto N, Handa H, Nishi S. Intracranial and intraspinal dissemination from a growth hormone-secreting pituitary tumor. Case report. J Neurosurg 1986;64(1):140–144
10. Kasperlik-Zaluska AA, Wislawski J, Kaniewska J, Zborzil J, Frankiewicz E, Zgliczyński S. Cytostatics for acromegaly. Marked improvement in a patient with an invasive pituitary tumour. Acta Endocrinol (Copenh) 1987;116(3):347–349
11. Nawata H, Higuchi K, Ikuyama S, et al. Corticotropin-releasing hormone- and adrenocorticotropin-producing pituitary carcinoma with metastases to the liver and lung in a patient with Cushing's disease. J Clin Endocrinol Metab 1990;71(4):1068–1073
12. Petterson T, MacFarlane IA, MacKenzie JM, Shaw MD. Prolactin secreting pituitary carcinoma. J Neurol Neurosurg Psychiatry 1992;55(12):1205–1206
13. Mixson AJ, Friedman TC, Katz DA, et al. Thyrotropin-secreting pituitary carcinoma. J Clin Endocrinol Metab 1993;76(2):529–533
14. Beauchesne P, Trouillas J, Barral F, Brunon J. Gonadotropic pituitary carcinoma: case report. Neurosurgery 1995;37(4):810–815, discussion 815–816
15. Kaltsas GA, Mukherjee JJ, Plowman PN, Monson JP, Grossman AB, Besser GM. The role of cytotoxic chemotherapy in the management of aggressive and malignant pituitary tumors. J Clin Endocrinol Metab 1998;83(12):4233–4238
16. Gollard R, Kosty M, Cheney C, Copeland B, Bordin G. Prolactin-secreting pituitary carcinoma with implants in the cheek pouch and metastases to the ovaries. A case report and literature review. Cancer 1995;76(10):1814–1820
17. McCutcheon IE, Pieper DR, Fuller GN, Benjamin RS, Friend KE, Gagel RF. Pituitary carcinoma containing gonadotropins: treatment by radical excision and cytotoxic chemotherapy: case report. Neurosurgery 2000;46(5):1233–1239, discussion 1239–1240
18. Lopes MB, Scheithauer BW, Schiff D. Pituitary carcinoma: diagnosis and treatment. Endocrine 2005;28(1):115–121
19. Kaltsas GA, Grossman AB. Malignant pituitary tumours. Pituitary 1998;1(1):69–81
20. Newlands ES, Stevens MF, Wedge SR, Wheelhouse RT, Brock C. Temozolomide: a review of its discovery, chemical properties, pre-clinical development and clinical trials. Cancer Treat Rev 1997;23(1):35–61
21. Stupp R, Mason WP, van den Bent MJ, et al; European Organisation for Research and Treatment of Cancer Brain Tumor and Radiotherapy Groups; National Cancer Institute of Canada Clinical Trials Group. Radiotherapy plus concomitant and adjuvant temozolomide for glioblastoma. N Engl J Med 2005;352(10): 987–996
22. Mirimanoff RO, Gorlia T, Mason W, et al. Radiotherapy and temozolomide for newly diagnosed glioblastoma: recursive partitioning analysis of the EORTC 26981/22981-NCIC CE3 phase III randomized trial. J Clin Oncol 2006;24(16):2563–2569
23. Hegi ME, Diserens AC, Gorlia T, et al. MGMT gene silencing and benefit from temozolomide in glioblastoma. N Engl J Med 2005;352(10):997–1003
24. Hagen C, Schroeder HD, Hansen S, Hagen C, Andersen M. Temozolomide treatment of a pituitary carcinoma and two pituitary macroadenomas resistant to conventional therapy. Eur J Endocrinol 2009;161(4):631–637
25. McCormack AI, McDonald KL, Gill AJ, et al. Low O6-methylguanine-DNA methyltransferase (MGMT) expression and response to temozolomide in aggressive pituitary tumours. Clin Endocrinol (Oxf) 2009;71(2):226–233
26. Berrocal A, Perez Segura P, Gil M, et al; GENOM Cooperative Group. Extended-schedule dose-dense temozolomide in refractory gliomas. J Neurooncol 2010;96(3):417–422
27. Tolcher AW, Gerson SL, Denis L, et al. Marked inactivation of O6-alkylguanine-DNA alkyltransferase activity with protracted temozolomide schedules. Br J Cancer 2003;88(7):1004–1011
28. Baer JC, Freeman AA, Newlands ES, Watson AJ, Rafferty JA, Margison GP. Depletion of O6-alkylguanine-DNA alkyltransferase

correlates with potentiation of temozolomide and CCNU toxicity in human tumour cells. Br J Cancer 1993;67(6):1299–1302
29. Fadul CE, Kominsky AL, Meyer LP, et al. Pituitary carcinomas respond to temozolomide. Neuro-oncol 2004;6:374
30. Zhu Y, Shahinian H, Maya MM, Bonert V, Lim S, Heaney A. Temodar: novel treatment for pituitary carcinoma. The Endocrine Society Annual Meeting 2004(138):43–45
31. Lim S, Shahinian H, Maya MM, Yong W, Heaney AP. Temozolomide: a novel treatment for pituitary carcinoma. Lancet Oncol 2006;7(6):518–520
32. Kovacs K, Horvath E, Syro LV, et al. Temozolomide therapy in a man with an aggressive prolactin-secreting pituitary neoplasm: Morphological findings. Hum Pathol 2007;38(1):185–189
33. Horvath E, Kovacs K, Scheithauer BW, Lloyd RV, Smyth HS. Pituitary adenoma with neuronal choristoma (PANCH): composite lesion or lineage infidelity? Ultrastruct Pathol 1994;18(6):565–574
34. Thodou E, Kontogeorgos G, Theodossiou D, Pateraki M. Mapping of somatostatin receptor types in GH or/and PRL producing pituitary adenomas. J Clin Pathol 2006;59(3):274–279
35. Neff LM, Weil M, Cole A, et al. Temozolomide in the treatment of an invasive prolactinoma resistant to dopamine agonists. Pituitary 2007;10(1):81–86
36. Moyes VJ, Alusi G, Sabin HI, et al. Treatment of Nelson's syndrome with temozolomide. Eur J Endocrinol 2009;160(1):115–119
37. Mohammed S, Kovacs K, Mason W, Smyth H, Cusimano MD. Use of temozolomide in aggressive pituitary tumors: case report. Neurosurgery 2009;64(4):E773–E774; discussion E774
38. Thearle MS, Freda PU, Bruce JN, Isaacson SR, Lee Y, Fine RL. Temozolomide (Temodar(R)) and capecitabine (Xeloda(R)) treatment of an aggressive corticotroph pituitary tumor. Pituitary 2009 Dec 4 [Epub ahead of print]
39. Amatori F, Di Paolo A, Del Tacca M, et al. Thymidylate synthase, dihydropyrimidine dehydrogenase and thymidine phosphorylase expression in colorectal cancer and normal mucosa in patients. Pharmacogenet Genomics 2006;16(11):809–816
40. Bush ZM, Longtine JA, Cunningham T, et al. Temozolomide as an adjuvant treatment for aggressive pituitary tumors: correlations of clinical outcomes with DNA methylation and MGMT expression. J Clin Endo Metab 2010;95:280–290
41. Laws ER Jr, Morris AM, Maartens N. Gliadel for pituitary adenomas and craniopharyngiomas. Neurosurgery 2003;53(2):255–269, discussion 259–260
42. Brem H, Ewend MG, Piantadosi S, Greenhoot J, Burger PC, Sisti M. The safety of interstitial chemotherapy with BCNU-loaded polymer followed by radiation therapy in the treatment of newly diagnosed malignant gliomas: phase I trial. J Neurooncol 1995;26(2):111–123
43. Brem H, Mahaley MS Jr, Vick NA, et al. Interstitial chemotherapy with drug polymer implants for the treatment of recurrent gliomas. J Neurosurg 1991;74(3):441–446
44. Jane JA Jr, Laws ER. Craniopharyngioma. Pituitary 2006;9(4):323–326
45. Laws ER Jr, Jane JA Jr. Craniopharyngioma. J Neurosurg Pediatr 2010;5(1):27–28, discussion 28–29
46. Linnert M, Gehl J. Bleomycin treatment of brain tumors: an evaluation. Anticancer Drugs 2009;20(3):157–164
47. Umezawa H, Ishizuka M, Maeda K, Takeuchi T. Studies on bleomycin. Cancer 1967;20(5):891–895
48. Umezawa H, Maeda K, Takeuchi T, Okami Y. New antibiotics, bleomycin A and B. J Antibiot (Tokyo) 1966;19(5):200–209
49. Mir LM, Tounekti O, Orlowski S. Bleomycin: revival of an old drug. Gen Pharmacol 1996;27(5):745–748
50. Takahashi H, Nakazawa S, Shimura T. Evaluation of postoperative intratumoral injection of bleomycin for craniopharyngioma in children. J Neurosurg 1985;62(1):120–127
51. Alén JF, Boto GR, Lagares A, de la Lama A, Gómez PA, Lobato RD. Intratumoural bleomycin as a treatment for recurrent cystic craniopharyngioma. Case report and review of the literature. Neurocirugia (Astur) 2002;13(6):479–485, discussion 485
52. Park DH, Park JY, Kim JH, et al. Outcome of postoperative intratumoral bleomycin injection for cystic craniopharyngioma. J Korean Med Sci 2002;17(2):254–259
53. Jiang R, Liu Z, Zhu C. Preliminary exploration of the clinical effect of bleomycin on craniopharyngiomas. Stereotact Funct Neurosurg 2002;78(2):84–94
54. Mottolese C, Stan H, Hermier M, et al. Intracystic chemotherapy with bleomycin in the treatment of craniopharyngiomas. Childs Nerv Syst 2001;17(12):724–730
55. Hader WJ, Steinbok P, Hukin J, Fryer C. Intratumoral therapy with bleomycin for cystic craniopharyngiomas in children. Pediatr Neurosurg 2000;33(4):211–218
56. Savas A, Arasil E, Batay F, Selcuki M, Kanpolat Y. Intracavitary chemotherapy of polycystic craniopharyngioma with bleomycin. Acta Neurochir (Wien) 1999;141(5):547–548, discussion 549
57. Savas A, Erdem A, Tun K, Kanpolat Y. Fatal toxic effect of bleomycin on brain tissue after intracystic chemotherapy for a craniopharyngioma: case report. Neurosurgery 2000;46(1):213–216, discussion 216–217
58. Sagoh M, Murakami H, Hirose Y, Mayanagi K. Occlusive cerebrovasculopathy after internal radiation and bleomycin therapy for craniopharyngioma—case report. Neurol Med Chir (Tokyo) 1997;37(12):920–923
59. Cavalheiro S, Sparapani FV, Franco JO, da Silva MC, Braga FM. Use of bleomycin in intratumoral chemotherapy for cystic craniopharyngioma. Case report. J Neurosurg 1996;84(1):124–126
60. Haisa T, Ueki K, Yoshida S. Toxic effects of bleomycin on the hypothalamus following its administration into a cystic craniopharyngioma. Br J Neurosurg 1994;8(6):747–750
61. Hargrave DR. Does chemotherapy have a role in the management of craniopharyngioma? J Pediatr Endocrinol Metab 2006;19(Suppl 1):407–412
62. Hukin J, Steinbok P, Lafay-Cousin L, et al. Intracystic bleomycin therapy for craniopharyngioma in children: the Canadian experience. Cancer 2007;109(10):2124–2131
63. Buckell M, Crompton MR, Robertson MC, Barnes GK. Lactate dehydrogenase in cerebral cyst fluids; total activity and isoenzyme distributions as an index of malignancy. J Neurosurg 1970;32(5):545–552
64. Jakacki RI, Cohen BH, Jamison C, et al. Phase II evaluation of interferon-alpha-2a for progressive or recurrent craniopharyngiomas. J Neurosurg 2000;92(2):255–260
65. Ikić D, Padovan I, Pipić N, et al. Treatment of squamous cell carcinoma with interferon. Int J Dermatol 1991;30(1):58–61
66. Ikić D, Padovan I, Pipić N, et al. Interferon therapy for basal cell carcinoma and squamous cell carcinoma. Int J Clin Pharmacol Ther Toxicol 1991;29(9):342–346
67. Yates AJ, Stephens RE, Elder PJ, Markowitz DL, Rice JM. Effects of interferon and gangliosides on growth of cultured human glioma and fetal brain cells. Cancer Res 1985;45(3):1033–1039
68. Sen GC, Lengyel P. The interferon system. A bird's eye view of its biochemistry. J Biol Chem 1992;267(8):5017–5020
69. Ierardi DF, Fernandes MJ, Silva IR, et al. Apoptosis in alpha interferon (IFN-alpha) intratumoral chemotherapy for cystic craniopharyngiomas. Childs Nerv Syst 2007;23(9):1041–1046
70. Yasuda M, Akiyama N, Miyamoto S, et al. Primary sellar lymphoma: intravascular large B-cell lymphoma diagnosed as a double cancer and improved with chemotherapy, and literature review of primary parasellar lymphoma. Pituitary 2010;13(1):39–47
71. Freda PU, Post KD. Differential diagnosis of sellar masses. Endocrinol Metab Clin North Am 1999;28(1):81–117
72. Gsponer J, De Tribolet N, Déruaz JP, et al. Diagnosis, treatment, and outcome of pituitary tumors and other abnormal intrasellar masses. Retrospective analysis of 353 patients. Medicine (Baltimore) 1999;78(4):236–269
73. Da Silva AN, Lopes MB, Schiff D. Rare pathological variants and presentations of primary central nervous system lymphomas. Neurosurg Focus 2006;21(5):E7
74. Gerstner ER, Batchelor TT. Primary central nervous system lymphoma. Arch Neurol 2010;67(3):291–297
75. Ferreri AJ, Abrey LE, Blay JY, et al. Summary statement on primary central nervous system lymphomas from the Eighth International Conference on Malignant Lymphoma, Lugano, Switzerland, June 12 to 15, 2002. J Clin Oncol 2003;21(12):2407–2414
76. Ferreri AJ, Reni M, Foppoli M, et al; International Extranodal Lymphoma Study Group (IELSG). High-dose cytarabine plus high-dose methotrexate versus high-dose methotrexate alone in patients with primary CNS lymphoma: a randomised phase 2 trial. Lancet 2009;374(9700):1512–1520

77. Shah GD, Yahalom J, Correa DD, et al. Combined immunochemotherapy with reduced whole-brain radiotherapy for newly diagnosed primary CNS lymphoma. J Clin Oncol 2007;25(30):4730–4735
78. Poortmans PM, Kluin-Nelemans HC, Haaxma-Reiche H, et al; European Organization for Research and Treatment of Cancer Lymphoma Group. High-dose methotrexate-based chemotherapy followed by consolidating radiotherapy in non-AIDS-related primary central nervous system lymphoma: European Organization for Research and Treatment of Cancer Lymphoma Group Phase II Trial 20962. J Clin Oncol 2003;21(24):4483–4488
79. Gavrilovic IT, Hormigo A, Yahalom J, DeAngelis LM, Abrey LE. Long-term follow-up of high-dose methotrexate-based therapy with and without whole brain irradiation for newly diagnosed primary CNS lymphoma. J Clin Oncol 2006;24(28):4570–4574
80. Abrey LE, Yahalom J, DeAngelis LM. Treatment for primary CNS lymphoma: the next step. J Clin Oncol 2000;18(17):3144–3150
81. DeAngelis LM, Seiferheld W, Schold SC, Fisher B, Schultz CJ; Radiation Therapy Oncology Group Study 93-10. Combination chemotherapy and radiotherapy for primary central nervous system lymphoma: Radiation Therapy Oncology Group Study 93-10. J Clin Oncol 2002;20(24):4643–4648
82. Batchelor T, Carson K, O'Neill A, et al. Treatment of primary CNS lymphoma with methotrexate and deferred radiotherapy: a report of NABTT 96-07. J Clin Oncol 2003;21(6):1044–1049
83. Gerstner ER, Carson KA, Grossman SA, Batchelor TT. Long-term outcome in PCNSL patients treated with high-dose methotrexate and deferred radiation. Neurology 2008;70(5):401–402
84. Pels H, Schmidt-Wolf IG, Glasmacher A, et al. Primary central nervous system lymphoma: results of a pilot and phase II study of systemic and intraventricular chemotherapy with deferred radiotherapy. J Clin Oncol 2003;21(24):4489–4495
85. Hoang-Xuan K, Taillandier L, Chinot O, et al; European Organization for Research and Treatment of Cancer Brain Tumor Group. Chemotherapy alone as initial treatment for primary CNS lymphoma in patients older than 60 years: a multicenter phase II study (26952) of the European Organization for Research and Treatment of Cancer Brain Tumor Group. J Clin Oncol 2003;21(14):2726–2731
86. Angelov L, Doolittle ND, Kraemer DF, et al. Blood-brain barrier disruption and intra-arterial methotrexate-based therapy for newly diagnosed primary CNS lymphoma: a multi-institutional experience. J Clin Oncol 2009;27(21):3503–3509
87. Glass J, Gruber ML, Cher L, Hochberg FH. Preirradiation methotrexate chemotherapy of primary central nervous system lymphoma: long-term outcome. J Neurosurg 1994;81(2):188–195
88. Cher L, Glass J, Harsh GR, Hochberg FH. Therapy of primary CNS lymphoma with methotrexate-based chemotherapy and deferred radiotherapy: preliminary results. Neurology 1996;46(6):1757–1759
89. Glass J, Shustik C, Hochberg FH, Cher L, Gruber ML. Therapy of primary central nervous system lymphoma with pre-irradiation methotrexate, cyclophosphamide, doxorubicin, vincristine, and dexamethasone (MCHOD). J Neurooncol 1996;30(3):257–265
90. Ferreri AJ, Reni M, Pasini F, et al. A multicenter study of treatment of primary CNS lymphoma. Neurology 2002;58(10):1513–1520
91. Khan RB, Shi W, Thaler HT, DeAngelis LM, Abrey LE. Is intrathecal methotrexate necessary in the treatment of primary CNS lymphoma? J Neurooncol 2002;58(2):175–178
92. Ferreri AJ, Reni M, Dell'Oro S, et al. Combined treatment with high-dose methotrexate, vincristine and procarbazine, without intrathecal chemotherapy, followed by consolidation radiotherapy for primary central nervous system lymphoma in immunocompetent patients. Oncology 2001;60(2):134–140
93. Guha-Thakurta N, Damek D, Pollack C, Hochberg FH. Intravenous methotrexate as initial treatment for primary central nervous system lymphoma: response to therapy and quality of life of patients. J Neurooncol 1999;43(3):259–268
94. Rubenstein JL, Fridlyand J, Abrey L, et al. Phase I study of intraventricular administration of rituximab in patients with recurrent CNS and intraocular lymphoma. J Clin Oncol 2007;25(11):1350–1356
95. Jennings MT, Gelman R, Hochberg F. Intracranial germ-cell tumors: natural history and pathogenesis. J Neurosurg 1985;63(2):155–167
96. Kyritsis AP. Management of primary intracranial germ cell tumors. J Neurooncol 2010;96(2):143–149
97. Liang L, Korogi Y, Sugahara T, et al. MRI of intracranial germ-cell tumours. Neuroradiology 2002;44(5):382–388
98. Ogawa K, Shikama N, Toita T, et al. Long-term results of radiotherapy for intracranial germinoma: a multi-institutional retrospective review of 126 patients. Int J Radiat Oncol Biol Phys 2004;58(3):705–713
99. Maity A, Shu HK, Janss A, et al. Craniospinal radiation in the treatment of biopsy-proven intracranial germinomas: twenty-five years' experience in a single center. Int J Radiat Oncol Biol Phys 2004;58(4):1165–1170
100. Merchant TE, Sherwood SH, Mulhern RK, et al. CNS germinoma: disease control and long-term functional outcome for 12 children treated with craniospinal irradiation. Int J Radiat Oncol Biol Phys 2000;46(5):1171–1176
101. Rogers SJ, Mosleh-Shirazi MA, Saran FH. Radiotherapy of localised intracranial germinoma: time to sever historical ties? Lancet Oncol 2005;6(7):509–519
102. Ogawa K, Toita T, Nakamura K, et al. Treatment and prognosis of patients with intracranial nongerminomatous malignant germ cell tumors: a multiinstitutional retrospective analysis of 41 patients. Cancer 2003;98(2):369–376
103. Matsutani M; Japanese Pediatric Brain Tumor Study Group. Combined chemotherapy and radiation therapy for CNS germ cell tumors—the Japanese experience. J Neurooncol 2001;54(3):311–316
104. Aoyama H, Shirato H, Ikeda J, Fujieda K, Miyasaka K, Sawamura Y. Induction chemotherapy followed by low-dose involved-field radiotherapy for intracranial germ cell tumors. J Clin Oncol 2002;20(3):857–865
105. da Silva NS, Cappellano AM, Diez B, et al. Primary chemotherapy for intracranial germ cell tumors: results of the third international CNS germ cell tumor study. Pediatr Blood Cancer 2010;54(3):377–383
106. Casali PG, Stacchiotti S, Sangalli C, Olmi P, Gronchi A. Chordoma. Curr Opin Oncol 2007;19(4):367–370
107. Yoneoka Y, Tsumanuma I, Fukuda M, et al. Cranial base chordoma—long term outcome and review of the literature. Acta Neurochir (Wien) 2008;150(8):773–778, discussion 778
108. Weinberger PM, Yu Z, Kowalski D, et al. Differential expression of epidermal growth factor receptor, c-Met, and HER2/neu in chordoma compared with 17 other malignancies. Arch Otolaryngol Head Neck Surg 2005;131(8):707–711
109. Tamborini E, Miselli F, Negri T, et al. Molecular and biochemical analyses of platelet-derived growth factor receptor (PDGFR) B, PDGFRA, and KIT receptors in chordomas. Clin Cancer Res 2006;12(23):6920–6928
110. Singhal N, Kotasek D, Parnis FX. Response to erlotinib in a patient with treatment refractory chordoma. Anticancer Drugs 2009;20(10):953–955
111. Casali PG, Messina A, Stacchiotti S, et al. Imatinib mesylate in chordoma. Cancer 2004;101(9):2086–2097
112. Casali PG, Stacchiotti S, Messina A, et al. Imatinib mesylate in 18 advanced chordoma patients. J Clin Oncol 2005;23(suppl):9012
113. Louis DN, Ohgaki H, Wiestler OD, et al. The 2007 WHO classification of tumours of the central nervous system. Acta Neuropathol 2007;114(2):97–109
114. Chamberlain MC. Adjuvant combined modality therapy for malignant meningiomas. J Neurosurg 1996;84(5):733–736
115. Chamberlain MC, Tsao-Wei DD, Groshen S. Temozolomide for treatment-resistant recurrent meningioma. Neurology 2004;62(7):1210–1212
116. de Robles P, McIntyre J, Kalra S, et al. Methylation status of MGMT gene promoter in meningiomas. Cancer Genet Cytogenet 2008;187(1):25–27
117. Muhr C, Gudjonsson O, Lilja A, Hartman M, Zhang ZJ, Långström B. Meningioma treated with interferon-alpha, evaluated with [(11)C]-L-methionine positron emission tomography. Clin Cancer Res 2001;7(8):2269–2276
118. Gupta V, Su YS, Samuelson CG, et al. Irinotecan: a potential new chemotherapeutic agent for atypical or malignant meningiomas. J Neurosurg 2007;106(3):455–462
119. Chamberlain MC, Tsao-Wei DD, Groshen S. Salvage chemotherapy with CPT-11 for recurrent meningioma. J Neurooncol 2006;78(3):271–276

120. Fuentes S, Chinot O, Dufour H, et al. Hydroxyurea treatment for unresectable meningioma. Neurochirurgie 2004;50(4): 461–467
121. Hahn BM, Schrell UM, Sauer R, Fahlbusch R, Ganslandt O, Grabenbauer GG. Prolonged oral hydroxyurea and concurrent 3D-conformal radiation in patients with progressive or recurrent meningioma: results of a pilot study. J Neurooncol 2005;74(2):157–165
122. Newton HB, Scott SR, Volpi C. Hydroxyurea chemotherapy for meningiomas: enlarged cohort with extended follow-up. Br J Neurosurg 2004;18(5):495–499
123. Mason WP, Gentili F, Macdonald DR, Hariharan S, Cruz CR, Abrey LE. Stabilization of disease progression by hydroxyurea in patients with recurrent or unresectable meningioma. J Neurosurg 2002;97(2):341–346
124. Schrell UM, Rittig MG, Anders M, et al. Hydroxyurea for treatment of unresectable and recurrent meningiomas. I. Inhibition of primary human meningioma cells in culture and in meningioma transplants by induction of the apoptotic pathway. J Neurosurg 1997;86(5):845–852
125. Schrell UM, Rittig MG, Anders M, et al. Hydroxyurea for treatment of unresectable and recurrent meningiomas. II. Decrease in the size of meningiomas in patients treated with hydroxyurea. J Neurosurg 1997;86(5):840–844
126. Wen PY, Yung WK, Lamborn KR, et al. Phase II study of imatinib mesylate for recurrent meningiomas (North American Brain Tumor Consortium study 01-08). Neuro-oncol 2009;11(6):853–860
127. Norden AD, Raizer JJ, Abrey LE, et al. Phase II trials of erlotinib or gefitinib in patients with recurrent meningioma. J Neurooncol 2010;96(2):211–217
128. Sinnott BP, Hatipoglu B, Sarne DH. Intrasellar plasmacytoma presenting as a non-functional invasive pituitary macro-adenoma: case report & literature review. Pituitary 2006;9(1):65–72
129. Palumbo A, Bertola A, Musto P, et al. Oral melphalan, prednisone, and thalidomide for newly diagnosed patients with myeloma. Cancer 2005;104(7):1428–1433
130. Palumbo A, Bringhen S, Caravita T, et al; Italian Multiple Myeloma Network, GIMEMA. Oral melphalan and prednisone chemotherapy plus thalidomide compared with melphalan and prednisone alone in elderly patients with multiple myeloma: randomised controlled trial. Lancet 2006;367(9513): 825–831
131. Facon T, Mary JY, Hulin C, et al; Intergroupe Francophone du Myélome. Melphalan and prednisone plus thalidomide versus melphalan and prednisone alone or reduced-intensity autologous stem cell transplantation in elderly patients with multiple myeloma (IFM 99-06): a randomised trial. Lancet 2007;370(9594): 1209–1218
132. Hulin C, Facon T, Rodon P, et al. Efficacy of melphalan and prednisone plus thalidomide in patients older than 75 years with newly diagnosed multiple myeloma: IFM 01/01 trial. J Clin Oncol 2009;27(22):3664–3670
133. Mateos MV, Hernández JM, Hernández MT, et al. Bortezomib plus melphalan and prednisone in elderly untreated patients with multiple myeloma: results of a multicenter phase 1/2 study. Blood 2006;108(7):2165–2172
134. Mateos MV, Hernández JM, Hernández MT, et al. Bortezomib plus melphalan and prednisone in elderly untreated patients with multiple myeloma: updated time-to-events results and prognostic factors for time to progression. Haematologica 2008;93(4):560–565
135. Rajkumar SV, Hayman S, Gertz MA, et al. Combination therapy with thalidomide plus dexamethasone for newly diagnosed myeloma. J Clin Oncol 2002;20(21):4319–4323
136. Rajkumar SV, Blood E, Vesole D, Fonseca R, Greipp PR; Eastern Cooperative Oncology Group. Phase III clinical trial of thalidomide plus dexamethasone compared with dexamethasone alone in newly diagnosed multiple myeloma: a clinical trial coordinated by the Eastern Cooperative Oncology Group. J Clin Oncol 2006;24(3):431–436
137. Gay F, Hayman SR, Lacy MQ, et al. Lenalidomide plus dexamethasone versus thalidomide plus dexamethasone in newly diagnosed multiple myeloma: a comparative analysis of 411 patients. Blood 2010;115(7):1343–1350
138. Jagannath S, Durie BG, Wolf JL, et al. Extended follow-up of a phase 2 trial of bortezomib alone and in combination with dexamethasone for the frontline treatment of multiple myeloma. Br J Haematol 2009;146(6):619–626

Index

Note: Page numbers followed by *f* and *t* indicate figures and tables, respectively.

A

Acromegaly
- endocrine evaluation, 63
- imaging, 129*f*
- radiation therapy, 201–202
- remission rates, 127–128
- reoperation, 128
- signs/symptoms, 126
- stereotactic radiosurgery (SRS), 220, 221*t*
- surgical management, 126–129

ACTH-producing microadenomas, imaging, 52*f*

Adenomas
- imaging, 51–53, 52*f*, 180*f*, 217*f*
- incidence, 124, 182*f*
- radiation therapy, 200–201
- surgical technique, 131–133
- surgical treatment, 124–133

Adnexal system assessment, 119

Adriamycin, 241

Amsler grid test, 116, 117*f*

Anatomy
- chondrosarcomas, 155–156
- chordomas, 155–156
- clinoidal meningiomas, 142
- parasellar region, 8–29
- sphenoid sinus, 13*f*
- suprasellar and third ventricular region, 47*f*
- tuberculum sellae meningiomas, 137
- visual adnexal structures, 83, 85
- visual afferent system, 67, 69
- visual efferent system, 69, 83

Angiography, 71*f*, 72*f*, 97*f*, 102*f*, 103*f*, 107*f*, 146–147

Anterior clinoid process, relationship to parasellar region, 35–36

Apoplectic adenomas, 58, 59*f*

Approaches, surgical
- bifrontal, 194–195
- cranio-orbitozygomatic (COZ)
  - for cavernous sinus meningiomas, 142–143
  - for clinoidal meningiomas, 143
  - electrode placement, 140*f*
  - lateral entry, 141–142, 141*f*
  - patient position, 139
  - reconstruction, 142
  - scalp incision, 140*f*
  - superior entry, 141, 141*f*
  - technique, 139–141
- endoscopic endonasal, 178–179, 179*f*
- endoscopic endonasal transclival, 180–181
- endoscopic endonasal transtuberculum/transplanum, 180
- endoscopic single-nostril endonasal, 6*f*
- frontotemporal, 2*f*
- orbitozygomatic (OZ), 193–194, 193*f*, 194*f*
- pterional, 150, 150*f*, 187–193, 188*f*, 189*f*, 190*f*, 191*f*, 192*f*, 193*f*
- subfrontal, 149–150, 149*f*, 195–196
- sublabial transsphenoidal, 2*f*, 178
- subtemporal, 1*f*, 150, 150*f*, 197
- supraorbital, 137–138, 137*f*, 196–197
  - incision, 136*f*
  - for meningiomas, 135–139
  - technique, 135–137
- transcallosal/transventricular, 151
- transnasal transsphenoidal, 13*f*, 126
- transsphenoidal, 127, 129, 151, 151*f*, 173
  - for pituitary adenomas, 131–133
  - *See also* Transsphenoidal surgery
- transpterygoid, 182–183
- *See also* Transcranial surgery

Arachnoid cysts, imaging, 55

Arterial relationships in parasellar region, 41–42

Astrocytomas, imaging, 53

B
B-scan, 72*f*
Bleomycin, 238–239
Botulinum toxin (Botox) injections, 108
Brachytherapy, early uses, 4

C
Carboplatin, 240
Cavernous sinus
  dissection of, 30*f*–32*f*, 33*f*–34*f*
  invasion, patterns of, 53*f*
  triangles, 40
Cavernous sinus meningiomas
  cranio-orbitozygomatic approach (COZ), 142–143
  endocrine evaluation, 142
  incidence, 142
  physical examination, 142
  radiation therapy, 204–205
Chemotherapy
  adriamycin, 241
  bleomycin, 238–239
  carboplatin, 240
  for chondrosarcomas, 166
  for chordomas, 240–241
  for craniopharyngiomas, 238–239
  cyclophosphamide, 240, 241
  erlotinib, 241
  etoposide, 240
  gefitinib, 241
  for germ cell tumors, 240
  hematopoietic cell transplantation (HCT), 242
  hydroxyurea, 241
  imatinib, 241
  interferon alfa-2a (IFN-a-2a), 239
  intrathecal, 240
  irinotecan (CPT-11), 241
  for meningiomas, 241
  methotrexate (MTX), 239–240
  for pituitary carcinomas, 236, 237*t*
  for pituitary lymphomas, 239–240
  for plasmacytomas, 241–242
  rituximab, 240
  temozolomide (TMZ), 236, 238, 241
  vincristine, 241
Chiasm, 42–45, 44*f*
Chondrosarcomas, 56, 57*f*
  anatomy, 155–156
  chemotherapy, 166
  epidemiology, 155
  imaging, 157–158, 157*f*
  incidence, 155
  pathology, 156
  radiation therapy, 165, 166*f*, 208–210, 209*t*
  recurrence, 165–166
  signs/symptoms, 156
  surgical approaches, 158–160, 161*t*
  surgical outcomes, 163, 164*t*, 165
  surgical technique, 160–163, 161*f*, 162*f*
  surgical treatment, 155–167
Chordomas, 56, 57*f*
  anatomy, 155–156
  chemotherapy, 166
  epidemiology, 155
  imaging, 157–158, 157*f*, 159*f*, 183*f*
  incidence, 155
  pathology, 156
  radiation therapy, 165, 166*f*, 208–210, 209*t*
  recurrence, 165–166
  signs/symptoms, 156
  surgical approaches, 158–160, 161*t*
  surgical outcomes, 163, 164*t*, 165
  surgical technique, 160–163, 161*f*, 162*f*
  surgical treatment, 155–167
Clinical target volume (CTV), 200
Clinoidal meningiomas
  anatomy, 142
  cranio-orbitozygomatic (COZ) approach, 143
  imaging, 143
  signs/symptoms, 143
  three types, 143, 143*f*
Clival masses, differential diagnosis of, 159*t*
Color vision assessment, 115–116
Computed tomography (CT)
  evaluation using, 50, 146, 157
  images, 57*f*, 100*f*, 120*f*, 147*f*, 162*f*, 164*t*
Conchae, 11*f*, 12
Conformal radiation therapy (CRT), 199
Confrontation testing, 86, 97*f*, 116
Contrast sensitivity assessment, 116
Conventional fractionated external beam radiation therapy (EBRT), 199
  conformal radiation therapy (CRT), 199
  indications, 200
  intensity-modulated radiation therapy (IMRT), 199
Cortisol levels, postoperative, 125
Cranio-orbitozygomatic (COZ) surgical approach
  for cavernous sinus meningiomas, 142–143
  for clinoidal meningiomas, 143
  electrode placement, 140*f*
  lateral entry, 141–142, 141*f*
  patient position, 139
  reconstruction, 142
  scalp incision, 140*f*
  superior entry, 141, 141*f*
  technique, 139–141
Craniopharyngiomas
  diagnosis, 146–147
  endocrinology, 147, 148*t*
  epidemiology, 146
  etiology/pathology, 145–146
  imaging, 54, 146–147, 147*f*, 152–153, 181*f*, 182*f*
  intercavitary radiation, 229–234
  operative approaches, 148–149, 149*t*
    pterional, 150, 150*f*

subfrontal, 149–150, 149*f*
subtemporal, 150, 150*f*
transcallosal/transventricular, 151
transsphenoidal, 151
ophthalmologic evaluation, 104*f*–107*f*
postoperative care, 152
rate of occurrence, 145
radiation therapy, 203–204
recurrence, 152–153
reoperation, 153
signs/symptoms, 146
stereotactic radiosurgery (SRS), 230–231, 230*f*, 231*f*
subtypes, 145
surgical outcomes, 152–153
surgical treatment, 145–153
treatment strategies, 148
Cushing disease
endocrine evaluation, 61, 63
imaging strategy, 50, 51, 124, 125
radiation therapy, 202
stereotactic radiosurgery (SRS), 217–218, 219*t*
surgical management, 124
Cyclophosphamide, 240, 241
Cyclotron, 5, 5*f*

D
Dermoid cysts, imaging, 55–56
Diaphragma sellae meningiomas
supraorbital approach, 138–139
three types, 138–139, 139*f*
Diaphragma sellae, relationship to sella, 24
Dural relationships, to parasellar region, 36–38

E
Elster's rule, 51
Endocrine evaluation
acromegaly, 63
cavernous sinus meningioma, 142
craniopharyngioma, 147, 148*t*
Cushing disease, 61–63
Rathke cleft cysts, 170–171, 171*t*
Endoscopic endonasal surgical approach, 6*f*, 178–179, 179*f*, 180–181
Endoscopic surgery, rise of, 5
Epidermoid cysts, imaging, 55–56, 55*f*
Erlotinib, 241
Esthesiometer, 99, 100*f*, 119
Etoposide, 240

F
Faden procedure, 108
Fractionation schedules, 199
Frontotemporal surgical approach, 2*f*
Fundus, 68*f*
Funduscopic examination, 70*f*, 75*f*, 76*f*, 79*f*, 81*f*, 89*f*, 91*f*, 119, 120*f*

G
Gamma knife,
invention of, 5
postoperative plan, 163*f*
Gefitinib, 241
Germ cell tumors (germinoma), 56, 58*f*, 206–208, 207*t*
Goldmann bowl, 93, 94
Granular cell tumors, imaging, 53

H
Hematopoietic cell transplantation (HCT), 242
Hertel exophthalmometer, 98, 99*f*, 119
Hess screen, 84*f*, 94, 95*f*, 97*f*, 98*f*, 102*f*, 109*f*, 110*f*, 111*f*, 113*f*
Hormone deficiency, 61, 62
Hydroxyurea, 241

I
Imaging
acromegaly, 129*f*
ACTH-producing microadenomas, 52
adenomas, 51–53, 52*f*, 180*f*, 217*f*
arachnoid cysts, 55
astrocytomas, 53
chondrosarcomas, 157–158, 157*f*
chordomas, 157–158, 157*f*, 159*f*, 183*f*
clinoidal meningiomas, 143
craniopharyngiomas, 54, 146–147, 147*f*, 152–153, 181*f*, 182*f*
Cushing disease, 50, 51, 124, 125
dermoid cysts, 55–56, 55*f*
granular cell tumors, 53
intracranial hypotension, 56, 58*f*
lymphocytic adnohypophysitis (LAH), 56, 58*f*
lymphocytic infundibuloneurohypophysitis (LIN), 56
meningiomas, 56, 57*f*
neurosarcoid, 58*f*
pars intermedia cysts, 55
pituicytomas, 53
pituitary abscess, bacterial, 56
pituitary apoplexy, 56, 58
pituitary gland, 51
plenum sphenoidale meningiomas, 181*f*
primary lymphoma, 54
Rathke cleft cysts, 55, 55*f*, 171–172, 171*f*
schwannomas, 56, 57*f*, 183*f*
tuberculum sellae meningiomas, 138*f*
Imatinib, 241
Intensity-modulated radiation therapy (IMRT), 199
Intercavernous venous connections, relationship to sella, 25–26, 25*f*
Interferon alfa-2a (IFN-a-2a), 239
Intracavitary radiation, for cystic craniopharyngiomas
additional treatment, 232
complications, 233
experiences, 229–230
follow-up, 231

Intracavitary radiation, for cystic craniopharyngiomas *(continued)*
rationale, 229
results, 231–234, 232*f*, 232*t*, 233*f*, 234*t*
stereotactic technique, 230–231, 230*f*, 231*f*
Intracranial hypotension, imaging, 56, 58*f*
Irinotecan (CPT-11), 241

L
Laryngoscope, video, 129*f*
Lymphocytic adenohypophysitis (LAH), imaging, 56, 58*f*
Lymphocytic infundibuloneurohypophysitis (LIN), imaging, 56

M
Maddox rod, 93, 93*f*, 118-119
Magnetic resonance (MR) angiography, 146–147
Magnetic resonance imaging (MRI), 68*f*
3.0-Tesla, sella protocol for, 51*t*
diffusion-weighted imaging (DWI), 51, 55*f*
dynamic keyhole technique, 50, 53*f*
Elster's rule, 51
evaluation using, 50–51
fluid-attenuated inversion recovery (FLAIR), 55
inferior petrosal sinus sampling (IPSS), 51, 125
normal anatomy, 50*f*
spoiled gradient (SPGR), 50
T1-weighted images (T1WIs), 50, 55*f*
enhanced, 51, 129*f*, 138*f*, 147*f*, 157*f*, 159*f*, 162*f*, 164*f*, 171, 172*f*, 181*f*, 182*f*, 183*f*, 224*f*, 232*f*, 233*f*
spin-echo, postcontrast, 52*f*
spoiled gradient (SPGR), postcontrast, 50*f*, 52*f*
unenhanced, 50*f*, 52*f*, 57*f*
T2-weighted images (T2WIs), 51, 52*f*, 57*f*, 59*f*, 147*f*, 157*f*, 171
use of contrast, 50
Magnetic resonance (MR) spectroscopy, 51
Marginal reflex distance (MRD), 98, 99*f*
Medial sphenoid meningiomas, radiation therapy, 204–205
Meningiomas
imaging, 56, 57*f*
surgical approaches, 135
cranio-orbitozygomatic (COZ), 139–142
supraorbital, 135–139
surgical treatment, 135–144
See also specific meningiomas
Methotrexate (MTX), 239-240
Microneurosurgery, origins of, 3
Middle clinoid process, relationship to parasellar region, 35–36
Middle fossa triangles, 40–41
Millimeter ruler, 98, 99*f*, 119

N
Nasal cavity, relationship to sella, 8–12
Nasal pathway, dissection of, 10*f*
Nasal septum, 11*f*, 12
Near card, 86*f*
Near vision assessment, 115
Nelson syndrome, stereotactic radiosurgery (SRS), 218, 220, 220*t*
Neural relationships, in parasellar region, 39–40
Neurosarcoid, imaging of, 58*f*
Neutral density filters, 87, 87*f*
Nonfunctioning pituitary adenoma
radiation therapy, 200–201
stereotactic radiosurgery (SRS), 217, 217*f*, 218*t*
surgical management, 131

O
Ocular malalignment assessment, 118–119
Ocular motor stability assessment, 117–118
Ocular motor systems assessment, 118
Operative monocular microscope (Nyle'n), 3*f*
Operative setup (Guiot and Hardy), 4*f*
Optic nerve, in sellar region, 44*f*
Optic nerve sheath meningiomas, radiation therapy, 205
Optic pathway meningiomas, radiation therapy, 205–206, 206*t*
Optic strut, relationship to parasellar region, 36
Opthalmologic evaluation, 61, 147
200 optotype E, 115*f*
Amsler grid test, 116, 117*f*
angiogram, 71*f*, 72*f*, 97*f*, 102*f*, 103*f*, 107*f*
assessment of
adnexal system, 119
color vision, 115–116
contrast sensitivity, 116
near vision, 115
ocular malalignment, 118–119
ocular motor stability, 117–118
ocular motor systems, 118
Snellen acuity, 115
stereo acuity, 116
visual field, 116–117
B-scan, 72*f*
cardinal positions, 84*f*, 95*f*, 96*f*, 98*f*, 102*f*, 109*f*, 110*f*, 111*f*, 112*f*, 113*f*
computed tomography (CT), 100*f*, 120*f*
confrontation testing, 86, 87*f*, 116
esthesiometer, 99, 100*f*, 119
funduscopic examination, 70*f*, 75*f*, 76*f*, 79*f*, 81*f*, 89*f*, 91*f*, 119, 120*f*
Goldmann bowl, 93, 94
Hertel exophthalmometer, 98, 99*f*, 119
Hess screen, 84*f*, 94, 95*f*, 97*f*, 98*f*, 102*f*, 109*f*, 110*f*, 111*f*, 113*f*
Maddox rod, 93, 93*f*, 118–119
marginal reflex distance (MRD), 98, 99*f*
millimeter ruler, 98, 99*f*, 119
MRI, 68*f*, 74*f*, 77*f*, 80*f*, 90*f*, 94*f*, 98*f*, 104*f*, 109*f*, 110*f*
near card, 86*f*

neutral density filters, 87, 87*f*
opthalmoscope, direct, 92, 92*f*, 117–118
optical coherence tomogram (OCT), 71*f*, 73*f*, 75*f*, 77*f*, 80*f*, 82*f*, 83*f*, 89*f*, 91*f*, 92, 104*f*, 106*f*, 107*f*, 119
patient history, 66–67
slit lamp, 98–99
supplies, 121
Titmus test, 116, 116*f*
upper lid range, 99, 99*f*
visual fields, 70*f*, 73*f*, 76*f*, 78*f*, 79*f*, 81*f*, 82*f*, 86–87, 88*f*, 102*f*, 104*f*, 105*f*, 106*f*
See also Visual system
Opthalmoscope, direct, 92, 92*f*, 117-118
Optical coherence tomogram (OCT), 71*f*, 73*f*, 75*f*, 77*f*, 80*f*, 82*f*, 83*f*, 89*f*, 91*f*, 92, 104*f*, 106*f*, 107*f*, 119
Orbitozygomatic (OZ) surgical approach, 193–194, 193*f*, 194*f*

P
Paraclinoid triangles, 41
Parasellar region, anatomy of, 28–42
Pars intermedia cysts, imaging, 55
Pituicytomas, imaging, 53
Pituitary abscess, bacterial, imaging, 56
Pituitary apoplexy, imaging, 56, 58
Pituitary gland
and the carotid artery, relationship to sella, 24–25
endoscopic view, 132*f*
imaging of, 51
incisions, 126*f*
relationship to sella, 24
subcranial relationships, 9*f*
Pituitary hypersecretion, 61–62
Pituitary stalk, 137*f*
Planning target volume (PTV), 200
Plenum sphenoidale meningiomas, imaging, 181*f*
Primary lymphoma, imaging, 54
Prolactinomas
radiation therapy, 202–203
stereotactic radiosurgery (SRS), 220, 222, 223*t*
surgical management, 129–130
treatment options, 130*f*
Proton therapy vs photon therapy, 200
Pterional surgical approach, 150, 150*f*, 187–193, 188*f*, 190*f*, 191*f*, 192*f*, 193*f*

R
Radiation therapy
clinical target volume (CTV), 200
conventional fractionated external beam radiation therapy (EBRT), 199
conformal radiation therapy (CRT), 199
indications, 200
intensity-modulated radiation therapy (IMRT), 199
dose limitations, 200
fractionation schedules, 199
gross tumor volume (GTV), 299
late effects
cerebrovascular events, 211
hypopituitarism, 210
radionecrosis, 211
second malignancy, 211
visual deficits, 210–211
planning target volume (PTV), 200
proton therapy vs photon therapy, 200
stereotactic radiosurgery (SRS), 199
gamma knife, 199
indications, 200
linear acclerator-based (LINAC), 199
proton beam units, 216
as specific treatment for
acromegaly, 201–202
cavernous sinus meningiomas, 204–205
chondrosarcomas, 165, 166*f*, 208–210, 209*t*
chordomas, 165, 166*f*, 208–210, 209*t*
craniopharyngiomas, 203–204
Cushing disease, 202
germ cell tumors, 206–208, 207*t*
medial sphenoid meningiomas, 204–205
nonfunctioning pituitary adenomas, 200–201
optic nerve sheath meningiomas, 205
optic pathway meningiomas, 205–206, 206*t*
pituitary carcinomas, 210
prolactinomas, 202–203
sellar metastases, 210
TSH-secreting adenomas, 203
tuberculum sellae meningiomas, 205
Radiosurgery, 4–5
Radium therapy, transnasal delivery of, 2*f*
Rathke cleft cysts (RCCs)
complications, 175
diagnosis, 170
endocrine evaluation, 170–171, 171*t*
imaging, 55, 55*f*, 171–172, 171*f*
operative approaches, 172–173
ophthalmologic evaluation, 79*f*–83*f*, 171, 171*t*
prevalence, 170
recurrence, 174
signs/symptoms, 170, 171*t*
surgical outcome, 173–174, 174*t*
surgical techniques, 173
surgical treatment, 170–175
Rituximab, 240
Roentgenography, 4–5

S
Schwannomas, imaging, 56, 57*f*, 183*f*
Sellar floor, 132*f*
Sellar and parasellar lesions
clinical manifestations, 61–62
evaluation, 61–63
management, 61–63
stereotactic radiosurgery (SRS), 224–225, 224*f*, 225*t*
Sellar and parasellar region
anatomy, 8–49
diagnosis for pathology, 50–59

Sellar and parasellar region *(Continued)*
early approaches, 1–3
historical perspective, 1–6
imaging anatomy, 51
imaging strategies, 50–51
radiologic evaluation, 50–59
superior view, 15*f*
Slit lamp, 98–99
Snellen acuity assessment, 115
Sphenoid bone
relationship to sella, 12–16
types, 14*f*
Sphenoid sinus
anatomy, 13*f*
anterior view, 20*f*
clival extensions of, 28*f*
endonasal approaches, 23*f*
endoscopic view, 132*f*
extensions of, 26, 27
inferior view, 17*f*
nasal pathway to, 18*f*
relationship to sella, 16–24
septa in, 19*f*
subcranial relationships, dissection showing, 22*f*
types, 16
Stereo acuity assessment, 116
Stereotactic radiosurgery (SRS), 165, 166*f*
devices, 216
gamma knife, 199, 216
linear accelerators (LINAC), 199, 216
proton beam units, 216
dosing, 216
remission, 222
side effects, 222–223, 225
techniques, 216
for treatment of
acromegaly, 220, 221*t*
craniopharyngiomas, 230–231, 230*f*, 231*f*
Cushing disease, 217–218, 219*t*
Nelson syndrome, 218, 220, 220*t*
nonfunctioning pituitary adenomas, 217, 217*f*, 218*t*
prolactinoma, 220, 222, 223*t*
sellar/parasellar meningiomas, 224–225, 224*f*, 225*t*
Steroids, perioperative use of, 125
Subfrontal surgical approach, 149–150, 149*f*, 195–196
Sublabial transsphenoidal surgical approach, 2*f*, 178
Subtemporal surgical approach, 1*f*, 150, 150*f*
Supraorbital surgical approach, 137–138, 137*f*, 196–197
Suprasellar and third ventricular region
anatomy, 47*f*
arterial relationships, 45–48
cranial nerves in, 42–45
neural relationships in, 43*f*
vascular relationships in, 46*f*
venous relationships, 48
ventricular and cisternal relationships, 42
Supraorbital flap, removal of, 137*f*
Surgical approaches. *See* Approaches, surgical
Surgical treatment
acromegaly, 126–129
adenomas, 124–133
cavernous sinus meningiomas, 142–143
chondrosarcomas, 155–167
chordomas, 155–167
clinoidal meningiomas, 143
craniopharyngiomas, 145–153
Cushing disease, 124–126
diaphragma sellae meningiomas, 138-139
meningiomas, 135–144
nonsecreting adenomas, 131
prolactinomas, 129–130
Rathke cleft cysts, 170–175
TSH-secreting adenomas, 130–131
tuberculum sellae meningiomas, 137-138
Synchrocyclotron, 5

T

Temozolomide (TMZ), 236, 238, 241
Thyroid-stimulating hormone (TSH)-secreting adenomas
radiation therapy, 203
signs/symptoms, 131
surgical management, 130–131
Titmus test, 116, 116*f*
Transcranial surgery
bifrontal approach, 194–195
orbitozygomatic (OZ) approach, 193–194, 193*f*, 194*f*
patient position, 188*f*, 195
preparation, 187
pterional approach, 187–193, 188*f*, 189*f*, 190*f*, 191*f*, 192*f*, 193*f*
subtemporal approach, 197
supraorbital keyhole approach, 196–197
unilateral subfrontal approach, 195–196
Transnasal route
to sella, 13*f*
to sphenoid sinus, 13*f*
Transpterygoid, 182–183
Transsphenoidal surgery
of the parasellar area
cavernous sinus, 182
clivus, 180
Meckel's cave, 182–183
retrosellar space, 180
suprasellar and anterior fossa, 180
reconstruction, 184
resurgence of, 4
of the sellar area
endoscopic endonasal, 178–179, 179*f*
microscopic endonasal, 178
microscopic sublabial, 178
Triangles, 37*f*–38*f*

Tuberculum sellae meningiomas
  anatomy, 137
  imaging, 138*f*
  radiation therapy, 205
  signs/symptoms, 137
  supraorbital approach, 137–138

V

Vincristine, 241
Visual field assessment, 70*f*, 73*f*, 76*f*, 78*f*, 79*f*, 81*f*, 82*f*, 86–87, 88*f*, 102*f*, 104*f*, 105*f*, 106*f*, 116–117
Visual system
  adnexal structures, 65
    anatomy, 83, 85
    assessment, 119
    evaluation, 98–99, 101
    rehabilitation, 108, 114
  afferent system, 65
    anatomy, 67, 69
    assessment, 115–117
    evaluation, 85–87, 92
    rehabilitation, 101, 103
  efferent system, 65
    anatomy, 69, 83
    assessment, 117–119
    evaluation, 92–94, 96, 98
    rehabilitation, 103, 108
  See also ophthalmologic evaluation